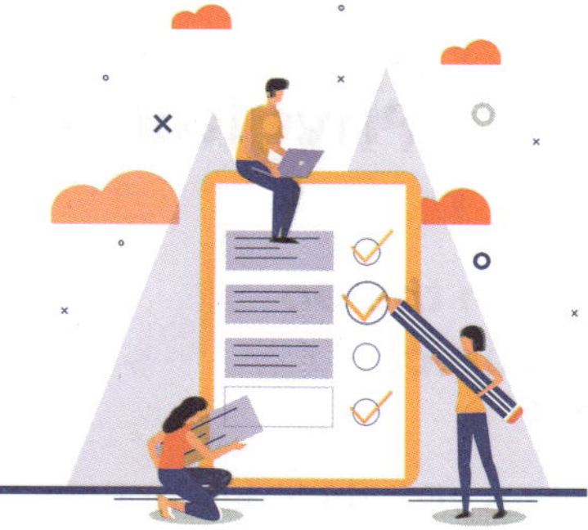

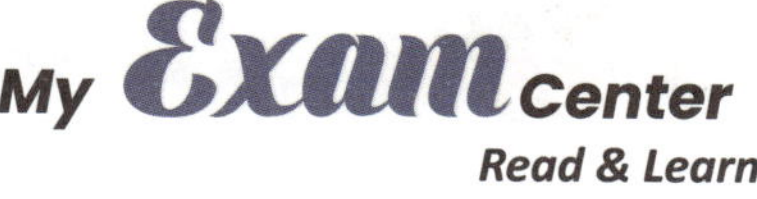

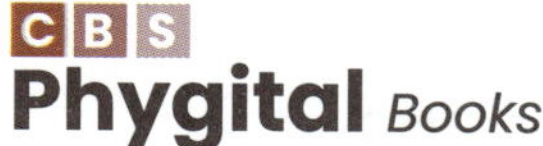

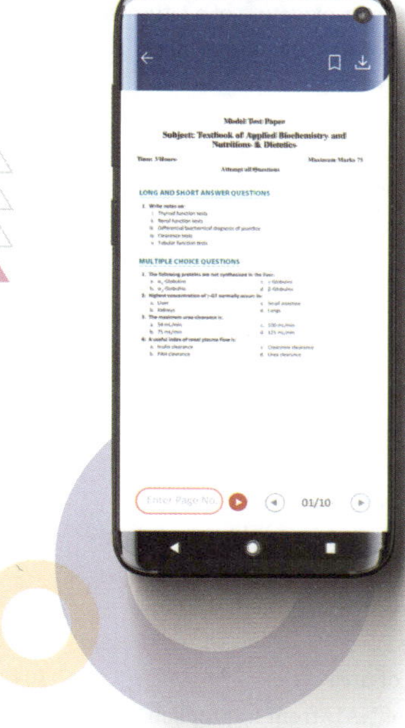

Solved Papers

Get Qs Bank covering the complete subject in the form of subjective exercises and extra exercises with their solutions

- **100+** Long Essay Questions
- **100+** Short Essay Questions

Unsolved Papers

Explore the pool of **20+** unsolved previous year exam papers of top Universities like Delhi University, RUHS, KUHS, CCS University, MGR University and many more (Semester-wise in PDF Format)

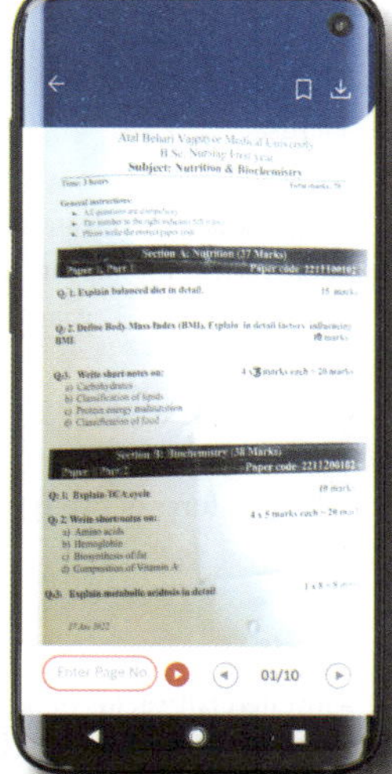

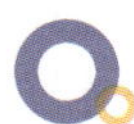

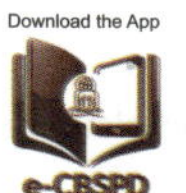

CBS Phygital Books >
Textbook of Applied Biochemistry and Nutrition & Dietetics PHYGITAL

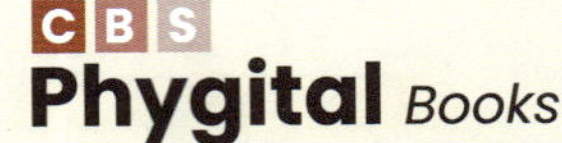

High Yield Topics

Revise on the Go

Get **50+** Topic-wise Selective Images & Tables with their description
for LMR and Quick reference, based on the topics of University examination

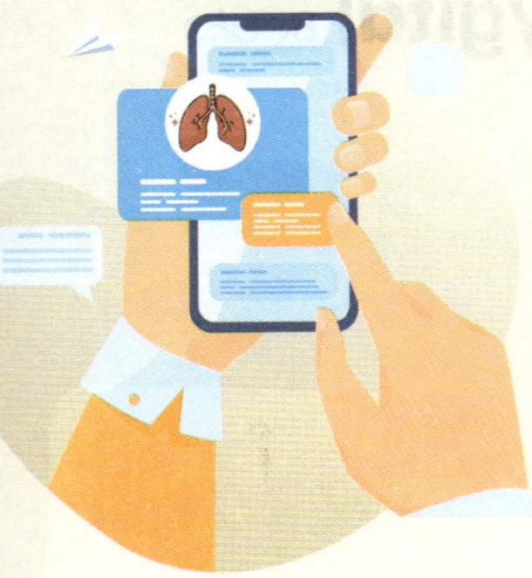

List of
High Yield
Topics

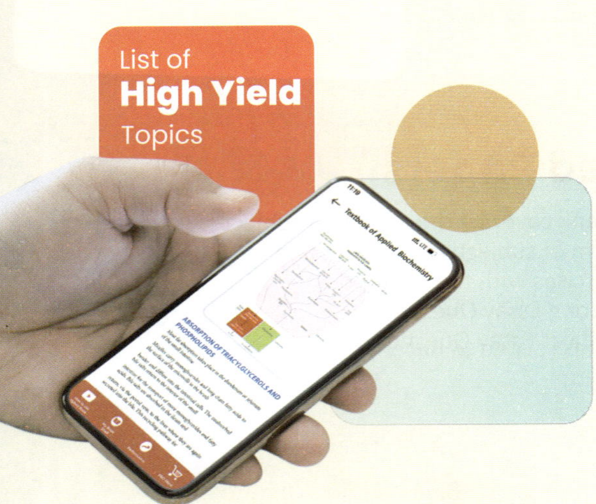

and many more...

Scan the QR Code
to Download the App

Download the App

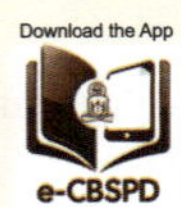
e-CBSPD

CBS Phygital Books >
**Textbook of Applied Biochemistry and
Nutrition & Dietetics PHYGITAL**

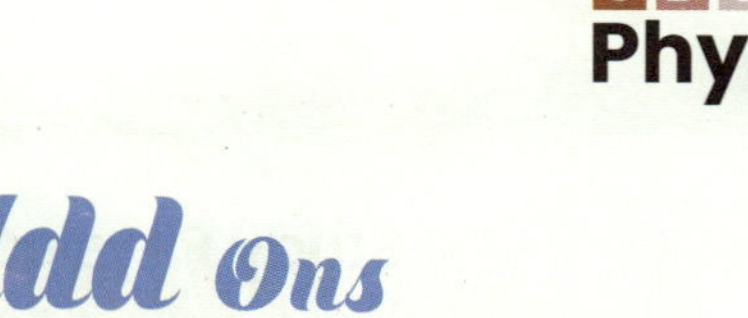

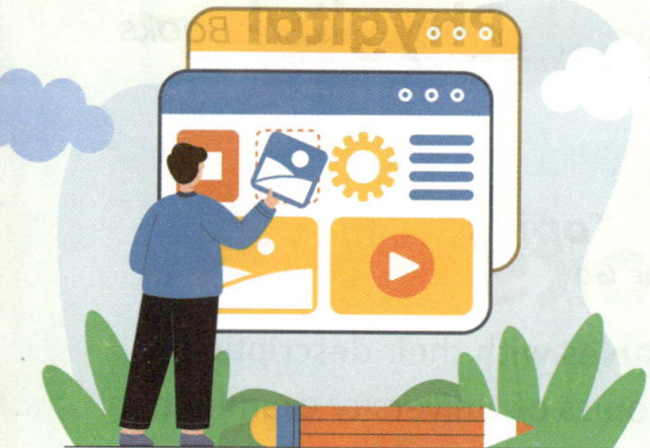

Add Ons

Dil Mange More Content

Don't settle for less, go beyond with Conceptual Videos, Recent Updates, E-books & much more...

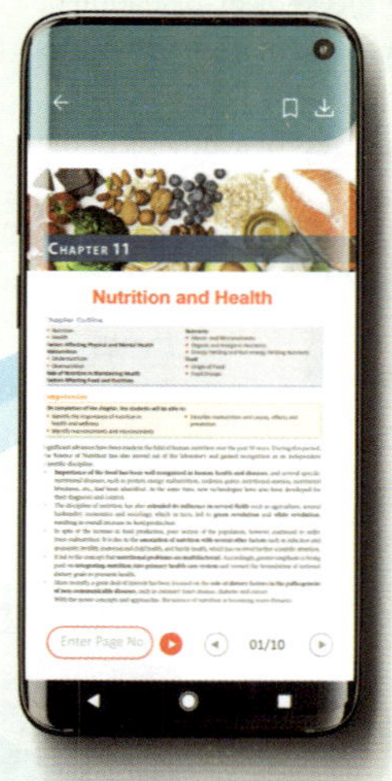

i. Recent Update

Regular updates related to **Recent advancement** and **Book Errata**

ii. E-book

Get PDFs of important chapters/sections (**Annexures/ Appendices**) of book

(This feature is for Institutions and pro-users)

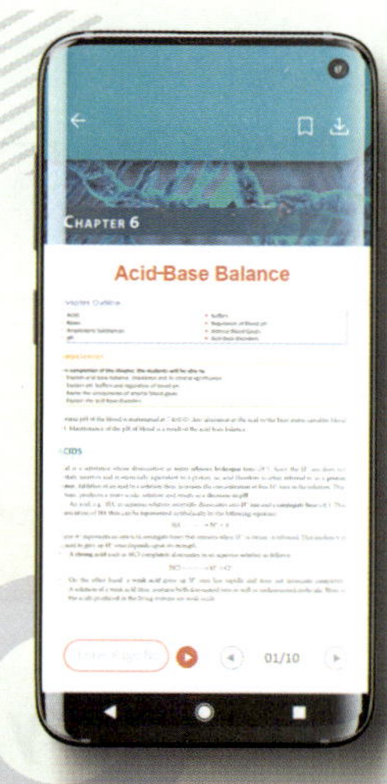

Study Physical+Digital with

CBS Phygital Books

(The *Hybrid* Edition)

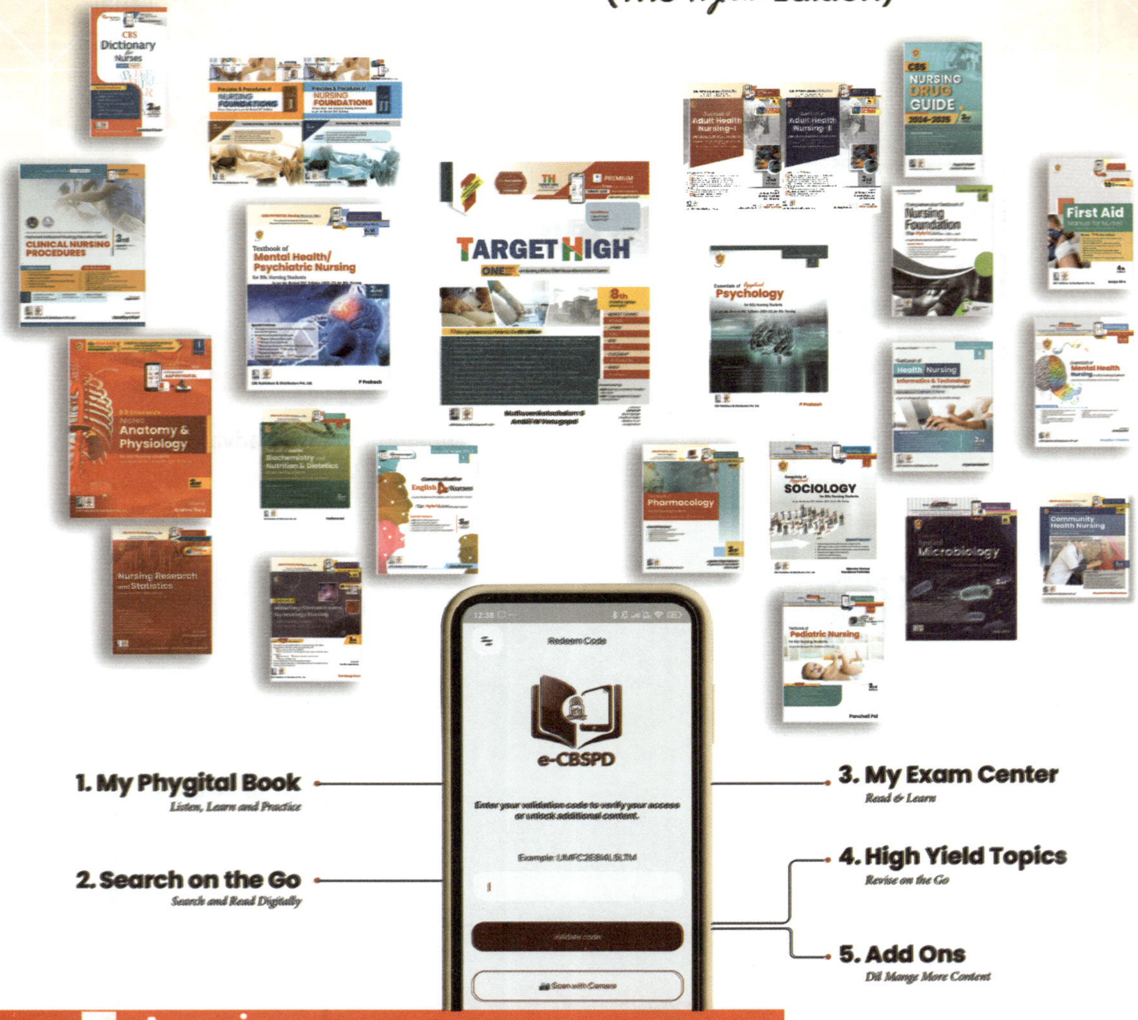

e-CBSPD

1. My Phygital Book
Listen, Learn and Practice

2. Search on the Go
Search and Read Digitally

3. My Exam Center
Read & Learn

4. High Yield Topics
Revise on the Go

5. Add Ons
Dil Mange More Content

5 Amazing Features

4-way approach of learning through

Digital Learning   **Easy Access**   **Futuristic Approach**   **Extra Knowledge**

Connect with us: 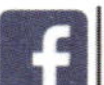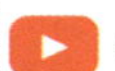 cbsnursingknowledgetree

Textbook of **Applied** Biochemistry and Nutrition & Dietetics

for BSc Nursing Students

As per the Revised INC Syllabus (2021-22)

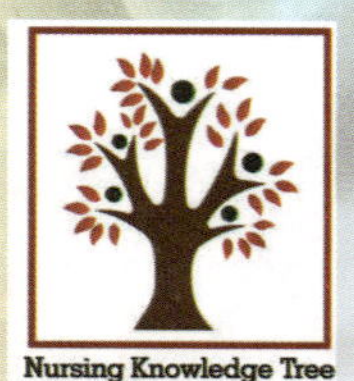

— **Second Edition** —

HARBANS LAL PhD, FACBI, FSOBSI, FIAO

Former Senior Professor & Head, Department of Biochemistry
Maharaja Agrasen Medical College, Agroha (Hisar), Haryana
Former Senior Professor, PGIMS, Rohtak, Haryana
Ex WHO Fellow

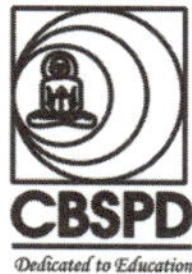

CBS Publishers & Distributors Pvt Ltd

• New Delhi • Bengaluru • Chennai • Kochi • Kolkata • Lucknow • Mumbai
• Hyderabad • Jharkhand • Nagpur • Patna • Pune • Uttarakhand

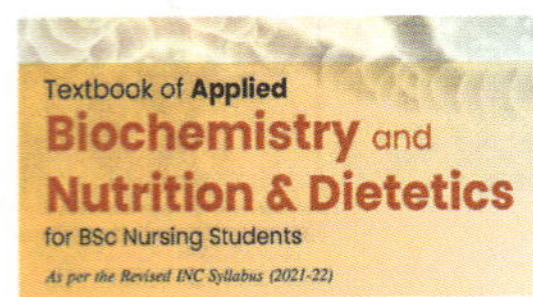

ISBN: 978-93-94525-75-7

Copyright © Harbans Lal

Reprint: 2026

Second Edition: 2025

First Edition: 2022

Published by **Satish Kumar Jain** and produced by **Varun Jain** for

CBS Publishers and Distributors Pvt Ltd

4819/XI Prahlad Street, 24 Ansari Road, Daryaganj, New Delhi 110 002, India.
Ph: +91-11-23289259, 23266861, 23266867   Website: www.cbspd.com
Fax: 011-23243014
e-mail: delhi@cbspd.com; cbspubs@airtelmail.in.

Corporate Office: 204 FIE, Industrial Area, Patparganj, Delhi 110 092
Ph: +91-11-4934 4934   Fax: 4934 4935
e-mail: feedback@cbspd.com

Branches

- **Bengaluru:** Seema House 2975, 17th Cross, K.R. Road, Banashankari 2nd Stage, Bengaluru-560 070, Karnataka
  Ph: +91-80-26771678/79   Fax: +91-80-26771680   e-mail: bangalore@cbspd.com

- **Chennai:** 7, Subbaraya Street, Shenoy Nagar, Chennai-600 030, Tamil Nadu
  Ph: +91-44-26680620, 26681266   Fax: +91-44-42032115   e-mail: chennai@cbspd.com

- **Kochi:** 68/1534, 35, 36-Power House Road, Opp. KSEB, Cochin-682018, Kochi, Kerala
  Ph: +91-484-4059061-65   Fax: +91-484-4059065   e-mail: kochi@cbspd.com

- **Kolkata:** Hind Ceramics Compound, 1st Floor, 147, Nilganj Road, Belghoria, Kolkata-700056, West Bengal
  Ph: +91-033-2563-3055/56   e-mail: kolkata@cbspd.com

- **Lucknow:** Basement, Khushnuma Complex, 7-Meerabai Marg (Behind Jawahar Bhawan), Lucknow-226001, Uttar Pradesh
  Ph: +0522-4000032   e-mail: tiwari.lucknow@cbspd.com

- **Mumbai:** PWD Shed, Gala No. 25/26, Ramchandra Bhatt Marg, Next to J.J. Hospital Gate No. 2, Opp. Union Bank of India, Noor Baug, Mumbai-400009, Maharashtra
  Ph: +91-22-66661880/89   Fax: +91-22-24902342   e-mail: mumbai@cbspd.com

Representatives

- **Hyderabad**   +91-9885175004
- **Nagpur**   +91-9421945513
- **Pune**   +91-9623451994
- **Jharkhand**   +91-9811541605
- **Patna**   +91-9334159340
- **Uttarakhand**   +91-9716462459

Printed at : Goyal Offset Works Pvt. Ltd. Haryana

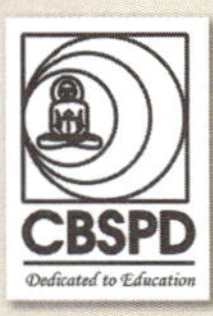

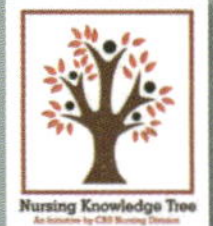

CBS Nursing Knowledge Tree

Extends its Tribute to

Florence Nightingale

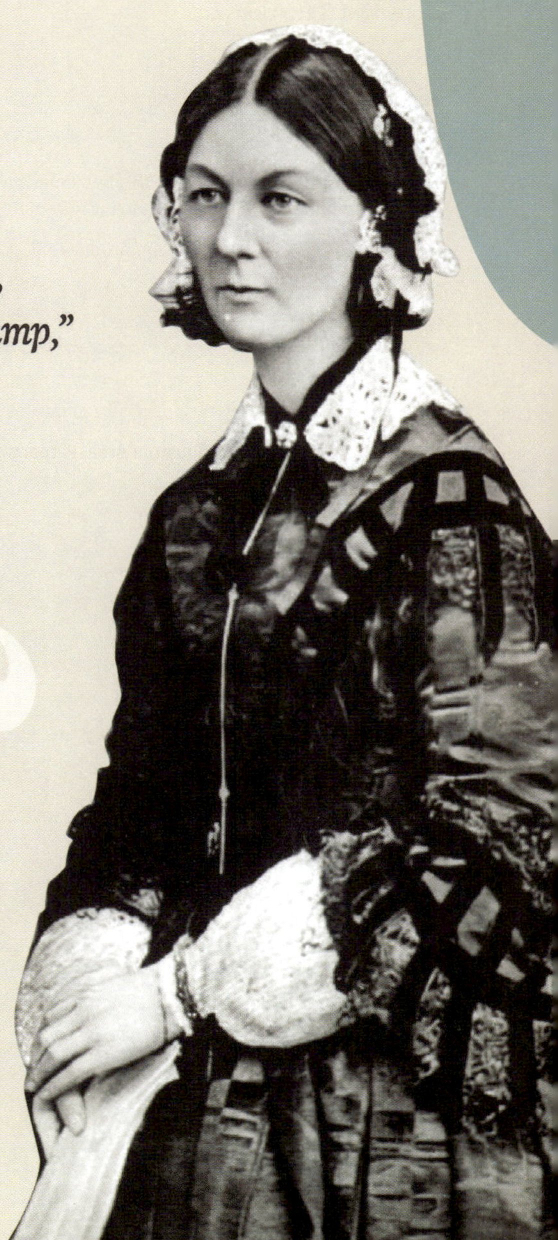

"

For glorifying the role of women as nurses,
For holding the title of " The Lady with the Lamp,"
For working tirelessly for humanity—
Florence Nightingale will always be
remembered for her
selfless and memorable services to the
human race.

"

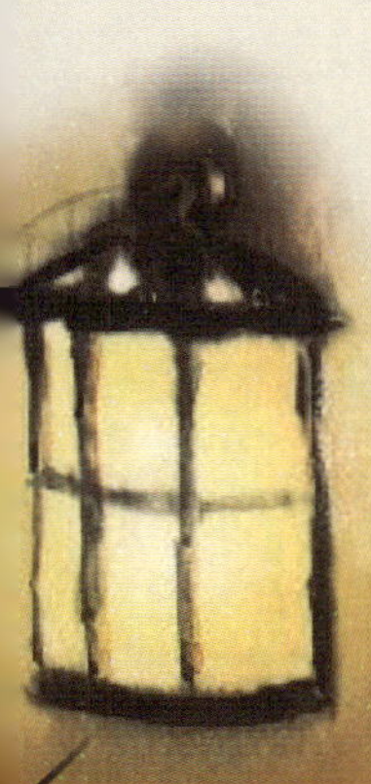

Florence Nightingale
(May 1820 – August 1910)

About the Author

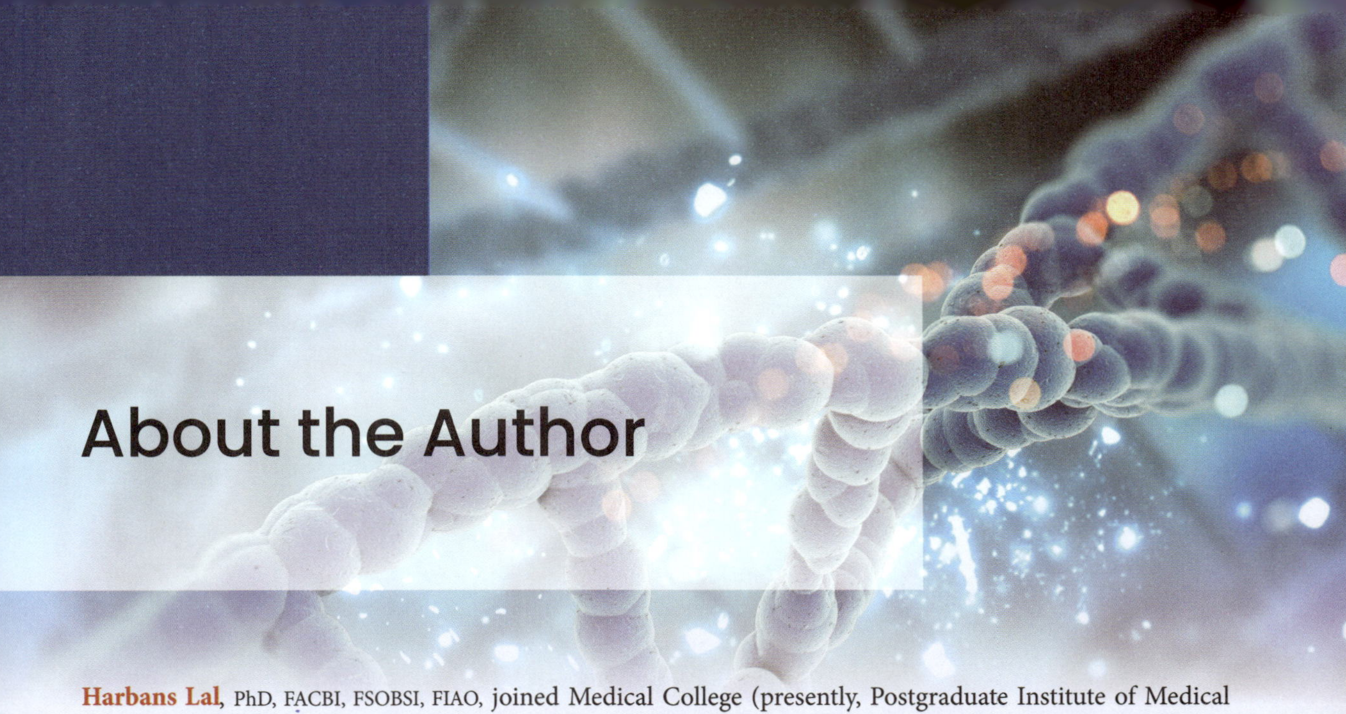

Harbans Lal, PhD, FACBI, FSOBSI, FIAO, joined Medical College (presently, Postgraduate Institute of Medical Sciences, Pt BD Sharma University of Health Sciences), Rohtak, Haryana, in 1976 as Lecturer in Biochemistry, and retired from there as Professor in 2009. Thereafter, he joined Maharaja Agrasen Medical College, Agroha (Hisar) as Senior Professor and Head of the Department of Biochemistry. The author has been teaching Biochemistry to Medical, Dental, Nursing, Physiotherapy and BSc MLT Students. He has also supervised a large number of PhD and MD students, written 12 textbooks and published more than 150 research papers in various national and international journals. He has also served as peer reviewer for several national and international research journals.

The author had been a visiting faculty at Louisiana State University Medical Center, New Orleans, USA; Department of Biosciences, MD University, Rohtak and SD Postgraduate Institute of Pharmaceutical Sciences, Pt. BD Sharma University of Health Sciences, Rohtak.

He is a life member of several scientific bodies, including Nutrition Society of India, Association of Clinical Biochemists of India, International Federation of Clinical Chemistry, Society of Biological Chemists of India, Society of Biological Scientists of India, Indian Science Congress Association, and Laboratory Animal Scientists Association.

He is also recipient of several national and international awards, including Nutrition Society of India's Young Scientists Award, World Health Organization Fellowship Award, Fellowship of the Association of Clinical Biochemists of India, Fellowship of the Society of Biological Scientists of India, Seth GS Medical College & KEM Hospital Oration Award, and the Best Teacher Award for Excellence in Teaching at Postgraduate Institute of Medical Sciences, Rohtak.

Preface to the Second Edition

It gives me immense pleasure to present the Second Edition of the **Textbook of Applied Biochemistry and Nutrition & Dietetics for BSc Nursing Students**. The book has been thoroughly revised and updated. Like the previous edition, the second edition of this book intends to convey the knowledge of time-old principles, which have been supplemented with modern developments. The figures, diagrams and tables incorporated in this edition, have been thoroughly updated and simplified. Information regarding Recommended Daily Allowances (RDA) for Indians has been updated as per the criteria of Indian Council of Medical Research-National Institute of Nutrition Expert Group 2020. The subject matter has been written in a simple, precise and lucid manner which will not only help the nursing students to grasp the basics of the subject but also prepare them for future integration with the clinical subjects in their journey to become knowledgeable nursing graduates. My endeavor always has been to keep the subject matter simple, relevant and easy to understand for the students.

Keeping aside some shortcomings that may have crept in, it is expected that the book will be welcomed by the teachers and the students of the various Nursing Colleges of India as well as of other countries, worldwide. Comments and constructive criticism, of course, will ensure further improvement of the book.

HARBANS LAL

hl.biopgimsr@gmail.com

Preface to the First Edition

A lot of encouragement and support of the faculty members and the students of several Nursing Colleges to my titles "Essentials of Biochemistry for BSc Nursing Students" and "Food & Nutrition", inspired me to present this book entitled **Textbook of Applied Biochemistry and Nutrition & Dietetics for BSc Nursing Students**. The book has been prepared as per **competencies-based new syllabus** prescribed by the **Indian Nursing Council**.

A major goal of this book is to provide the basic idea of applied biochemistry as well as applied nutrition and dietetics to the BSc Nursing students in a concise and interesting manner.

All the chapters have been thoroughly revised and updated, and the text in each chapter has been supplemented with suitable tables, outlined flowcharts and figures. Some important questions have also been included at the end of each chapter under the Assess Yourself segment.

HARBANS LAL

hl.biopgimsr@gmail.com

Acknowledgments

I express my sincere thanks and acknowledgments to the Director, National Institute of Nutrition (ICMR), Hyderabad, for allowing me to use RDA for Indians as per recommendations of the ICMR-NIN Group 2020.

I extend my special thanks to **Mr Satish Kumar Jain** (Chairman) and **Mr Varun Jain** (Managing Director), M/s CBS Publishers and Distributors Pvt Ltd for their wholehearted support in publication of this book.

I sincerely thank the entire CBS team for bringing out the book with utmost care and attractive presentation. I would like to thank Ms Nitasha Arora (Assistant General Manager – Publishing) and Dr Anju Dhir (Sr. Product Manager cum Commissioning Editor) for their publishing support. I would also like to extend my thanks to Ms Surbhi Gupta (Sr. Editor cum Team Lead), Mr Ashutosh Pathak (Assistant Production Manager cum TL) and all the production team members for devoting laborious hours in editing, designing and typesetting the book.

All the suggestions and critical evaluation by readers and academicians are highly appreciated.

Special Features of the Book

Learning Objectives in the beginning of every chapter help readers understand the purpose of the chapter.

Chapter Outline gives a glimpse of the content covered in the chapter.

Key Terms are added in each chapter to help understand difficult scientific terms in easy language.

TABLE 6.1: Normal blood values for some of the parameters related to ABG

Parameter	Normal value
pH	7.35–7.45
pCO_2	35–45 mm Hg
HCO_3^-	22–26 mEq/L
Base excess	–2.0–3.0 mmol/L

Numerous **Tables** have been used in the chapters to facilitate learning in a quick way.

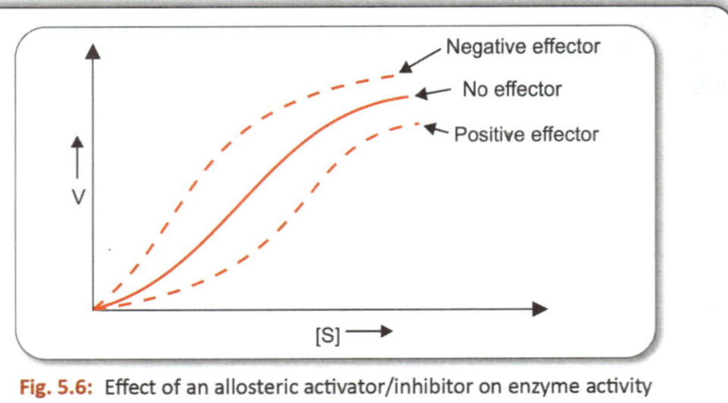

Fig. 5.6: Effect of an allosteric activator/inhibitor on enzyme activity

The book is well illustrated with relevant colorful **Figures** to add value to the content.

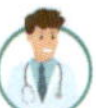 Clinical Correlation

Refsum Disease

Genetic **deficiency of α-hydroxylase enzyme** *(a monooxygenase) results in an increase in* **phytanic acid** *in the serum and its accumulation in several tissues. This in turn leads to a neurological disorder called* **Refsum disease.**

Clinical Correlation boxes cover applied aspects of clinical situations.

 Hapten

Low molecular weight substances, such as amino acids, sugars and small polymers that by themselves are not able to initiate antibody formation but can combine with specific carrier molecules (e.g., a protein) and induce a specific antibody response, are called **haptens**.

Special boxes are used to highlight the important facts in the chapters wherever required.

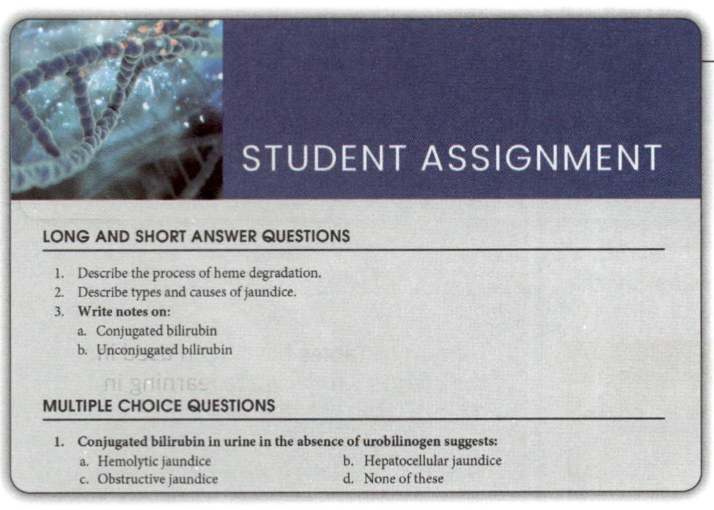

At the end of chapters, **Student Assignment** section is given which contains long and short answer questions and multiple choice questions to help students attain mastery over the subject.

Syllabus

Placement: BSc Nursing (II Semester)   **Time:** Theory 40 Hours

Applied Biochemistry

Description: The course is designed to assist the students to acquire knowledge of the normal biochemical composition and functioning of human body, its alterations in disease conditions and to apply this knowledge in the practice of nursing.

Unit	Time (Hrs)	Learning Outcomes	Content	Teaching/Learning Activities	Assessment Methods
I	8 (T)	Describe the metabolism of carbohydrates and its alterations	**Carbohydrates** • Digestion, absorption and metabolism of carbohydrates and related disorders • Regulation of blood glucose • Diabetes Mellitus—type 1 and type 2, symptoms, complications and management in brief • Investigations of diabetes mellitus ▪ OGTT—Indications, procedure, interpretation and types of GTT curve ▪ Mini GTT, extended GTT, GCT, IV GTT ▪ HbA1c (Only definition) • Hypoglycemia—Definition and causes	• Lecture cum discussion • Explain using charts and slides • Demonstration of laboratory tests	• Essay • Short answer • Very short answer
II	8 (T)	Explain the metabolism of lipids and its alterations	**Lipids** • Fatty acids—Definition, classification • Definition and clinical significance of MUFA and PUFA, essential fatty acids, trans fatty acids • Digestion, absorption and metabolism of lipids and related disorders • Compounds formed from cholesterol • Ketone bodies (name, types and significance only) • Lipoproteins—types and functions (metabolism not required) • Lipid profile • Atherosclerosis (in brief)	• Lecture cum discussion • Explain using charts and slides • Demonstration of laboratory tests	• Essay • Short answer • Very short answer

Contd...

Unit	Time (Hrs)	Learning Outcomes	Content	Teaching/Learning Activities	Assessment Methods
III	9 (T)	• Explain the metabolism of amino acids and proteins • Identify alterations in disease conditions	**Proteins** • Classification of amino acids based on nutrition, metabolic rate with examples • Digestion, absorption and metabolism of protein and related disorders • Biologically important compounds synthesized from various amino acids (only names) • Inborn errors of amino acid metabolism – only aromatic amino acids (in brief) • Plasma protein—types, function and normal values • Causes of proteinuria, hypoproteinemia, hypergammaglobinemia • Principle of electrophoresis, normal and abnormal electrophoretic patterns (in brief)	• Lecture cum discussion • Explain using charts, models and slides	• Essay • Short answer • Very short answer

IV	4 (T)	Explain clinical enzymology in various disease conditions	**Clinical Enzymology**
			• Isoenzymes—Definition and properties
			• Enzymes of diagnostic importance in
			  ■ Liver diseases—ALT, AST, ALP, GGT
			  ■ Myocardial infarction—CK, cardiac troponins, AST, LDH
			  ■ Muscle diseases—CK, aldolase
			  ■ Bone diseases—ALP
			  ■ Prostate cancer—PSA, ACP
				• Lecture cum discussion
				• Explain using charts and slides
					• Essay
					• Short answer
					• Very short answer

V	3 (T)	Explain acid base balance, imbalance and its clinical significance	**Acid Base Maintenance** • pH—definition, normal value • Regulation of blood pH—blood buffer, respiratory and renal • ABG—normal values • Acid base disorders—types, definition and causes	• Lecture cum discussion • Explain using charts and slides	• Short answer • Very short answer
VI	2 (T)	Describe the metabolism of hemoglobin and its clinical significance	**Heme Catabolism** • Heme degradation pathway • Jaundice—type, causes, urine and blood investigations (Van den Berg test)	• Lecture cum discussion • Explain using charts and slides	• Short answer • Very short answer
VII	3 (T)	Explain different function tests and interpret the findings	**Organ Function Tests (Biochemical Parameters and Normal Values Only)** • Renal • Liver • Thyroid	• Lecture cum discussion • Visit to lab • Explain using charts and slides	• Short answer • Very short answer
VIII	3 (T)	Illustrate the immunochemistry	**Immunochemistry** • Structure and functions of immunoglobulin • Investigations and interpretation – ELISA	• Lecture cum discussion • Explain using charts and slides • Demonstration of laboratory tests	• Short answer • Very short answer

Applied Nutrition and Dietetics

Placement: BSc Nursing (II Semester) **Time:** Theory 45 Hours
Lab: 15 Hours

Description: The course is designed to assist the students to acquire basic knowledge and understanding of the principles of Nutrition and Dietetics and apply this knowledge in the practice of Nursing.

Unit	Time (Hrs)	Learning Outcomes	Content	Teaching/Learning Activities	Assessment Methods
I	2 (T)	Define nutrition and its relationship to health	**Introduction to Nutrition** *Concepts* • Definition of nutrition and health • Malnutrition—under nutrition and over nutrition • Role of nutrition in maintaining health • Factors affecting food and nutrition *Nutrients* • Classification • Macro and micronutrients • Organic and inorganic • Energy yielding and non-energy yielding *Food* • Classification—food groups • Origin	• Lecture cum discussion • Charts/slides	• Essay • Short answer • Very short answer
II	3 (T)	Describe the classification, functions, sources and recommended daily allowances (RDA) of carbohydrates	**Carbohydrates** • Composition—starches, sugar and cellulose • Recommended daily allowance (RDA) • Dietary sources • Functions	• Lecture cum discussion • Charts/slides • Models • Display of food items	• Essay • Short answer • Very short answer
		Explain BMR and factors affecting BMR	**Energy** • Unit of energy—Kcal • Basal metabolic rate (BMR) • Factors affecting BMR		
III	3 (T)	Describe the classification, functions, sources and RDA of proteins	**Proteins** • Composition • Eight essential amino acids • Functions • Dietary sources • Protein requirements—RDA	• Lecture cum discussion • Charts/slides • Models • Display of food items	• Essay • Short answer • Very short answer
IV	2 (T)	Describe the classification, functions, sources and RDA of fats	**Fats** • Classification—saturated and unsaturated • Calorie value • Functions • Dietary sources of fats and fatty acids • Fat requirements—RDA	• Lecture cum discussion • Charts/slides • Models • Display of food items	• Essay • Short answer • Very short answer

Contd...

Unit	Time (Hrs)	Learning Outcomes	Content	Teaching/Learning Activities	Assessment Methods
V	3 (T)	Describe the classification, functions, sources and RDA of vitamins	**Vitamins** • Classification—fat soluble and water soluble • Fat soluble—vitamins A, D, E, and K • Water soluble—thiamine (vitamin B1), riboflavin (vitamin B2), nicotinic acid, pyridoxine (vitamin B6), pantothenic acid, folic acid, vitamin B12, ascorbic acid (vitamin C) • Functions, dietary sources and requirements—RDA of every vitamin	• Lecture cum discussion • Charts/slides • Models • Display of food items	• Essay • Short answer • Very short answer
VI	3 (T)	Describe the classification, functions, sources and RDA of minerals	**Minerals** • Classification—major minerals (Calcium, phosphorus, sodium, potassium and magnesium) and trace elements • Functions • Dietary sources • Requirements—RDA	• Lecture cum discussion • Charts/slides • Models • Display of food items	• Short answer • Very short answer

VII	7 (T)
	8 (L)
		Describe and plan balanced diet for different age groups, pregnancy, and lactation	**Balanced Diet**
			• Definition, principles, steps
			• Food guides—basic four food groups
			• RDA—definition, limitations, uses
			• Food exchange system
			• Calculation of nutritive value of foods
			• Dietary fiber
			Nutrition Across Life Cycle
			• Meal planning/menu planning—definition, principles, steps
			• Infant and young child feeding (IYCF) guidelines—breastfeeding, infant foods
			• Diet plan for different age groups—children, adolescents and elderly
			• Diet in pregnancy—nutritional requirements and balanced diet plan
			• Anemia in pregnancy—diagnosis, diet for anemic pregnant women, iron and folic acid supplementation and counseling
			• Nutrition in lactation—nutritional requirements, diet for lactating mothers, complementary feeding/weaning
				• Lecture cum discussion
				• Meal planning
				• Lab session on
				  ■ Preparation of balanced diet for different categories
				  ■ Low cost nutritious dishes
					• Short answer
					• Very short answer

Contd...

Unit	Time (Hrs)	Learning Outcomes	Content	Teaching/Learning Activities	Assessment Methods
VIII	6 (T)	Classify and describe the common nutritional deficiency disorders and identify nurses' role in assessment, management and prevention	**Nutritional Deficiency Disorders** • Protein energy malnutrition—magnitude of the problem, causes, classification, signs and symptoms, severe acute malnutrition (SAM), management and prevention and nurses' role • Childhood obesity—signs and symptoms, assessment, management and prevention and nurses' role • Vitamin deficiency disorders—vitamin A, B, C and D deficiency disorders—causes, signs and symptoms, management and prevention and nurses' role • Mineral deficiency diseases—iron, iodine and calcium deficiencies—causes, signs and symptoms, management and prevention and nurses' role	• Lecture cum discussion • Charts/slides • Models	• Essay • Short answer • Very short answer
IX	4 (T) 7 (L)	Principles of diets in various diseases	**Therapeutic Diets** • Definition, objectives, principles • Modifications—consistency, nutrients • Feeding techniques • Diet in diseases—obesity, diabetes mellitus, CVD, underweight, renal diseases, hepatic disorders constipation, diarrhea, pre- and post-operative period	• Lecture cum discussion • Meal planning • Lab session on preparation of therapeutic diets	• Essay • Short answer • Very short answer
X	3 (T)	Describe the rules and preservation of nutrients	**Cookery Rules and Preservation of Nutrients** • Cooking—methods, advantages and disadvantages • Preservation of nutrients • Measures to prevent loss of nutrients during preparation • Safe food handling and storage of foods • Food preservation • Food additives and food adulteration • Prevention of Food Adulteration Act (PFA) • Food standards	• Lecture cum discussion • Charts/slides	• Essay • Short answer • Very short answer

Contd…

Unit	Time (Hrs)	Learning Outcomes	Content	Teaching/Learning Activities	Assessment Methods
XI	4 (T)	Explain the methods of nutritional assessment and nutrition education	**Nutrition Assessment and Nutrition Education** • Objectives of nutritional assessment • Methods of assessment—clinical examination, anthropometry, laboratory and biochemical assessment, assessment of dietary intake including food frequency questionnaire (FFQ) method • Nutrition education—purposes, principles and methods	• Lecture cum discussion • Demonstration • Writing nutritional assessment report	• Essay • Short answer • Evaluation of nutritional assessment report
XII	3 (T)	Describe nutritional problems in India and nutritional programs	**National Nutritional Programs and Role of Nurse** • Nutritional problems in India • National nutritional policy • National nutritional programs—Vitamin A supplementation, Anemia Mukt Bharat Program, Integrated Child Development Services (ICDS), Mid-day Meal Scheme (MDMS), National Iodine Deficiency Disorders Control Program (NIDDCP), Weekly Iron Folic Acid Supplementation (WIFS) and others as introduced • Role of nurse in every program	• Lecture cum discussion	• Essay • Short answer • Very short answer
XIII	2 (T)	• Discuss the importance of food hygiene and food safety • Explain the acts related to food safety	**Food Safety** • Definition, food safety considerations and measures • Food Safety Regulatory Measures in India—Relevant Acts • Five keys to safer food • Food storage, food handling and cooking • General principles of food storage of food items (E.g., milk, meat) • Role of food handlers in food borne diseases • Essential steps in safe cooking practices	• Guided reading on related acts	• Quiz • Short answer

Contents

Section A Applied Biochemistry

Section B Applied Nutrition and Dietetics

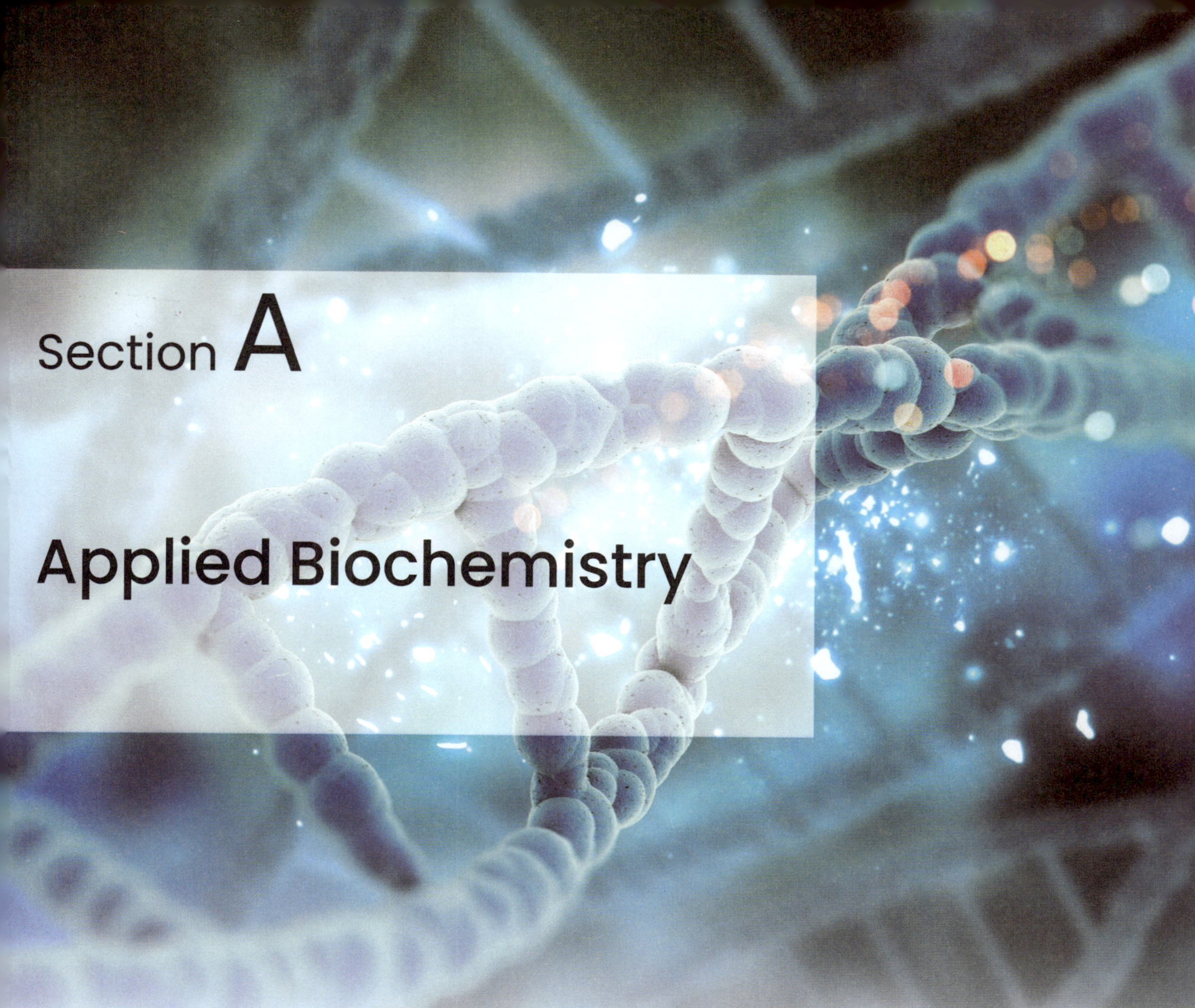

SECTION OUTLINE

Introduction to Biochemistry and its Significance in Nursing

LEARNING OBJECTIVES

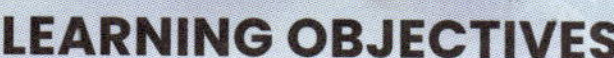

After the completion of the chapter, the readers will be able to:
- Understand the history of biochemistry.
- Discuses applications and significance of biochemistry in nursing.
- Find out the purpose of studying biochemistry.
- Interpret the postnatal counseling and psychological support.

CHAPTER OUTLINE

- Introduction
- History of Biochemistry
- Biochemistry and Molecular Biology
- Applications of Biochemistry

- Biochemistry as the Scientific Basis of Medicine
- Significance of Biochemistry in Nursing
- Aim of the Course

KEY TERMS

Biochemical techniques: The use of microorganisms and enzymes in the laboratory methods to study biochemical processes.

Human biochemistry: The application of chemistry in the study of biological processes going on in the human body at the cellular and molecular level.

Metabolic disorder: A disorder that negatively alters the body's processing and distribution of macronutrients such as proteins, fats, and carbohydrates.

Molecular biology: The study of the structure and function of molecules and macromolecular systems associated with biological processes, especially the molecular basis of inheritance and protein synthesis.

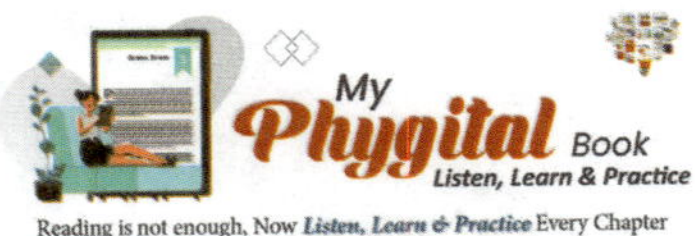

INTRODUCTION

Biochemistry, sometimes called **biological chemistry**, is the study of chemical processes within the body/cell relating to the living organisms.

HISTORY OF BIOCHEMISTRY

- The dawn of biochemistry may have been the **discovery of the first enzyme** diastase (these days also called amylase) in 1833 by Payen.
- Thereafter, Buchner contributed the first demonstration of a complex biochemical process outside a cell in 1896, i.e., **alcoholic fermentation** in cell extracts of yeast.
- Although the term "biochemistry" seems to have been first used in 1882, it is generally accepted that the formal coinage of biochemistry occurred in 1903 by Neuberg, a German chemist.
- Since then biochemistry has advanced, especially after the mid-20th century, with the **development of the new techniques** such as chromatography, X-ray diffraction, Nuclear Magnetic Resonance (NMR) spectroscopy, radioisotopic labeling and electron microscopy, etc. These techniques allowed for the discovery and detailed **analysis of many molecules** and **metabolic pathways** of the cell such as glycolysis and the Krebs cycle (citric acid cycle), etc.

BIOCHEMISTRY AND MOLECULAR BIOLOGY

Another significant historic event in **biochemistry** is the discovery of the gene and its role in the **transfer of information in the cell**. This part of biochemistry is called **molecular biology**.

- In the 1950s, Watson, Crick, Franklin and Wilkins were instrumental in solving the **structure of DNA** (deoxyribonucleic acid) and suggesting its relationship with the **genetic transfer of information**.
- In 1958, Beadle and Tatum showed that **one gene produces one enzyme**.
- In 1988, Pitchfork was the first person convicted of murder with **DNA evidence**, which led to the growth of the use of molecular biology **in forensic science**.
- More recently, Fire and Mello discovered the role of **ribonucleic acid interference** (RNAi) in the **silencing of gene** expression.

Thus, depending upon the exact definition of the terms used, molecular biology can be thought of a branch of biochemistry or biochemistry as a tool to investigate and study molecular biology.

APPLICATIONS OF BIOCHEMISTRY

These days biochemistry has become so successful at explaining the living processes in almost **all the areas of life sciences**, viz. agriculture, nutrition and medicine.

- In **agriculture**, biochemists investigate and try to discover the ways to improve crop cultivation, yield and nutritive values of the food grains, vegetables and fruits.
- In **nutrition**, they study how to maintain health and the effects of nutritional deficiencies.
- In **medicine**, biochemists investigate the causes and cure of diseases.

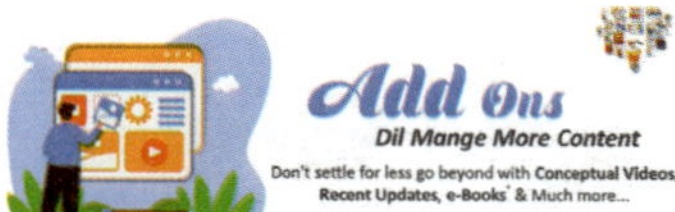

BIOCHEMISTRY AS THE SCIENTIFIC BASIS OF MEDICINE

Biochemistry is beyond all other branches of science and forms a scientific basis of medicine.

- **Human biochemistry** focuses on the biochemistry of human beings and their medical illnesses. For example, there are more than twenty different chemical reactions known to be involved, in sequence, in the conversion of glucose to carbon dioxide and water but we are now able to say that a particular one is affected by the available supply of insulin.
- **Clinicians** think of biochemistry, chiefly as a collection of analytical procedures whose results they find **useful in diagnosis**, e.g., the diagnosis of **hyperglycemia** or **renal glycosuria** is dependent on blood glucose determination; **gout** on the estimation of uric acid; **hyperparathyroidism** on serum calcium concentration while **nephrosis** with respect to the estimation of serum proteins, etc.

SIGNIFICANCE OF BIOCHEMISTRY IN NURSING

A review of the application of biochemistry in nursing needs to mention **many therapeutic agents** whose existence was first demonstrated in laboratory experiments. Moreover, these preparations, in usable forms, were first achieved by **biochemical techniques**, e.g., the hormone insulin, all the vitamins and many other products of therapeutic significance. If an infant is always vomiting after giving milk, she or he probably, has **galactose intolerance**. Similarly, if an infant is born with **jaundice**, her or his liver is not fully functional. When color of the infant's urine turns dark, probably he/she suffers from an amino acid **metabolic disorder**. Anemic children, older, elder or geriatric persons can be explained with biochemistry, e.g., intake of iron (Fe), hemolytic disorder (**G6PD deficiency** or **pyruvate kinase deficiency**) or a chronic renal disease. Many such conditions thus, can be explained on the **basis of biochemistry**.

AIM OF THE COURSE

The course for students of BSc Nursing is designed to assist them to acquire knowledge of the normal biochemical composition and functioning of human body, its alterations in disease conditions and to apply this knowledge in the practice of nursing.

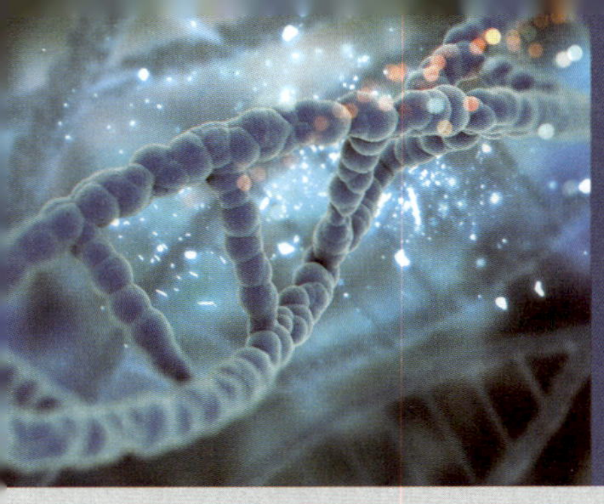

LONG AND SHORT ANSWER QUESTIONS

1. Discuss applications of biochemistry.
2. Write a short note on significance of biochemistry in nursing.

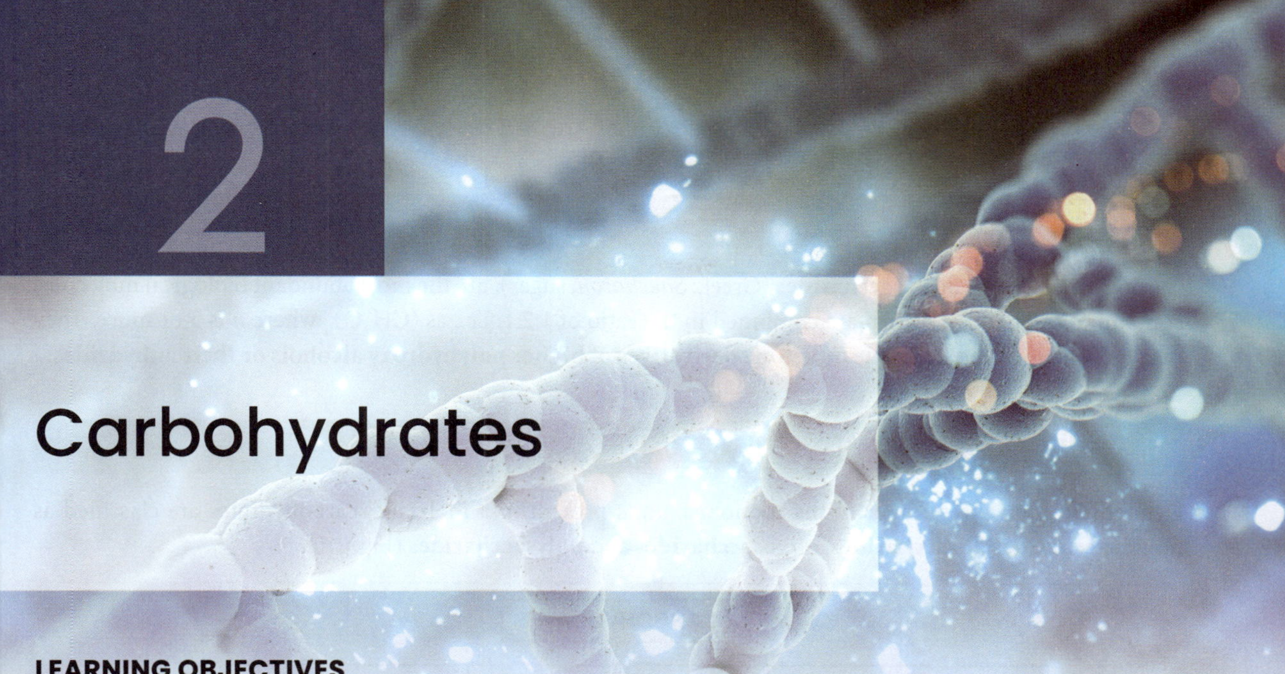

2

Carbohydrates

LEARNING OBJECTIVES

After the completion of the chapter, the readers will be able to:
- Describe the uses and metabolism of carbohydrates and its alterations.
- Learn the metabolism of glucose and glycogen.
- Understand diabetes mellitus.

CHAPTER OUTLINE

- Introduction
- Classification of Carbohydrates
- Uses of Carbohydrates
- Metabolism of Carbohydrates
- Metabolism of Glucose
- Glycolysis
- Gluconeogenesis
- Tricarboxylic Acid Cycle
- Glycogen Metabolism
- Pentose Phosphate Pathway
- Metabolism of Fructose and Galactose
- Regulation of Blood Glucose
- Diabetes Mellitus

KEY TERMS

Amylopectin: It is a polysaccharide made up of many units of glucose linked together by linear 1-4 glycosidic linkages and 1-6 glycosidic linkages.

Derived sugars: Modification of sugar molecules by addition or substitution other than hydroxyl group.

Enolase: A cytosolic metalloenzyme responsible for the conversion of 2-phosphoglycerate into phosphoenolpyruvate, the second to last step in glycolysis.

Glycogen primer: It is a protein "primer" that is termed as glycogenin, which is required for the initiation of glycogen synthesis. During this process, uridine-diphosphate-glucose (UDPG) is used as source of glucose by the enzyme glucuronyltransferase.

Ketoacidosis: High levels of ketones that cause the blood to become more acidic; it is a severe life-threatening condition requiring immediate treatment.

INTRODUCTION

Carbohydrates, also called **saccharides** (Greek: *Sakcharon*, sugar), are the most abundant biological molecules containing C, H and O, which are combined in the ratio of 1:2:1, i.e., as $(CH_2O)_n$ where n is 3 or more. They may be defined as the **aldehyde or ketone derivatives of higher polyhydroxy alcohols or their anhydrides.**

CLASSIFICATION OF CARBOHYDRATES

Depending upon the number of the monomer units present in a molecule, carbohydrates are classified as **monosaccharides**, **disaccharides**, **oligosaccharides** and **polysaccharides** (Fig. 2.1).

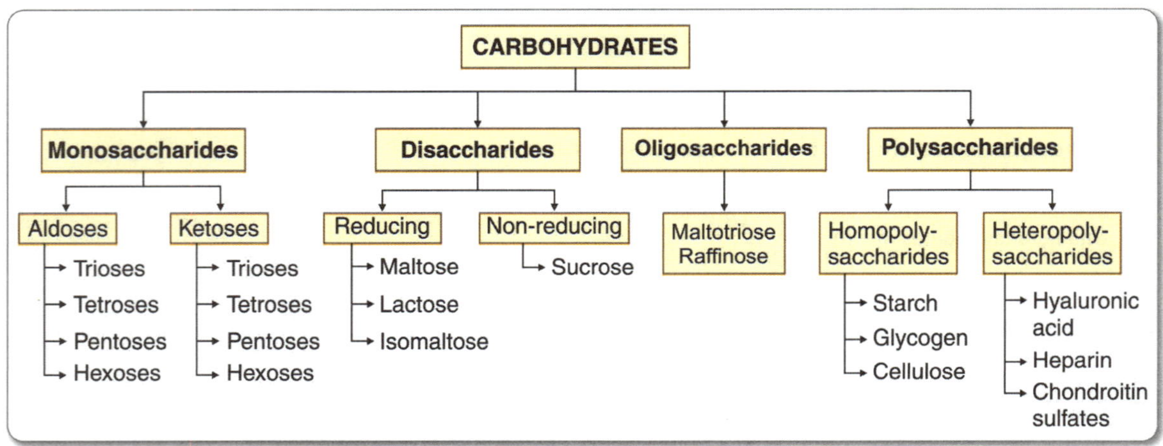

Fig. 2.1: Classification of carbohydrates

Monosaccharides

Monosaccharides are **simple sugars,** which can join in several ways to form di, oligo and polysaccharides. These are the aldehyde or ketone derivatives of the straight chain polyhydroxy alcohols which contain 3 or more carbons.

Classification of the Monosaccharides

Monosaccharides are divided into different groups, according to:
- **Chemical nature** of their carbonyl group or
- **Number of carbon atoms** in the chain (Table 2.1).

TABLE 2.1: Classification of monosaccharides

Monosaccharides	Number of carbons	Aldoses	Ketoses
Trioses	3	Glyceraldehyde	Dihydroxyacetone
Tetroses	4	Erythrose	Erythrulose
Pentoses	5	Ribose	Ribulose
Hexoses	6	Glucose	Fructose

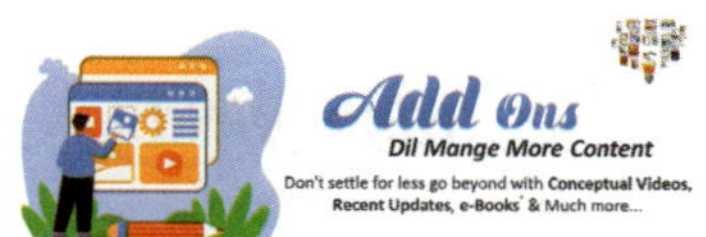

According to chemical nature of the carbonyl group: *According to the chemical nature of the carbonyl group, monosaccharides are divided into two groups as aldoses and ketoses:*

1. *Aldoses:* The sugar is an aldose when it has an **aldehyde (–CHO) group** on carbon-1, e.g., glucose.
2. *Ketoses:* The sugar is a ketose when it has a **ketone (–CO)** group at carbon-2, e.g., fructose.

Some of the ketoses are named by inserting '-**ul**' before the suffix '-**ose**' in the name of the corresponding aldose, e.g., **erythrulose**. It is a ketose corresponding to erythrose, which is an aldose.

According to number of carbon atoms: *According to the number of carbon atoms, monosaccharides are designated as trioses, tetroses, pentoses, hexoses, etc.:*

- *Trioses:* Trioses are the smallest monosaccharides with **three carbon atoms,** e.g., **glyceraldehyde** (an aldotriose) and **dihydroxyacetone** (a ketotriose). Both, are of physiological significance, as their phosphate esters, i.e., glyceraldehyde-3-phosphate and dihydroxyacetone phosphate, occur as intermediates of glycolysis.
- *Tetroses:* Tetroses have **four carbon atoms,** e.g., **erythrose** (an aldotetrose) and **erythrulose** (a ketotetrose). Erythrose, as erythrose-4-phosphate, occurs as an intermediate in hexose monophosphate (HMP) shunt.
- *Pentoses*: Pentoses contain **five carbon atoms**, e.g., **ribose** (an aldopentose) and **xylulose** (a ketopentose). Both of these occur as intermediates of the HMP shunt. Ribose is also a constituent of nucleotides found in ribonucleic acids (RNAs).
- *Hexoses:* Hexoses contain **six carbon atoms**, e.g., **glucose** (an aldohexose) and **fructose** (a ketohexose). Glucose, commonly known as dextrose, is used as a source of energy in the body. Galactose is a constituent of milk sugar lactose. Fructose is a constituent of the common sugar sucrose.

Monosaccharides of biological importance are exhibited in Figure 2.2.

Derived Sugars

Several derivatives of monosaccharides, such as acids, alcohols, amino acid derivatives and methyl glycosides also occur in the body.

Acids

Oxidation of carbon-1 of an aldose **converts** its **aldehyde group to the carboxyl group** and **forms an acid** which is called **aldonic acid**, e.g., D-gluconic acid.

On the other hand, **oxidation of the primary alcoholic group at carbon 6** of an aldose produces **uronic acid**, e.g., D-glucuronic acid (Fig. 2.3).

Alcohols

Sugars reduce under mild conditions and produce cyclic polyhydroxyalcohols called **alditols**, e.g., **ribitol** (a component of FMN and FAD) and **xylitol** (a sweetener used in the formation of gums and candies).

Amines

Amino sugars such as **glucosamine** and **galactosamine** are formed when the **–OH group at carbon-2 is substituted by** the **–NH$_2$ group** (Fig. 2.4).

Some of the amino sugars also occur as their acetylated derivatives. Several derivatives of the amino sugars are found in glycosaminoglycans such as in hyaluronic acid, chondroitin sulfates, erythromycin, etc. **N-acetylneuraminic acid** and its derivatives are called **sialic acids.** They are important constituents of **glycoproteins** and **glycolipids.**

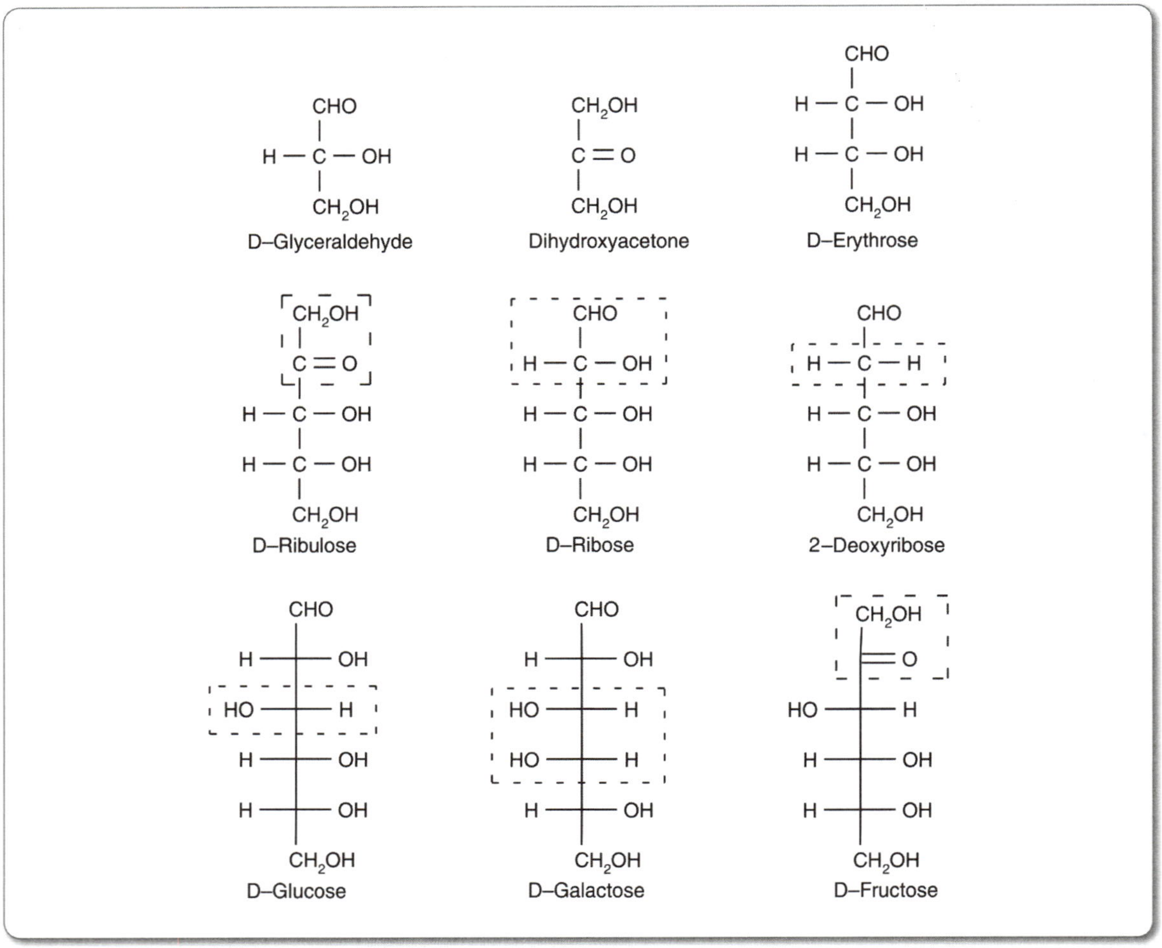

CHO
|
H — C — OH
|
CH_2OH

D–Glyceraldehyde

CH_2OH
|
C = O
|
CH_2OH

Dihydroxyacetone

CHO
|
H — C — OH
|
H — C — OH
|
CH_2OH

D–Erythrose

CH_2OH
|
C = O
|
H — C — OH
|
H — C — OH
|
CH_2OH

D–Ribulose

CHO
|
H — C — OH
|
H — C — OH
|
H — C — OH
|
CH_2OH

D–Ribose

CHO
|
H — C — H
|
H — C — OH
|
H — C — OH
|
CH_2OH

2–Deoxyribose

CHO
H —— OH
HO —— H
H —— OH
H —— OH
CH_2OH

D–Glucose

CHO
H —— OH
HO —— H
HO —— H
H —— OH
CH_2OH

D–Galactose

CH_2OH
O
HO —— H
H —— OH
H —— OH
CH_2OH

D–Fructose

Fig. 2.2: Some monosaccharides of biological importance

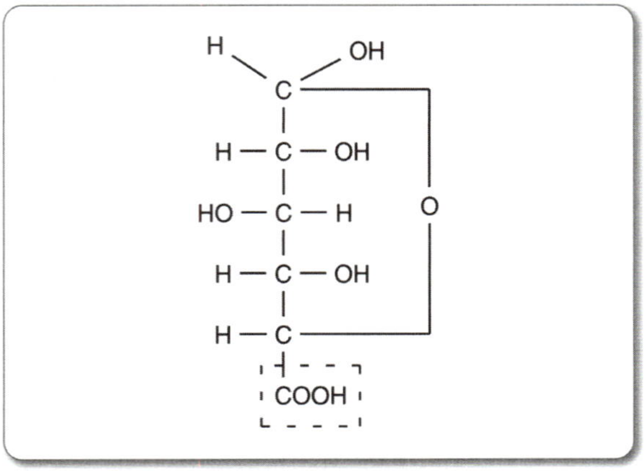

H   OH
C
|
H — C — OH
|
HO — C — H   O
|
H — C — OH
|
H — C
|
COOH

Fig. 2.3: D-glucuronic acid

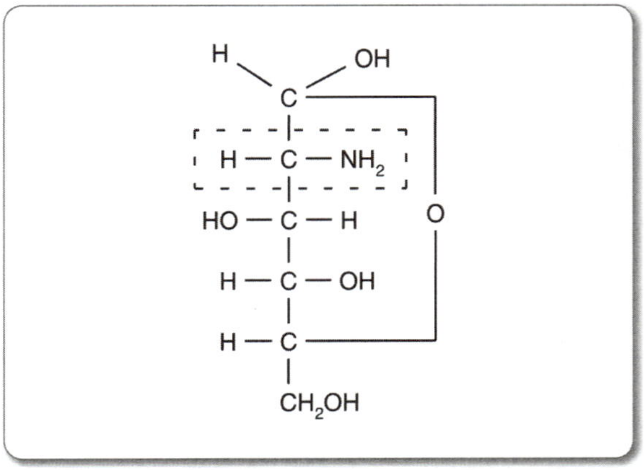

H   OH
C
|
H — C — NH_2
|
HO — C — H   O
|
H — C — OH
|
H — C
|
CH_2OH

Fig. 2.4: Glucosamine

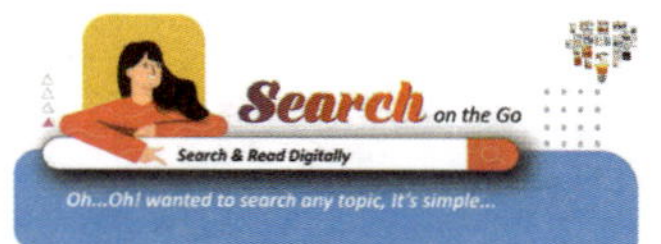

Glycosides

When **carbon-1 of a sugar molecule reacts with an alcohol** such as methanol, it **yields** a compound called **methyl glycoside.** Methyl glycosides are **found in glycosaminoglycans.**

Disaccharides

Disaccharides consist of **two** similar or dissimilar **monosaccharides** which are **linked** together **by a glycosidic bond.** **Maltose, lactose** and **sucrose** are the disaccharides, which have biological importance.

Maltose

Maltose [α-D glucopyranosyl-(1,4) α-D glucopyranose] consists of two α-D glucopyran units which are linked together by **α-1, 4-glycosidic linkage.** Accordingly, in maltose, the –OH group at carbon 4 of a glucose molecule is linked to the –OH group at the carbon l (the anomeric carbon) of the other glucose molecule. This in turn leaves a free **–OH at** the anomeric carbon, i.e., **carbon-l,** of the first glucose molecule suggesting that **maltose is a reducing disaccharide** (Fig. 2.5).

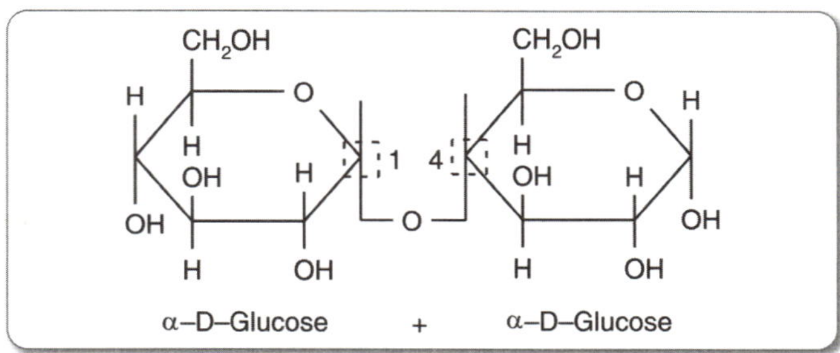

Fig. 2.5: Maltose

Maltose is usually obtained as one of the hydrolyzed products of some polysaccharides such as starch and glycogen. **Maltose** is **hydrolyzed** to its consituent monosaccharides, i.e., **two glucose units,** by the enzyme **maltase** in the intestinal lumen.

Lactose

Lactose [β-D-galactopyranosyl-(1,4) β-D glucopyranose] consists of a molecule each of β-**D galactopyranose** and **β-D-glucopyranose,** which are **linked together by β-1, 4-glycosidic linkage.** The glycoside bond links **carbon-1 of galactose to carbon-4 of glucose.** This in turn, leaves a **free anomeric carbon on the glucose residue.** Thus, **lactose is a reducing disaccharide** (Fig. 2.6).

Fig. 2.6: Lactose

Lactose is found in milk, hence it is also called **milk sugar**. It is synthesized in the mammary glands during lactation from where it is secreted into milk.

Lactose is hydrolyzed by the intestinal enzyme **lactase** (β-D-galactosidase) to its constituent monosaccharides, i.e., **glucose** and **galactose.**

Sucrose

Sucrose [α-D-glucopyranosyl - (1, 2) - β-D-fructofuranose] consists of one molecule each of **α-D glucopyranose** and **β-D fructofuranose** which are linked by **β-1, 2-glycosidic linkage** (Fig. 2.7).

Since the carbonyl groups of both the monosaccharides, i.e., **carbon-1 of glucose and carbon-2 of fructose participate in the formation of the glycosidic bond** and that as such **there is no free carbonyl carbon on any of its monosaccharide,** hence **sucrose is a non-reducing sugar.**

Sucrose, also known as **invert sugar,** is most abundant disaccharide, which is **found in plants**. It is also referred to as **table sugar** or **cane sugar**. It is **hydrolyzed to** its monosaccharides, i.e., **glucose** and **fructose by** the intestinal enzyme **sucrase,** which is also referred to as **invertase.**

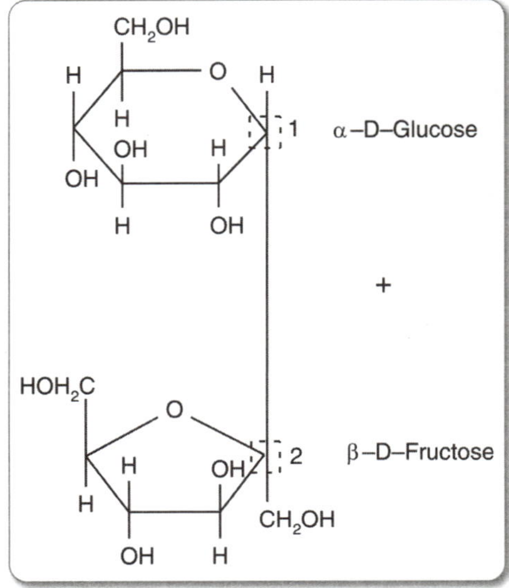

Fig. 2.7: Sucrose

Oligosaccharides

Oligosaccharides are the carbohydrates built by the linking of more than two (generally **three to ten**) **monosaccharide units** by O-glycosidic bonds, e.g., maltotriose, raffinose, etc. Most of these are not digested in human beings. High extent of O-linked oligosaccharides occur in mucin.

Oligosaccharides are usually attached to proteins at the sequences that form surface loops or turns. Some oligosaccharides also play structural roles. A single protein may contain several N- and O-linked oligosaccharide chains. Glycosylation may affect structure, stability or activity of a protein.

Polysaccharides

Polysaccharides, also called **glycans,** are **polymers of** a large number (usually **more than ten**) of **monosaccharides**, which are linked together by glycosidic bonds. They are sparingly soluble in cold water but form a colloidal solution in hot water. Polysaccharides are neither sweet in taste nor have reducing properties.

Polysaccharides are classified as homopolysaccharides and heteropolysaccharides.

Homopolysaccharides

Homopolysaccharides or **homoglycans** are the polymers of the **identical** monosaccharide units. Common homopolysaccharides of biological significance are **starch, glycogen** and **cellulose (polymers of glucose),** and **inulin (a polymer of fructose).**

Starch

Starch is stored as reservoir of carbohydrate in cereals (wheat, maize, etc.) and tubers (potato, etc.), in **plants**. Starch consists of two polysaccharides units called α-**amylose** and **amylopectin.** Starch has both α-**1 → 4** and α-**1 → 6** linkages (Fig. 2.8).

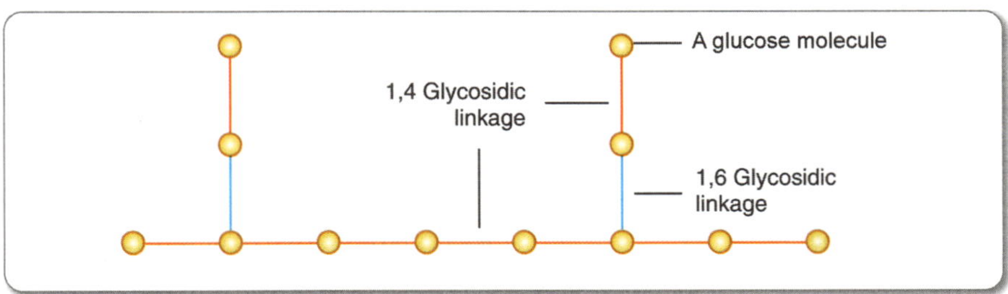

Fig. 2.8: Starch

α-*Amylose* is a **linear** polymer of glucose. In amylose, glucose residues are linked together by α-**(1 → 4) glycosidic bonds**.

Amylopectin is a **branched polymer of glucose.** It has both, α-1 → 4 linkages (in the straight chain) as well as α-1 → 6 linkages (at the branching point). Branching occurs after every 24–30 glucose residues.

Starch is a major source of carbohydrate in human diet. **Amylase,** present in the saliva and the pancreatic juice, randomly hydrolyses α-1 → 4 **glycosidic bonds** of starch and degrades it to a mixture of **maltose, maltotriose and dextrins.**

Glycogen

Glycogen is a **polysaccharide that is found in animals.** It is also called **animal starch.** Although, glycogen is found in all the cells, it is most prevalent in muscle and liver.

Glycogen has both α-1 → 4 **as well as** α-1 → 6 **glycosidic linkages.** It is a highly branched structure and, compared to starch, branching occurs more frequently in glycogen, i.e., after every 10–12 glucose residues (Fig. 2.9).

In the liver, glycogen is used as a readily available source of glucose during starvation.

Differences between starch and glycogen

Table 2.2 lists various differences between starch and glycogen.

Cellulose

Cellulose is a **component** of plant cell wall. **It is a linear polymer having** β-D glucosyl- (1 → 4) α-D **glucose repeating units. Cellulose thus has** β-1(1 → 4) **glycosidic linkages.**

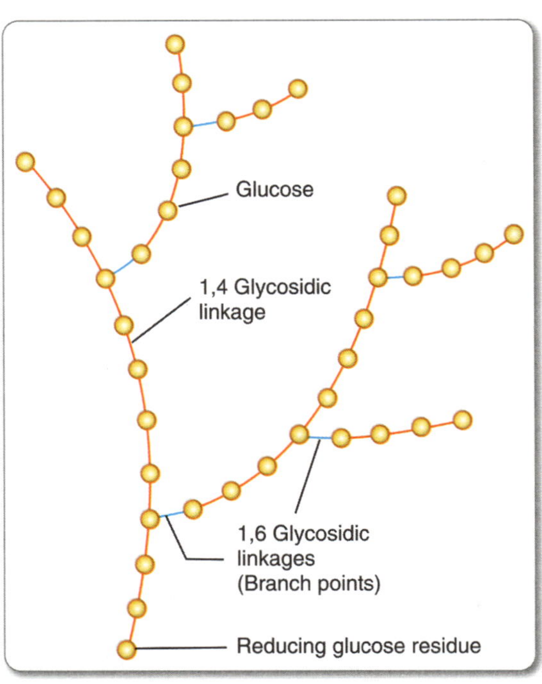

Fig. 2.9: Glycogen

TABLE 2.2: Differences between starch and glycogen

Starch	Glycogen
It is a plant reserve food that is mostly stored in seeds.	It is an animal reserve food that is mainly stored in the liver and muscle.
It is less branched. Branching occurs after nearly 20–30 glucose units.	It is highly branched. Branching occurs after nearly 10–12 glucose units.
It consists of two types of structures, referred to as amylose and amylopectin.	No such structures are present.
It is sparingly soluble in cold water and forms a paste in hot water.	It forms an opalescent solution in water.
It gives violet color with iodine	It gives brown to red color with iodine.

Cellulose cannot be digested by human beings because we lack cellulases, i.e., the enzymes which are responsible for hydrolyzing β-(1 → 4) linkages. Cellulose, though cannot be utilized by human beings, it forms a considerable part of the vegetarian food and adds to the bulk of feces.

Inulin

Inulin **is a linear** homopolymer of β-D fructose. **It is found in the bulbs of dahlia, onion and garlic. Inulin is not utilized by human beings but is of biological significance since it is used in the determination of glomerular filtration rate (GFR).**

Dextrans

Dextrans are highly branched homopolymers of glucose having 1 → 6, 1 → 4 **and** 1 → 3 **glycoside linkages.** Various microorganisms grown in a sucrose media produce dextrans. These have molecular weight between 1 and 4 millions. Dextrans are used for intravenous infusion, as volume expanders, in the treatment of Hypovolemic shock.

Chitin

Chitin is present in the exoskeleton of insects. It is composed of **N-acetylglucosamine residues**, which are **linked by β-1 → 4 glycosidic linkages.**

Heteropolysaccharides

Heteropolysaccharides, also called **heteroglycans**, consist of repeating disaccharide units, which bear negatively charged groups. These are present in the connective tissue, e.g., cartilage, tendon, skin and blood vessel walls. Heteropolysaccharides are linked to proteins and are also called **glycosaminoglycans**. **Glycosaminoglycan-protein** complexes are also referred to as **proteoglycans.**

Glycosaminoglycans

Most important glycosaminoglycans are **hyaluronic acid, chondroitin sulfates, heparin,** etc.

Hyaluronic Acid

Hyaluronic acid is composed of repeating units of **D-glucuronic acid and N-acetyl-D-glucosamine**. This polysaccharide chain is the longest of the glycosaminoglycans (GAG) and is different from other GAGs as hyaluronic acid is the only GAG which is nonsulfated. Hyaluronic acid not covalently attached to protein and

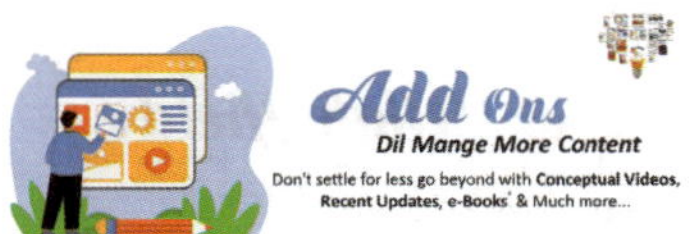

is not limited to animal tissues but is also found in bacteria. It is an important GAG component of **connective tissue, synovial fluid and vitreous humor** of the eye. Viscoelastic behavior of hyaluronate solution makes them excellent biological shock absorbers and lubricants.

Chondroitin Sulfates

Chondroitin sulfates contain **glucuronic acid and N-acetylgalactosamine with sulfate** on the hydroxyl group of either carbon-4 (chondroitin-4-sulfate) or carbon-6 (chondroitin-6-sulfate). Chondroitin sulfates are the major components of the cartilage, where chondroitin sulfates bind collagens, and hold fibers in a tight and strong network. These are also found in **aorta, tendons and ligaments**.

- **Dermatan Sulfate:** It is derived from chondroitin by enzymatic epimerization of carbon-5 of glucuronate residues to iduronate residues. Thus, dermatan sulfate contains **L-iduronic acid** (with variable amounts of glucuronic acid) and **N-acetylgalactosamine**. It is found in **skin, blood vessels, tendon** and **heart valves**.

- **Heparan Sulfate:** These are not constructed of identical disaccharides but exhibit structural diversity. It consists of **glucuronic or iduronic acid and glucosamine**. Some glucosamines are acetylated, and may have N- and O-sulfate groups. It is a ubiquitous cell-surface component as well as extracellular substance in **blood vessel walls and brain**. Heparan sulfates, which function directly at the cell surface, interact with a variety of proteins, including important growth factors and their receptors (such as fibroblast growth factors and their receptors). The formation of ternary complexes of heparan sulfate with fibroblast growth factors and fibroblast growth factor receptors, initiate signaling processes.

- **Keratan Sulfates:** It is the most heterogeneous group of glycosaminoglycans as its sulfate content is variable. It contains smaller amounts of **fucose, mannose, N-acetylglucosamine and sialic acid**. The repeating disaccharide, generally, is N-acetylglucosamine and galactose. Sulfate content is variable and may be present on hydroxyl group at carbon-6. Keratan sulfates are linked to proteins either by an N-linkages (keratan sulfate I) or O-linkages (keratan sulfate II). Keratan sulfate I is found in **cornea** while keratan sulfate II occurs in **loose connective tissue** proteoglycan aggregates with chondroitin sulfate.

Heparin

Heparin consists of **glucuronic or iduronic acid and glucosamine**. Most of its glucosamine units are N-sulfated. Sulfate is also bound to the hydroxyl group on carbon-2 of uronic acid residues and carbon-3 or carbon-6 of glucosamine. It is a highly charged polymer found in the **intracellular granules of mast cells** that occurs in arterial walls, especially **in the liver, lungs and skin**. Heparin is widely used, clinically, to **inhibit blood clotting**, e.g., in postsurgical patients.

USES OF CARBOHYDRATES

- Carbohydrates are the main source of **energy** in the body. Brain cells and RBCs are entirely dependent on glucose as the energy source. Energy production from carbohydrates is 4 kcal/g.
- **Starch** is the storage form of energy **in plants** and **glycogen in animals**. During fasting, these stored carbohydrates release glucose.
- Carbohydrates can be **converted to** other biomolecules like **fat**.
- Glycoproteins and glycolipids are **components of cell membranes** and receptors. All the plasma proteins except albumin contain oligosaccharide chains.

- Carbohydrates form **structural basis of many organisms**, e.g., cellulose of plants; exoskeleton of insects, cell wall of microorganisms and mucopolysaccharides as ground substances in higher organisms.

METABOLISM OF CARBOHYDRATES

Principal sources of carbohydrates include starch from cereals, pulses, potatoes, rice, etc.; lactose from milk **and sucrose** from table sugar. Glucose may not form an essential part of a diet, since all the dietary carbohydrates are readily converted to glucose in the body.

Digestion of Carbohydrates

Digestion of carbohydrates begins in the mouth where salivary amylase hydrolyses starch into smaller polysaccharides and maltose. Chewing stimulates the production of saliva and mixes salivary amylase with the food. Only about 5% of the starch is broken down by the time the food is swallowed. When carbohydrate enters the stomach, acidity of the stomach stops the action of salivary amylase by denaturing the enzyme.

As stomach contents enter small intestine, the pancreas secretes pancreatic amylase through the pancreatic duct into the small intestine. Pancreatic amylase continues the digestion of starch, breaking it into maltose. Meanwhile, brush border disaccharidases; break various disaccharides into monosaccharides (Table 2.3).

Dietary fiber moves to the large intestine where bacteria partially ferment these undigested carbohydrates, and produce gas and a few short-chain fatty acids. Soluble fiber softens the stool and makes it easier to pass. Insoluble fiber resists bacterial activity and passes unchanged to add bulk to stool.

TABLE 2.3: Role of enzymes in the digestion of carbohydrates

Enzyme	Site of action	Catalytic action
Salivary amylase	Mouth	Starch/Glycogen → Partially hydrolyzed dextrins, oligosaccharides, isomaltose and maltose
Pancreatic amylase	Small intestine	Partially hydrolyzed dextrins/oligosaccharides → Dextrins, maltose, isomaltose, maltotriose
α-Dextrinase	Small intestine	α-Limit dextrins → Maltotriose, glucose
Disaccharidases	Small intestine	
Sucrase		Sucrose → Glucose and fructose
Lactase		Lactose → Glucose and galactose
Maltase		Maltose/Maltotriose → Glucose
Isomaltase		Isomaltose → Glucose

Absorption of Monosaccharides

Different monosaccharides are absorbed into the mucosal cell lining the small intestine by two mechanisms. Whereas **fructose is absorbed by facilitated diffusion, glucose and galactose are absorbed by active transport.** Glucose is also absorbed by the sodium-linked glucose transporter called SLGT-1.

In the villi, absorbed monosaccharides pass through the intestinal mucosal cells and enter the liver *via* the portal vein. Within the liver, galactose and fructose are also converted to glucose.

METABOLISM OF GLUCOSE

Fates and Sources of Glucose in the Body

Glucose is the major **monosaccharide,** which enters the **liver**. Thereafter, it is converted to glycogen and **stored in the liver and muscle.** It is also **oxidized** in the liver to **produce energy** (Fig. 2.10).

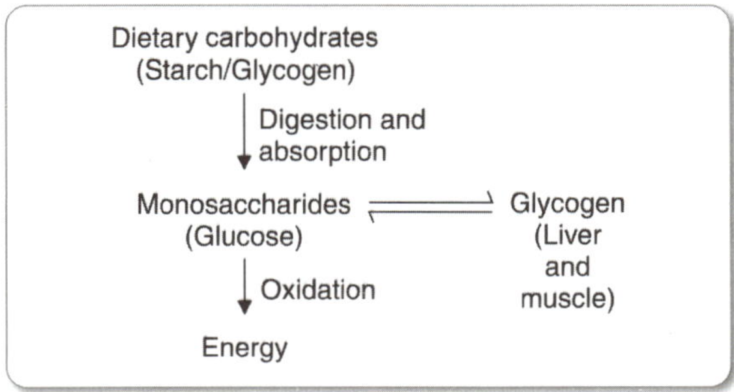

Fig. 2.10: Metabolic fates of glucose

Various metabolic **pathways,** which **utilize glucose, include glycolysis, glycogenesis and pentose phosphate pathway.**

On the other hand, **gluconeogenesis** and **glycogenolysis** are the **pathways** which generate **glucose.**

GLYCOLYSIS

Glycolysis is also called as **Embden-Meyerhof Parnas pathway** or **Embden-Meyerhof Pathway.** It is a process of **catabolism** of **glucose** either in the presence of oxygen, such as in the liver (**aerobic glycolysis**), or lack of oxygen, such as in skeletal muscle (**anaerobic glycolysis**).

Glycolytic enzymes are present in the extra-mitochondrial compartment of the cell. Although aerobic glycolysis occurs in most of the tissues, like liver and kidney, anaerobic glycolysis occurs only in muscle (Fig. 2.11).

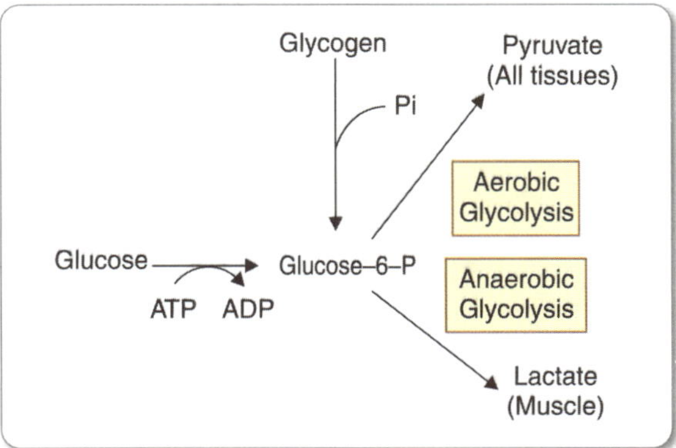

Fig. 2.11: Differences between aerobic and anaerobic glycolysis

Various reactions of the glycolytic pathway are shown in Figure 2.12.

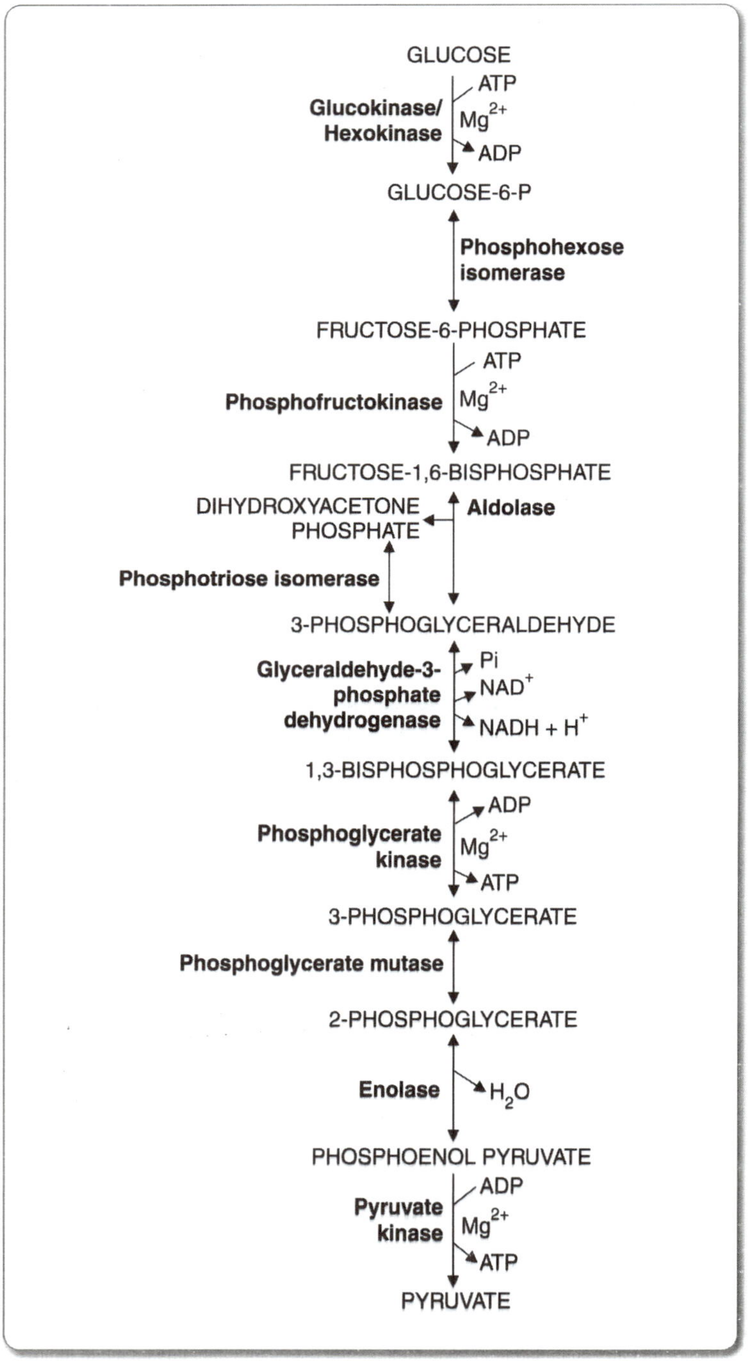

GLUCOSE
Glucokinase/Hexokinase — ATP, Mg^{2+}, ADP
GLUCOSE-6-P
Phosphohexose isomerase
FRUCTOSE-6-PHOSPHATE
Phosphofructokinase — ATP, Mg^{2+}, ADP
FRUCTOSE-1,6-BISPHOSPHATE
DIHYDROXYACETONE PHOSPHATE — Aldolase
Phosphotriose isomerase
3-PHOSPHOGLYCERALDEHYDE
Glyceraldehyde-3-phosphate dehydrogenase — Pi, NAD^+, $NADH + H^+$
1,3-BISPHOSPHOGLYCERATE
Phosphoglycerate kinase — ADP, Mg^{2+}, ATP
3-PHOSPHOGLYCERATE
Phosphoglycerate mutase
2-PHOSPHOGLYCERATE
Enolase — H_2O
PHOSPHOENOL PYRUVATE
Pyruvate kinase — ADP, Mg^{2+}, ATP
PYRUVATE

Fig. 2.12: Metabolism of glucose *via* aerobic glycolysis

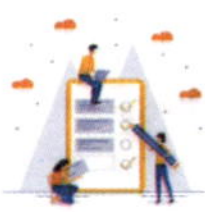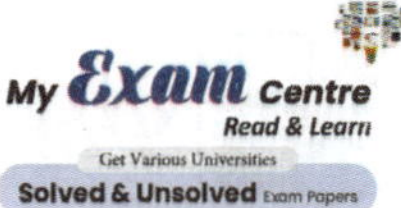

- **Phosphorylation of Glucose: Glucose** is activated, irreversibly, to **glucose-6-phosphate** by **glucokinase** or **hexokinase**, in the presence of ATP and Mg^{2+} (Fig. 2.13).

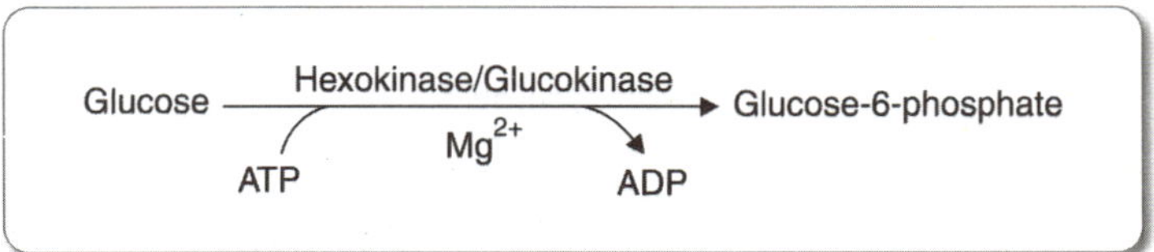

Fig. 2.13: Phosphorylation of glucose

Hexokinase is allosterically inhibited by glucose-6-phosphate and has high affinity (low K_m) for glucose. This enzyme is present in **all the extrahepatic tissues.**

In the liver, in the fed state, this reaction is catalyzed **by glucokinase** which is an inducible enzyme. Its activity is induced by glucose since it has low affinity (high K_m) for glucose and its function is to remove glucose from blood in the fed state.

- **Glucose-6-phosphate** is isomerized, in a freely reversible reaction, to **fructose-6-phosphate** by the enzyme **phosphohexose isomerase.**

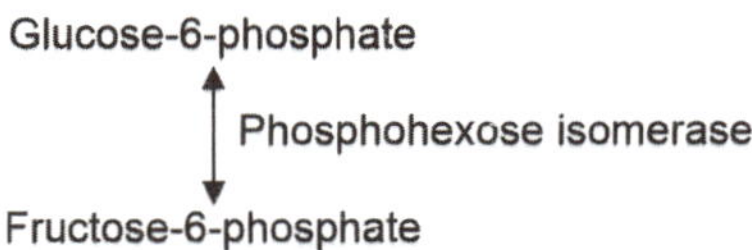

- **Fructose-6-phosphate** is then phosphorylated, by an allosteric enzyme **phosphofructokinase**, to form **fructose-1,6-bisphosphate.**

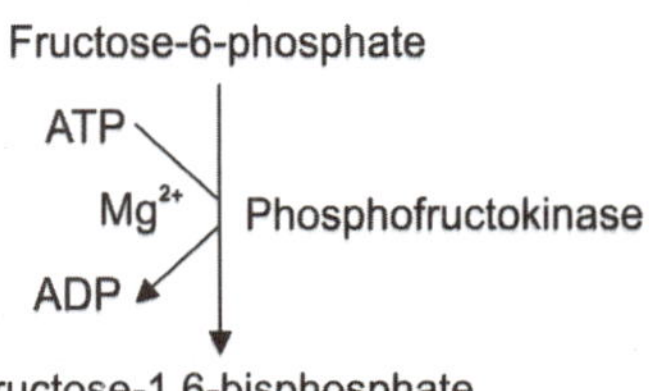

This is an irreversible reaction. It requires ATP, which acts as a co-substrate as well as an allosteric inhibitor of the enzyme.

- **Fructose-1,6-bisphosphate** (a hexose) is cleaved by **aldolase** to **3-phosphoglyceraldehyde** (glyceraldehyde-3-phosphate) and **dihydroxyacetone phosphate**, the two trioses.

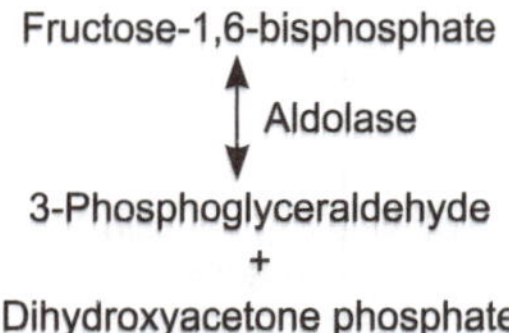

- Subsequently, only 3-phosphoglyceraldehyde enters the pathway. Hence, **dihydroxyacetone phosphate** is also converted to **3-phosphoglyceraldehyde** by the enzyme **phosphotriose isomerase.**

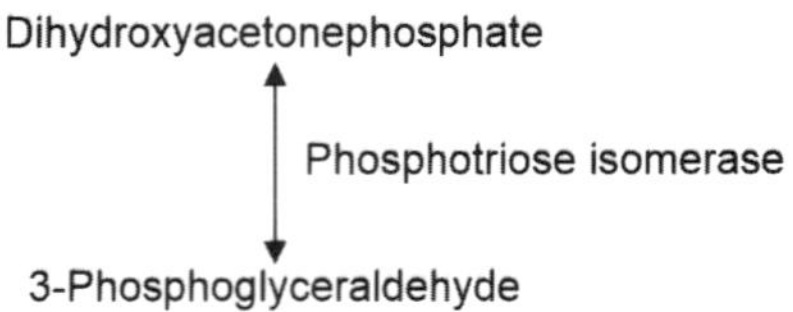

Glycerol can also enter the glycolytic pathway through this reaction.

- In the presence of NAD$^+$ and inorganic phosphate (Pi), **glyceraldehyde-3-phosphate dehydrogenase** oxidizes 3-phosphoglyceraldehyde to **1,3-bisphosphoglycerate**.

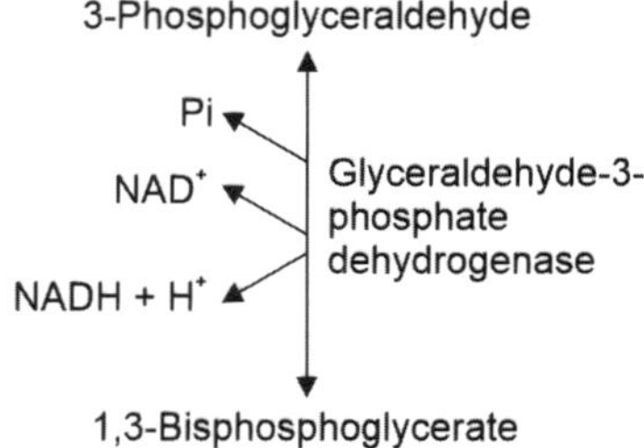

- In the next step, **1,3-bisphosphoglycerate** is converted to **3-phosphoglycerate**. This reaction is catalyzed by the enzyme **phosphoglycerate kinase**.

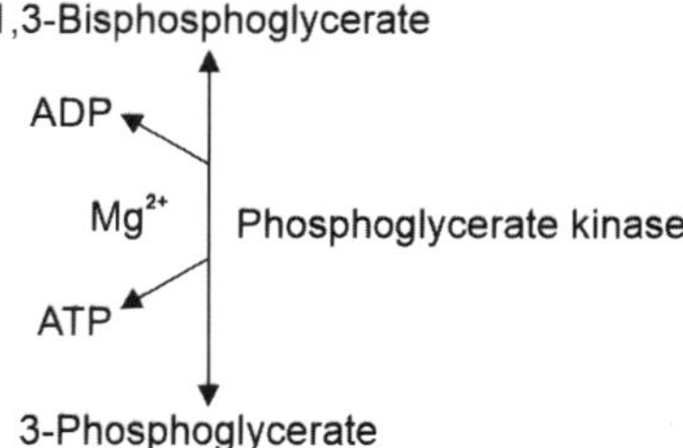

In this reaction, there is production of ATP. It is called substrate-level production of ATP (i.e. **substrate level phosphorylation**).

> **Arsenic Acid as Inhibitor of Glycolysis**
> Arsenic acid inhibits phosphorylation at this step and thus, ATP production.

- Thereafter, **3-phosphoglycerate** is converted to **2-phosphoglycerate** by the enzyme phosphoglycerate mutase.

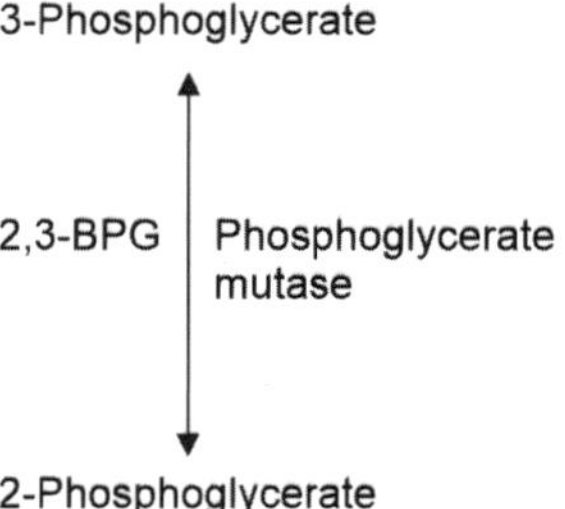

2,3-bisphosphoglycerate (2,3-BPG) acts as coenzyme for this reaction.

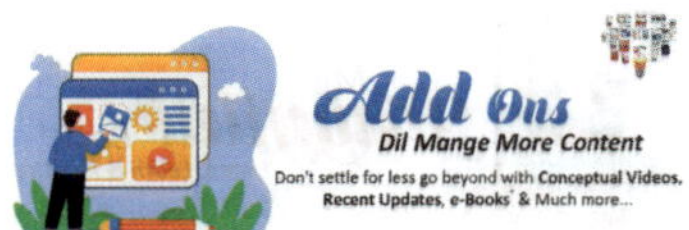

- **Enolase** converts **2-phosphoglycerate** to a high-energy compound called **phosphoenolpyruvate.**

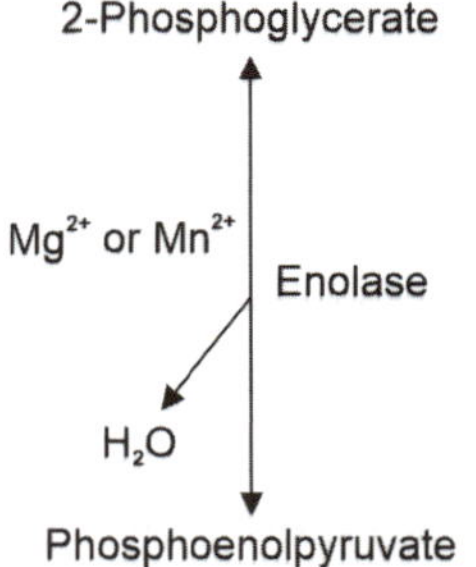

Enolase requires Mg^{2+} or Mn^{2+} for its activity but is inhibited by fluoride.

> **Use of Fluoride as Anticoagulant**
> **Fluoride** inhibits this reaction, therefore, fluoride is added to the blood, as a preservative when blood is collected for glucose estimation.

- Subsequently, **phosphoenolpyruvate** is converted to **pyruvate,** irreversibly. This reaction is catalyzed by the enzyme pyruvate kinase. It also phosphorylates ADP to ATP.

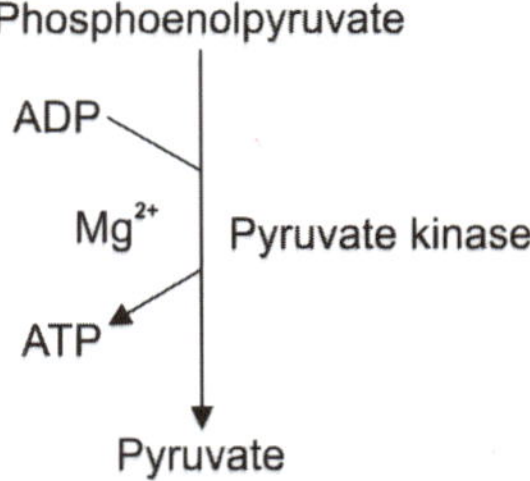

Deficiency of pyruvate kinase leads to hemolytic anemia.

Regulation of Glycolysis

There are three irreversible steps which are catalyzed by hexokinase, phosphofructokinase and pyruvate kinase. These are the sites of the regulation of glycolysis.

Insulin stimulates these enzymes and increases utilization of glucose by glycolysis. On the other hand, **glucagon inhibits** this process.

Fate of Pyruvic Acid

- **Oxidative Decarboxylation to Acetyl CoA:** *Under aerobic conditions,* **pyruvate** is transported into mitochondria where it is oxidatively decarboxylated to **acetyl CoA** by the enzyme **pyruvate dehydrogenase complex** (Fig. 2.14).

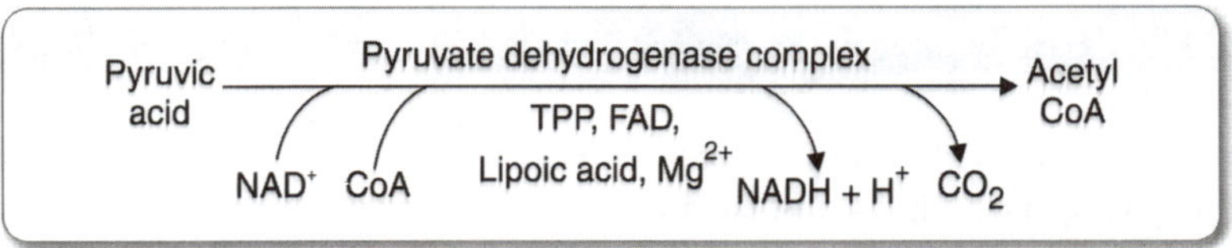

Fig. 2.14: Conversion of pyruvate to acetyl CoA

Pyruvate dehydrogenase complex requires five coenzymes, i.e., **TPP, CoA, NAD⁺, FAD** and **lipoic acid**. Insulin stimulates its activity, whereas it is inhibited by acetyl CoA, NADH and increased ATP/ADP ratio.

> **Pyruvate Dehydrogenase Complex and Lactic Acidosis**
> Pyruvate dehydrogenase complex is inhibited by arsenate and mercuric ions as well as by dietary deficiency of thiamin. Inhibition of the enzyme results in accumulation of pyruvate and lactate, resulting in **lactic acidosis.** This in turn may manifest several neurological disturbances.

- **Reduction to Lactate:** *Under anaerobic conditions* **pyruvate** is reduced to **lactate**. This reaction is catalyzed by the enzyme **lactate dehydrogenase** which requires NADH + H⁺.

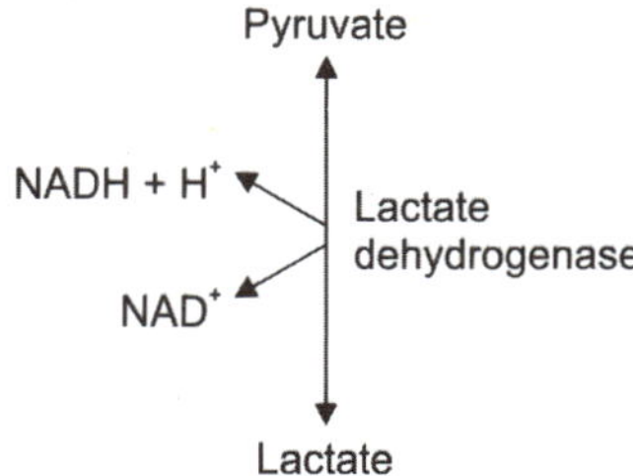

Tissues such as skeletal muscle, when function under hypoxic conditions, produce a large amount of lactic acid.

ATP Production in Glycolysis

The number of ATP produced during glycolysis varies, depending upon the condition.

- *Under Anaerobic Conditions:* Since each of the energy-yielding steps, i.e., conversion of 1,3-bisphosphoglycerate to 3-phosphoglycerate and phosphoenolpyruvate to pyruvate produce one ATP, **total** 2 ATP are produced per molecule of triose or **4** molecules of **ATP per** molecule of **hexose** (Fig. 2.15).

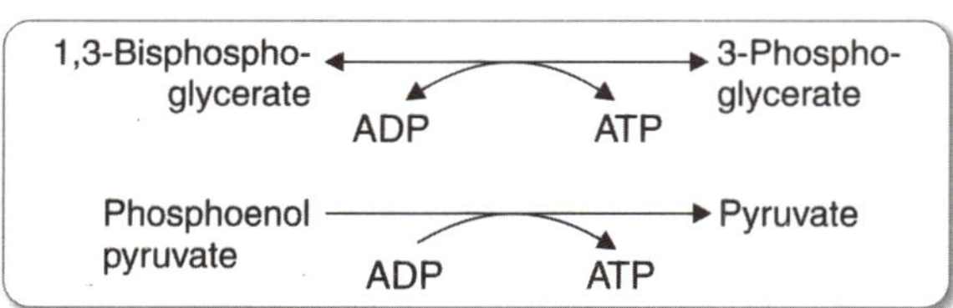

Fig. 2.15: Energy-yielding steps in glycolysis

As 2 ATP are used in the initial two reactions of the process, i.e., conversion of glucose to glucose-6-phosphate and fructose-6-phosphate to fructose-1,6-bisphosphate, **net energy yield** per molecule of glucose is **2 ATP**.

- *Under Aerobic Conditions:* Under aerobic condition, NADH produced during the conversion of 3-phosphoglycerate to 1,3-bisphosphoglycerate enters electron transport chain and forms 2.5. Thus, additionally, 5 ATP are produced per molecule of glucose. Total yield under aerobic conditions, therefore, is 9 ATP while the **net yield** is **7 ATP**.

GLUCONEOGENESIS

Gluconeogenesis (neoglucogenesis) is the process of the **formation of glucose** from various **non-carbohydrate sources,** such as the glucogenic amino acids, lactate, glycerol and propionate. Gluconeogenesis takes place in the fasting state or on a low carbohydrate diet, particularly in the liver and some other tissues, which are solely dependent on glucose for their energy demand. It does not occur in muscle.

Gluconeogenesis thus, enables maintenance of blood glucose when all the dietary glucose has been absorbed and oxidized. This process is essential since blood glucose level has to be maintained to support metabolism of the tissues that use glucose as the primary substrate such as the brain, red blood cells and lens.

As discussed above, there are three **irreversible reactions in the glycolytic pathway** (Fig. 2.16).

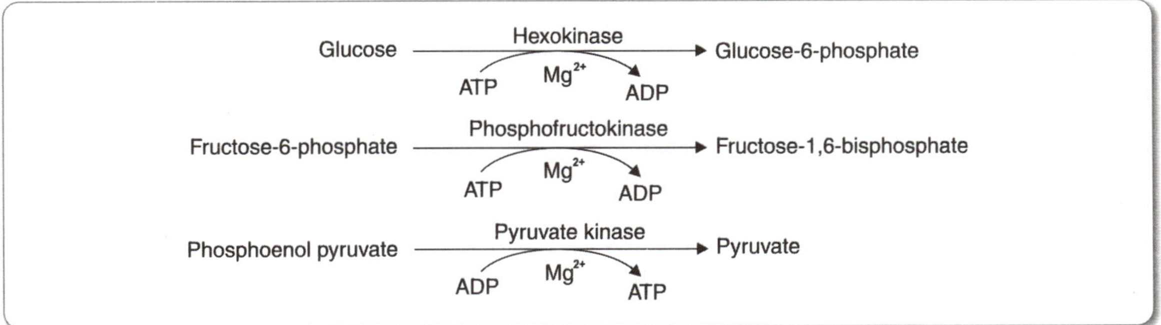

Fig. 2.16: Irreversible reactions in the glycolytic pathway.

Gluconeogenesis is not reversal of glycolysis, since these reactions are bypassed by an alternate set of reactions, which include:

Conversion of Pyruvate to Phosphoenolpyruvate

For the reversal of the pyruvate to phosphoenolpyruvate, **pyruvate** is first converted to **oxaloacetate** by the enzyme **pyruvate carboxylase,** in mitochondria.

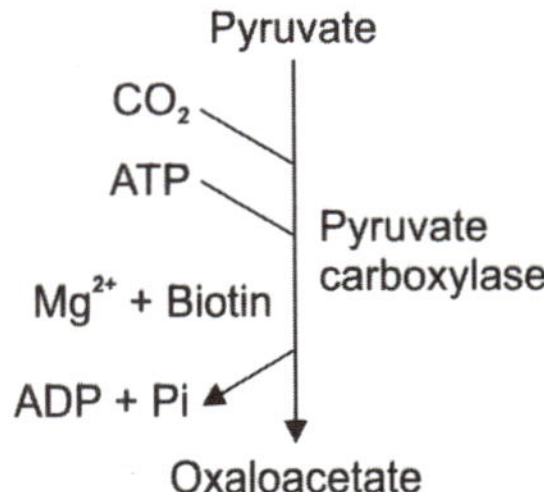

Thereafter, malate dehydrogenase converts oxaloacetate to malate, which is freely transported across the mitochondrial membrane. Malate thus, comes out from the mitochondria to the cytosol where it is converted back to oxaloacetate by the same enzyme. This also reduces NAD^+ to $NADH + H^+$. This enzyme thus, not only transports oxaloacetate (*via* malate) but also reducing equivalents from mitochondria into cytosol. Reactions of gluconeogenesis thus occur in the cytosol as well as mitochondria.

In the cytosol, **oxaloacetate** is converted to **phosphoenolpyruvate** by the enzyme **phosphoenolpyruvate carboxykinase** (PEP-carboxykinase).

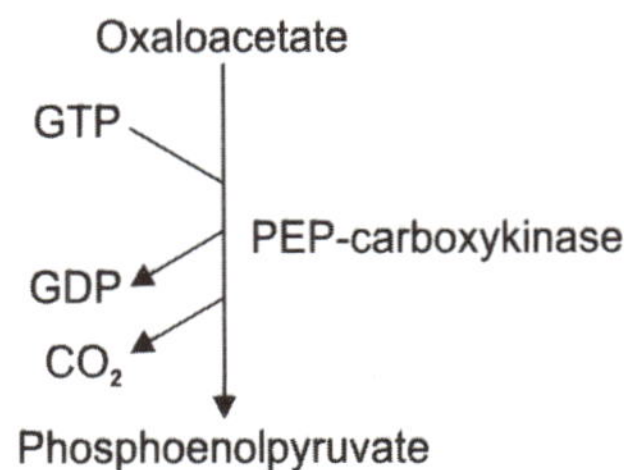

Conversion of Fructose-1,6-Bisphosphate to Fructose-6-Phosphate

Fructose-1,6-bisphosphate is converted to fructose-6-phosphate by the enzyme **fructose-1,6-bisphosphatase.**

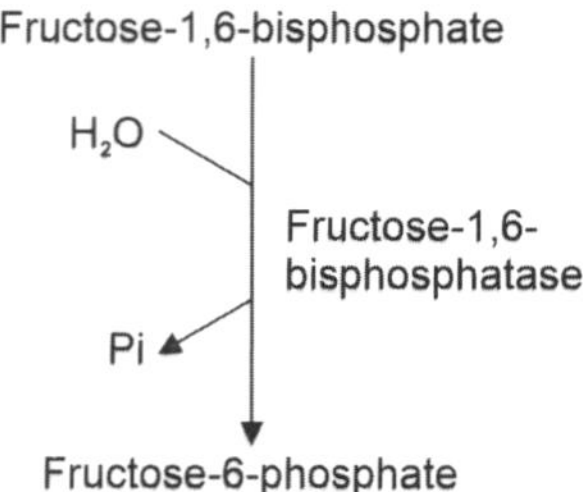

Conversion of Glucose-6-Phosphate to Glucose

Glucose-6-phosphate is converted to glucose by the enzyme **glucose-6-phosphatase.** This enzyme is not found in the muscle and adipose tissue.

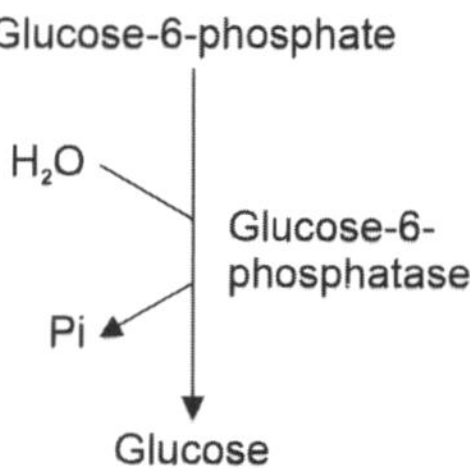

Substrates for Gluconeogenesis

Lactate

Lactate is produced during the process of anaerobic glycolysis. For its conversion to glucose, firstly, **lactate** is oxidized to **pyruvate**. This reaction is catalyzed by the enzyme **lactate dehydrogenase**, which requires NAD^+.

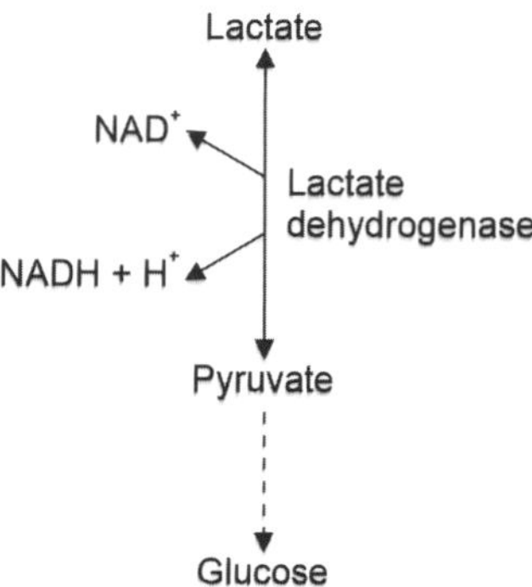

The direction of LDH reaction depends on the relative intracellular concentrations of pyruvate and lactate, and on the ratio of $NADH/NAD^+$, in the cell. The formation of lactate is the major fate of pyruvate in several tissues such as red blood cells, lens and cornea of the eye, etc.

Subsequently, pyruvate is converted to glucose by the **reversal of the glycolytic reactions.**

Glycogenic Amino Acid

In the liver, various glucogenic amino acids transfer their α-amino group by transamination and release carbon skeletons, which form intermediates of the citric acid cycle (Table 2.4).

These citric acid cycle intermediates in turn can form glucose by reversal of the glycolytic reactions *via* pyruvate.

TABLE 2.4: Formation of the citric acid cycle intermediates from glucogenic amino acids

Amino acids	Citric acid cycle intermediate formed
Gly, Ala, Ser, Thr, Cys, Trp and HO-Pro	Pyruvate
Arg, His, Glu, Gln and Pro	α-Ketoglutarate
Phe and Tyr	Fumarate
Val, Ile and Met	Succinyl CoA

Glycerol

Glycerol is produced as a result of lipolysis in the adipose tissue. **Glycerol kinase** converts it to α-**glycerol phosphate** in the liver, which is later reduced by a dehydrogenase to **dihydroxy-acetone phosphate** and can enter glycolysis at this point (Fig. 2.17).

Propionate

Oxidation of fatty acids containing odd number of carbon atoms, in addition to acetyl CoA, produces a molecule of **propionyl CoA,** particularly in ruminants. In human beings, propionyl CoA is obtained from Ile, Val and Thr. It is converted to **D-methylmalonyl CoA** by **propionyl CoA carboxylase**. D-Methylmalonyl CoA is then converted to **L-methylmalonyl CoA** and finally, by an isomerase to **succinyl CoA,** which is an intermediate of the citric acid cycle. Succinyl CoA in turn can be converted to glucose *via* pyruvate (Fig. 2.18).

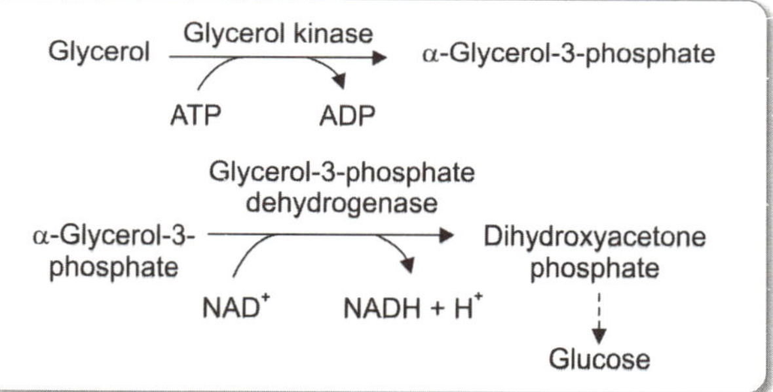

Fig. 2.17: Conversion of glycerol to glucose

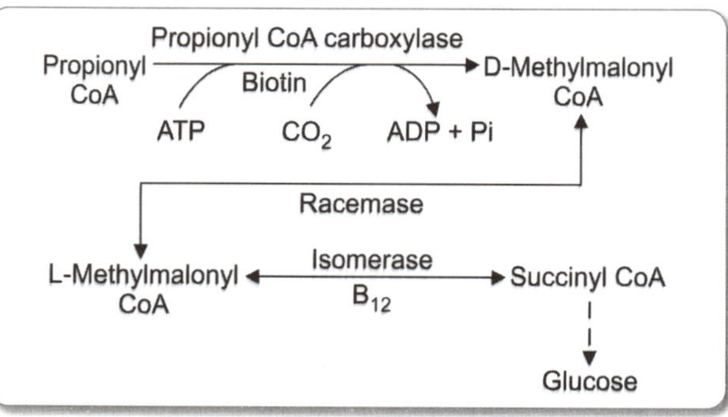

Fig. 2.18: Conversion of propionyl CoA to glucose

TRICARBOXYLIC ACID CYCLE

Tricarboxylic acid cycle is also called **citric acid cycle** or the **Krebs cycle.** It is a process of **oxidation of acetyl CoA** (active acetate) to CO_2 and H_2O.

During the course of the oxidation of acetyl CoA, reducing equivalents are produced, which enter respiratory chain and generate a large amount of ATP. Reactions of the Krebs cycle are shown in Figure 2.19.

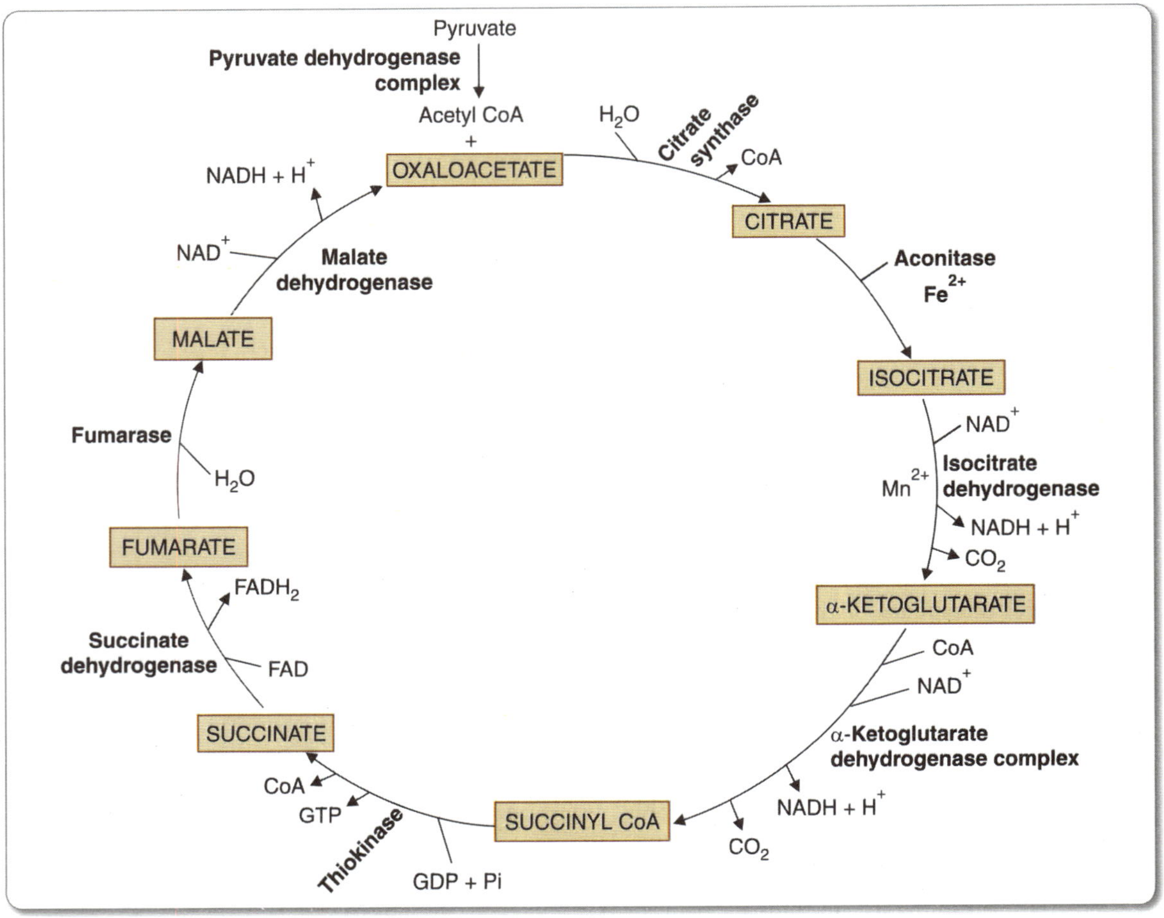

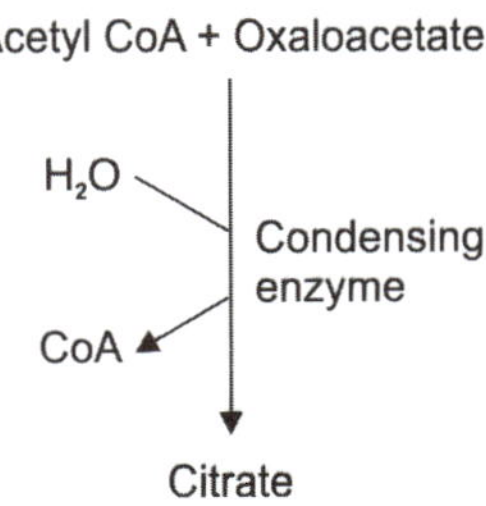

Fig. 2.19: Tricarboxylic acid cycle

- In the first step, **acetyl CoA** (formed from pyruvate under aerobic condition) combines with **oxaloacetate** and forms citric acid (a tricarboxylic acid).

This reaction is catalyzed by the enzyme **citrate synthase,** also called the **condensing enzyme.**

- **Citrate** is then rearranged to **cis-aconitate**, which is subsequently changed to isocitrate. Both of these steps are catalyzed by **aconitase.**

Inhibition of Aconitase by Fluoroacetate
Aconitase, which converts citrate to isocitrate is **inhibited by fluoroacetate.**

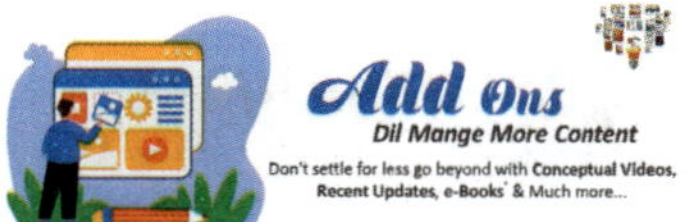

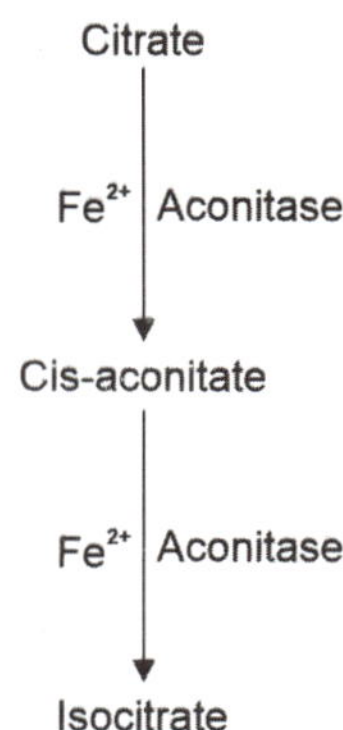

- In the presence of **isocitrate dehydrogenase, isocitrate** is converted to oxalosuccinate, which is subsequently decarboxylated to α-**Ketoglutarate**.

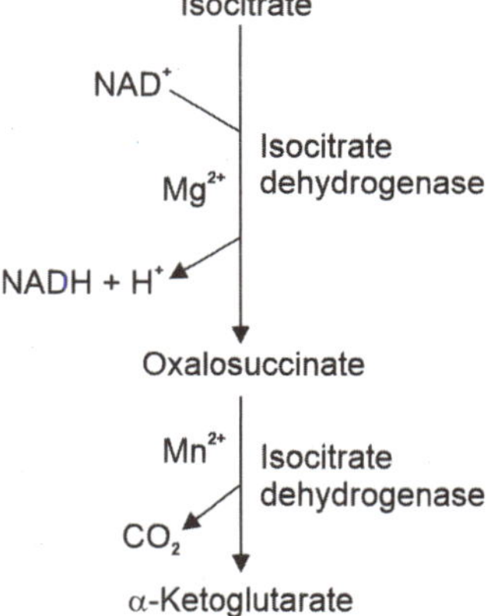

- **α-Ketoglutarate** undergoes oxidative decarboxylation and gets converted to **succinyl CoA.**

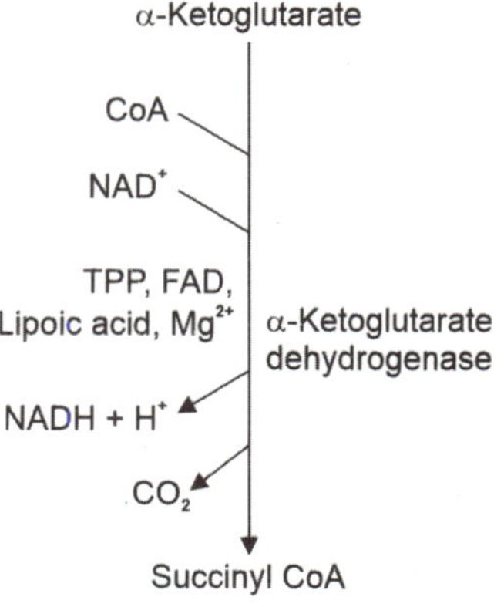

This reaction is similar to the conversion of pyruvate to acetyl CoA. α-**Ketoglutarate dehydrogenase complex,** which also requires five coenzymes, i.e., TPP, NAD⁺, FAD, coenzyme A and lipoic acid, catalyzes this reaction.

- **Succinyl CoA** is converted to **succinate,** by the enzyme **succinate thiokinase**.

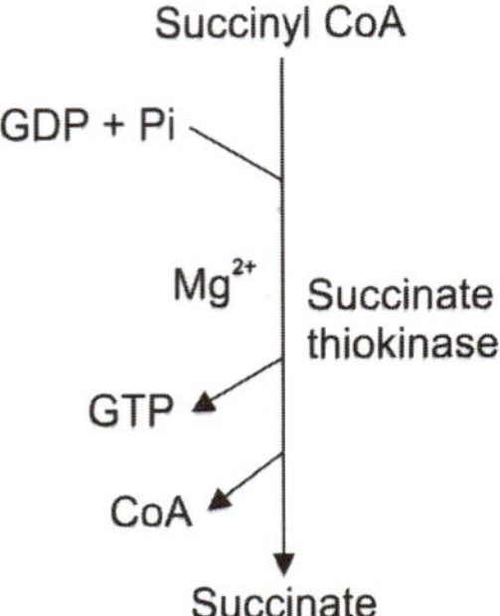

During this reaction, a molecule of GTP is formed. This is known as **substrate level phosphorylation, as a high-energy** molecule is formed at the substrate level.

- **Succinate** is converted to **fumarate,** by the enzyme **succinate dehydrogenase.**

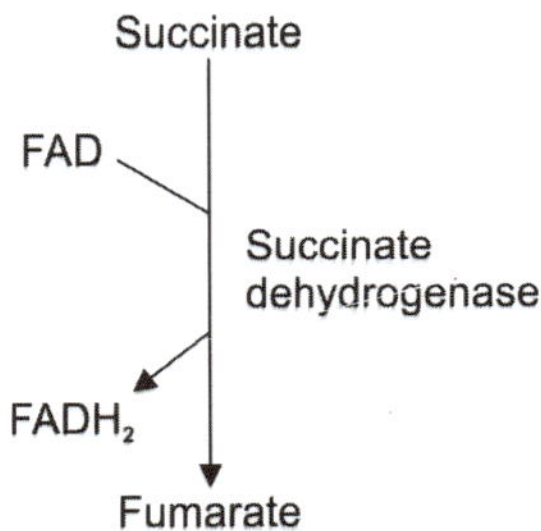

Due to structural similarities between malonate and succinate, **malonate inhibits** succinate dehydrogenase, **competitively.**

- With the addition of a molecule of water, by the enzyme fumarase (fumarate hydratase), fumarate is converted to L-malate.

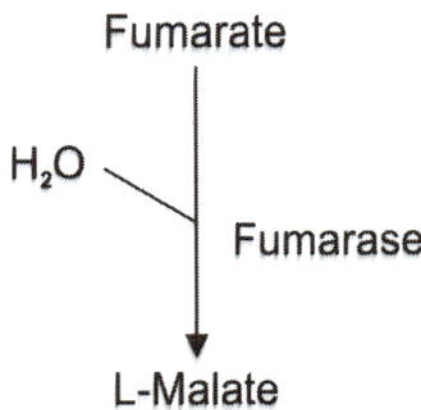

- Finally, **malate dehydrogenase,** in the presence of NAD⁺, converts **malate** to **oxaloacetate.**

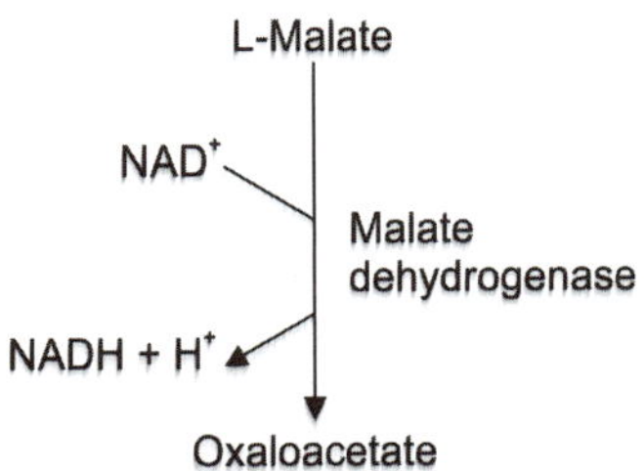

Energy Yield from Tricarboxylic Acid Cycle

As a result of oxidation of one molecule of acetyl CoA in the Krebs cycle, three molecules of NAD^+ and one molecule of FAD are reduced.

Reducing equivalents from $NADH + H^+$ enter respiratory chain and result in the production of 2.5 molecules of ATP. Similarly, $FADH_2$ yields 1.5 ATP. Besides, there is also substrate level production of GTP.

Thus, **total ATP yield**, per molecule of acetyl CoA, is **10 ATP** (Table 2.5).

As mentioned above, conversion of pyruvate to acetyl CoA also generates $NADH + H^+$ and gives 2.5 ATP. Thus, total number of ATP produced from oxidation of pyruvate is 12.5.

TABLE 2.5: Energy production in citric acid cycle

Reaction	Reducing equivalents produced as	Number of ATP produced
Isocitrate → α-Ketoglutarate	$NADH + H^+$	2.5
α-Ketoglutarate → Succinyl CoA	$NADH + H^+$	2.5
Succinyl CoA → Succinate	–	1
Succinate → Fumarate	$FADH_2$	1.5
Malate → Oxaloacetate	$NADH + H^+$	2.5
	Total	**10**

Since 2 molecules of pyruvate are formed from one molecule of glucose, therefore, in addition to energy yield during aerobic glycolysis (7 ATP) a molecule of glucose also produces 25 ATP *via* the Krebs cycle. Thus, a total of 32 ATP are obtained when a molecule of glucose is completely oxidized to CO_2 and H_2O under aerobic conditions, i.e., *via* glycolysis and Krebs cycle.

Biological Significance of Tricarboxylic Acid Cycle

Citric acid cycle has a **dual role**, i.e., it is important in oxidation as well as synthetic processes. It is thus **amphibolic** in nature.

It is **catabolic** for the oxidation of carbohydrates, lipids and proteins, as they are completely oxidized to CO_2 and H_2O, and release energy.

It is also important in the **anabolic** reactions, as various intermediates of the cycle can be used for the biosynthesis of the nonessential amino acids. Various intermediates of the cycle are also potentially glucogenic and thus, can give rise to glucose in liver and kidney (Fig. 2.20).

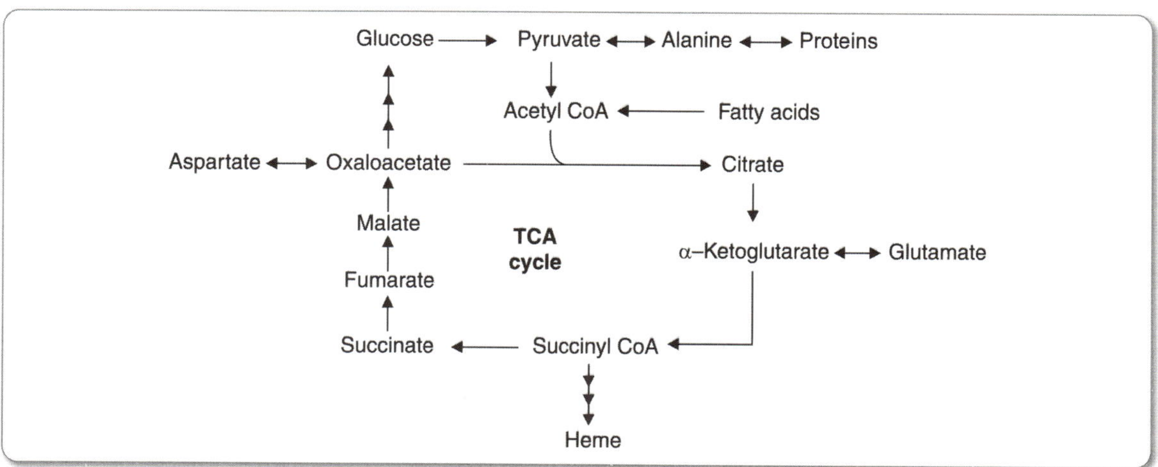

Fig. 2.20: Biological significance of tricarboxylic acid cycle.

GLYCOGEN METABOLISM

Glycogen Synthesis

Glycogen synthesis (**Glycogenesis**) is the process of the **conversion of glucose to glycogen**. Although, it is operative in several tissues, liver and muscle are the main organs for the synthesis of glycogen. Glycogenesis is stimulated by insulin.

Various reactions of glycogenesis are shown in Figure 2.21.

- **Glucose** is first activated (phosphorylated) to **glucose-6-phosphate.**

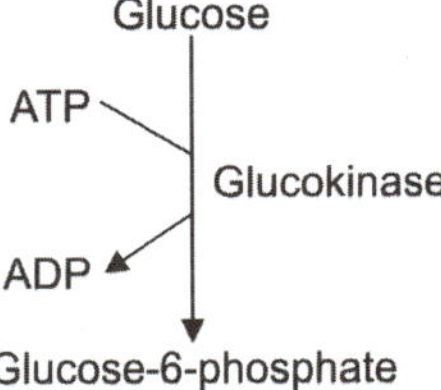

In the liver, **glucokinase** converts most of the glucose into glucose-6-phosphate, in the fed state. This is an inducible enzyme and has greater specificity for its substrate.

In the muscle and other tissues, this reaction is catalyzed by **hexokinase.**

- **Glucose-6-phosphate** is epimerised to form **glucose-1-phosphate,** by the enzyme **phosphoglucomutase.**

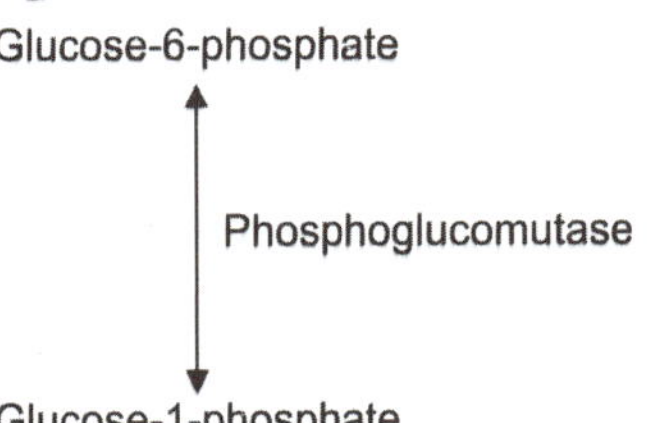

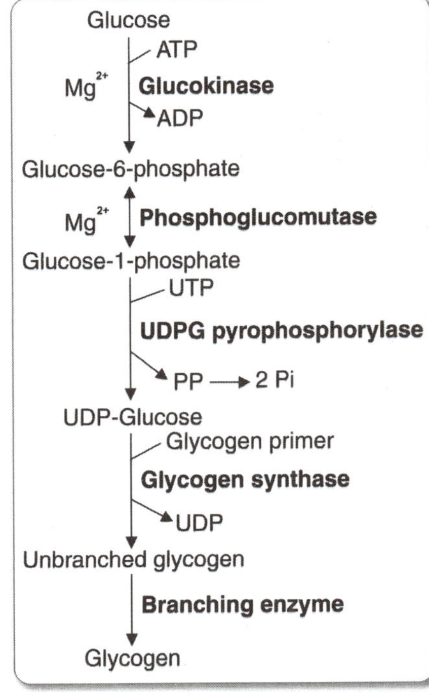

Fig. 2.21: Glycogenesis

- **Glucose-1-phosphate** reacts with UTP and gets converted to **uridine diphosphate glucose** (UDP-Glu). This reaction is catalyzed by **UDPG pyrophosphorylase** (glucose-1-phosphate uridyltransferase).

  Pyrophosphate, so released during this process, is immediately hydrolyzed to two molecules of **inorganic phosphate,** by **pyrophosphatase.**

- From **UDP-Glu,** glucose is transferred to the **glycogen primer** (i.e., the preformed oligosaccharide). This reaction is catalyzed by the enzyme **glycogen synthase.**

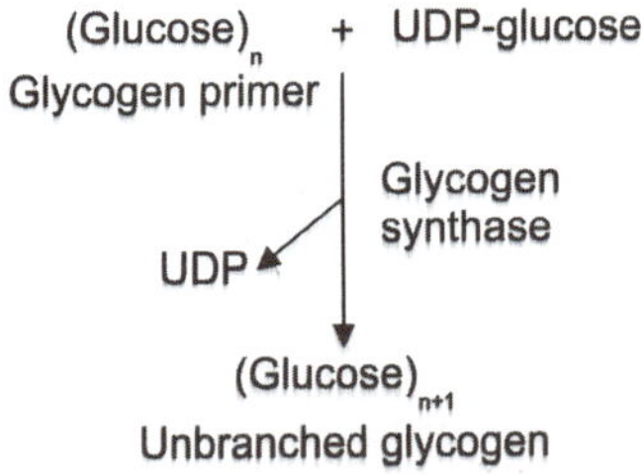

Glycogen primer is formed on a protein known as glycogenin.

The incoming glucose is linked to the primer at the non-reducing end, by 1,4-α-glycosidic linkage and results in elongation of the pre-existing branch. This results in the formation of an **unbranched glycogen**.

Both, glycogen primer and UDP-Glu are the substrates for glycogen synthase, which is a key enzyme of glycogenesis.

- Once the straight chain containing nearly 11 glucose residues is formed, **branching enzyme** removes a block of 7–8 glycosyl residues from the growing chain and transfers it to the neighboring chain (Fig. 2.22).

This branch point again grows with the addition of the glucose molecules at the $1 \rightarrow 4$ linkage. This in turn results in the formation of a highly branched glycogen structure.

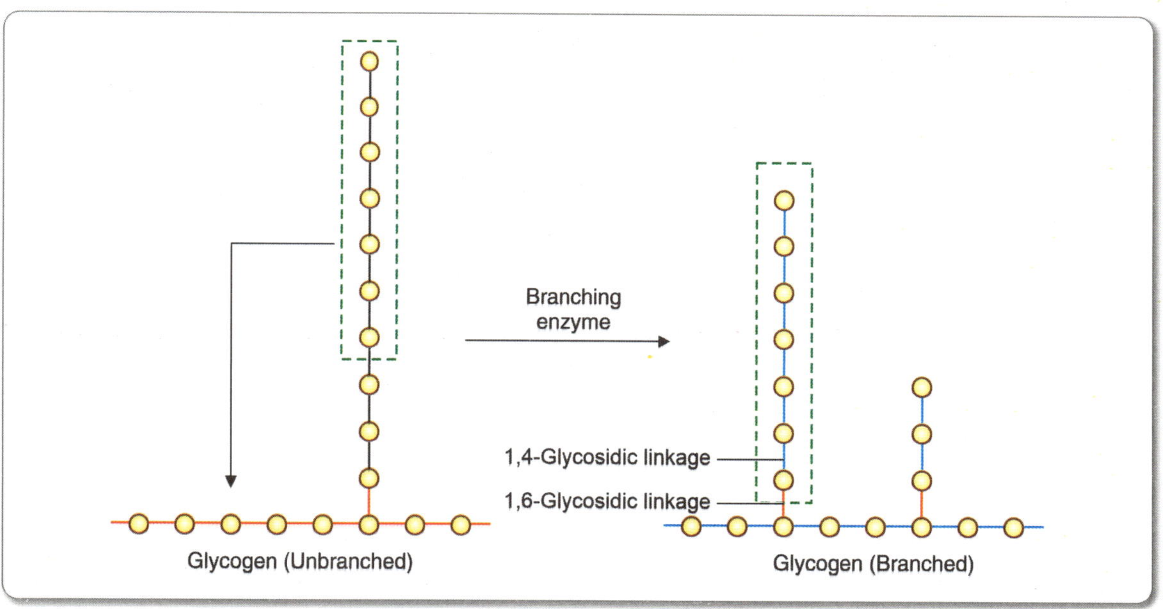

Fig. 2.22: Formation of a branch point by the branching enzyme during glycogenesis

Degradation of Glycogen

Glycogen breakdown (**glycogenolysis**) is the process of the conversion of **glycogen** to either **glucose-6-phosphate** in muscle or **free glucose** in **liver** and **kidney**.

- In the first step, glucose molecules are sequentially removed from **glycogen** as **glucose-1-phosphate**. This reaction is catalyzed by the enzyme **phosphorylase**. It is the rate limiting step of this pathway.

Phosphorylase hydrolyzes the α-1,4-glycosidic bonds and removes glucose units, as glucose-1-phosphate, until nearly four glucose residues are left. After the action of phosphorylase, **glycogen** is partially hydrolyzed, leaving **limit dextrin**.

$$\text{(Glucose)}_n \ \text{Glycogen}$$

Pi $\searrow$ | Phosphorylase

$$\text{(Glucose)}_{n-1} + \text{Glucose–1–phosphate}$$

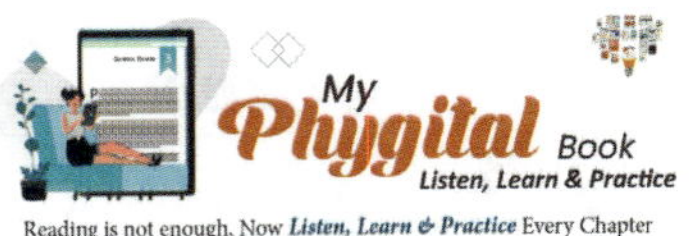

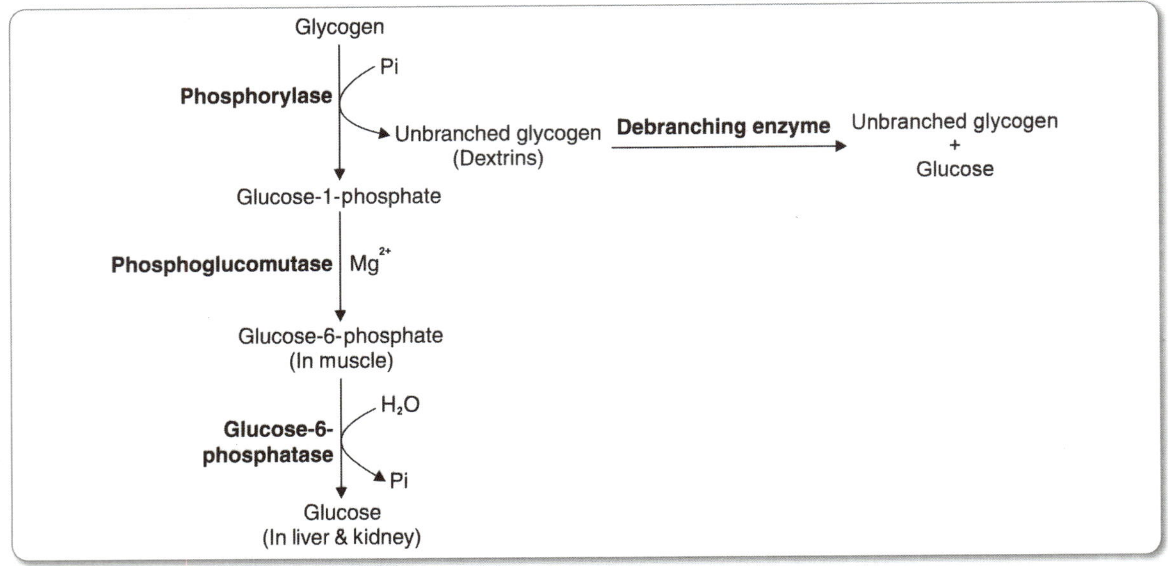

Fig. 2.23: Glycogenolysis

- Limit dextrin is further hydrolyzed by the debranching enzyme to glucose-1-phosphate and free glucose (Fig. 2.23).

  Debranching enzyme is a bifunctional enzyme. Its first unit has **glycosyltransferase,** i.e., $1 \rightarrow 4$ α-D-glucontransferase [α-$(1 \rightarrow 4)$ transglycosylase], **activity** in which a strand of three glucosyl residues is removed from the four glucosyl residue branch of the molecule and is attached to the nonreducing end of another branch. This reaction forms a new $\alpha(1 \rightarrow 4)$ linkage and thus, three more glucose units become available for the phosphorylase reaction.

  The $\alpha(1 \rightarrow 6)$ bond, which is linking the leftover glucosyl residue on the branch point to the main chain, is hydrolyzed by the second unit of the debranching enzyme that is referred to as **amylo-α-1,6-glucosidase**. This glucosyl residue is released as free glucose, rather than as glucose-1-phosphate, leaving the unbranched glycogen molecule (Fig. 2.24).

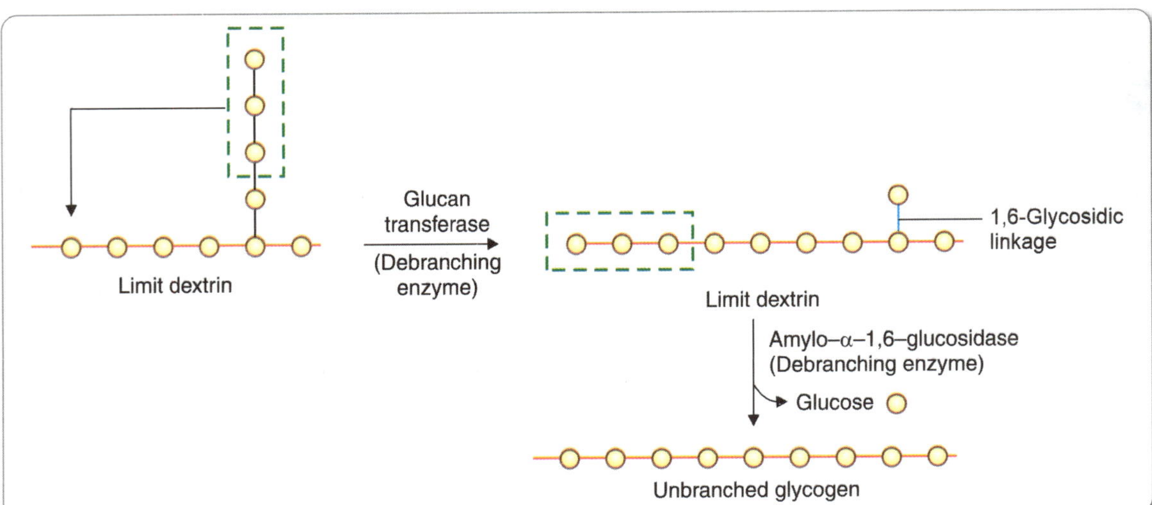

Fig. 2.24: Removal of a branch point by the debranching enzyme during glycogenolysis

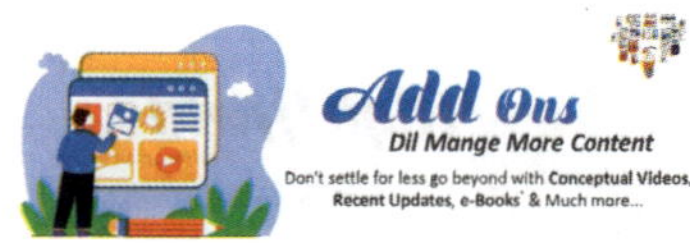

Clinical Correlation

Glycogen Storage Diseases

This is a group of inherited disorders that are associated with glycogen metabolism where an abnormal type or quantity of the glycogen is deposited in different tissues.

According to the deficiency of the enzyme involved, there are several types of glycogen storage diseases. Though >15 types of glycogen storage disorders are known to occur, three of these are most common in children. These are referred to as von Gierke disease (type I), Cori disease or Forbes disease (type III) and Andersen disease (type IV) (Table 2.6).

TABLE 2.6: Glycogen storage diseases

Type	Glycogen storage disease	Deficient enzyme	Features
I	Von Gierke's disease	Glucose-6-phosphatase	Liver, renal and intestinal epithelial cells are loaded with glycogen. There also occurs hypoglycemia, lactic acidosis, ketosis, hyperlipidemia and hyperuricemia.
II	Pompe disease	Lysosomal acid maltase	Accumulation of glycogen in the lysosomes. It is fatal and may result in heart failure.
III	Limit dextrinosis/Forbes disease or Cori's disease	Debranching enzyme	Accumulation of the branched polysaccharide in liver, muscle, heart and leucocytes.
IV	Amylopectinosis or Anderson's disease	Branching enzyme	Accumulation of the polysaccharide having few branch points. Death may occur due to liver or cardiac failure within first year of life.
V	McArdle's syndrome	Muscle phosphorylase	Muscle has abnormally high glycogen content. There is diminished exercise tolerance with little or no lactate in blood after exercise.
VI	Her's disease	Liver phosphorylase	High glycogen content in liver. There is also a tendency towards hypoglycemia.

Cooperative and repetitive actions of phosphorylase and debranching enzyme result in complete hydrolysis of glycogen.

During glycogenolysis, glucose-1-phosphate and glucose are liberated in the ratio of approximately 10:1.

- **Glucose-1-phosphate**, produced as a result of the action of phosphorylase, is converted to **glucose-6-phosphate** by the enzyme **phosphoglucomutase**.

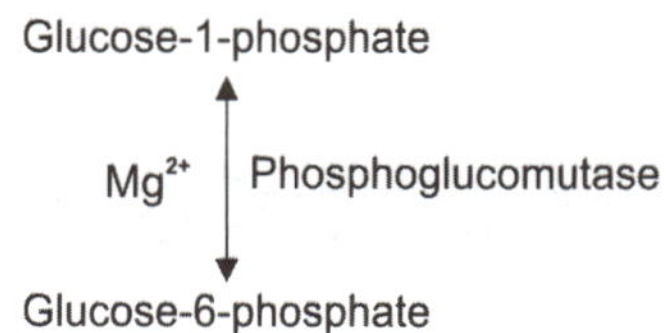

In the muscle, glucose-6-phosphate is the end product of glycogen breakdown and is used in the glycolytic pathway to liberate energy that is required during exercise. Thus, glycogenolysis is followed by glycolysis, due to the absence of the enzyme glucose-6-phosphatase in the muscle.

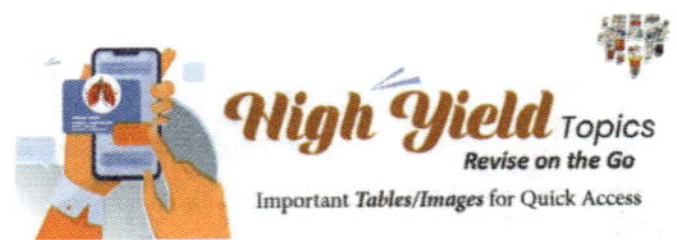

- In liver and kidney, glucose-6-phosphate is further hydrolyzed to **glucose.** This reaction is catalyzed by **glucose-6-phosphatase.**

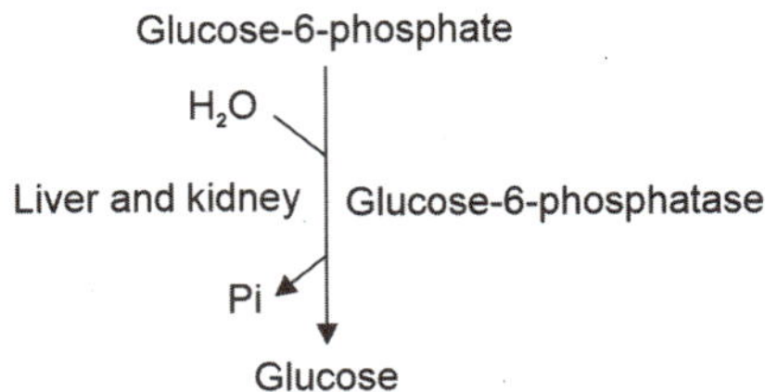

Glycogen, which is stored **in the liver,** is thus converted to free glucose and is used to **maintain blood glucose level** in a hypoglycemic state.

In the muscle, end product of glycogen breakdown, during glycolysis, is glucose-6-phosphate and not glucose. This is due to **absence of the enzyme glucose-6-phosphatase.** This, glucose-6-phosphate, is used for energy production during exercise *via* anaerobic glycolysis and results in the production of lactate.

Lactic acid is transported to the liver and reforms glucose by the process of gluconeogenesis, and becomes available for the muscle and other tissues. This is called **Cori cycle.**

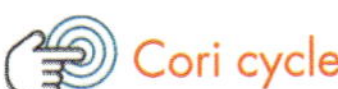 Cori cycle

Process of the transport of lactate from the muscle to the liver, for its conversion into glucose, which again goes to the muscle and reforms glycogen, for its re-utilization during exercise is called lactic acid cycle or Cori cycle. It results in the net exchange of glycogen via glucose-6-phosphate and lactate in the two tissues, i.e., the muscle and the liver (Fig. 2.25).

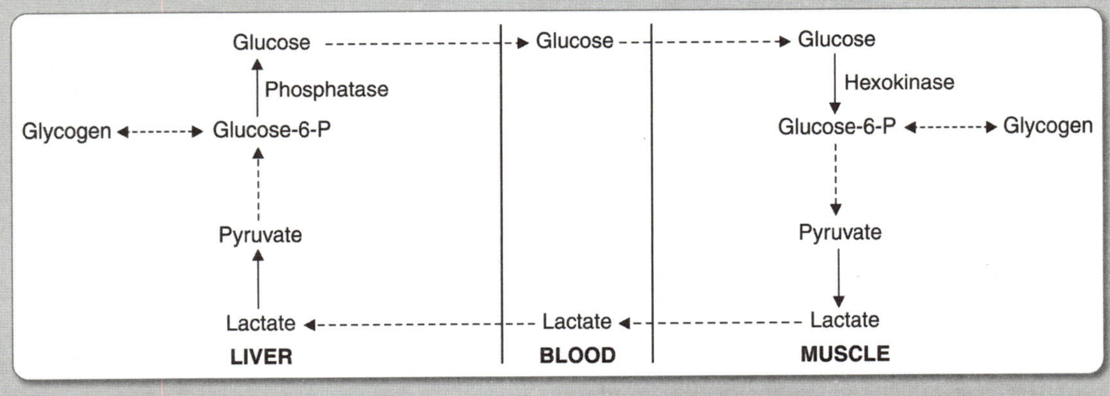

Fig. 2.25: Cori cycle

PENTOSE PHOSPHATE PATHWAY

Pentose phosphate pathway, also called **hexose monophosphate shunt (HMP shunt)**, is the second major pathway for the metabolism of glucose. Enzymes for this pathway are localized in the cytosol, while reducing equivalents are accepted by $NADP^+$, instead of NAD^+. This pathway is operative in many tissues such as liver, erythrocytes, lactating mammary glands, testes and adipose tissue. Rate of the HMP shunt reactions is increased by insulin.

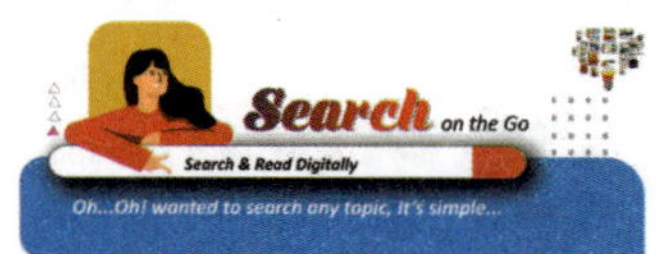

In the overall process, six molecules of glucose are utilized to give six molecules of CO_2 and six molecules of pentoses. The pentoses are subsequently, rearranged to give four molecules of fructose-6-phosphate and two molecules of glyceraldehyde-3-phosphate. Two trioses also form a hexose by the reversal of glycolysis thus, regenerating five molecules of hexoses (Fig. 2.26).

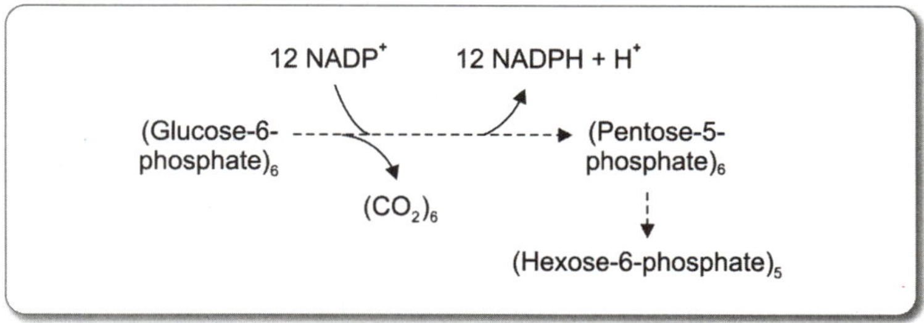

Fig. 2.26: HMP shunt—an overview

- Firstly, **glucose** is activated to **glucose-6-phosphate**, by the enzyme **hexokinase.**

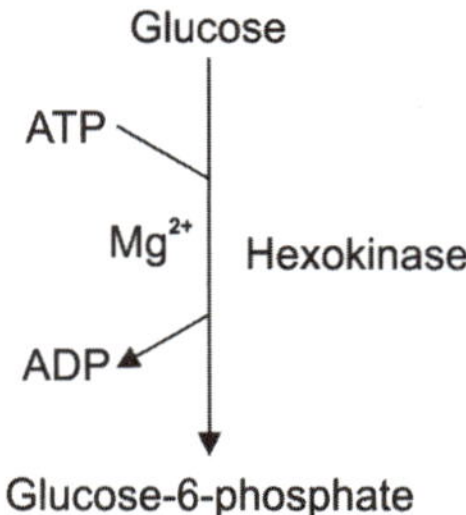

- Thereafter, **glucose-6-phosphate** is changed to **6-phosphogluconolactone** and subsequently, to **6-phosphogluconate**, by the enzyme **glucose-6-phosphate dehydrogenase.** This enzyme is induced by insulin.
  During this process $NADP^+$ is reduced to $NADPH + H^+$ (Fig. 2.27).

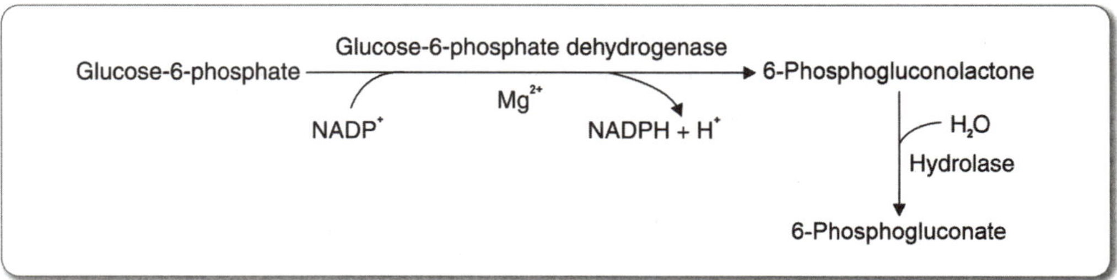

Fig. 2.27: Conversion of glucose-6-phosphate to 6-phosphogluconate in HMP shunt

- In the next reaction, a hexose is converted to a pentose. In this process, **6-phosphogluconate** is oxidized by the enzyme **6-phosphogluconate dehydrogenase**, to form an intermediate, called **3-keto-6-phospho-gluconate.** This reaction also generates $NADPH + H^+$.

  Subsequently, by the enzyme **6-phosphogluconate decarboxylase,** a carbon is removed from **3-keto-6-phosphogluconate,** as CO_2, leaving a **pentose** called **ribulose-5-phosphate** (Fig. 2.28).

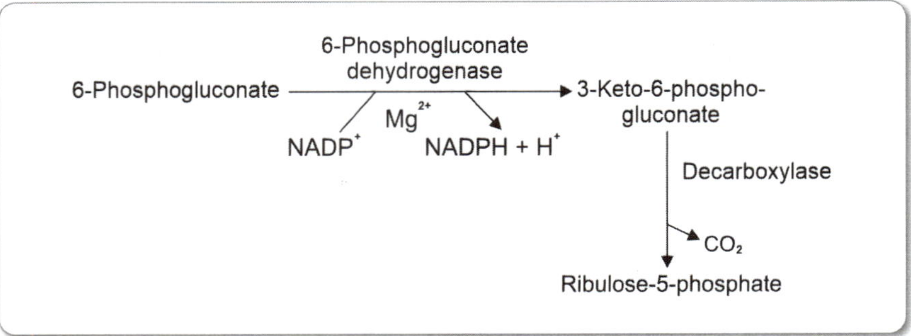

Fig. 2.28: Conversion of 6-phosphogluconate to ribulose-5-phosphate in HMP shunt

These two enzymes, i.e., glucose-6-phosphate dehydrogenase and 6-phosphogluconate dehydrogenase, are the regulatory enzymes of this shunt.

- In the second stage of the shunt, ribulose-5-phosphate changes to other pentoses.
  Ribulose-5-phosphate is changed to **ribose-5-phosphate,** by the enzyme **ribose-5-phosphate ketoisomerase,** and to **xylulose-5-phosphate** by the enzyme **ribulose-5-phosphate epimerase** (Fig. 2.29).

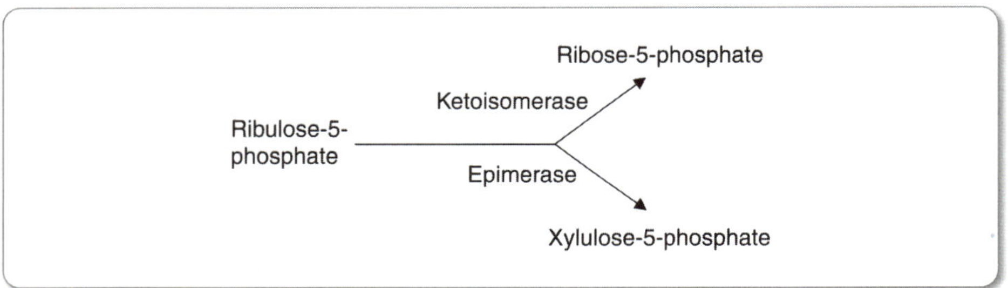

Fig. 2.29: Conversion of ribulose-5-phosphate to other pentoses in HMP shunt

- In the next reaction, carbon skeletons of the two pentoses are rearranged. In this process two pentoses are converted to a hexose and a tetrose (Fig. 2.30).
  Firstly, **a transketolase** transfers a ketol group (the first 2 carbon atoms) from **xylulose-5-phosphate** to **ribose-5-phosphate**, forming **sedoheptulose-7-phosphate** and **glyceraldehyde-3-phosphate.** Transketolase requires TPP as a coenzyme.

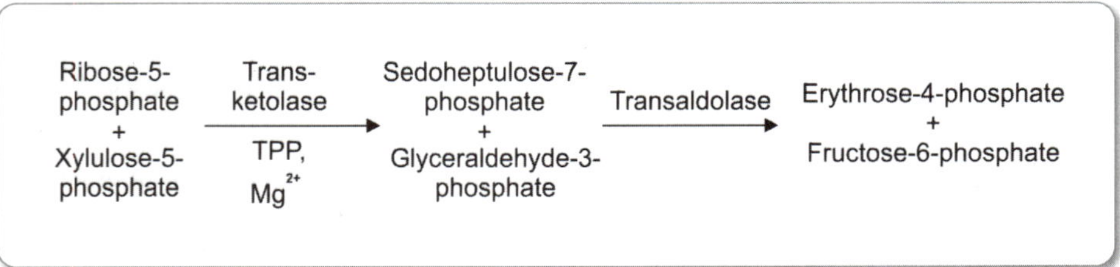

Fig. 2.30: Conversion of pentoses to a hexose and a tetrose in HMP shunt

Subsequently, an aldol group (3 carbons moiety) is transferred by the enzyme **transaldolase,** from **sedoheptulose-7-phosphate** to **glyceraldehyde-3-phosphate**, forming **fructose-6-phosphate** and **erythrose-4-phosphate.**

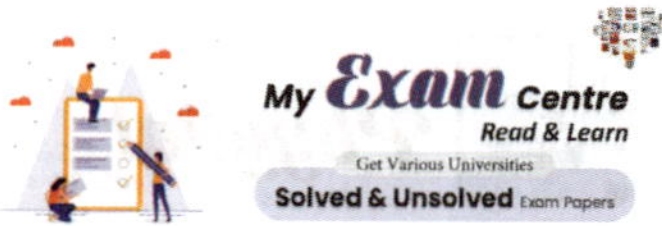

- In the next reaction, **transketolase** transfers a ketol group (2 carbons moiety) from **xylulose-5-phosphate** to **erythrose-4-phosphate**, forming **fructose-6-phosphate** and **glyceraldehyde-3-phosphate**. It converts a pentose and a tetrose to a hexose and a triose (Fig. 2.31).

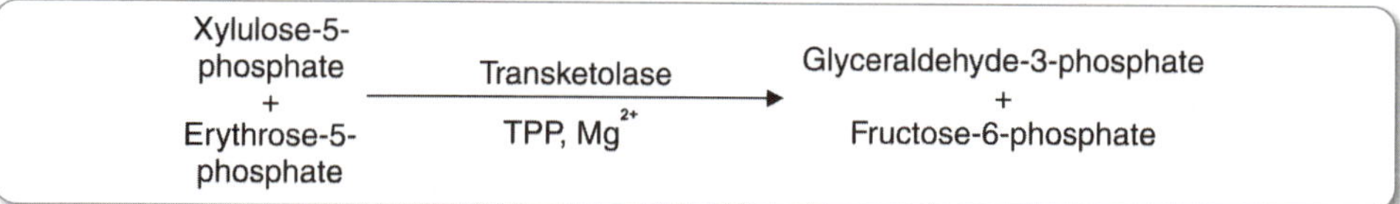

Fig. 2.31: Conversion of a pentose and a tetrose to a hexose and a triose in HMP shunt

Reactions of the pentose phosphate pathway are outlined in Figure 2.32.

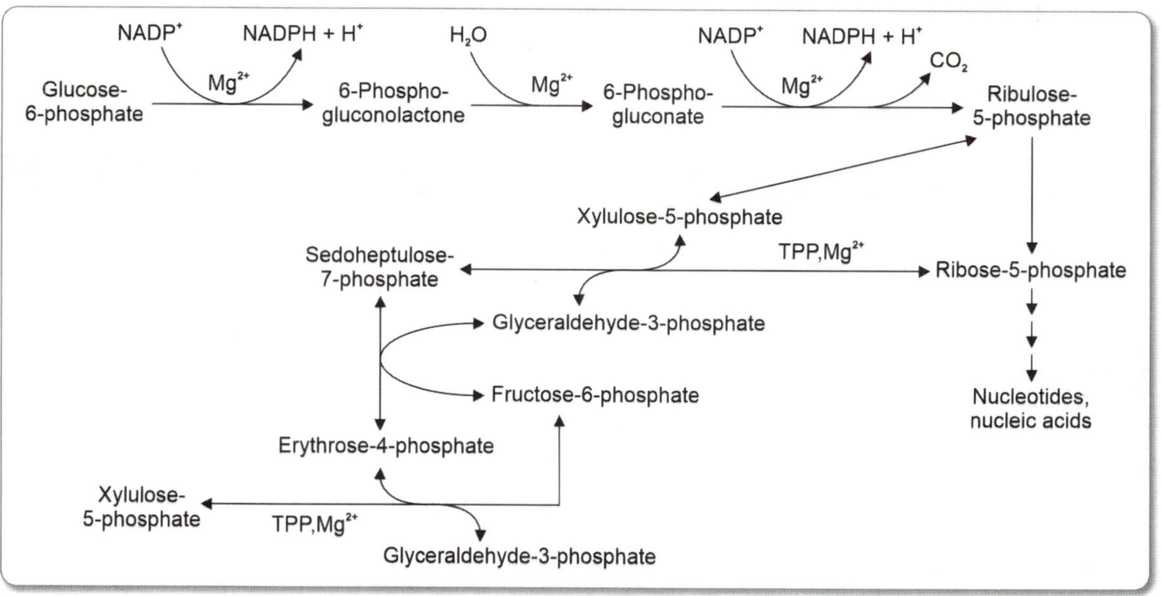

Fig. 2.32: Outline of HMP shunt

Biological Importance of Pentose Phosphate Pathway

In the Liver

- **Generation of NADPH:** Two molecules of NADP are reduced to NADPH, per molecule of glucose-6-phosphate, in the pentose phosphate pathway. **NADPH,** so produced, is used for the various anabolic reactions, such as synthesis of fatty acids and cholesterol.
- **Source of pentoses:** Pentose phosphate pathway is also important source of **pentoses,** which are required for the biosynthesis of nucleic acids (Fig. 2.33).

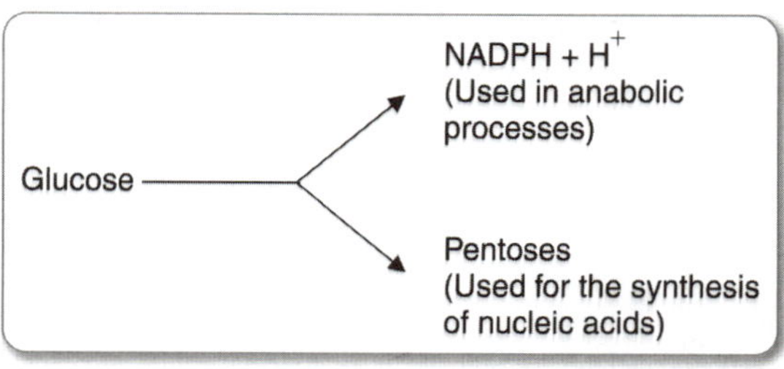

Fig. 2.33: Biological significance of HMP shunt in the liver

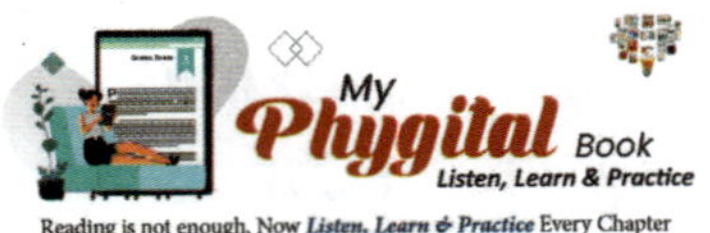

In Erythrocytes

NADPH is utilized by glutathione reductase in the erythrocytes, to maintain the reduced state of glutathione and prevent their hemolysis. This reaction is important for the detoxification of H_2O_2 which is produced in the erythrocytes. If accumulates, H_2O_2 decreases their life span and causes hemolysis (Fig. 2.34).

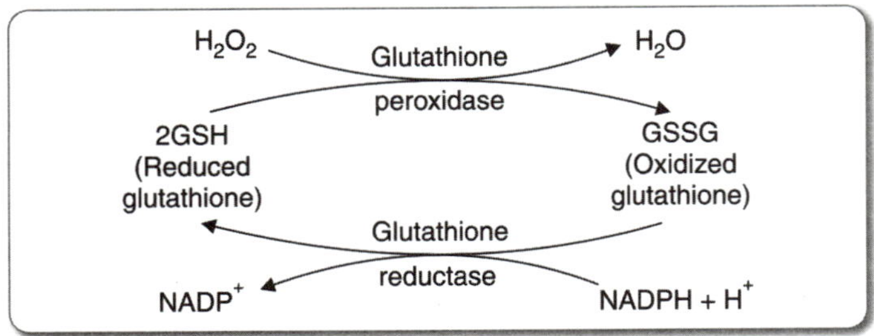

Fig. 2.34: Significance of NADPH in RBCs

METABOLISM OF FRUCTOSE AND GALACTOSE

Although, glucose is the most widely used monosaccharide, fructose and galactose are also important fuels and can be funneled into the glycolytic pathway.

Metabolism of Fructose

Fructose can enter the glycolytic pathway by any of the two routes:

- Most of the ingested fructose is metabolized by **the liver**, using the fructose-1-phosphate pathway. The first step is the phosphorylation of fructose to **fructose-1-phosphate** by **fructokinase**.

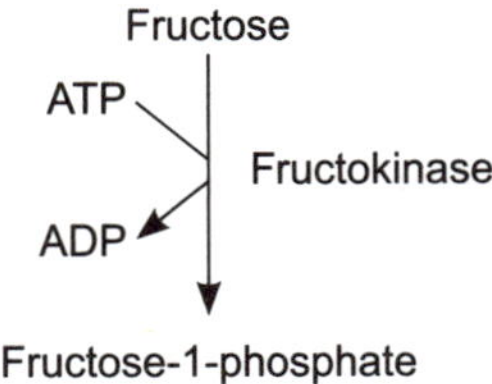

Fructose-1-phosphate is then **splitted into glyceraldehyde and dihydroxyacetone phosphate**, an intermediate in glycolysis. This aldol cleavage is catalyzed **by a specific fructose-1-phosphate aldolase.**

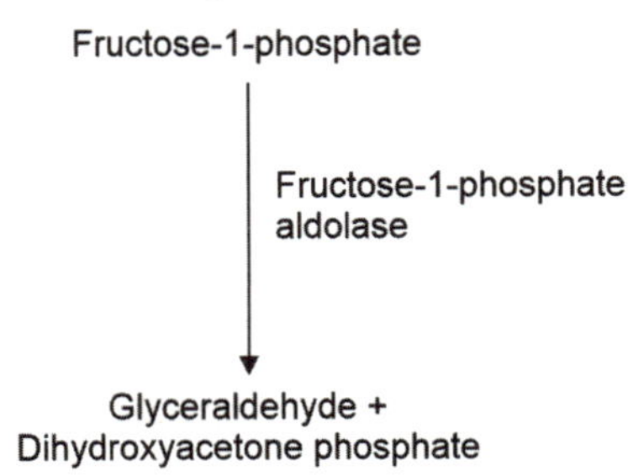

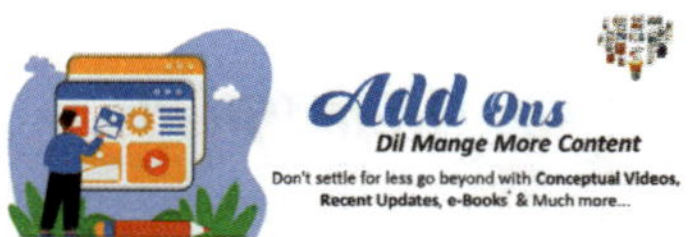

Glyceraldehyde is then **phosphorylated by triose kinase to glyceraldehyde-3-phosphate**, a glycolytic intermediate.

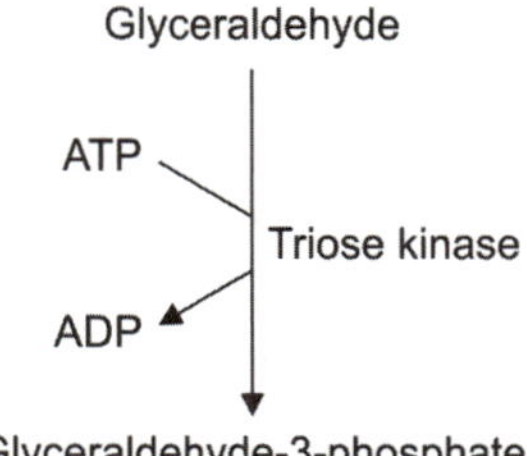

- In **other tissues**, fructose can be phosphorylated to **fructose-6-phosphate by hexokinase.**

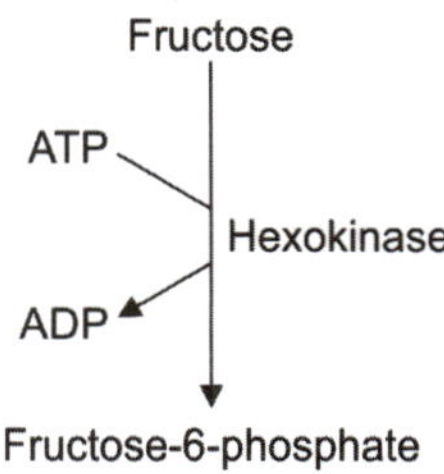

> **Fructose Intolerance**
> In hereditary **fructose intolerance**, fructose cannot be converted to glucose because of a **defect in** the gene encoding **fructose-1,6-bisphosphate aldolase**. Nutrition therapy involves the elimination of fructose and sucrose from the diet.

Metabolism of Galactose

Galactose is converted into glucose-6-phosphate in four steps:

1. The first reaction is the phosphorylation of **galactose to galactose-1-phosphate by galactokinase.**

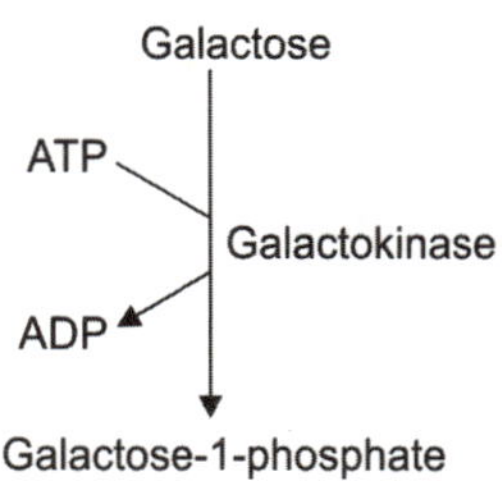

2. Galactose-1-phosphate then acquires uridyl group from uridine diphosphate glucose (UDP-glucose), an intermediate in the synthesis of glycosidic linkages, in glycogenesis. This reaction is catalyzed by **galactose-1-phosphate uridyl transferase,** and **produces UDP-galactose** and glucose-1-phosphate.

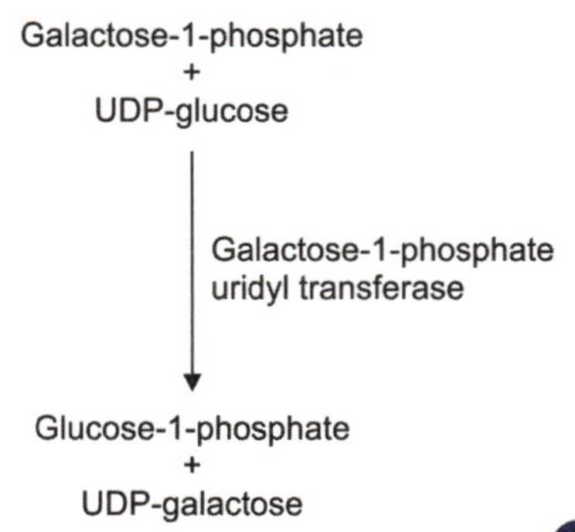

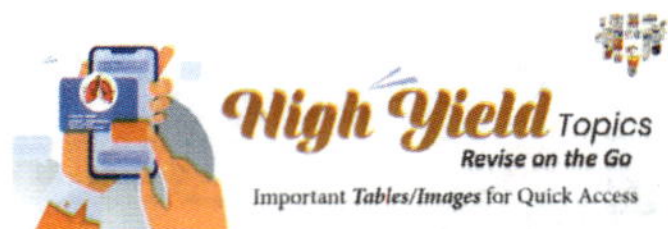

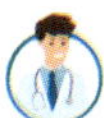

Clinical Correlation

Galactosemia

The disruption of galactose metabolism is referred to as **galactosemia**. *The most common form of galactosemia is an inherited* **deficiency** *of* **galactose-1-phosphate uridyl transferase** *activity. Afflicted infants fail to thrive and vomit or have diarrhea after consuming milk. In addition, enlargement of the liver and jaundice are common, sometimes progressing to cirrhosis. The blood galactose level is markedly elevated and galactose is also found in the urine. The absence of the enzyme transferase in red blood cells is a definite diagnostic criterion.*

Cataract is formed since the transferase is not active in the lens of the eye and in the presence of aldol reductase the accumulating galactose is reduced to galactitol. Since galactitol is osmotically active, water diffuses into the lens, instigating the formation of cataract.

The most common treatment is to remove galactose (and lactose) from the diet. Although elimination of galactose from the diet prevents liver disease and cataract development, the majority of patients still suffer from central nervous system malfunction. Female patients also display ovarian failure.

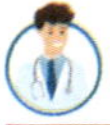

Clinical Correlation

Lactose Intolerance

Many adults are unable to metabolize the milk sugar lactose and experience gastrointestinal disturbances, if they consume milk. This condition is referred to as **lactose intolerance** *or hypolactasia. It is most commonly caused by a* **deficiency of the enzyme lactase**, *which cleaves lactose into glucose and galactose. The lactose is a good energy source for micro-organisms in the colon and they ferment it to lactic acid while also generating methane and hydrogen gas. The gas produced creates uncomfortable feeling of gut distension and flatulence. The lactate produced by the microorganisms is osmotically active and draws water into the intestine, resulting in diarrhea. If severe enough, the gas and diarrhea hinder the absorption of other nutrients such as fat and protein. The simplest treatment is to avoid the consumption of milk and milk products (containing lactose).*

3. The galactose moiety of UDP-galactose is then epimerized to UDP-glucose by **UDP-galactose-4-epimerase**.

   This is a reversible reaction and is important in the reverse direction also, for the conversion of **UDP-glucose** into UDP-galactose. UDP-galactose is essential for the synthesis of galactosyl residues in complex polysaccharides and glycoproteins, if the amount of galactose in the diet is inadequate to meet these needs.

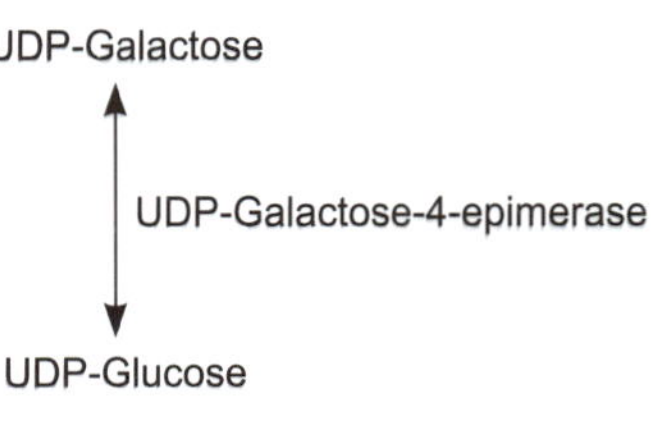

4. Finally, glucose-1-phosphate (formed from galactose) is isomerized to **glucose-6-phosphate, by phosphoglucomutase**.

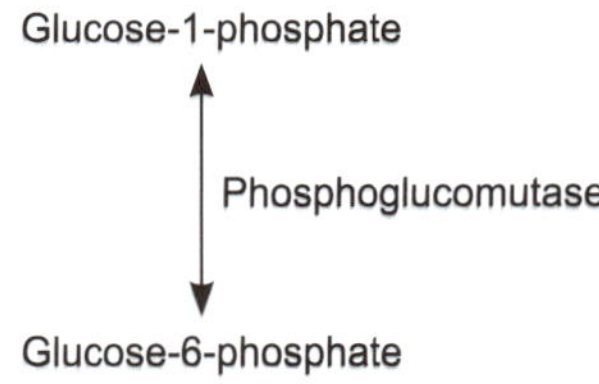

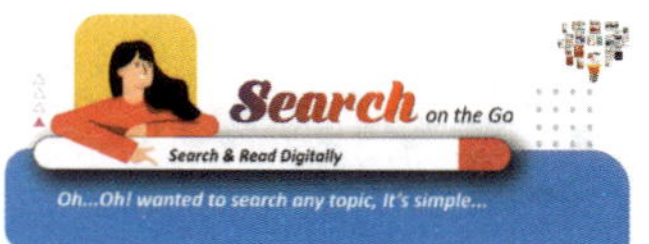

REGULATION OF BLOOD GLUCOSE

Blood glucose level is maintained within the **normal** physiological **range** of **60–90 mg/100 mL** in the fasting (postabsorptive) state by various **hormones** and by the **kidney.**

By Hormones

Several hormones regulate blood glucose concentration. While insulin lowers blood glucose, various other hormones increase blood glucose level (Fig. 2.35).

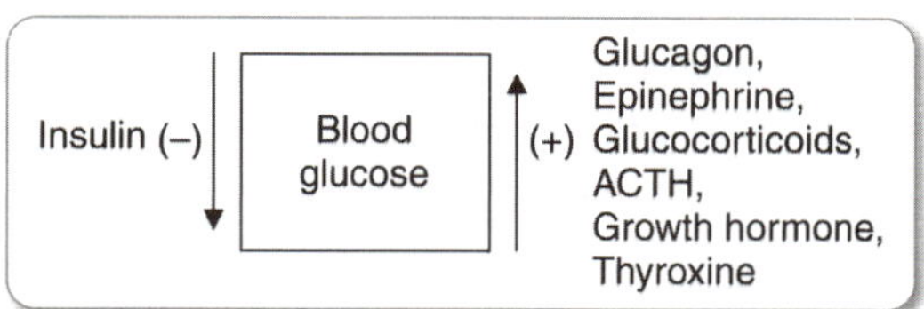

Fig. 2.35: Regulation of blood glucose by hormones

Hormone which has Hypoglycemic Action

Insulin is the only hormone which has hypoglycemic action. It is released into the blood stream under the direct influence of hyperglycemia. It is a polypeptide containing 2 chains and is produced by β-**cells of the islets of Langerhans** of the pancreas.

Insulin **lowers blood glucose** concentration by increasing uptake of glucose by the extrahepatic tissues. Insulin also **promotes glycolysis** and **glycogenesis**, both in the liver and the muscle. At the same time, insulin also **suppresses glycogenolysis** in the liver and the kidney. Besides, insulin also suppresses **gluconeogenesis.**

Insulin also **stimulates synthesis of various enzymes** such as glucose-6-phosphate dehydrogenase, 6-phosphogluconate dehydrogenase, ATP-citrate lyase, etc. Insulin also **represses synthesis** of pyruvate carboxylase; PEP-carboxykinase and fructose-1,6-bisphosphatase.

Insulin also **promotes transport of amino acids** across the cell membrane and thus **stimulates protein synthesis.**

Insulin also **inhibits ketogenesis** and **promotes lipogenesis.**

Hormones which have Hyperglycemic Action

Several hormones have hyperglycemic action. These are called diabetogenic hormones and include **glucagon, epinephrine, glucocorticoids, growth hormone** and **thyroxine.**

- *Glucagon*: Glucagon is produced by α-**cells** of the **islets of Langerhans** of pancreas. Its synthesis is stimulated under the influence of hypoglycemia. It acts only in the liver and **promotes glycogenolysis.** It also promotes **gluconeogenesis** from amino acids and lactate.

- *Epinephrine*: Epinephrine, also called **adrenaline**, is secreted by **adrenal medulla**. It is a hormone in the **first line of defense** against hypoglycemia. It is a derivative of tyrosine.
  Epinephrine **promotes glycogenolysis**, both in the liver and muscle. Epinephrine also promotes **gluconeogenesis** in the liver. It **also inhibits release of insulin** from the pancreas and decreases transport and utilization of glucose in different tissues. At the same time, epinephrine also **stimulates secretion of glucagon.**

- *Glucocorticoids*: Glucocorticoids are steroids secreted by **adrenal cortex.** They are antagonists to insulin. Cortisol is a major glucocorticoid present in blood. It **stimulates protein catabolism** in the **muscle** and **promotes gluconeogenesis** in the **liver.** It also **stimulates lipolysis** and **inhibits glucose oxidation,** by the liver. Cortisol also facilitates actions of other hyperglycemic hormones (permissive effects) such as glucagon, epinephrine and growth hormone, which further inhibit uptake and utilization of glucose by the peripheral tissues.

- **Growth hormone: Anterior pituitary** secretes growth hormone. Its secretion is stimulated under the influence of hypoglycemia. Prolonged administration of the growth hormone **stimulates secretion of insulin.** As a result of increased insulin secretion, β-cells are exhausted producing diabetes-like situation. Growth hormone also **decreases glucose uptake** and **utilization by muscle.** It also **promotes lipolysis in the adipose tissue.**
- **Thyroxine:** It is secreted by **the thyroid gland.** It **stimulates intestinal absorption of glucose** and promotes **glycogenolysis** as well as **gluconeogenesis** in the liver. Thyroxine also causes **destruction of insulin.** Hyperthyroidism is generally associated with hyperglycemia and mild diabetes.

By Kidney

Kidney also regulates blood **glucose** concentration, which is continuously **filtered by the glomeruli** and is completely **reabsorbed by the renal tubules.** However, when blood glucose concentration exceeds 180 mg/dL (renal threshold value); tubules fail to reabsorb all the filtered glucose, some of which starts appearing in the urine.

DIABETES MELLITUS

Blood glucose concentration in a normal adult remains in the range of 60–90 mg/100 mL. When the value exceeds 100 mg/dL, it is called **hyperglycemia.** Persistent hyperglycemia may be a result of **diabetes mellitus.** Diabetes mellitus is characterized by persistent **hyperglycemia** with or without glycosuria (**glucosuria).** This is the commonest endocrine disease caused by the **deficiency in secretion** and/or **action of insulin.** Besides insulin, several diabetogenic hormones also influence blood glucose concentration.

Diabetes mellitus is defined as a state of **chronic hyperglycemia,** which may be a result of genetic and/or environmental factors. It is a multifactorial disease. There are two major clinical classes of diabetes mellitus which are referred to as:

- Type 1 diabetes mellitus, also referred to as Insulin Dependent Diabetes Mellitus (IDDM), and
- Type 2 diabetes mellitus, also referred to as Noninsulin Dependent Diabetes Mellitus (NIDDM).

Type 1 Diabetes Mellitus

Type 1 diabetes mellitus, also called **insulin dependent diabetes mellitus (IDDM)** or **juvenile-onset diabetes** because it usually appears in the childhood or in **young age group** (commonly <40 years of age). There is absolute deficiency of insulin, due to a gradual **depletion of β-cells** of the pancreas, which may get destroyed by some autoimmune process.

Type 1 diabetes mellitus is characterized by **hyperglycemia, hyperlipoproteinemia** (raised chylomicron and VLDL) and **severe ketoacidosis.** This, in turn, suggests that besides defects in carbohydrate metabolism, there are also abnormalities in fat and protein metabolism in such patients.

Hyperglycemia in type 1 diabetes mellitus is a result of **inability** of the insulin-dependent tissues, **to take up glucose** as well as due to **accelerated hepatic gluconeogenesis** from amino acids (derived from muscle protein).

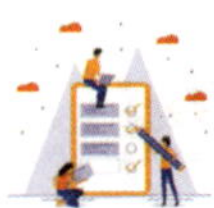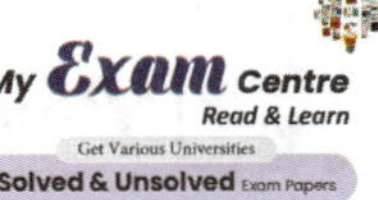

Increased lipolysis (in the **adipose tissue)** and **accelerated fatty acid oxidation** (in the **liver**) result in **ketoacidosis.**

Insulin deficiency also **reduces lipoprotein lipase** activity, thereby resulting in **hyperchylomicronemia.**

Patients with type 1 diabetes mellitus can usually be recognized by abrupt appearance of **polyuria** (frequent urination), **polydipsia** (excessive thirst) and **polyphagia** (excessive hunger), often triggered by the stress or some other illness. These symptoms are usually accompanied with fatigue, weight loss and weakness.

Its diagnosis is confirmed by **high fasting blood glucose,** commonly accompanied with **ketoacidosis.** Insulin injection though does not cure the disease, it promotes glucose uptake by the tissues and inhibits gluconeogenesis, lipolysis and proteolysis.

Life span of the patient is reduced as a result of the degenerative complications, such as kidney malfunction, nerve impairment and cardiovascular disease.

Hyperglycemia may also lead to blindness through retinal degeneration and glycosylation of the lens proteins which in turn may also cause cataract.

Type 2 Diabetes Mellitus

Majority of the diabetic patients (over 80%) suffer from type 2 diabetes mellitus, also called **non-insulin dependent diabetes mellitus (NIDDM).** It is also called **maturity-onset-diabetes** since it usually occurs in the middle age group (usually >40 years of age), particularly in those who are obese. Occurrence of the disease is almost completely determined by the genetic factors. Type 2 diabetes mellitus develops gradually, without obvious symptoms. Metabolic alterations are milder than type 1 diabetes mellitus.

Type 2 diabetes mellitus is characterized by **hyperglycemia,** often with **hypertriglyceridemia**. In spite of high level of insulin, glucose levels are poorly controlled because of the lack of normal response to insulin. **Insulin resistance** in these patients may be due to increased expression of the tumor necrosis factor-α, in the adipocytes of obese individuals. Hyperglycemia is mainly a result of the **poor peripheral utilization of glucose**, especially in muscle.

Ketoacidosis does not develop because adipocytes remain sensitive to the effect of insulin.

Rapid *De novo* synthesis of fatty acids and VLDL lead to **hypertriglyceridemia** without hyperchylomicronemia.

Blood glucose concentration is much higher than normal, particularly after a meal.

Weight reduction and dietary modifications often correct hyperglycemia of type 2 diabetes mellitus. **Hypoglycemic agents** such as **sulphonylureas,** may be required to achieve a satisfactory fall in blood glucose level.

Salient features of two types of diabetes mellitus are shown in Table 2.7.

Complications of Diabetes Mellitus
Metabolic complications of the uncontrolled diabetes include ketoacidosis and coma in IDDM, hyperosmolar nonketotic coma in NIDDM, or hypoglycemia due to insulin overdose.

Long-term complications of the disease **include acute myocardial infarction** (diabetic patients often present with painless acute myocardial infarction, i.e., silent MI), due to accelerated atherosclerosis and coronary heart disease, **nephropathy, retinopathy, neuropathy, infections** and **delayed wound healing.**

Diabetic Ketoacidosis

Diabetic ketoacidosis is a common feature observed **in patients with insulin-dependent diabetes mellitus.** This is due to the severe deficiency of insulin with excess of glucagon and other hyperglycemic hormones such as epinephrine, cortisol and growth hormone.

Plasma free fatty acid concentration is increased. This in turn leads to increased production of ketone bodies by the liver.

There is also **marked hyperglycemia, ketonemia, ketonuria** and **water and electrolyte imbalance**.

Various features of the disease can be corrected by insulin administration.

TABLE 2.7: Salient features of two types of diabetes mellitus

Features	IDDM	NIDDM
Type of diabetes	Juvenile onset (Type I)	Maturity onset (Type II)
Prevalence	About 20%	About 80%
Age of onset	<40 years	>40 years
Body habitués	Normal to wasted (weight loss)	Obese
Plasma insulin	Low (due to β-cell destruction)	Normal to high (insulin resistance)
Plasma glucagon	High (suppressible)	High (resistant)
Acute complications	Ketoacidosis	Hyperosmolar coma (ketoacidosis is rare)
Insulin therapy	Responsive	Resistant
Oral hypoglycemic agents	Unresponsive	Responsive

Investigations of Diabetes Mellitus

Oral Glucose Tolerance Test

Indications

The normal value for blood glucose remains in the range of 60–90 mg/100 mL. When the value exceeds 100 mg/dL, it is called **hyperglycemia**. Persistent hyperglycemia may be a result of **diabetes mellitus**, which can be diagnosed by **glucose tolerance test (GTT)**.

The glucose tolerance test is a laboratory test in which glucose is given and blood samples are taken at different intervals, to determine how quickly it is cleared from the blood. GTT is usually used to test for diabetes, insulin resistance, impaired β-cell function, and sometimes, reactive hypoglycemia and acromegaly, or some rare disorders of carbohydrate metabolism.

Oral glucose tolerance test (OGTT) is performed by giving a load of glucose, orally. It is helpful in confirming the diagnosis of diabetes in those patients whose fasting blood glucose concentration is in the upper normal limit, with transient or sustained glycosuria without the symptoms of diabetes, or with family history of the disease.

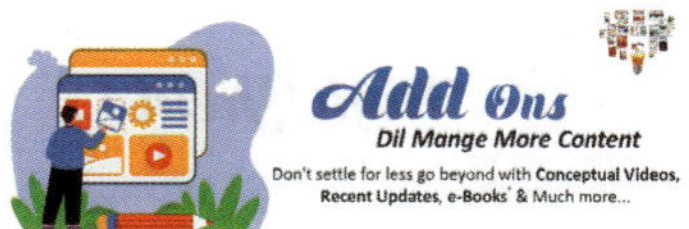

Procedure

For OGTT, fasting venous blood sample (after 12–16 hours of fast) is drawn, in a fluoride-oxalate tube. Thereafter, 75 g of glucose (about 1 g/kg body weight) is given in nearly 200–300 mL of water. Blood samples are redrawn after every 30 minutes, till 2–2½ hours. Urine specimen may also be collected simultaneously. Each blood sample is analyzed for glucose and sometimes insulin levels are also assessed. The intervals and number of samples vary according to the purpose of the test. Thereafter, glucose tolerance curve is plotted (Fig. 2.36).

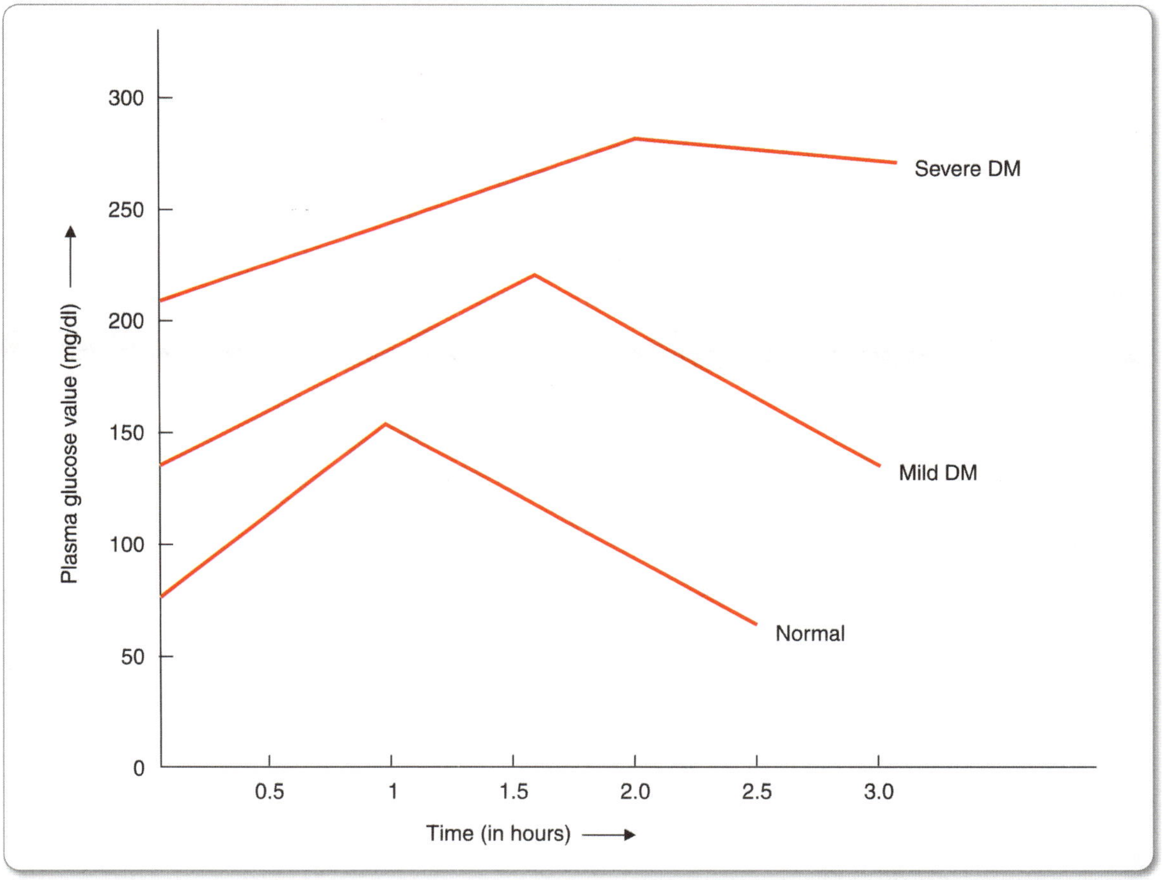

Fig. 2.36: Types of oral glucose tolerance test (GTT) curves

Interpretation and Types of GTT

Fasting blood glucose concentration, maximum blood glucose value after a glucose load, and the rate at which it returns towards the fasting value, give an idea about the disease.

Normal GTT—For a normal individual, fasting blood glucose value should be within the normal limit. It is increased by about 50% within 60 minutes and thereafter returns toward fasting after 2 hours. Glycosuria is not observed in any of the urine sample.

Any deviation from the above is referred to as an abnormal glucose tolerance curve.

GTT in a Diabetic Patient

In a patient with diabetes mellitus, fasting blood glucose level is above normal. In addition, the rise in blood glucose with time may be higher and the level may not return towards fasting. In addition, glucose may be present in urine.

> ***Renal glycosuria:*** If glucose tolerance curve is normal but there is glucose in urine, it is referred to as renal glycosuria.

Mini GTT

International Committee of Diabetologists has recommended the estimation of blood glucose in the overnight fasting and postprandial samples (2 hours after 75 g of a glucose load) to confirm the diagnosis of diabetes mellitus. It is referred to as mini GTT and is sufficient to diagnose or exclude all forms of diabetes mellitus.

Accordingly, an individual is said to be **normal** if fasting blood glucose value is <100 mg/100 mL and the 2-hours' value is below 140 mg/100 mL. A fasting value of 126 mg/100 mL or higher and the 2 hours' value of >200 mg/100 mL is diagnostic of **diabetes mellitus**. Fasting value between 100–125 mg/100 mL and/or the 2 hours' value between 140 and 200 mg/100 mL is referred to as **impaired glucose tolerance** (Table 2.8).

TABLE 2.8: Criteria for the evaluation of mini GTT

GTT	Fasting plasma glucose (mg/dL)	Two hours value after 75 g of glucose (mg/dL)
Normal	<100	<140
Impaired GT	100–125	≥140 – ≤199
Diabetes mellitus	≥126	≥200

Extended GTT

Extended GTT gives clue about symptoms which one may have experienced may be due to low blood sugar. The test also provides information about our body's production of a hormone called insulin. Thus, extended GTT has been used for a variety of purposes, such as detecting reactive hypoglycemia, defining subsets of hypothalamic obesity, or insulin-resistance or deficiency.

For **extended GTT**, blood samples are to be collected at **30, 60, 120** and **180 minutes** for glucose, insulin and C-peptide. One **may even need to extend the test up to 5 hours**.

Glucose Challenge Test

Glucose challenge test (GCT) also measures body's response to glucose. It is done during pregnancy to screen gestational diabetes, the diabetes that develops during pregnancy.

The GCT is done in two steps. It can be done at any time of day, not on an empty stomach. First one is asked to drink a sugary solution (50 g of glucose). One hour later, the blood sugar level is measured. It is used to screen for gestational diabetes and the test is, generally, done between weeks 24 and 28 of pregnancy. However, it can be done as early as during the first prenatal visit if one is at high risk of gestational diabetes due to obesity, a personal history of gestational diabetes, a family history of diabetes or other factors. Abnormal test results early in pregnancy might indicate that one has pre-existing type 2 diabetes, that was not previously recognized, rather than gestational diabetes.

A blood sugar value >140 mg/dL identifies approximately 80% of women with gestational diabetes.

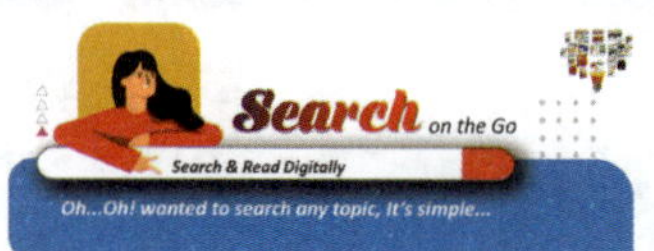

Intravenous GTT

Intravenous glucose tolerance test (IV GTT) aids in evaluating the time to onset of diabetes among persons expressing anti-islet autoantibodies. Most commonly, glucose (25 g/dL) is injected into vein at 0.5 g/kg body weight (maximum 35 g), over 5 minutes and insulin levels are measured before, and 1 and 3 minutes after the glucose infusion. Blood samples for glucose determinations are drawn immediately before glucose injection and thereafter every 10 minutes for 1 hour.

It is rarely used to diagnose diabetes but is used for research purposes only.

Glycated-hemoglobin

Glycated-hemoglobin (HbA1c) reflects the average blood sugar concentration for a time period of 6–8 weeks and remains unaffected by the short-term fluctuations in blood sugar. Compared with repeated daily blood sugar test, HbA1c helps in evaluating the adequacy of diabetic control. An elevated HbA1c level may signal the need for a change in insulin regimen or meal plan. However, target HbA1c goal may vary depending on age and various other factors. HbA1c can be measured by ion exchange method or HPLC.

> *Reference range*
> 4–6%

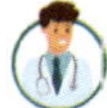 ## Clinical Correlation

Interpretation og HbA1c
- **High levels** of glycated-hemoglobin are directly linked to the microvascular complications, like retinopathy and nephropathy. High HbA1c are also seen in iron deficiency anemia, probably because of high proportion of old erythrocytes.
- **Decreased levels** may be seen in hemolytic disease or in other conditions with reduced red cell survival.

Hypoglycemia

Hypoglycemia refers to a condition when plasma glucose concentration is below 40 mg/dL. It is a common and potentially dangerous complication of insulin treatment, particularly, in tightly-controlled diabetes. Insulinoma (benign adenoma of pancreatic islets) can also cause hypoglycemia. Estimating plasma insulin concentration, which is raised during fasting, helps in the diagnosis of hypoglycemia.

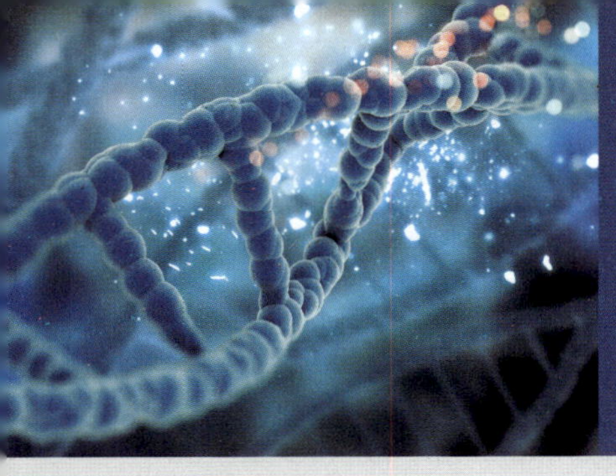

LONG AND SHORT ANSWER QUESTIONS

1. Define carbohydrate. Give its classification.
2. What are polysaccharides? Classify them.
3. Differentiate between starch and glycogen.
4. Outline reactions of the citric acid cycle. Give energetics of the cycle and explain the amphibolic role of this cycle.
6. Outline pentose phosphate pathway reactions. Discuss significance of the pathway in different tissues.
7. Give outline of glycolysis. What are its regulatory steps? What is the energy yield of this pathway?
8. Define glycogenolysis. Outline reactions of this pathway.
9. What is glycogenesis? Give reactions of glycogenesis.
10. **Explain:**
    a. Why aerobic glycolysis releases more energy than anaerobic glycolysis?
    b. How glycolysis can be reversed?
    c. Citric acid cycle and its energetics.
11. **Discuss:**
    a. Regulation of blood glucose
    b. Glycogenolysis
    c. Metabolism of fructose
    d. Metabolism of galactose
12. **Write notes on:**
    a. Diabetes mellitus
    b. Glycogenesis
    c. Gluconeogenesis
    d. Glycogen storage diseases
    e. Energetics of the citric acid cycle
    f. Oxidation of pyruvate to acetyl CoA
    g. von Gierke disease
    h. Cori cycle
    i. Digestion and absorption of carbohydrates
    j. Differentiate between type 1 and type 2 diabetes mellitus
    k. Galactosemia
    l. Lactose intolerance
    m. Lactose intolerance
    n. Diabetic ketoacidosis
    o. Oral glucose tolerance test
    p. Extended GTT
    q. Intravenous GTT
    r. Glycated hemoglobin
    s. Hypoglycemia
    t. Glucose challenge test
    u. Inulin
    v. Homopolysaccharides
    w. Heteropolysaccharides
    x. Oral glucose tolerance test
    y. Mini GTT

MULTIPLE CHOICE QUESTIONS

1. **Which of the following is a nonreducing sugar?**
   - a. Sucrose
   - b. Maltose
   - c. Glucose
   - d. Lactose

2. **Sucrose has glucose and ____________.**
   - a. Maltose
   - b. Fructose
   - c. Glycogen
   - d. Galactose

3. **Aldose sugar is converted to ketose sugar by:**
   - a. Oxidoreductase
   - b. Aldolase
   - c. Decarboxylase
   - d. Isomerase

4. **Enzyme that hydrolyzes sucrose is:**
   - a. Invertase
   - b. Amylase
   - c. Lactase
   - d. Maltase

Notes

3

Lipids

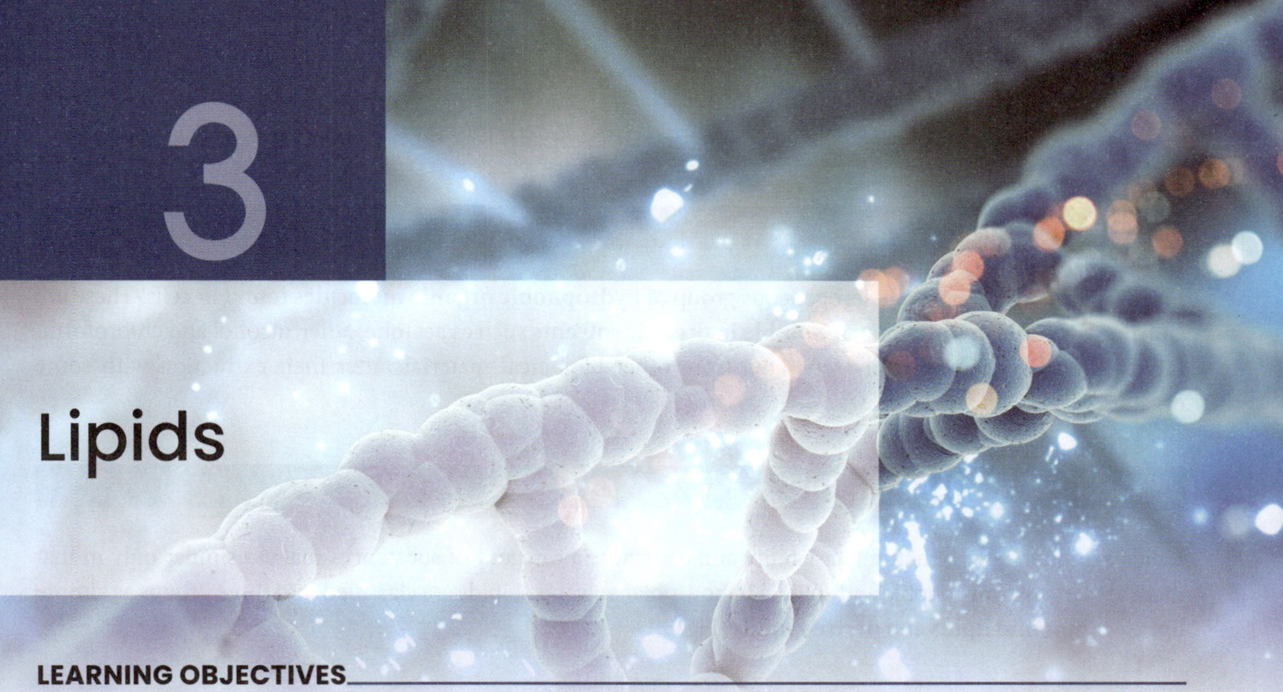

LEARNING OBJECTIVES

After the completion of the chapter, the readers will be able to:
- Explain the classification and uses of lipids and its alterations.
- Explain the types, metabolism, synthesis of fatty acids.
- Understand the role of liver in lipid metabolism.
- Describe cholesterol, its biosynthesis and its compounds.
- Know about ketone bodies, lipoproteins and lipid profile.

CHAPTER OUTLINE

- Introduction
- Classification of Lipids
- Fatty Acids
- Triacylglycerols
- Prostaglandins
- Phospholipids
- Steroids
- Uses of Lipids
- Digestion and Absorption of Lipids
- Metabolism of Fatty Acids
- Synthesis of Fatty Acids
- Metabolism of Triacylglycerols
- Role of Liver in Lipid Metabolism
- Cholesterol
- Ketone Bodies
- Lipoproteins
- Lipid Profile

KEY TERMS

Cerebrosides: Neutral compounds that consist of ceramide (sphingosine and FA) and a monosaccharide bound by a β-glycosidic bond to the C1 of sphingol; these are important components of animal muscle and nerve cell membranes.

Chylomicrons: Large triglyceride-rich lipoproteins produced in enterocytes from dietary lipids.

Halogenation: A chemical reaction which introduces one or more halogens into an unsaturated hydrocarbon chain.

Rancidity: A condition in which aerial oxidation of unsaturated fat present in food gives it an unpleasant flavor and odor, making the food undesirable for consumption.

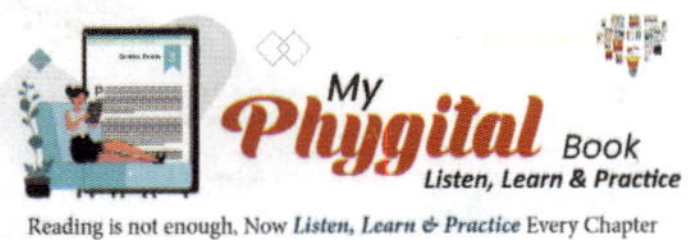

INTRODUCTION

Lipid (Greek: *lipos,* fat) is a heterogeneous group of **hydrophobic organic molecules** found in cells. These are **sparingly soluble in water** but are **soluble in organic solvents** such as acetone, ether, alcohol and chloroform. Lipids, therefore, can be easily separated from other biological materials after their extraction with some organic solvent.

CLASSIFICATION OF LIPIDS

Lipids exhibit greater structural variability and constitute a category of substances that are similar only in that these are largely hydrophobic and soluble in non-polar solvents. Lipids are classified into three groups as **simple lipids, compound lipids** and **derived lipids** (Fig. 3.1).

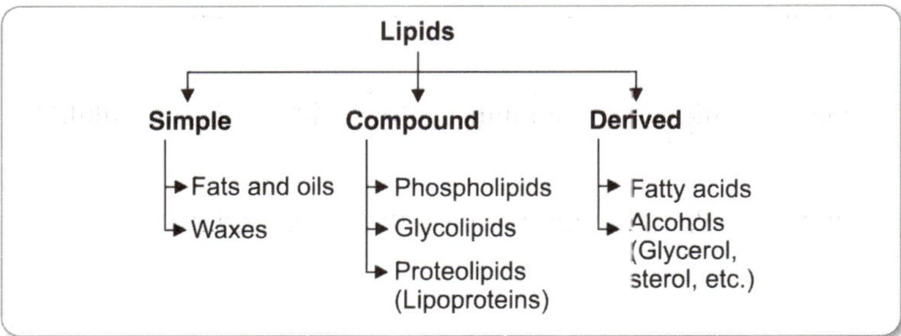

Fig. 3.1: Classification of lipids

Simple Lipids

Simple lipids are **esters of fatty acids** with **alcohol.** These include neutral fats, oils and waxes.

- **Neutral fats and oils** are the mixtures of triacylglycerols (**triglycerides**) whose fatty acid composition may vary with source. Fats and oils differ only in the way that **fats** are **solid** while **oils** are **liquid** at room temperature.
- **Neutral fats** are obtained from animal sources. These have, comparatively, more number of saturated fatty acids and higher melting points.
- On the other hand, **oils** are obtained from plant seeds. Oils are usually rich in unsaturated fatty acids and have low melting points.
- Esters of long chain fatty acids with high molecular weight like monohydroxy aliphatic alcohols are called **waxes**. Waxes are used in the manufacturing of wax-polishes.

Compound Lipids

In addition to **fatty acids** and **alcohol, compound lipids** also contain an **amphipathic group.** For example, lipids conjugated with phosphoric acid are called **phospholipids.**

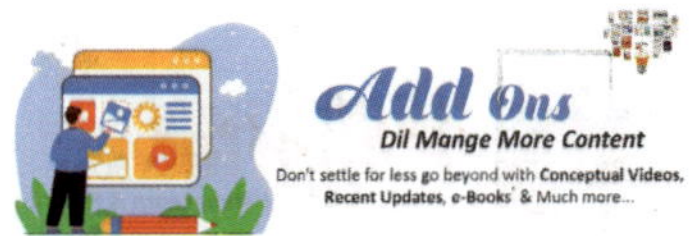

Derived Lipids

Derived lipids are obtained after hydrolysis of simple and compound lipids. These include **fatty acids, glycerol,** etc.

FATTY ACIDS

Fatty acids are the carboxylic acids with a long hydrocarbon side chain that may be saturated or unsaturated (having one or more double bonds).

- Major source of the circulating free fatty acids is adipose tissue.
- After intraplasmic hydrolysis of the triacylglycerols, in chylomicrons and very low-density lipoproteins, free fatty acids enter plasma and serve an important source of energy for many tissues.
- Since free fatty acids have limited solubility in water, they are transported in plasma bound to albumin, which has specific binding sites for free fatty acids.
- Most of the naturally occurring fatty acids have even number of carbon atoms, since these are synthesized from acetyl CoA, i.e., from two carbon units.

Classification of Fatty Acids

According to their chain length, fatty acids are divided into three groups, referred to as:

1. **Short-chain fatty acids**, which contain 4–8 carbon atoms,
2. **Medium-chain fatty acids**, which contain 10–14 carbon atoms, and
3. **Long-chain fatty acids**, which contain 16 or more carbon atoms.

All types of fatty acids have different physicochemical properties and are metabolized in the body in different ways. In plants and higher animals, predominant fatty acids are those containing 16 and 18 carbon atoms, e.g., palmitic acid, oleic acid, linoleic acid, stearic acid, etc.

Saturated and Unsaturated Fatty Acids

Saturated Fatty Acids

Saturated fatty acids have a suffix '-**anoic**' after the name of the hydrocarbon chain, e.g., octadecanoic acid, a saturated fatty acid having 18 carbon atoms.

- Saturated fatty acids are highly flexible molecules and can assume a wide range of conformations because there is relatively free rotation around the C–C bond.
- These are commonly found in fats which are obtained from the animal source, such as butter.
- Saturated fatty acids of common biological significance are listed in Table 3.1.

Unsaturated Fatty Acids

Unsaturated fatty acids have a suffix '-**enoic**' after the name of the hydrocarbon chain, e.g., octadecenoic acid, an unsaturated fatty acid having 18 carbon atoms and one double bond. It is also called oleic acid.

Unsaturated fatty acids **may have one or more double bonds**.

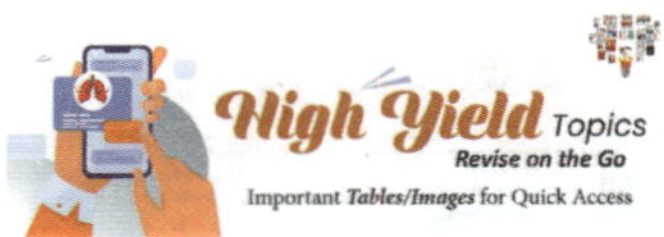

Monounsaturated Fatty Acids

Monounsaturated fatty acids (MUFA) have one double bond. They are, usually, liquid at room temperature. Oils from palm, groundnut, cottonseed, sesame and olive, are rich in monounsaturated fatty acids as compared to other oils, e.g., oleic acid.

TABLE 3.1: Saturated fatty acids of biological significance

Fatty acids	Number of carbons	Formula	Sources
Acetic acid	2	CH_3-COOH	Fermentation of carbohydrates
Butyric acid	4	$CH_3-(CH_2)_2-COOH$	Butter
Caproic acid	6	$CH_3-(CH_2)_4-COOH$	Butter, fat from plant sources
Caprylic acid	8	$CH_3-(CH_2)_6-COOH$	- do -
Capric acid	10	$CH_3-(CH_2)_8-COOH$	- do -
Lauric acid	12	$CH_3-(CH_2)_{10}-COOH$	Coconut oil
Myristic acid	14	$CH_3-(CH_2)_{12}-COOH$	- do -
Palmitic acid	16	$CH_3-(CH_2)_{14}-COOH$	Animal and plant fats
Stearic acid	18	$CH_3-(CH_2)_{16}-COOH$	- do -
Arachidic acid	20	$CH_3-(CH_2)_{18}-COOH$	Peanut oil

Polyunsaturated Fatty Acids

Polyunsaturated fatty acids (PUFA) have more than one double bond in the molecule and are liquid at room temperature. Polyunsaturated fatty acids help reduce cholesterol, and lower the risk of a heart disease. Soybean oil, corn oil, safflower oil, walnuts and sunflower seeds are good sources of polyunsaturated fatty acids, which are present only in plant foods, e.g., linoleic acid.

Nomenclature of an Unsaturated Fatty Acid

Widely used convention to represent an unsaturated fatty acid is to indicate the number of carbon atoms, followed by the number of the double bonds with their positions in the hydrocarbon chain. For example, octadecanoic acid, a fatty acid with 18 carbon atoms with one double bond which is present after carbon atom number 9 (i.e. between carbon atoms number 9 and 10), is represented as 18:1; 9 (Fig. 3.2).

$$\overset{18}{CH_3} - (CH_2)_7 - CH = \overset{10}{CH} - \overset{9}{(CH_2)_7} - \overset{1}{COOH}$$

Fig. 3.2: Oleic acid—an unsaturated fatty acid

An unsaturated fatty acid may be identified either by the delta or the omega system of nomenclature.

Delta System of Nomenclature

According to the delta (δ) system of nomenclature, carbon atoms in the fatty acid chain are numbered from the carboxy-terminal end. This carbon atom (–COOH) is labeled as carbon atom number 1. The carbon atom next to the carboxyl group, i.e., the α-carbon atom, is referred to as carbon atom number 2, and so on.

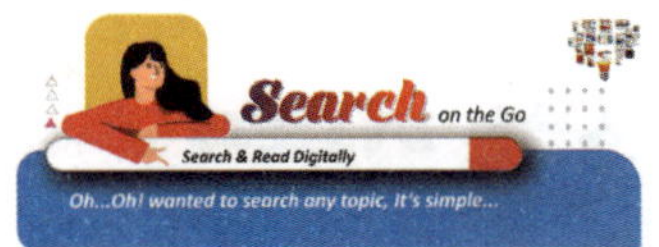

Accordingly, an unsaturated fatty acid is represented by:

- A number, showing the number of carbon atoms, followed by the symbol colon (:) and another number, which represents the number of double bonds.
- This number is further followed by the symbol semicolon (;) and some other numbers which indicate positions of the double bonds. For example, linoleic acid, a fatty acid with 18 carbon atoms and two double bonds, which are present after carbon atom numbers 9 and 12, is represented as 18:2;9,12 (Fig. 3.3).

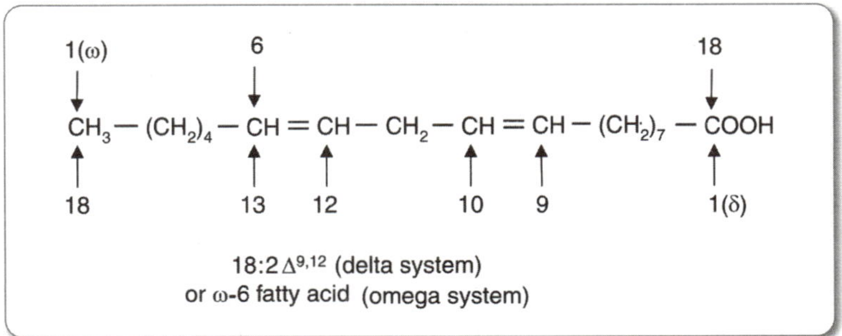

Fig. 3.3: Linoleic acid

Omega System of Nomenclature

According to the omega (ω) system of nomenclature, carbon atoms are numbered from the methyl end. This carbon is referred to as the omega (ω) carbon. Accordingly, an unsaturated fatty acid is represented by:

- The omega symbol (ω), followed by a number.
- The number followed by the symbol ω represents the number of the carbon atom immediately after which the first double bond appears from the methyl end. For example, in linoleic acid, since the first double bond from the ω-end is present after the sixth carbon atom, the linoleic acid is, thus, referred to as ω-6 fatty acid (Fig. 3.4).

Fig. 3.4: Omega system of nomenclature of a fatty acid

Polyunsaturated Fatty Acids

Unsaturated fatty acids having two or more double bonds are referred to as polyunsaturated fatty acids (PUFA). These are obtained from plant seed oils, e.g., soybean oil, sunflower oil, groundnut oil, etc.

Significance of PUFA

- PUFA are **essential components of cell membranes**. While ω-6 PUFAs are predominant in all cells, the nerve tissue has high levels of long chain ω-3 PUFA.

- An appropriate balance of the two PUFAs, namely, linoleic and α-linolenic acids in the diets is **essential for the functioning of vascular, immune, nervous and renal systems and for early human development.**
- The lipid lowering and other physiological effects of individual members of the PUFAs vary widely. As compared to linoleic acid, α-**linolenic (ω-3) acid** is more beneficial **for prevention of inflammation** and accumulation of fatty material in blood vessels (**atherosclerosis**) and clotting of blood (**thrombosis**). The long chain n-3 PUFA of fish oils and micro algae have greater antiatherogenic, antithrombotic and anti-inflammatory effects than alpha-linolenic (ω-3) acid of plant foods.
- These are also **important for vision and brain growth.** Therefore, pregnant women should consume foods that are rich in ALA and long chain ω-3 PUFA from fish and fish oils.
- PUFAs, particularly, ω-**3 PUFA increase insulin sensitivity and increase peripheral glucose utilization,** and **decrease adiposity**, hence, are anti-atherogenic.
- The **n-6 PUFA decreases plasma cholesterol** as well as **HDL cholesterol** level (only at high intake).

Essential Fatty Acids

α-Linoleic acid (an omega-6 fatty acid) and linolenic acid (an omega-3 fatty acid) are referred to as **essential fatty acids (EFA)**. However, if diet lacks α-linoleic acid, arachidonic acid (which is also an omega-6 fatty acid) becomes dietary essential. EFA form essential component of the diet, and are necessary for growth and normal health. These are not synthesized in our body and serve a number of important functions, like:

1. Synthesis of **prostaglandins**.
2. Serve as structural element of **mitochondrial membrane**.
3. Help in the prevention of **fatty liver**.
4. Important **role in vision**.

Trans Fatty Acids

Trans (*trans*) fatty acids are isomers of the normal cis (*cis*) fatty acids, produced when PUFAs are hydrogenated, such as in the production of margarine and vegetable shortening.

- Trans fatty acids are usually **found in commercially fried** and **processed foods**, and are **even more hazardous than the dietary cholesterol.**
- Trans fatty acids are **formed from the chemical process, by hydrogenation**, which converts liquid oils into semi-solid form.
- Our **body is unable to metabolize trans fatty acids**, causing them to accumulate.
- While saturated fat (found in butter, cheese, red meat, and coconut and palm oils) raises serum cholesterol level, trans fatty acids are still more harmful, since they **increase LDL-cholesterol** (bad cholesterol) and **decrease HDL-cholesterol** (good cholesterol).
- WHO recommends that trans fatty acids **should, preferably, not be consumed**. However, total intake of trans fatty acids should not exceed 1% of energy intake.

TRIACYLGLYCEROLS

Triacylglycerols (also called **triglycerides**) or *neutral fats* are **fatty acid triesters of glycerol** (glycerin) which is a trihydric alcohol.

- Glycerol with one molecule of fatty acid is called **monoacylglycerol (MAG)**, with two molecules of fatty acids a **diacylglycerol (DAG)**, and with three molecules of fatty acids a **triacylglycerol (TAG; Fig. 3.5)**.

Fig. 3.5: Glycerol and a triacylglycerol

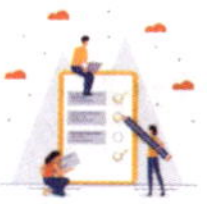
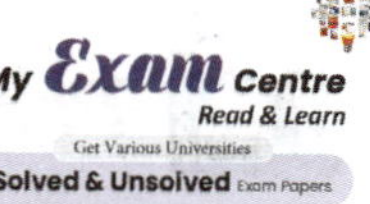

- A molecule of triacylglycerol may contain three similar or dissimilar fatty acids which may be saturated and/or unsaturated. All natural fats and oils, invariably, are mixed triacylglycerols. Plant oils are usually rich in unsaturated fatty acids.
- Triglycerides are named according to the presence of the fatty acid residues attached to glycerol, e.g., 1-palmitoyl-2-arachidonoyl-3-stearoylglycerol is a triacylglycerol which has palmitic acid at carbon-1, arachidonic acid at carbon-2 and stearic acid at carbon-3 of glycerol. Generally, with the primary alcoholic group of a triacylglycerol, i.e., at α-positions (at carbon-1 and carbon-3 of glycerol), there are saturated fatty acids while at carbon-2 there is an unsaturated fatty acid.
- Triacylglycerols are transported in plasma in chylomicrons and very low density lipoproteins.

Properties of Triacylglycerols

- **Triacylglycerol** is the **storage form of energy** in the body. In animals, fat cells (adipocytes) are important for the synthesis and storage of triacylglycerols. Average fat content of a normal human being is about 21% in men and 26% in women. This in turn may allow them to survive for 2–3 months.
- TAG are **hydrolyzed** by **lipases** to **free fatty acids** and **glycerol** (Fig. 3.6).

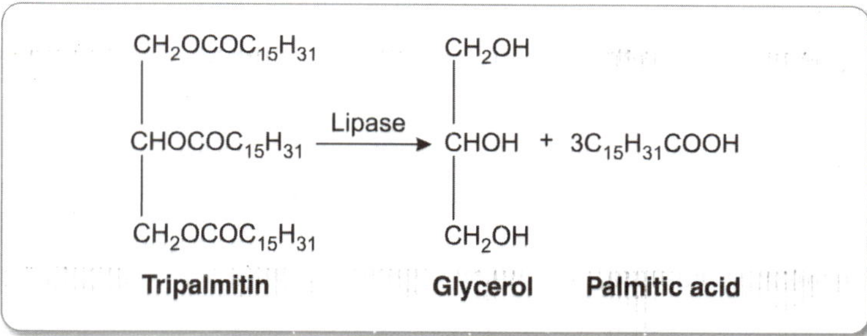

Fig. 3.6: Hydrolysis of a triacylglycerol by lipase

- Naturally occurring fat, particularly from animal sources, develop unpleasant odor and taste, if stored for a long period under moist conditions. This is called **rancidity**. Antioxidants, e.g., vitamin E, can prevent development of rancidity.
- **Unsaturated fatty acids** found in triacylglycerols **accept halogens** such as iodine, at the double bond. This process is termed **halogenation**. It is a measure of the degree of unsaturation.

PROSTAGLANDINS

Prostaglandins and the related compounds thromboxanes and leukotrienes are collectively referred to as **eicosanoids**. These are synthesized from polyunsaturated fatty acids with 20 carbons. Arachidonic acid is the immediate precursor of the predominant class of prostaglandins in man. Prostaglandins exist in virtually every mammalian tissue and act as local hormones.

There are three classes of prostaglandins (PG) referred to as **A, E and F**. They are distinguished by the functional group on the cyclopentane ring. A series has α, β-unsaturated ketone, E series contain β-hydroxy ketone while F series has 1, 3-diol. Subscript indicates number of double bonds in the side chain.

Prostaglandins of series 2 are derived from arachidonic acid and are the principal prostaglandins in man. They are of great significance, biologically. They are natural mediators of inflammation. Synthetic prostaglandins are very effective in inhibiting gastric acid secretion in patients with peptic ulcer. PGE_2 and PGF_2 have been used to induce parturition. PGI_2 inhibits platelet aggregation.

PHOSPHOLIPIDS

Phospholipids are a heterogeneous group of compounds, which contain one or more phosphoric acid residues and a polar group that may be a nitrogenous base, an amino acid or a polyhydroxy alcohol. In addition, phospholipids also contain one or two long chain fatty acids.

These are **amphipathic in nature,** i.e., they contain both, a **hydrophilic head** and a long **hydrophobic tail**.

- **Hydrophilic domain** interacts with the aqueous environment and contains a phosphate group plus an alcohol, e.g., serine, choline, etc.
- **Hydrophobic domain** forms the nonaqueous environment and contains a long chain fatty acid or fatty acid-derived hydrocarbon chain.

Physiological Role of Phospholipids

- Phospholipids are predominant lipids of a **cell membrane**. Membrane phospholipids also function as a reservoir for intracellular messengers. They also serve as anchor for some proteins in a cell membrane.
- Phospholipids are also **component of lung surfactants**.
- These are also **essential components of the bile** and help in regulation of serum cholesterol.

Classification of Phospholipids

Phospholipids are classified into several groups (Table 3.2).

TABLE 3.2: Classification of phospholipids

Glycerophospholipids	Sphingolipids
• Lecithin (Phosphatidylcholine) • Cephalins (Phosphatidylethanolamine and phosphatidylserine) • Phosphatidylinositols • Cardiolipins and plasmalogens	• Sphingomyelins • Cerebrosides • Gangliosides

Glycerophospholipids

Phospholipids which are the **derivatives of glycerol** are called glycerophospholipids or **phosphoglycerides**. These are major components of a biological membrane and are the derivatives of **phosphatidic acid**.

Phosphatidic acid consists of a molecule of glycerol, two fatty acids and a molecule of phosphoric acid. When phosphoric acid is attached at carbon 3 of glycerol, it is referred to as glycerol-3-phosphate. Its carbon-1 and 2 are esterified with two fatty acids. Usually, a saturated fatty acid is attached at carbon-1 (α-carbon) while a polyunsaturated fatty acid is attached at carbon-2 (β-carbon) of glycerol.

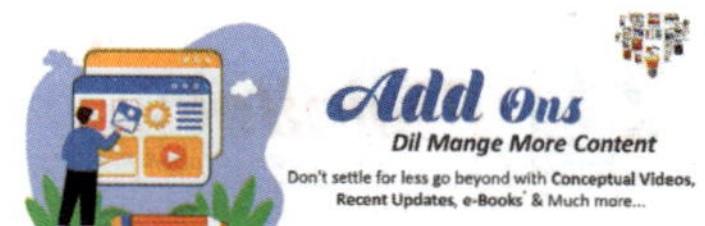

Phosphoryl group of phosphatidic acid may be linked either to a nitrogenous compound such as ethanolamine, choline, serine or to some other group like inositol. Various glycerophospholipids include phosphatidylethanolamine (cephalin), phosphatidylcholine (lecithin), phosphatidylinositol, etc.

Lecithins

Lecithins contain **choline** (a nitrogenous base) at carbon-3. These are the surface active agents and help in emulsification of fat. Lecithins are widely distributed in the brain, nerve cells, sperm and egg yolk. Various hydrolytic enzymes, known as phospholipases, act at different sites of glycerophospholipids and hydrolyze them. For example, phospholipase A_2 removes a fatty acid from carbon-2 and forms lysophospholipid, called lysolecithin.

Cephalins

Cephalins are glycerophospholipids where (instead of choline present in the lecithin) either **ethanolamine** or **serine** is present as a nitrogenous base. Cephalins are present in erythrocyte membrane, brain and many other tissues.

Phosphatidylinositols

Phosphatidylinositols are the glycerophospholipids containing inositol instead of a nitrogenous base. These are found mainly in the brain.

Plasmalogens

Plasmalogens are the glycerophospholipids in which carbon-1 of **glycerol** is linked to **an unsaturated fatty acid** by an ether linkage (in the cis-configuration) rather than a saturated fatty acid linked by the ester linkage. Plasmalogens are present in cardiac and skeletal muscles and semen.

Sphingolipids

Sphingolipids do not contain glycerol but are the derivatives of an unsaturated amino alcohol, which is referred to as **sphingosine**. Sphingolipids have 18 carbon atoms and one double bond.

N-Acyl derivatives of sphingosine are called **ceramides**. These are the parent compounds of most of the sphingolipids, e.g., sphingomyelins, cerebrosides and gangliosides.

Sphingomyelins

Sphingomyelins are ceramides which contain either phosphocholine or phosphoethanolamine, and are called sphingophospholipids. Myelin sheath, that surrounds and electrically insulates many nerve cell axons, is rich in sphingomyelin.

Cerebrosides

Cerebrosides are glycosphingolipids. They contain **ceramide**, which is **attached to** a **sugar residue,** such as a galactose or glucose. Hence, cerebrosides are ceramide monosaccharides. Most prevalent cerebrosides are **galactocerebrosides** and **glucocerebrosides**.

A number of the cerebrosides are found in white matter of the brain and in the myelin sheath of nerves. These are named with respect to the presence of the fatty acid, e.g., a galactosylceramide called **cerebron** contains cerebronic acid. Similarly, **nervon** has an unsaturated derivative of lignoceric acid which is referred to as nervonic acid.

Gangliosides

Gangliosides are the most complex glycolipids. These are **ceramides which contain oligosaccharides** including **hexosamines** (glucosamine or galactosamine) and at least one molecule of **N-acetylneuraminic acid** (NANA or sialic acid).

Gangliosides are present in large amount in ganglion cells of the central nervous system, particularly, in the nerve endings. More than 60 gangliosides are known to occur. Each one of it has different oligosaccharide head groups. Gangliosides are designated as GM_1, GM_2, GM_3, etc.

STEROIDS

The most common steroid is **cholesterol.** It is a derivative of **cyclopentanoperhydrophenanthrene ring** also called **steroid nucleus,** which consists of four fused, non-polar rings which are labelled as A, B, C, and D.

Cholesterol is the most abundant steroid found in animals. It has **27 carbons,** a **hydroxyl group** at **carbon 3,** a **double bond** between **carbons 5 and 6, two methyl groups** at **carbons 18 and 19,** and a **side chain at carbon 17** (Fig. 3.7).

Because of the presence of the OH group, cholesterol is called a steroid alcohol (sterol). Due to the presence of this group, cholesterol can form ester with the long chain fatty acids, called cholesterol esters.

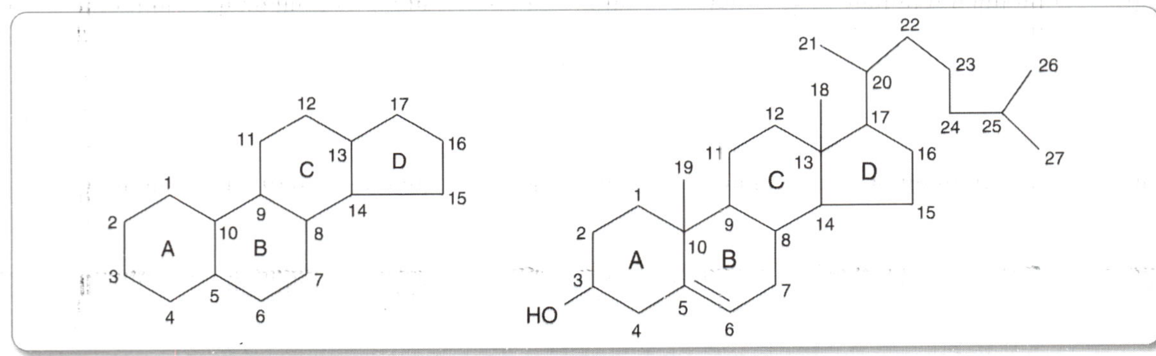

Fig. 3.7: Structure of the steroid ring and cholesterol

USES OF LIPIDS

- **Storage form of energy:** Triacylglycerols stored in adipose tissue release free fatty acids during fasting and starvation
- **Structural components of biomembranes** (phospholipids and cholesterol)
- **Metabolic regulators** (steroid hormones and prostaglandins)
- **Act as surfactants, detergents** and **emulsifying agents** (amphipathic lipids)
- **Act as electric insulators** in myelin sheath of nervous system
- **Provide insulation** against changes in external temperature (subcutaneous fat)
- **Give shape** and **contour** to the body
- **Protect internal organs** by providing a cushioning effect (pads of fat)—loss of these fat pad lead to visceroptosis.

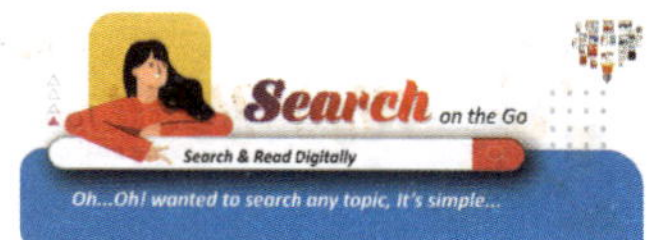

- **Help in absorption of fat soluble vitamins** (A, D, E and K)
- **Improve taste** and **palatability of food**.

DIGESTION AND ABSORPTION OF LIPIDS

Digestion of Triacylglycerols and Phospholipids

Digestion of triglycerides is initiated in the mouth with chewing and by the action of the **lingual lipase**. Thereafter, with the action of **gastric lipase**, and churning and contraction by the stomach, nearly 30% of the dietary triglycerides get degraded to diglycerides and free fatty acids, within 2–3 hours. Contents from the stomach pass into the small intestine. Presence of the fat in the small intestine stimulates the release of two hormones, i.e., cholecystokinin (CCK) and secretin from the duodenal cells. CCK signals the gallbladder to contract and release bile, down the bile duct and into the duodenum. Bile contains large quantities of bile salts and lecithin. Secretin signals the pancreas to release pancreatic juice which is rich in pancreatic lipase.

Bile emulsifies fat and breaks fat globules (clumps of triglycerides) into small pieces and keep them suspended in solution. This in turn increases total surface area for the action of **pancreatic lipase**. Pancreatic lipase hydrolyzes all the accessible triglycerides, within minutes, into monoglycerides and free fatty acids. Bile salts surround the hydrolyzed products of fat digestion and form water soluble globules with a fatty core, called **micelles.** Micelles transport monoglycerides and free fatty acids through the watery intestinal environment to the brush border of the intestinal mucosal cells for absorption.

Similarly, **phospholipases** hydrolyze phospholipids and release monoglycerides, free fatty acids, phosphate and a nitrogenous substance (Table 3.3).

TABLE 3.3: Sites and actions of various digestive enzymes on the hydrolysis of lipids

Enzyme	Site of action	Action of the enzyme
Lingual lipase	Mouth	Triglycerides → Fatty acids, monoglycerides, glycerol (important in neonates)
Lipase/Colipase	Pancreas	Triglycerides → Fatty acids, monoglycerides, glycerol
Phospholipase A/B	Pancreas	Lecithin → Fatty acid, lysolecithin
Cholesterol esterase	Pancreas	Cholesterol esters → Cholesterol, fatty acids
Retinyl ester hydrolase	Pancreas	Retinyl esters → Retinol, fatty acids
Monoglyceride lipase	Small intestine	Monoglycerides → Glycerol, fatty acids
Lecithinase	Small intestine	Lecithin → Fatty acids, glycerol, phosphoric acid, choline

Absorption of the Digestion Products of Lipids

Most fat absorption takes place **in the duodenum or jejunum of the small intestine**.

Micelles carry monoglycerides and long chain fatty acids to the surface of the microvilli in the brush border and diffuse into the intestinal cells. The unabsorbed bile salts return to the interior of the small intestine for the transport of more monoglycerides and fatty acids. Bile salts are absorbed in the ileum and return, *via* the portal vein, to the liver where they are again secreted into the bile. This recycling pathway for bile, i.e., from the liver to the intestine and from the intestine to the liver is called **enterohepatic circulation.**

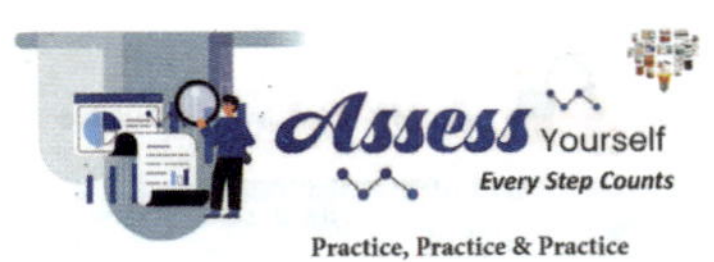

As monoglycerides and fatty acids pass into the intestinal cells, they reform triglycerides. Most of the triglycerides as well as cholesterol and phospholipids combine with apoproteins and form **chylomicrons.** Chylomicrons make their way to the central lacteal of the villi where they enter the lymph system, to be propelled through the thoracic duct, and emptied into vein in the neck (Fig. 3.8).

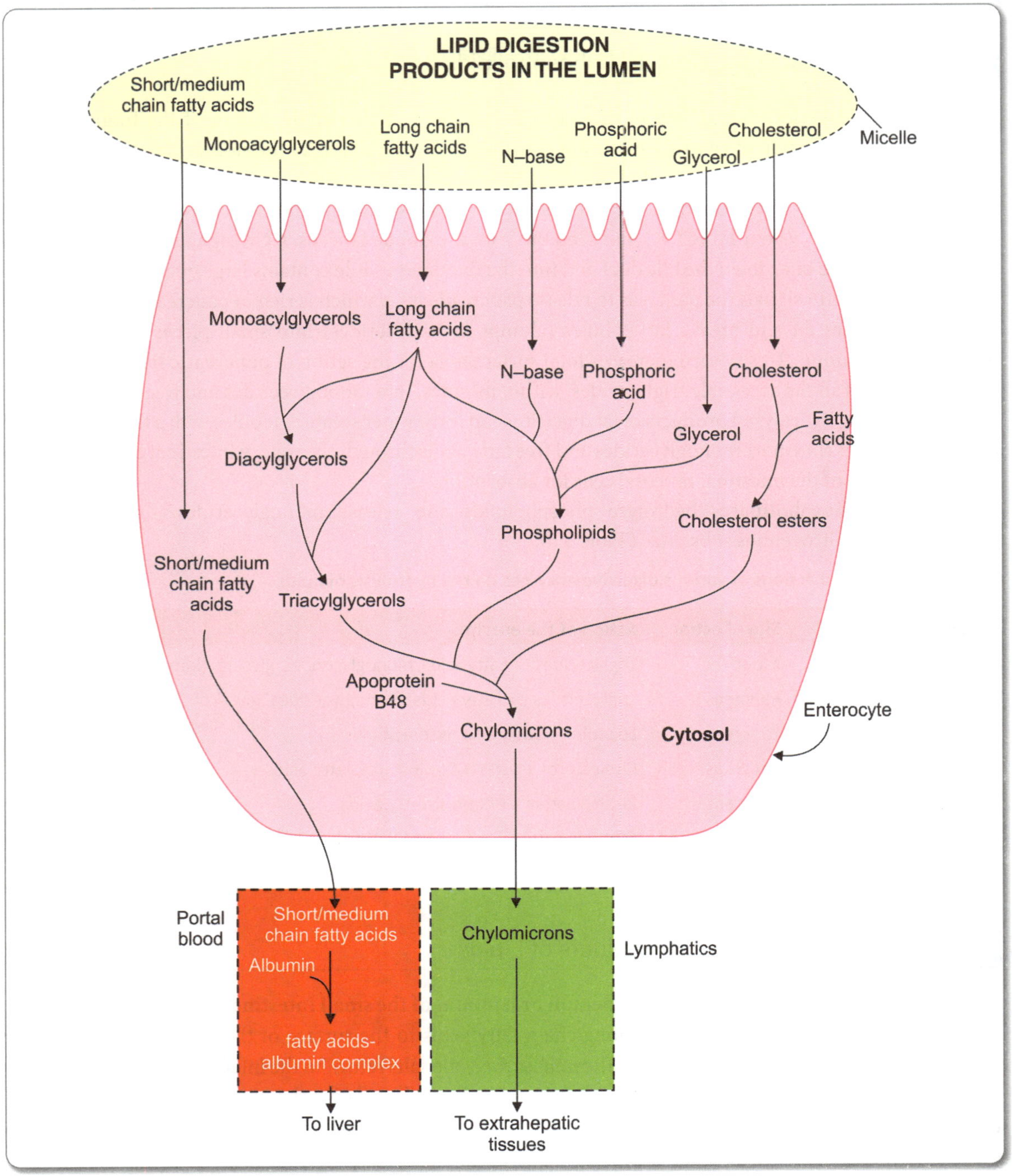

Fig. 3.8: Absorption of the digestion products of lipids

Glycerol, and medium and short chain fatty acids are absorbed directly into the blood stream. Dietary fat begins to appear in the bloodstream after 1–2 hours of meal, with a peak after 3–5 hours. It is generally cleared by 10 hours.

> **Role of Bile Salts in the Absorption of Fat**
> Absorption of fat is drastically reduced in the absence of bile salts. As a result of it, bulk of the unabsorbed fat is excreted in the stool. The production of stool with an abnormally high amount of fat is referred to as **steatorrhea**. Steatorrhea may follow diseases of malabsorption such as **cystic fibrosis**, radiation therapy or digestive tract surgery. In such conditions, triglycerides with medium chain fatty acids are often given in the diet. This is due to the reason that medium chain fatty acids are comparatively more water soluble than long chain fatty acids and thus can be emulsified more readily. Breast milk is a rich source of medium and short chain fatty acids.

Digestion and Absorption of Sterols

Sterols remain, mostly, unchanged by digestion. Their absorption is also relatively poor. Cholesterol gets esterified prior to its absorption. Dietary fat increases absorption of cholesterol whereas plant sterols and dietary fiber decrease cholesterol absorption.

METABOLISM OF FATTY ACIDS

Breakdown of Fatty Acids

Major pathway for the catabolism of fatty acids occurs in the mitochondria. This pathway is called β–**oxidation** and was proposed by **Knoop.**

β-Oxidation

In this process, **oxidation** of fatty acids **occurs at the β-carbon atom** (carbon-3) and two carbon fragments are successively removed from the carboxyl end of fatty acyl CoA. This in turn results in the **elimination of two terminal carbon atoms as acetyl CoA,** thereby leaving fatty acyl CoA that has two carbons less than the original fatty acid (Fig. 3.9).

Activation of Fatty Acid

A long chain fatty acid (fatty acid containing >12 carbons) enters a cell where it is converted to its CoA derivative, by the enzyme long-chain fatty acyl CoA synthetase (thiokinase) in the cytosol.

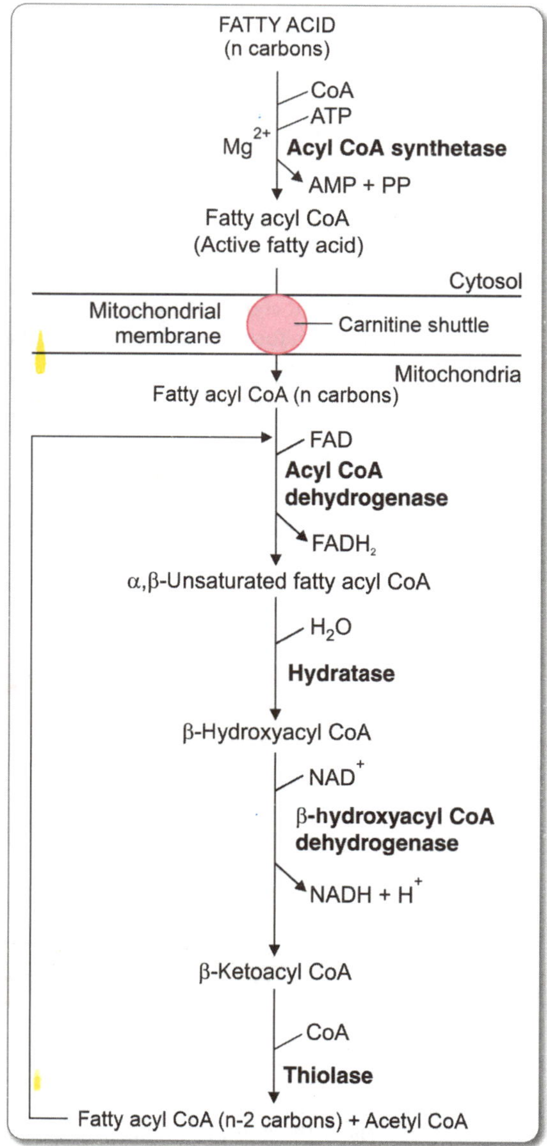

Fig. 3.9: The process of β-oxidation of a fatty acid

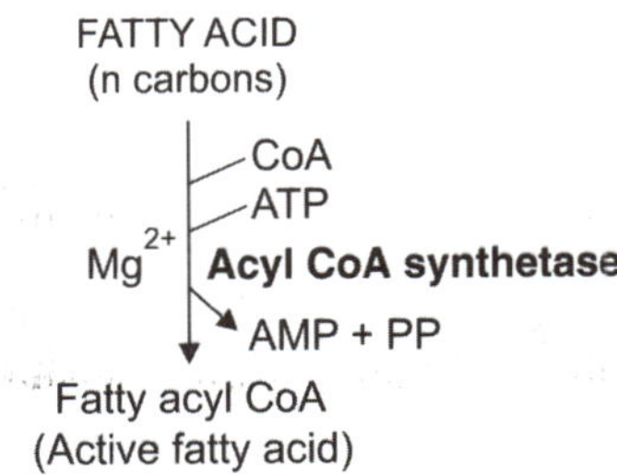

Transport of Active Fatty Acid into Mitochondria

The process of β-**oxidation** occurs in the mitochondrial matrix. Thus, fatty acid must be transported across the mitochondrial membrane. Short chain fatty acids can cross the inner mitochondrial membrane and are activated to their CoA derivatives within the mitochondria. However, it is impermeable to a long chain fatty acid. A long chain fatty acid is transported, from cytosol to the mitochondrial matrix, with the help of a specialized carrier called **carnitine.** This process is called **carnitine shuttle** (Fig. 3.10).

Carnitine Shuttle

In this process, an acyl group is first transferred from the cytosolic CoA to carnitine, by the enzyme carnitine palmitoyltransferase-I (CPT-I). This enzyme is associated with the outer mitochondrial membrane and is also referred to as carnitine acyltransferase-I (CAT-I). This reaction forms acylcarnitine and releases CoA. Thereafter, acylcarnitine is transported into the mitochondrial matrix, by a protein called carnitine acyltranslocase. Finally, CPT-II (CAT-II), which is present in the inner mitochondrial membrane, catalyzes transfer of the acyl group, from acylcarnitine to CoA, into the mitochondrial matrix and releases carnitine.

Carnitine is obtained from meat. A small amount of it can also be synthesized in the liver and kidney, from lysine and methionine. Carnitine deficiency can be observed in patients with a liver disease, malnutrition or in strict vegetarians. Congenital deficiency of CPT-I or CPT-II may also be observed. Such a deficiency can result in the decreased ability to use long chain fatty acids by the tissues.

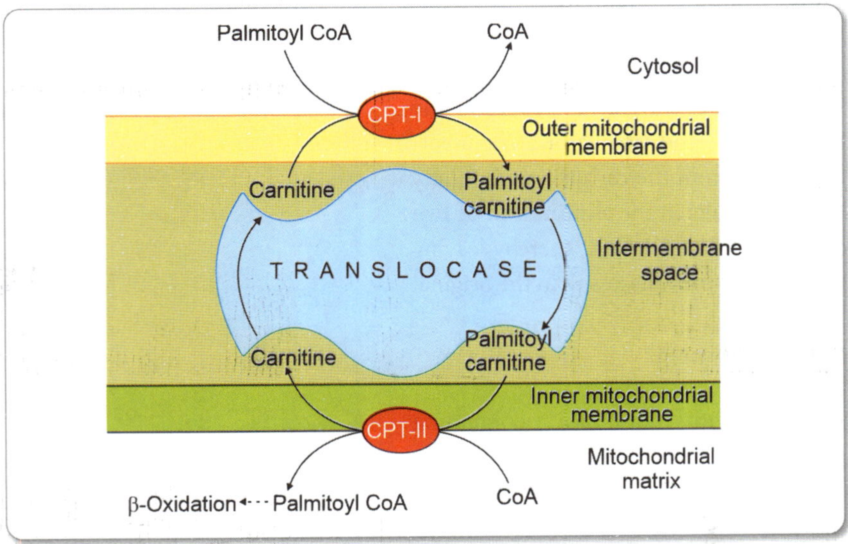

Fig. 3.10: Role of carnitine in the transport of fatty acid from cytosol to mitochondria

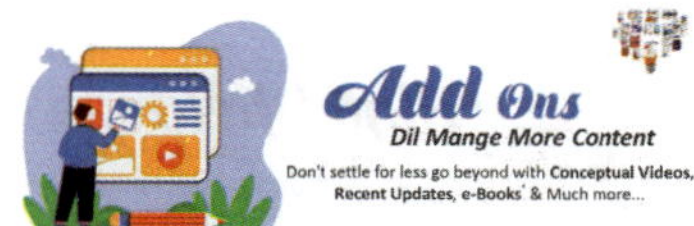

Process of β-oxidation

The process of β-oxidation consists of four reactions, which result in shortening of the fatty acid chain by two carbons. It includes:

- **Oxidation:** After activation of the fatty acid such as palmitic acid, and its entry into the mitochondrial matrix, flavoprotein containing **acyl CoA dehydrogenase removes two hydrogens** from the α- and β-positions of the fatty acyl CoA and **produces FADH$_2$.** The fatty acyl CoA is changed to α, β-unsaturated fatty acyl CoA (enoyl CoA).

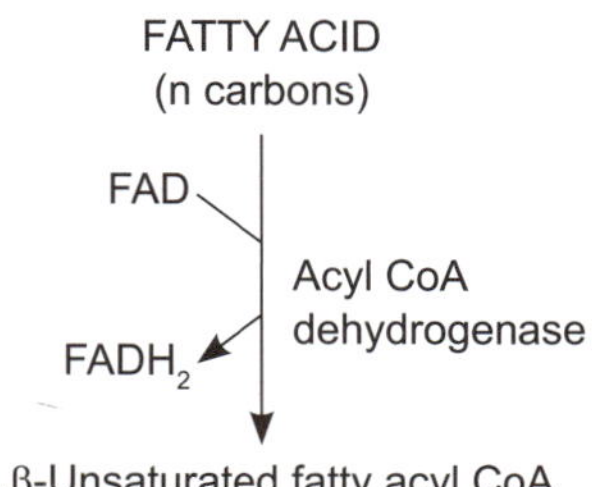

- **Hydration:** In the next step, **enoyl CoA hydratase adds a molecule of water** at the double bond and converts the enoyl CoA to β-hydroxyacyl CoA.

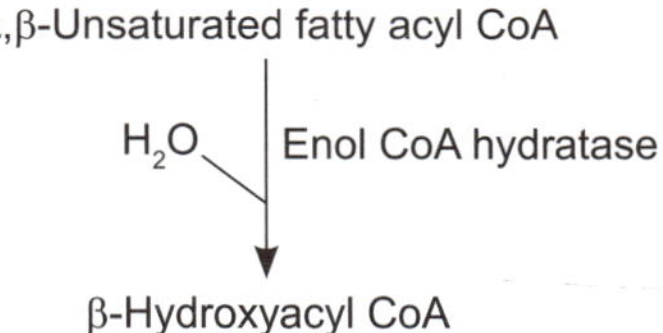

- **Oxidation:** Thereafter, β-**hydroxyacyl CoA dehydrogenase oxidizes** β-**hydroxyacyl CoA** to β-ketoacyl CoA.

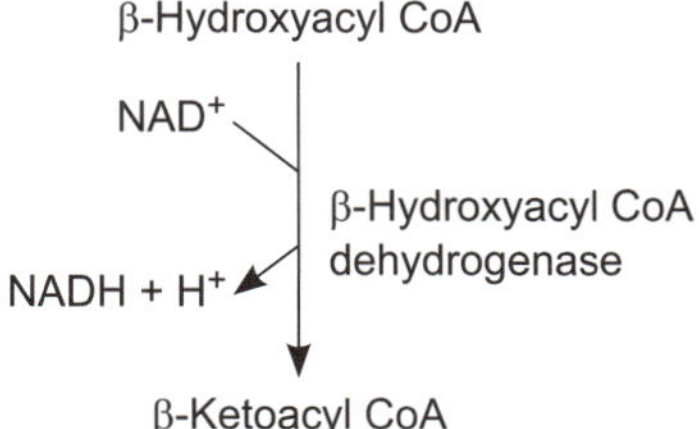

- **Cleavage:** In the last step, acyl CoA: acyltransferase, also called **thiolase,** in the presence of CoA results in thiolytic **cleavage of the** β-**ketoacyl CoA** into acetyl CoA and fatty acyl CoA which has two carbons less than the original fatty acyl CoA.

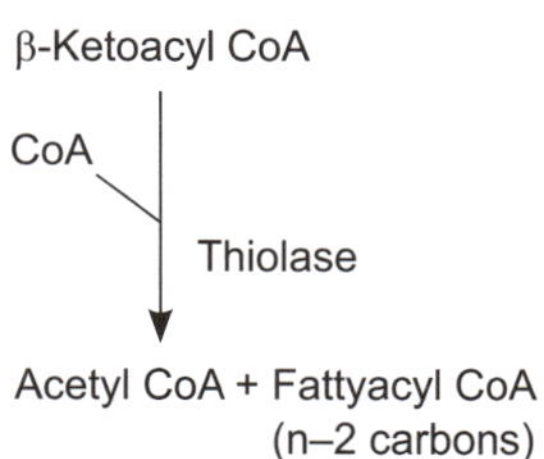

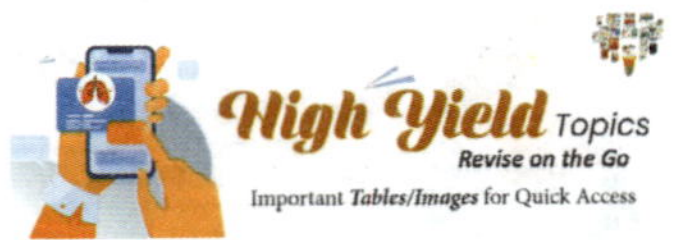

These four steps are repeated, i.e., the fatty acyl CoA again undergoes above four sets of reactions, starting with acyl CoA dehydrogenase. Each cycle produces acetyl CoA, $FADH_2$ and NADH. Thus, the fatty acid is sequentially degraded to acetyl CoA.

Energy Production from β-Oxidation

When a molecule of **palmitic acid ($C_{15}H_{31}COOH$)** undergoes β-oxidation, it **releases 8 molecules of acetyl CoA** in seven rounds. In every round, one molecule, each of $FADH_2$ and NADH + H⁺ are produced, which in turn generate 1.5 and 2.5 ATP, respectively.

Thus, a total of 28 ATP are produced during this process. In addition, each molecule of acetyl CoA, when oxidized *via* the citric acid cycle, produces 10 ATP. Therefore, additionally, 80 ATP are produced from 8 molecules of acetyl CoA. Hence, a total of **108 ATP** are produced from one molecule of palmitic acid.

As two high energy phosphate bonds are hydrolyzed from one molecule of ATP, which is changed to AMP, thus a total of 2 ATP are used during activation of the fatty acid.

Therefore, there is a **net yield of 106 ATP** when one molecule of palmitic acid (fatty acid with 16 carbons) is completely oxidized.

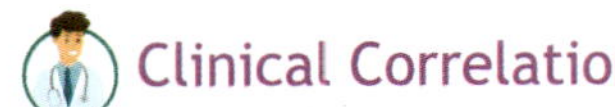

Clinical Correlation

Sudden Infant Death Syndrome (SIDS)

Medium-chain fatty acyl CoA dehydrogenase deficiency *leads to an autosomal recessive disorder, which is referred to as* **sudden infant death syndrome (SIDS) or Reye's syndrome**. *This in turn reduces fatty acid oxidation. Features of the disease include vomiting, lethargy and coma, accompanied with the hypoketotic hypoglycemia and dicarboxylic aciduria. Symptoms appear after more than 12 hours of fast and are more complicated on prolonged starvation, usually within 2 years of life. Treatment includes a carbohydrate rich diet.*

Oxidation of Fatty Acids with Odd Number of Carbon Atoms

β-Oxidation of a saturated fatty acid with odd number of carbon atoms proceeds in the same way as a saturated fatty acid with even number of carbons, until final three carbons are reached. Thus, **in addition to acetyl CoA, it also produces a molecule of propionyl CoA** (containing 3 carbons), which is used as follows:

- Firstly, propionyl CoA is carboxylated by the enzyme propionyl CoA carboxylase, to D-methylmalonyl CoA. This enzyme requires biotin (Fig. 3.11).

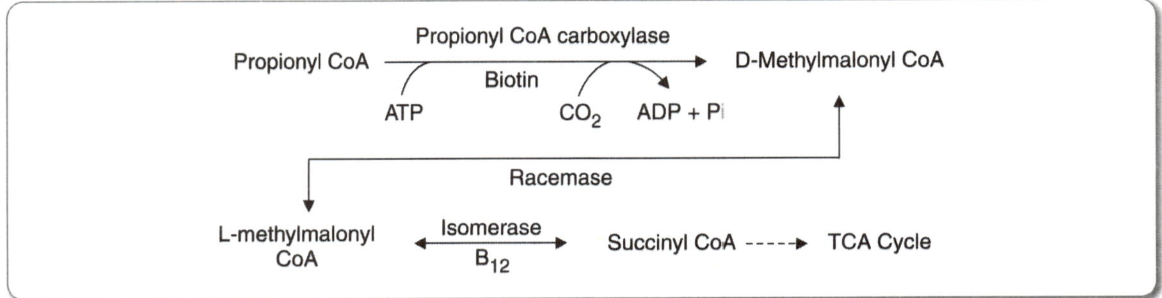

Fig. 3.11: Conversion of propionyl CoA to succinyl CoA

- D-methylmalonyl CoA is then converted to L-methylmalonyl CoA, by the enzyme methylmalonyl CoA racemase.

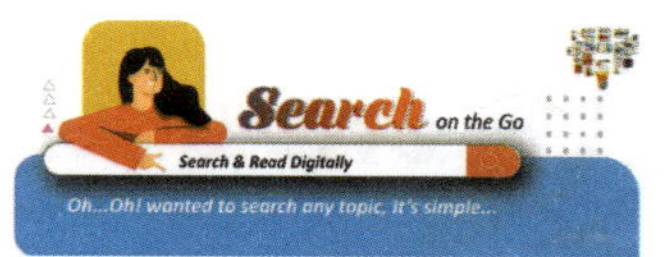

- Finally, L-methylmalonyl CoA is converted to succinyl CoA by the enzyme methylmalonyl CoA mutase. This enzyme requires deoxyadenosylcobalamin (coenzyme form of vitamin B_{12}).

Oxidation of Unsaturated Fatty Acids

Unsaturated fatty acids are activated, transported across the inner mitochondrial membrane and **undergo β-oxidation,** by the process similar to that of a saturated fatty acid. However, since the double bonds of the naturally occurring unsaturated fatty acids are found in cis-configuration (compared to those produced during β-oxidation, which have trans-configuration) hence, **three additional enzymes are required** for their oxidation. These include:

- **Enoyl CoA isomerase,**
- **Dienoyl CoA reductase, and**
- **3,2-Enoyl CoA isomerase**

Thus, in addition to the other enzymes of β-oxidation, these three enzymes are also required for the oxidation of unsaturated fatty acids (Fig. 3.12).

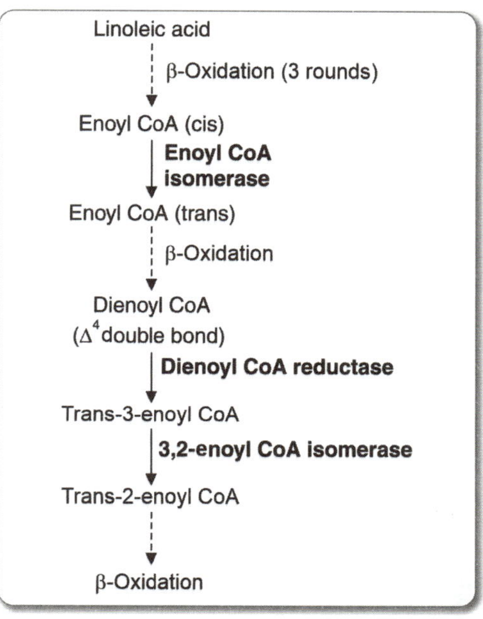

Fig. 3.12: Oxidation of an unsaturated fatty acid

Alternate Oxidative Pathways

α-Oxidation of Fatty Acids

Fatty acids are also oxidized by another process, called α-oxidation, in microsomes, in the liver and brain.

- During α-oxidation, a fatty acid is metabolized by α-hydroxylation, followed by dehydrogenation and decarboxylation (Fig. 3.13).
- **In this process,** there is **sequential removal of a carbon atom as CO_2, from the carboxyl end** of the fatty acid. This process neither produces CoA intermediates nor generates ATP.

ω-Oxidation of Fatty Acids

In this process, oxidation of the medium and long chain fatty acids occurs from both the ends.

- Firstly, the **end methyl group (–CH_3) of the acyl chain,** called ω-**carbon, is oxidized** and forms a dicarboxylic acid. This reaction is catalyzed by the enzyme ω-**hydroxylase,** which requires cytochrome P_{450}.

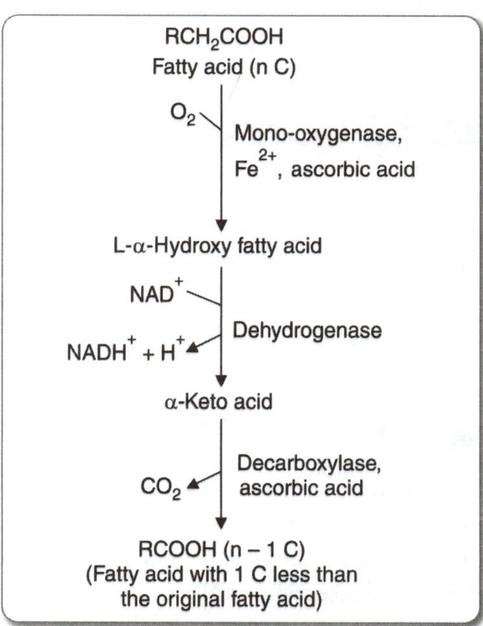

Fig. 3.13: The process of α-oxidation of a fatty acid

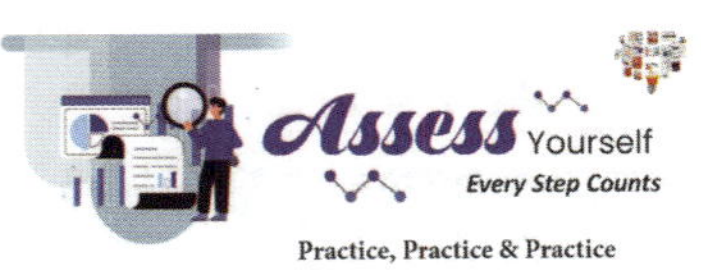

- This **dicarboxylic acid** thereafter, **undergoes β-oxidation from both the ends**, simultaneously (Fig. 3.14).

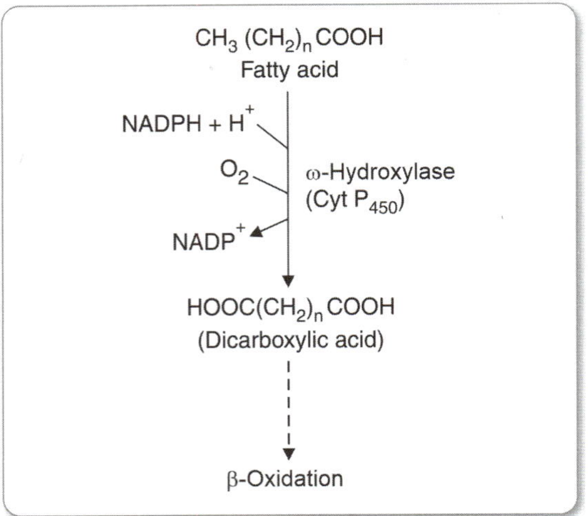

Fig. 3.14: The process of ω-oxidation of a fatty acid

Clinical Correlation

Refsum Disease

Genetic **deficiency of** α-**hydroxylase enzyme** *(a monooxygenase) results in an increase in* **phytanic acid** *in the serum and its accumulation in several tissues. This in turn leads to a neurological disorder called* **Refsum disease.**

Metabolic Fates of Acetyl CoA

Acetyl CoA is mainly **used** in the **Krebs cycle.**

Besides **Krebs cycle,** acetyl CoA can also be used for the **synthesis of fatty acids** and **cholesterol.** A small quantity of it is also converted to **ketone bodies** in the liver (Fig. 3.15).

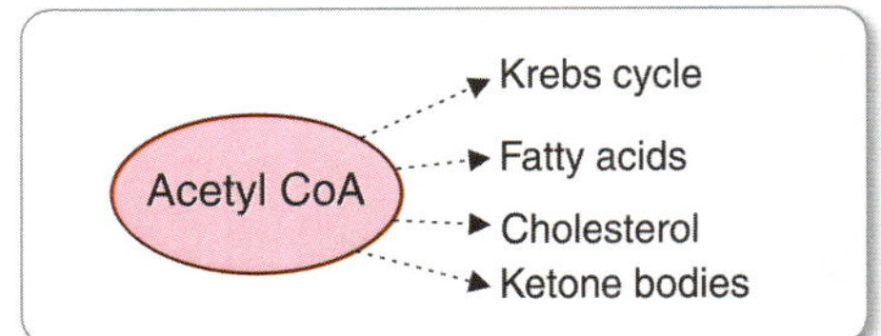

Fig. 3.15: Metabolic fates of acetyl CoA

SYNTHESIS OF FATTY ACIDS

Mammals can synthesize a major portion of the saturated as well as monounsaturated fatty acids. First, a saturated, straight chain, 16 carbon containing fatty acid, i.e., palmitic acid is synthesized, which is subsequently changed to other fatty acids.

The process of fatty acid synthesis is called **de novo synthesis**. In human beings, fatty acid synthesis occurs, primarily in the cytosol, in the liver, lactating mammary glands and to a lesser extent in the adipose tissue.

De Novo Synthesis of Fatty Acids

Acetyl CoA, which is produced in the mitochondria, first comes out of the mitochondria to the cytosol, where fatty acid synthesis occurs. Mitochondrial membrane, however, is impermeable to CoA. Thus, first step in fatty acid synthesis is the transport of the acetate, from mitochondria to the cytosol. For this purpose, **acetyl CoA condenses with oxaloacetate and forms citrate. Citrate is then translocated from mitochondria to the cytosol,** where it is cleaved **by the enzyme ATP-citrate lyase and releases acetyl CoA and oxaloacetate, in the cytosol** (Fig. 3.16).

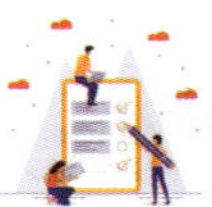
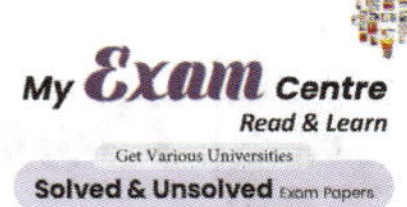

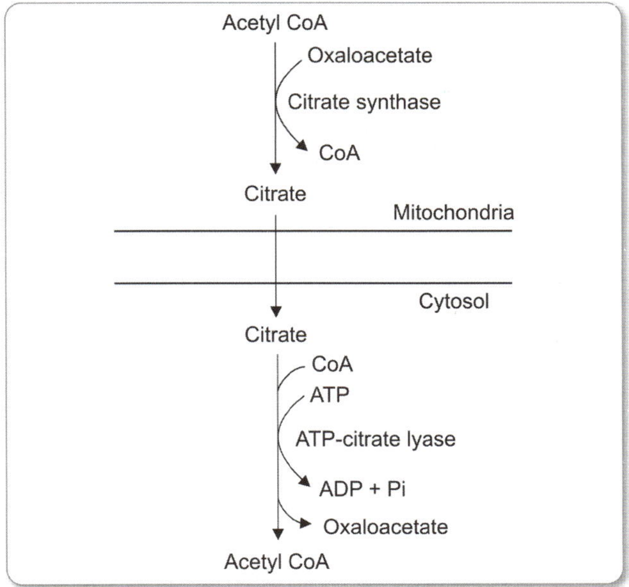

Fig. 3.16: Transport of acetyl CoA from mitochondria to cytosol

Conversion of Acetyl CoA to Malonyl CoA

Acetyl CoA is used in fatty acid synthesis after its carboxylation and conversion to malonyl CoA. In the cytosol, **acetyl CoA** is carboxylated **to malonyl CoA** by a biotin-containing enzyme, referred to as **acetyl CoA carboxylase.** This coenzyme is covalently linked to the lysyl residue of the enzyme, which requires ATP and CO_2 (as HCO_3^-).

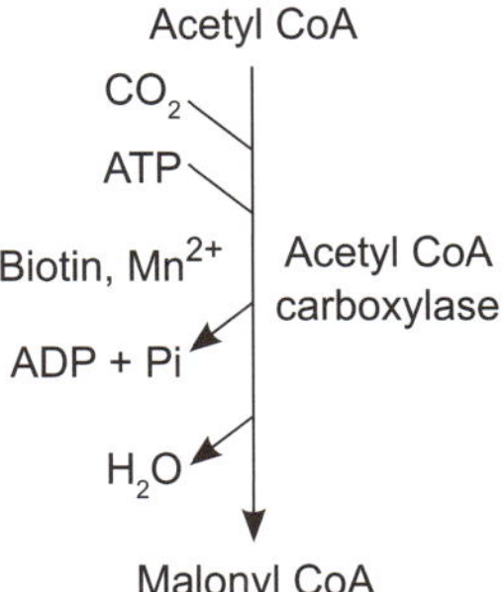

Prolonged consumption of high calorie diet increases synthesis of the enzyme **acetyl CoA carboxylase** while fasting or low calorie diet decreases its synthesis.

Synthesis of Palmitic Acid

An enzyme referred to as fatty acid synthase catalyzes the remaining reactions of fatty acid synthesis, in eukaryotes. It is a multifunctional, dimeric enzyme, composed of the two identical subunits. Its each monomer is a multicatalytic polypeptide with seven different enzyme activities plus a domain that covalently binds a molecule of 4′-phosphopantotheine. During fatty acid synthesis, 4′-phosphopantotheine carries acetyl and acyl units on its terminal thiol (–SH) groups.

In prokaryotes, fatty acid synthase is a multienzyme complex and the 4′-phosphopantotheine domain is present on a separate protein, referred to as acyl carrier protein (ACP).

Individually, different enzyme activities of the fatty acid synthase complex are designated as **acetyl CoA-ACP acetyl transacylase, malonyl CoA-ACP transacylase,** β-ketoacyl-ACP synthase (**condensing enzyme**), β-ketoacyl ACP **reductase,** β-hydroxyacyl ACP **dehydratase** and enoyl-ACP **reductase. These enzyme activities** are separate catalytic domains that are present on each subunit of the multicatalytic fatty acid synthase complex.

Fatty acid synthase contains **two-SH groups,** called **pantotheinyl-SH group,** which is referred to as the **ACP-SH,** and the **thiol-SH group** that is designated as the **CYS-SH.**

- Fatty acid synthesis starts with the **transfer of** the **molecule of acetate, from acetyl CoA to the ACP-SH.** This reaction is catalyzed by the **acetyl CoA-ACP acetyl transacylase domain** of the fatty acid synthase complex.

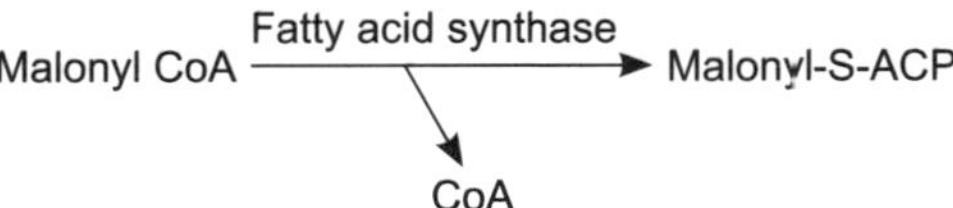

This two-carbon fragment is transferred to the **CYS-SH,** which is a temporary holding site.

- At the same time, **malonyl CoA-ACP transacylase** domain of the fatty acid synthase **transfers three carbon malonate unit from malonyl CoA** to the vacant **-SH** group of ACP.

- In the next step, malonyl group loses CO_2 and transfers the acetyl group, by β-ketoacyl ACP synthase domain of the fatty acid synthase, which in turn causes **condensation of the two acetyl group on the CYS–SH** and forms **a four carbon acetoacetyl unit that is attached to the ACP domain.**

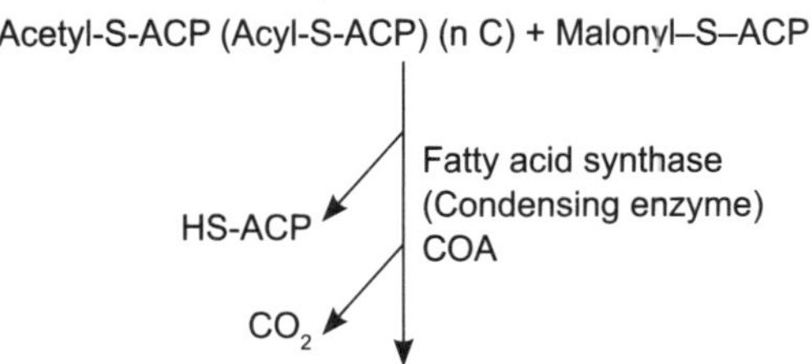

- β-Ketoacyl ACP **reductase** domain of the fatty acid synthase reduces keto group of the **acetoacetyl-S-ACP to β-Hydroxybutyryl-S-ACP** (β-Hydroxyacyl-S-ACP).

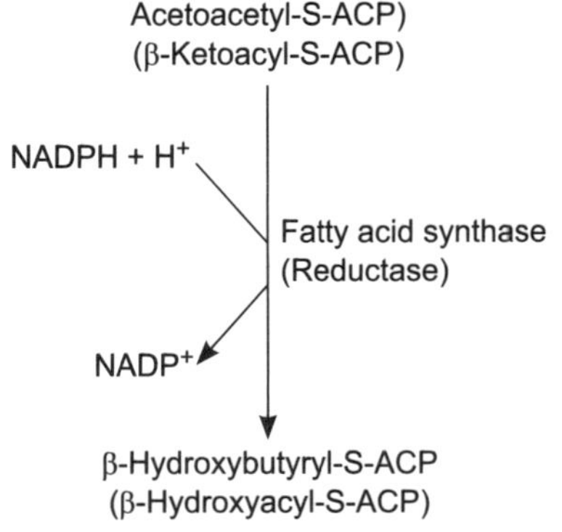

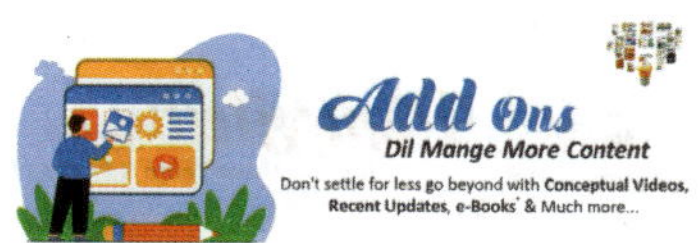

- β-Hydroxyacyl-ACP **dehydratase domain** of the fatty acid synthase removes a molecule of H_2O from β-**Hydroxyacyl-S-ACP** and introduces a double bond in it, to form crotonyl-S-ACP (α,β-unsaturated acyl-S-ACP).

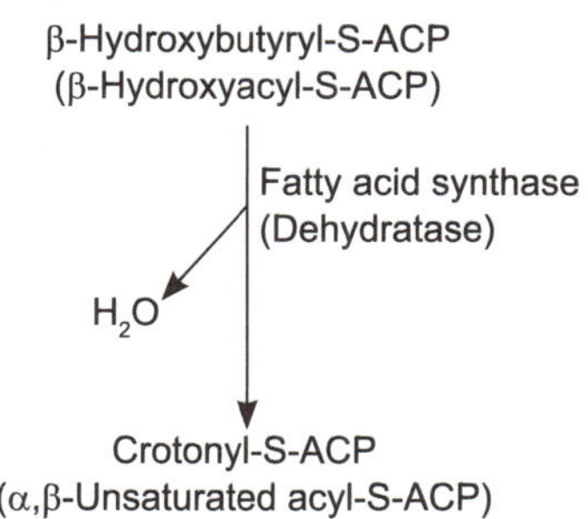

- **Crotonyl-S-ACP is reduced by the enoyl-ACP reductase domain** of the fatty acid synthase and is converted **to butyryl-S-ACP** (acyl-S-ACP).

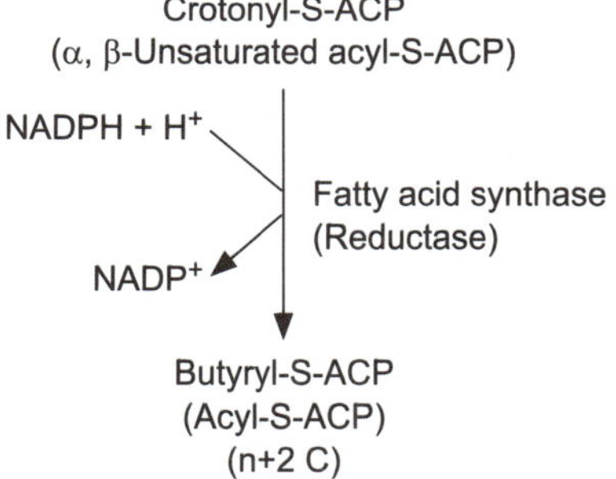

As a result of these reactions, a four carbon compound is formed, whose three terminal carbons are fully saturated and remain attached to ACP.

These steps are again repeated, beginning with the transfer of the butyryl chain to the CYS-SH. This cycle of the reactions is repeated five more times, each time incorporating two carbon units which are derived from malonyl CoA and are attached to the growing fatty acid chain at the carboxyl end. When the chain length reaches 16 carbons, the process is terminated with the formation of palmitoyl-S-ACP. Thereafter, **palmitoyl thioesterase cleaves the thioester bond with the release of palmitate** (Fig. 3.17).

Palmitoyl-S-ACP $\xrightarrow{\text{Thioesterase}}$ Palmitate

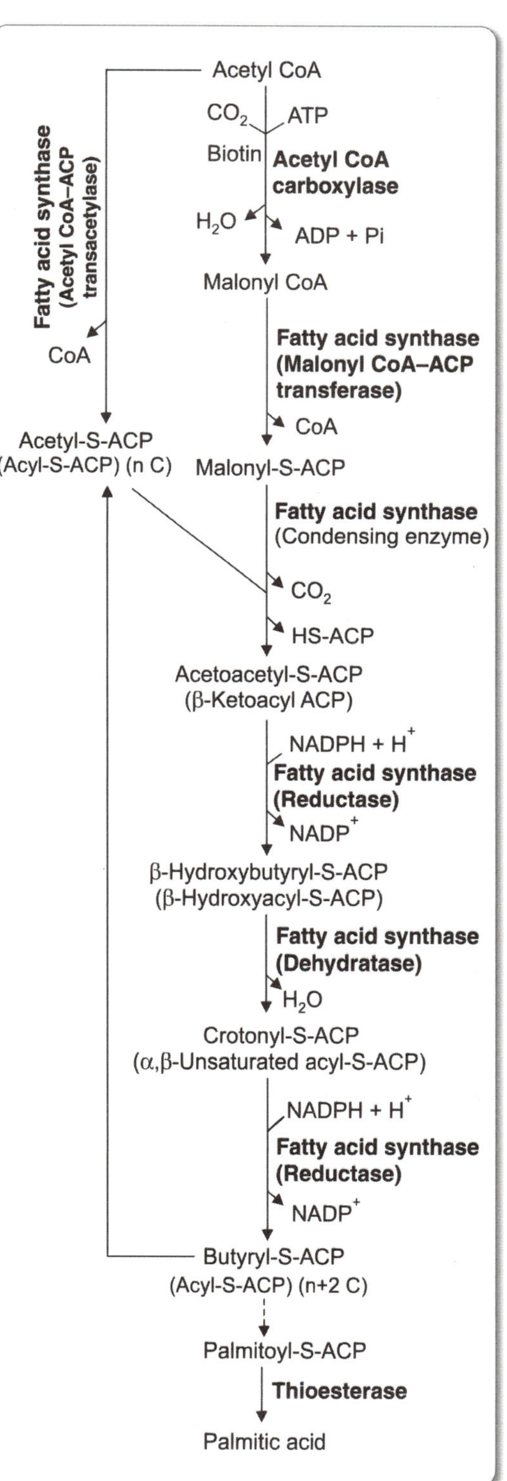

Fig. 3.17: The process of **de novo** synthesis of palmitic acid.

Reducing equivalents (NADPH + H$^+$), which are used in the biosynthesis of fatty acids, are derived from the pentose phosphate pathway.

The overall reaction is:

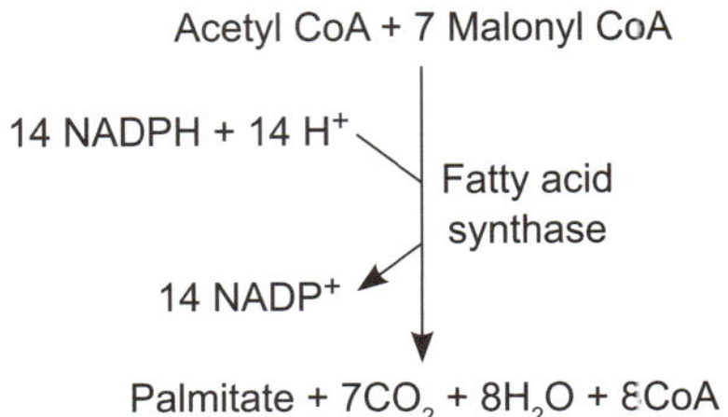

Regulation of Fatty Acid Synthesis

The rate-limiting step in the synthesis of fatty acids is the conversion of acetyl CoA to malonyl CoA. This reaction is catalyzed by the enzyme acetyl CoA carboxylase which is stimulated by citrate.

Citrate, allosterically, **activates acetyl CoA carboxylase,** while a **long chain fatty acyl CoA** acts **as an allosteric inhibitor.**

Insulin also **stimulates** activity of **this enzyme**. A high carbohydrate diet increases production of acetyl CoA, which in turn increases the citrate pool. Thus, a high carbohydrate diet leads to increased fatty acid synthesis. Insulin also reduces cAMP level, inhibits activation of the hormone sensitive lipase and favors lipogenesis.

On the other hand, **glucagon** increases cAMP level, activates lipase activity and **inhibits fatty acid synthesis**. Glucagon thus, promotes release of fatty acids from the adipose tissue (lipolysis) and opposes lipogenesis.

Fatty acid synthase is also a key enzyme of the palmitate biosynthesis. **A high carbohydrate diet** or a **fat free diet stimulates** fatty acids synthase activity. On the other hand, **high fat diet, fasting** and **glucagon** decrease enzyme synthesis.

Phosphorylated sugars, e.g., **glucose-6-phosphate**, also **activate** this enzyme.

Synthesis of Other Fatty Acids

Palmitate, produced by the fatty acid synthase catalyzed reactions can be modified by:

- Chain elongation, and/or
- Desaturation.

Chain Elongation

Chain elongation of a fatty acid occurs in the mammalian system by the addition of two carbon units in the mitochondria and the endoplasmic reticulum.

In the Mitochondria

Chain elongation in the mitochondria takes place by the successive addition of acetyl CoA, as two carbon units, where both NADH as well as NADPH can be used as a source of the reducing equivalents.

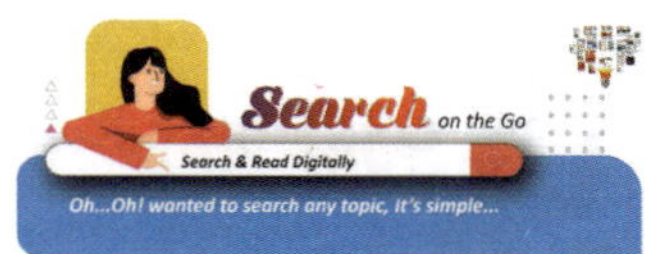

This is the process of the **reversal of β-oxidation** with the exception that NADPH-linked enoyl CoA reductase replaces FAD-linked acyl CoA dehydrogenase.

Firstly, **acyl CoA condenses with acetyl CoA** and **forms β-ketoacyl CoA,** which is subsequently reduced to β-hydroxyacyl CoA. Removal of a molecule of water converts β-hydroxyacyl CoA to α, β-unsaturated fatty acyl CoA (enoyl CoA), which is finally reduced to the higher member of the fatty acid (Fig. 3.18)

In the Endoplasmic Reticulum

The process of chain elongation in the endoplasmic reticulum is **similar to the process of de novo synthesis of fatty acid,** as occur in the cytosol. It utilizes malonyl CoA as a source of two carbon unit but elongation occurs **as a CoA derivative of the fatty acid rather than the ACP-derivative.**

In most of the tissues, chain elongation in the endoplasmic reticulum converts palmitate to stearate.

Brain, however, has additional elongation capabilities, allowing it to produce very long chain fatty acids (up to 24-carbon atoms). These fatty acids are required for the synthesis of complex lipids, within the brain.

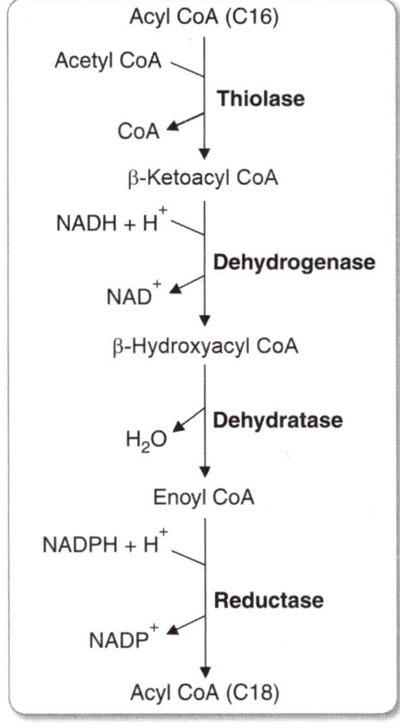

Fig. 3.18: Chain elongation of a fatty acid in mitochondria

Desaturation

Desaturation of a fatty acid (addition of the cis double bond) occurs in higher animals, in the endoplasmic reticulum, **by desaturases,** which are the mixed function oxidases. Desaturation reaction requires NADPH and O_2 (Fig. 3.19).

Several polyunsaturated fatty acids can be synthesized through additional desaturation and elongation. Human beings, however, lack the ability to introduce a double bond prior to carbon-9, i.e., between carbon-9 and the ω-carbon of the chain.

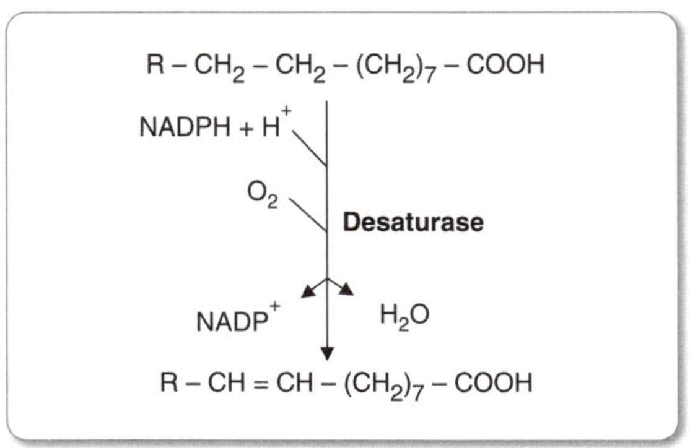

Fig. 3.19: Desaturation of a fatty acid

METABOLISM OF TRIACYLGLYCEROLS

Synthesis of Triacylglycerols

Fatty acids are stored in the liver and adipose tissue in collaboration with glycerol, as triacylglycerols. The process of biosynthesis of triacylglycerol is called **lipogenesis**.

Lipogenesis occurs mainly in the liver and the adipose tissue. It requires activation of free fatty acid and α-glycerol phosphate and the re-esterification of glycerol phosphate (Fig. 3.20).

- **Activation of fatty acid:** Free fatty acid, in the presence of ATP and CoA, is activated to fatty acyl CoA (acyl CoA) by the family of fatty acyl CoA synthetases (thiokinases).
- **Synthesis of glycerol phosphate:** There are two pathways for the production of glycerol phosphate:
    - L-α-glycerol-3-phosphate is formed by the reduction of dihydroxyacetone phosphate, an intermediate of glycolysis. This reaction is catalyzed by glycerol-3-phosphate dehydrogenase.
    - Alternatively, in the tissues such as **liver, lactating mammary glands, kidney and intestinal mucosa**, glycerol can be directly converted, to L-α-glycerol-3-phosphate, by the enzyme glycerol kinase.

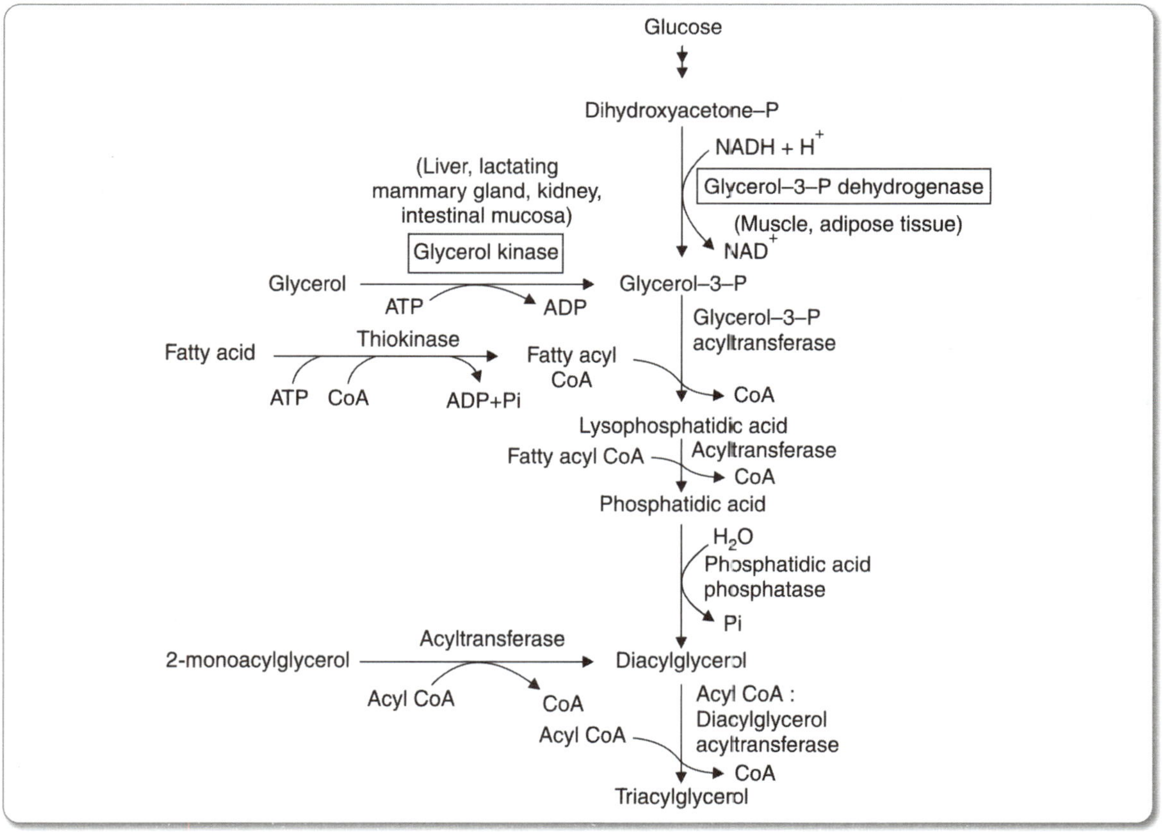

Fig. 3.20: The process of synthesis of the triacylglycerols

- **Synthesis of triacylglycerol**: After activation of the fatty acid and the synthesis of L-α-glycerol phosphate, triacylglycerol is synthesized by the re-esterification of L-α-glycerol phosphate:

- Firstly, a molecule of acyl CoA combines with α-glycerol phosphate and forms 1-acylglycerol-3-phosphate (lysophosphatidic acid). This reaction is catalyzed by the enzyme glycerol-3-phosphate acyltransferase.
- Thereafter, 1-acylglycerol-3-phosphate is converted to 1,2-diacylglycerolphosphate (phosphatidic acid) by the enzyme 1-acylglycerol-3-phosphate acyltransferase, also called lysophosphatidyl acyl-transferase.
- Phosphatidic acid is then hydrolyzed to 1,2-diacylglycerol by the enzyme phosphatidic acid phosphohydrolase, also called phosphatidic acid phosphatase.

  In many tissues such as intestine, liver, kidney, aorta and lactating mammary glands, especially in the intestinal mucosa, 1,2-diacylglycerol is also formed from 2-monoacylglycerol, since monoacylglycerol is directly absorbed in the intestinal mucosa. This reaction is catalyzed by the enzyme monoacylglycerol acyltransferase.
- Finally, diacylglycerol is esterified to form triacylglycerol. This reaction is catalyzed by the enzyme diacylglycerol acyltransferase.

  Generally, palmitic acid is present at position 1 while oleic acid may be found at positions 2 and 3 of the triacylglycerol, in adipose tissue, in human beings.

Breakdown of Triacylglycerols

Only a little amount of triacylglycerol is stored **in the liver**. Most of it is exported, packed with cholesteryl esters, cholesterol, phospholipids and apolipoproteins, as **very low density lipoprotein** (VLDL).

Triacylglycerol is stored **in adipose tissue**, in the cytosol of the cell. It serves as depot fat, which is ready for mobilization, when body requires fuel.

Fatty acids that are stored in the adipose tissue in the form of **triacylglycerols** are mainly **oxidized for energy**. Mobilization of the stored fat requires hydrolytic release of the fatty acids and glycerol, from triacylglycerols. The enzyme called hormone-sensitive lipase, which removes fatty acids from carbon-1 and/or 3 of a triacylglycerol, initiates this process. Additional lipases, which are specific for diacylglycerols and monoacylglycerols, remove the remaining fatty acids (Fig. 3.21).

Utilization of these fatty acids, however, vary from tissue to tissue, depending upon the metabolic status of the tissue. Impairment in fatty acid oxidation may lead to hypoglycemia.

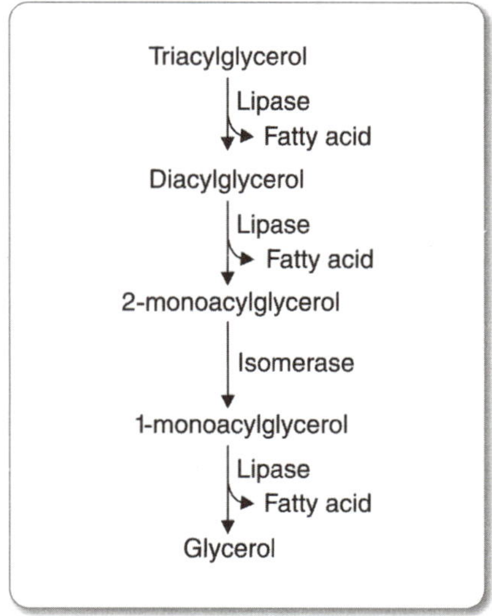

Fig. 3.21: Breakdown of triacylglycerols

ROLE OF LIVER IN LIPID METABOLISM

- Liver is the primary tissue for *de novo* **synthesis of fatty acids**. This pathway occurs in the absorptive period because dietary calorie intake exceeds energy expenditure and fatty acid synthesis is favored by the availability of substrate.

- **Triacylglycerol synthesis** is favoured in the liver because fatty acyl CoA is available, both from *de novo* synthesis from acetyl CoA and from hydrolysis of the triacylglycerols component of chylomicron remnants, which are removed from the blood by hepatocytes.

- The liver **packages triacylglycerols into VLDL** particles that are secreted into blood for use by extrahepatic tissues, particularly adipose tissue and muscle. VLDLs are produced in the liver. These are composed predominantly of triacylglycerols (approximately 60%) and their function is to carry this lipid from the liver to the peripheral tissues. VLDLs are secreted directly into the blood by the liver as nascent VLDL particles containing apo B-100.

- **Chylomicron remnants** are rapidly **removed from the circulation by the liver** whose cell membrane contains lipoprotein receptors that recognize apo E. Chylomicron remnants bind to these receptors and are taken into the hepatocytes by receptor-mediated endocytosis. Their cholesteryl esters and triacylglycerols are hydrolyzed and metabolized in the liver.

- Liver, in addition to intestine, adrenal cortex, and reproductive tissues, **makes** the largest contribution to the body's **cholesterol** pool. Liver also plays a central role in the **regulation of the body's cholesterol** homeostasis. For example, cholesterol enters the liver pool and is eliminated from the liver as free cholesterol in the bile or converted to bile salts that are secreted into the intestinal lumen. It also serves as a component of plasma lipoproteins, which are transported to the peripheral tissues.

- **Bile acids are synthesized** in the liver. The most common resulting compounds are cholic acid and chenodeoxycholic acid, called primary bile acids. Before the bile acids leave the liver, these are conjugated to a molecule of either glycine or taurine.

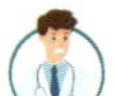

Clinical Correlation

Fatty Liver

*Fatty liver, also known as **fatty liver disease** (FLD) or **steatosis hepatitis**, is a reversible condition where large vacuoles of triacylglycerols accumulate in liver cells via the process of steatosis. Despite having multiple causes, fatty liver can be considered a single disease that occurs worldwide in those with excessive alcohol intake and who are obese (with or without effects of insulin resistance). The condition is also associated with other diseases that influence fat metabolism. Eating fatty food does not, by itself, produce fatty liver.*

Although fatty liver is commonly associated with alcohol intake or metabolic syndrome (diabetes, hypertension and dyslipidemia) but can also be due to any one of these causes which include metabolic (abetalipoproteinemia, glycogen storage diseases, acute fatty liver of pregnancy, lipodystrophy); nutritional (malnutrition, severe weight loss, gastric bypass); drugs and toxins (methotrexate, glucocorticoids, environmental hepatotoxins, e.g., phosphorus, toxic mushroom); or other causes (inflammatory bowel disease, HIV).

The diagnosis of steatosis is made when fat in the liver exceeds 5–10% by weight. The patient may have an enlarged liver or minor elevation of liver enzyme tests. The treatment of fatty liver is related to the cause. It is important to remember that simple fatty liver may not require treatment. The benefit of weight loss, dietary fat restriction and exercise in obese patients is inconsistent. Reducing or eliminating alcohol intake can improve fatty liver due to alcohol toxicity. Controlling blood sugar may reduce the severity of fatty liver in patients with diabetes.

Lipotropic Factors

A lipotropic factor is defined as a substance which prevents or removes an accumulation of excess of fat in the liver. These include choline, betaine and other related compounds, choline precursors, such as methionine and inositol. In addition to playing important role in the mobilization and utilization of dietary fat, lipotropic factors act as the body's natural emulsifiers, holding blood lipids in solution and resisting lipid deposition within the cardiovascular system. Sufficient lipotropic factors can also keep homocysteine levels in check to support cardiovascular health, including the health of the arterial walls and blood lipids.

The body is able to synthesize lipotropic factors when given all the ingredients, i.e., choline, inositol, betaine, folic acid and B vitamins.

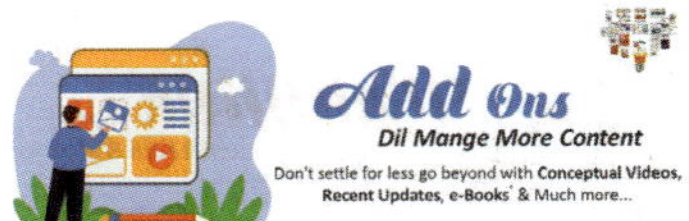

These new structures are called **bile salts**. Bile salts are more effective detergents than bile acids because of their enhanced amphipathic nature. Bile salts provide the only significant mechanism for cholesterol excretion, both as a metabolic product of cholesterol and as a solubilizer of cholesterol in bile.

- The **oxidation of fatty acids** derived from adipose tissue is the major source of energy in hepatic tissue, during prolonged fasting.
- The liver is also unique to **synthesize** and release **ketone bodies** (primarily 3-hydroxybutyrate) to the blood, for use as fuel by peripheral tissues.

CHOLESTEROL

Cholesterol is derived **from diet**. It is **also synthesized in various tissues** in the body. About 50% of the normal intake of dietary cholesterol is absorbed by the small intestine while the rest of it is excreted in the feces.

Nearly 0.3 g of **cholesterol is absorbed** from the diet, daily. Ingested cholesterol is absorbed with other lipids and is incorporated into chylomicrons and VLDL. More than 80% of it is esterified in the intestinal mucosa and is transported with lipoproteins.

Cholesterol is **excreted from the body** either as fecal neutral sterol or as bile acid. About 600–750 mg of cholesterol is lost each day as bile acids, 500–600 mg in fecal neutral sterols, 75–100 mg is shed by the skin and nearly 35–50 mg is converted into steroid hormones.

Cholesterol **content in normal human blood** varies from 130 mg to 220 mg/100 mL, being equally distributed between plasma and erythrocytes. Only about 30% of the circulating cholesterol occurs **free**, while the remaining of it exists in the form of **cholesterol esters**. Usually, a long chain fatty acid is attached to the –OH group (by an ester linkage), on carbon 3 of the ring A of cholesterol.

An adult man contains about 1 g of cholesterol/kg body weight. Nearly 25% of cholesterol is present in the membrane of the nervous system, as a major **component of myelin sheath**. It is also a major **component of plasma membrane. Cholesterol** is also a metabolic **precursor** of various substances such as **steroid hormones** (glucocorticoids and mineralocorticoids), **vitamin D** and **bile acids and salts**.

Egg, meat and milk are the important dietary sources of cholesterol. It is also synthesized in the body by nearly all cells. The amount of cholesterol synthesized each day, in man, is at least twice to that of ingested in the diet.

Biosynthesis of Cholesterol

A large quantity of cholesterol (about 1 g/day) is synthesized in the extramitochondrial compartment of the cell. Important sites for cholesterol biosynthesis include liver, skin, intestine, adrenal cortex and reproductive tissues, including ovaries, testes and placenta.

All the carbon atoms of **cholesterol** are derived **from acetate** (acetyl CoA), which is obtained from several sources such as oxidation of long chain fatty acids, ketogenic amino acids and glucose (*via* pyruvate).

De novo synthesis of cholesterol takes place in the body, as shown in Figure 3.22.

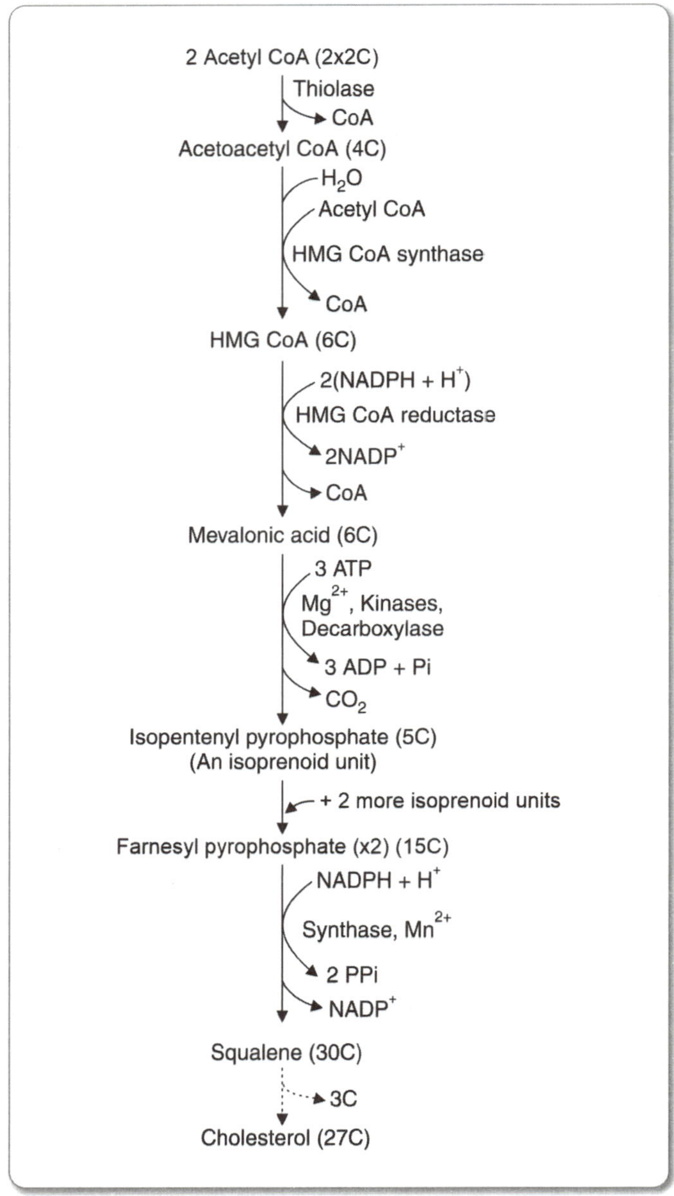

Fig. 3.22: *De novo* synthesis of cholesterol

Regulation of Cholesterol Biosynthesis

Dietary cholesterol, feedback inhibition and its disposal from the liver, regulate cholesterol synthesis.

- **Dietary cholesterol:** Rate of de novo synthesis of cholesterol is inversely related to the amount of dietary cholesterol. When dietary cholesterol intake is reduced, cholesterol synthesis is increased in the liver and the intestine, to meet needs of the other tissues.

  On the other hand, when dietary cholesterol intake is increased, its synthesis is reduced.

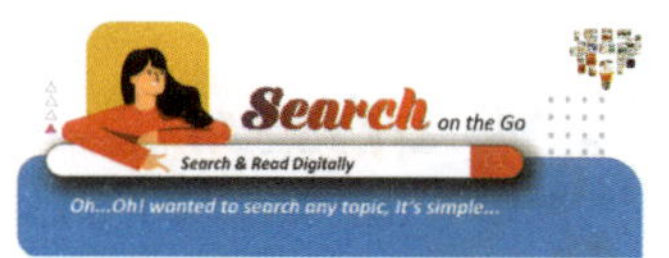

- **Feed back inhibition:** Cholesterol inhibits its own synthesis by feedback inhibition. The enzyme HMG CoA reductase regulates cholesterol synthesis. Cholesterol inhibits the activity of HMG CoA reductase, by suppressing its synthesis and promoting inactivation.
- **Disposal by the liver:** Liver removes cholesterol by different processes:
  - **Esterification of cholesterol:** Both, HDL and lecithin:cholesterol acyltransferase (LCAT) are important for the removal of cholesterol from the body.
    - ◆ LCAT is a plasma enzyme which is produced mainly by the liver. It transfers one fatty acid from carbon 2 of lecithin to the 3-hydroxy group of cholesterol. This reaction is freely reversible and utilizes cholesterol, which is present in HDL.

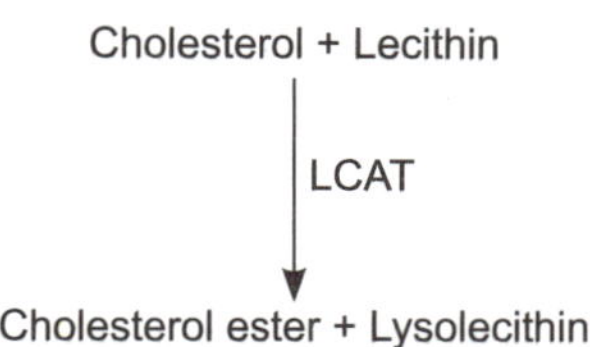

  - ◆ Cholesterol esters, so formed, diffuse into the core of the HDL particle where they are transported from the tissues and plasma, to the liver, which is the only organ that is capable of metabolizing and excreting cholesterol.

    This is referred to as the **reverse transport of cholesterol** since HDL provides the vehicle for the transport of cholesterol, from the peripheral tissues to the liver.

    In a normal healthy adult, on a low cholesterol diet, about 1300 mg of cholesterol is returned to the liver, each day.
  - **Excretion of cholesterol:** Free cholesterol as well as bile acids/salts are excreted in the bile.
  - **Incorporation of cholesterol into VLDL:** In the liver, cholesterol is incorporated into VLDL and is secreted into circulation.

Compounds Formed from Cholesterol

Free cholesterol is present in abundance, **in bile**. It is also present in large amounts, **in the myelin structure of the brain.** Cholesterol also occurs in the esterified form **in the cell membrane.**

Cholesterol is also a precursor of several compounds, i.e., **bile acids, steroid hormones** and **vitamin D** (Fig. 3.23).

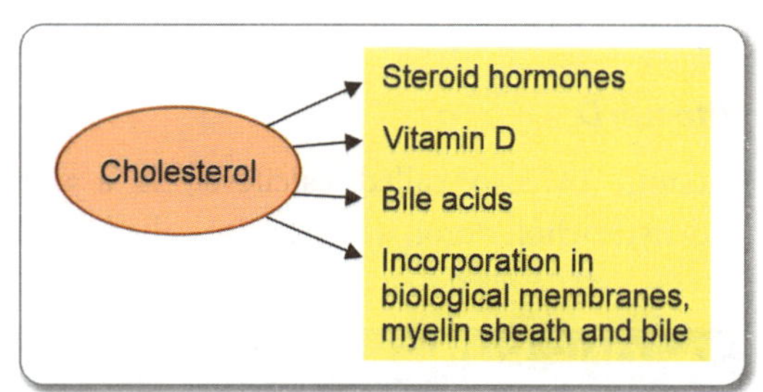

Fig. 3.23: Compounds formed from cholesterol

Bile Acids

Bile acids contain 24 carbons with two or three hydroxyl groups and a side chain that has a carboxyl group, which is not fully ionized at physiological pH. These are amphipathic in nature.

Primary Bile Acids

Bile acids are synthesized in the liver, from cholesterol. Most common bile acids which are synthesized in the liver, are called **cholic acid and chenodeoxycholic acid.** These are also referred to as **primary bile acids.** In the liver, these compounds get conjugated with a molecule of either glycine or taurine (derived from cystine) by an amide bond, which is formed between the carboxyl group of the bile acid and the amino group of glycine/taurine. These conjugates, i.e., **glycocholate and glycochenodeoxycholate** as well as **taurocholate and taurochenodeoxycholate** are referred to as **bile salts**. Normally, the ratio of glycine to taurine conjugates is approximately 3:1. Because of their enhanced amphipathic nature, bile salts are more effective detergents than bile acids.

Secondary Bile Acids

Bile salts enter small intestine, where bacteria remove glycine and taurine and regenerate bile acids. These bacteria also remove a hydroxyl group from primary bile acids, producing **deoxycholic acid** (from cholic acid) and **lithocholic acid** (from chenodeoxycholic acid). These compounds are called **secondary bile acids**.

Mixture of primary and secondary bile acids and salts is observed, primarily, in the ileum. These are actively transported from the intestinal mucosal cells into the portal blood and are removed by liver parenchymal cells. Liver again converts both, primary and secondary bile acids into bile salts by conjugation with glycine and taurine, and secrets them into bile.

This process of secretion of bile salts into bile, their passage through the duodenum, where some of them are re-converted to bile acids, and their subsequent return to the liver is termed *enterohepatic circulation*.

Bile salts have detergent properties and are essential for digestion and absorption of lipids.

Steroid Hormones

Steroid hormones are also derived from cholesterol. Cholesterol is first converted to pregnenolone, which is subsequently used for the synthesis of steroid hormones, in specific tissues. Steroid hormones are divided into two groups:

1. **Sex and progestational hormones**
2. **Hormones of the adrenal cortex**

Hormones secreted by the adrenal cortex are grouped as **glucocorticoids** and **mineralocorticoids**. Principal **glucocorticoid** is **cortisol** (hydrocortisone), which act predominantly in intermediary metabolism of carbohydrates, lipids and proteins. Principal **mineralocorticoid** is **aldosterone** which predominantly regulates the metabolism of sodium and potassium.

Vitamin D

Vitamin D, also called calciferol, is a steroid alcohol (sterol). It is synthesized in the skin from 7-dehydrocholesterol, which is also called provitamin D.

KETONE BODIES

Acetoacetate, β-hydroxybutyrate and **acetone** are collectively referred to as **ketone bodies** (acetone bodies). The process of the **formation of ketone bodies** is called **ketogenesis.**

In a normal man, concentration of the ketone bodies is usually <3 mg/100 mL of blood. In certain conditions such as during prolonged starvation or impaired glucose oxidation, like diabetes mellitus, when fat becomes the source of energy and lipolysis is accelerated, there is increased production of acetyl CoA. This, in turn, cannot be fully utilized through Krebs cycle (due to lack of oxaloacetate) and is converted to ketone bodies.

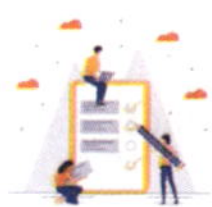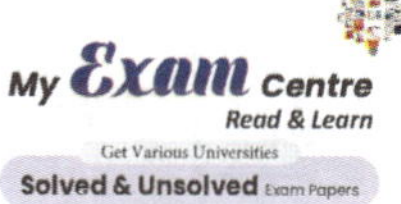

Clinical condition resulting from the **increased synthesis of ketone bodies** is called **ketosis**. Ketone bodies are diffused into the **blood. Increased** concentration of ketone bodies in the blood is called **ketonemia**. This in turn also results in their increased excretion in the urine, which is referred to as **ketonuria**.

Formation of ketone bodies occurs in the mitochondria, in the liver since liver has a highly active system for the production of acetoacetate, which is the principal ketone body.

Utilization of Ketone Bodies

Acetoacetate and β-hydroxybutyrate, which are produced by the liver, can be used as a source of energy in the peripheral tissues such as kidney and muscle. Although glucose is the major fuel for brain in the well-nourished state but during starvation even brain starts utilizing ketone bodies.

The process of the oxidation of ketone bodies is called **ketolysis**.

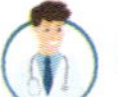 ## Clinical Correlation

Ketosis

Both, acetoacetate and β-hydroxybutyrate are the strong acids. Slowly they deplete the alkali reserve of the body and cause **metabolic acidosis**. *Hence, this condition is also called* **ketoacidosis**.

Ketosis occurs **in severe diabetes, starvation** *or* **on high fat-low carbohydrate diet**.

Under normal conditions, acetone formation is negligible but when acetoacetate accumulates, such as in severe diabetic ketoacidosis, the amount of acetone in the blood increases to the extent that it can be detected in the breath of the patient.

In the patients with insulin dependent diabetes mellitus, major metabolic derangements include marked hyperglycemia, ketonemia and ketonuria. It may also be associated with water and electrolyte imbalance.

LIPOPROTEINS

Lipids as are not soluble in the aqueous plasma, hence these are transported in the body in association with proteins. These protein-lipid complexes are called **lipoproteins** or proteolipids. Lipoproteins **are globular micelle like particles consisting of** nonpolar core of **triacylglycerols** and **cholesterol esters,** which are surrounded by the amphiphilic coating that consists of **proteins, cholesterol** and **phospholipids**.

Various lipoproteins can be separated according to their density by ultracentrifugation. Lipoproteins can also be separated according to their protein content, by electrophoresis (Table 3.4).

TABLE 3.4: Physical properties and chemical composition of human serum lipoproteins

	Chylomicrons	VLDL	IDL	LDL	HDL
Density (g/mL)	<0.95	<1.006	1.006–1.019	1.019–1.063	>1.063
S_f	>400	20–400	12–20	0–12	3.0–9.0
Electrophoretic mobility	Origin	Pre-β	Fast-β	β	α
Protein concentration (%)	2–4	8–12	15–20	20–25	40–45
Free cholesterol (%)	1–3	5–10	7–8	7–10	3–5
Cholesterol esters (%)	2–4	10–15	18–22	35–40	12–18
Triacylglycerols (%)	85–90	50–65	25–30	6–10	4–6
Phospholipids (%)	8–10	16–20	18–22	20–24	25–30

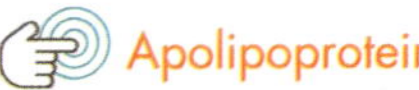 Apolipoproteins

Protein components of lipoproteins are called apolipoproteins *or* **apoproteins.** *Apolipoproteins serve as the structural components of lipoproteins, provide recognition sites for cell surface receptors and serve as activators for enzymes involved in lipoprotein metabolism.*

Various apolipoproteins are divided into different classes from A to E. At least nine types are known to occur in human serum lipoproteins. These are referred to as AI, AII, B-48, B-100, CI, CII, CIII, D and E. All of them except B-100 are water soluble.

Apolipoprotein B-100 (apo B-100) is one of the largest monomeric protein, which is synthesized by the liver and is present in the LDL.

Classification of Lipoproteins

Lipoproteins are classified into different groups as follows:

Chylomicrons

Chylomicrons are very large particles which are secreted into lymphatics by mucosal cells of small intestine. About 90% of their mass is triglycerides, which together with cholesterol esters and fat soluble vitamins form a core of the particle. Its surface layer is made of free cholesterol, phospholipids and apoproteins (apo B-48, apo AI and apo AIV).

Functions of Chylomicrons

Chylomicrons are triglycerides-rich particles that are assembled in the intestinal mucosal cells. They carry dietary triacylglycerols, cholesterol, and cholesteryl esters to peripheral (extrahepatic) tissues.

Very Low Density Lipoproteins

Very low density lipoproteins (VLDL), also called **pre-β-lipoproteins**, are large particles which are secreted into the blood stream, by the hepatocytes. Fifty to sixty percent of their mass is triacylglycerols. VLDL contains relatively more cholesterol esters than chylomicrons. Their surface coat contains free cholesterol and phospholipids, a single molecule of apo B-100 and other apoproteins. VLDL is transformed into **intermediate density lipoproteins (IDL).**

These are referred to as IDL (also called LDL_1) since their density as well as lipid composition are in between the VLDL and the LDL. Major apoproteins of IDL are apo C and apo B-100. IDL is either removed by liver or converted to LDL_2, also called low density lipoproteins (LDL).

Functions of VLDL

VLDL particles are composed of triacylglycerols like chylomicrons but their function is to transport lipids from liver to the peripheral tissues.

Low Density Lipoproteins

Low density lipoprotein **(LDL)** particles have a density range of 1.019–1.063. It contains a single molecule of apo B-100 and carries about 75% of total cholesterol, in human plasma.

Functions of LDL

Primary function of LDL is to transport cholesterol from liver to the extrahepatic tissues.

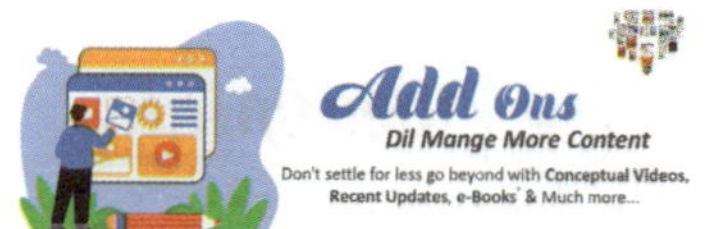

High Density Lipoproteins

High density lipoprotein (HDL) fraction is very heterogeneous. It is commonly separated into two major groups called HDL_2 (d 1.063–1.125) and HDL_3 (d 1.125–1.21). Further, there occur at least two types of HDL_2 and three types of HDL_3. Major apoproteins found in HDL include apo AI, apo AII, apo AIV, apo C, apo D and apo E.

The HDL particles are synthesized in the liver and **are released into the blood stream,** by exocytosis. In the liver, HDL is degraded and releases cholesterol, which is either repacked in the lipoproteins or is converted to bile acids and secreted into bile, for its removal from the body (Fig. 3.24).

Elevated levels of HDL in plasma thus, protect the body against atherosclerosis.

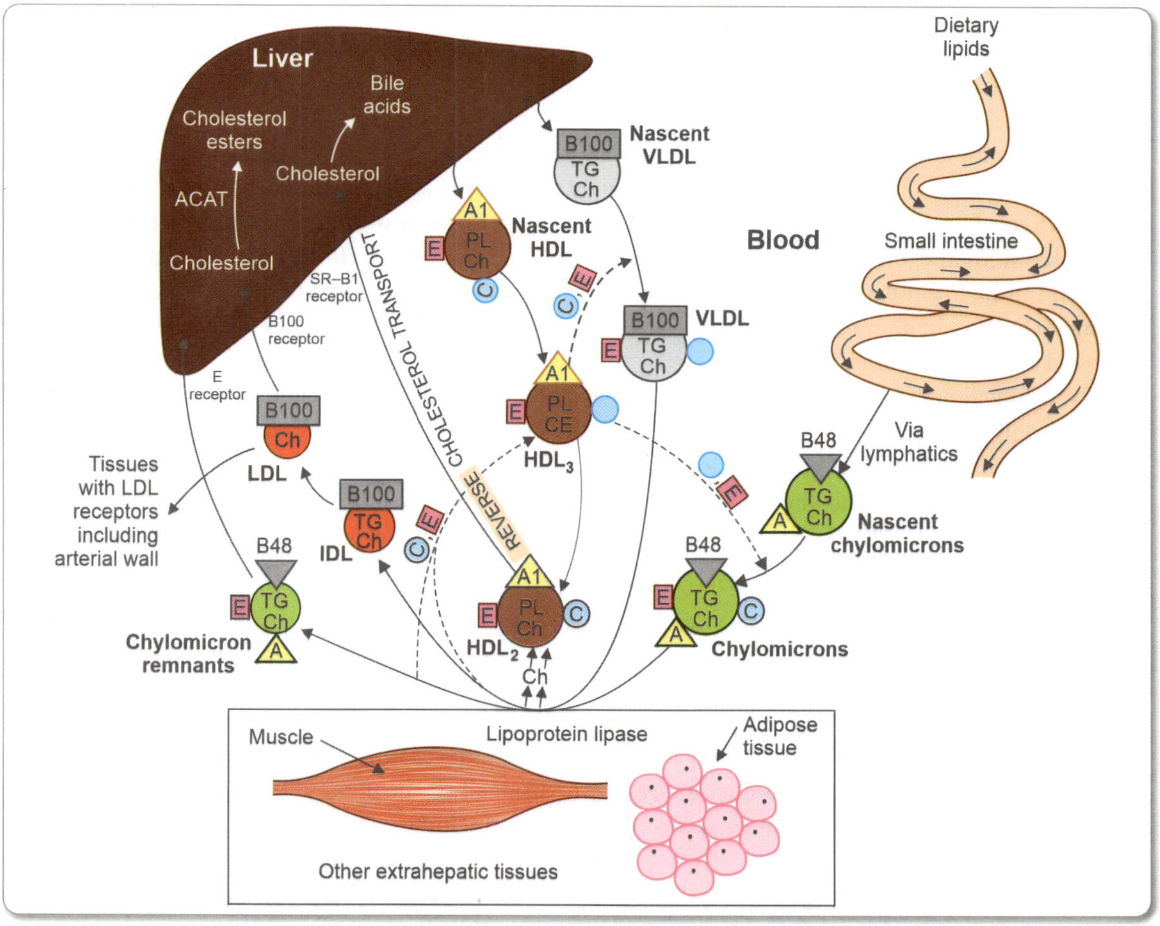

Fig. 3.24: Metabolism of lipoproteins

Abbreviations: ACAT, acylcholesterol acyltransferase; CE, cholesterol esters; Ch, cholesterol; PL, phospholipids; TG, triacylglycerols.

Functions of HDL

The HDL performs several functions:

- HDL **serves as a circulating reservoir of apo C-II**, which in turn is transferred to the chylomicrons and VLDL as an activator of lipoprotein lipase.

- It **removes free cholesterol from the extrahepatic tissues** and esterifies it with the help of lecithin: cholesterol acyltransferase (LCAT), which is present in plasma. HDL thus, transports cholesterol from the extrahepatic tissues to liver.
- HDL **transfers cholesteryl esters to VLDL** and LDL, in exchange of triacyglycerols and phospholipids from there.
- HDL also **carries cholesteryl esters to the liver**.

LIPID PROFILE

Lipid profile refers to the estimation of various fractions of lipids present in serum, which include, mainly, **total cholesterol, LDL-cholesterol, HDL-cholesterol** and **triglycerides in serum. Serum lipids** and lipoproteins **should be measured after a 10 hours fast** because chylomicrons normally are present in plasma up to 10 hours after a meal.

- Serum begins to appear hazy when the level of triglycerides reaches above 200 mg/dL. Chylomicrons can be readily detected because they form a white supernatant layer, after refrigeration. **For differentiation of disorders of lipoproteins, triglycerides and total cholesterol are routinely measured**. The measurement of plasma total cholesterol is a first line screening test. **Most of the cholesterol present in plasma is found in LDL.** Similarly, **plasma triglycerides concentration** is a measure of the **sum of total of VLDL and IDL.** To obtain a more accurate picture of lipid metabolism, we measure or calculate cholesterol present in the LDL or HDL fractions.
- The fasting lipid profile, i.e., the **concentration of total cholesterol, LDL-cholesterol, HDL-cholesterol and triglycerides,** provides information about the main **lipid markers of cardiovascular risk. LDL-cholesterol to HDL-cholesterol ratio** indicates the balance between cholesterol transport to and from peripheral tissues. A **ratio above 5 indicates increased cardiovascular risk**.
  - Dividing the value of triglycerides by 5, gives the concentration of VLDL-cholesterol in plasma.

$$\textbf{VLDL-cholesterol} \text{ (mg/dL)} = \text{Triglycerides}/5$$

  - LDL-cholesterol concentration in plasma can also be calculated from the value of total cholesterol, triglycerides and HDL-cholesterol, by the equation, called Friedewald equation, as follows:

$$\textbf{LDL-cholesterol} \text{ (mg/dL)} = \text{Total cholesterol} - [\text{HDL cholesterol} + \text{Triglycerides}/5]$$

- A large number of specialized investigations, including ultracentrifugation, apolipoprotein estimation and enzymes, and molecular genetic studies may occasionally be helpful.
- **Other biochemical** cardiovascular risk factors or **markers include troponins, myoglobin, homocysteine** and **C-reactive protein**.
  - In about 95% of the patients with **primary hypercholesterolemia, plasma cholesterol concentration is** usually **raised**, as the abnormality is due to a combination of dietary factors and a number of genetic abnormalities in handling cholesterol.
  - **In patients with familial hypertriglyceridemia, plasma triglycerides concentration in VLDL is increased** since this condition is associated with defects either in the production or in the catabolism of VLDL.
  - **In familial combined hyperlipidemia,** there may be increase **in plasma LDL only, plasma VLDL only, or both.**

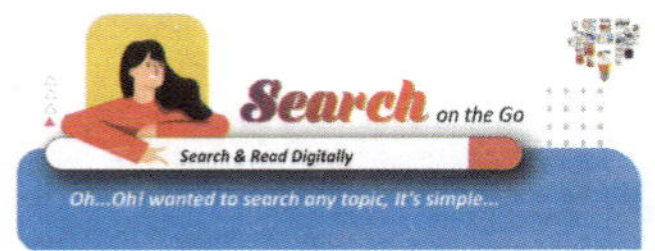

Clinical Correlation

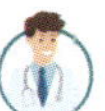

Atherosclerosis

*Atherosclerosis (***arteriosclerosis***) is a disease of arterial wall. It is characterized by the accumulation **of cholesterol** and its esters in cells, which are derived from monocyte-macrophage line smooth muscle cells. This in turn results in the formation of **atherosclerotic plaque, which narrows the blood vessels** and serves as the site of thrombus formation (Fig. 3.25).*

High calorie diet or diet rich in saturated fat and cholesterol, hypercholesterolemia, sedentary life style, stress and strain, obesity, hypertension and smoking are important contributory factors favorable in the development of atherosclerosis.

Risk of developing the disease is directly related to the concentration of the LDL-cholesterol, in plasma. *It is also inversely related to the plasma concentration of HDL-cholesterol. Therefore, **LDL-cholesterol** is called **bad cholesterol** while **HDL-cholesterol** is referred to as **good cholesterol**.*

*Drugs like **cholestyramine** bind bile salts and promote their excretion in stool. This in turn **increases the rate of bile salt synthesis** and LDL uptake by the liver. **Lovastatin**, the drug that is used in the treatment of **hyperlipidemia**, is an **inhibitor of the enzyme HMG CoA reductase**. Hence, it decreases endogenous synthesis of cholesterol and stimulates LDL uptake (via LDL receptors) by the tissues.*

Dietary recommendations

1. **Reduce the intake of fat**. *Not >30% of total energy intake should come from fat.*
2. **Limit intake of visible fat**. *Not >10% calories/day should come from visible fat.*
3. **Reduce the intake of cholesterol**. *Dietary cholesterol should be <300 mg/day.*
4. **Trans fatty acids intake should limit** *to <1% calories/day.*
5. **Increase ω-3 fatty acid intake** *from dietary or supplementary fish oils.*
6. **Eat five** *or* **more servings of fruits** *and vegetables/day.*
7. **Reduce salt intake**.

Other Life Style Interventions

In addition to dietary advice, other life style interventions include:

– **Promotion of physical activity**, *e.g., adults should perform at least 30 minutes of moderate activity (brisk walking), at least 5 days/week.*
– **Limit sedentary activities,** *and give up smoking.*

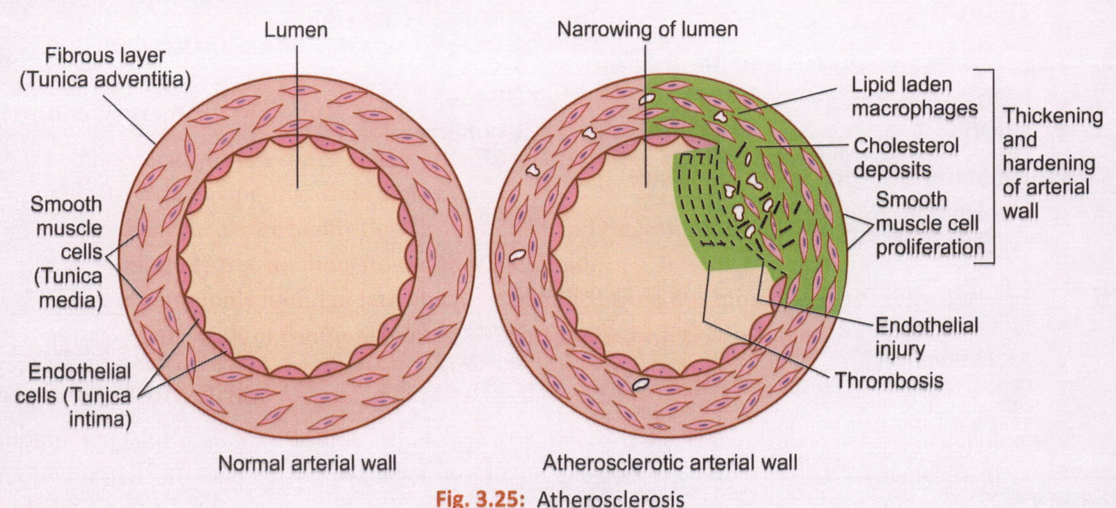

Fig. 3.25: Atherosclerosis

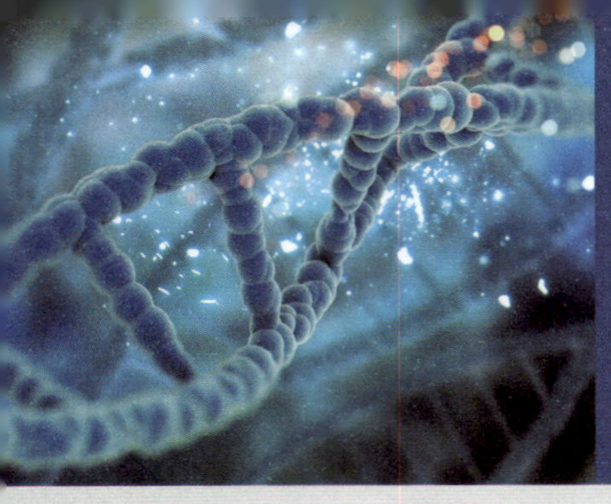

STUDENT ASSIGNMENT

LONG AND SHORT ANSWER QUESTIONS

1. What are fatty acids? Classify them. Write biological significance of polyunsaturated fatty acids.
2. Outline β-oxidation of fatty acids. How much energy is produced when a molecule of palmitic acid is oxidized to acetyl CoA?
3. Outline *De novo* synthesis of fatty acids. What is the source of reducing equivalents? How *De novo* fatty acid synthesis differs from fatty acid elongation in the mitochondria and the endoplasmic reticulum?
4. Outline cholesterol synthesis. Add a note on its relationship with atherosclerosis.
5. **Describe briefly:**
   a. Classification of fatty acids
   b. Compounds formed from cholesterol
6. **Write notes on:**
   a. Ketone bodies
   b. Atherosclerosis
   c. Sudden infant death syndrome
   d. Refsum disease
   e. Diabetic ketoacidosis
   f. PUFA
   g. MUFA
   h. Essential fatty acids
   i. Lipoproteins

MULTIPLE CHOICE QUESTIONS

1. **Linoleic acid is:**
   a. An ω-3 fatty acid
   b. An ω-6 fatty acid
   c. An ω-9 fatty acid
   d. A saturated fatty acid

2. **Triglycerides are released from the liver in:**
   a. HDL
   b. LDL
   c. VLDL
   d. Chylomicrons

3. **Which of the following is ω-6 fatty acid:**
   a. Linolenic acid
   b. Linoleic acid
   c. Lysergic acid
   d. Arachidonic acid

4. **Which of the following is referred to as eicosanoid:**
   a. Linolenic acid
   b. Linoleic acid
   c. Arachidonic acid
   d. Oleic acid

ANSWER KEY

1. b   **2.** c   **3.** b   **4.** c

4

Proteins

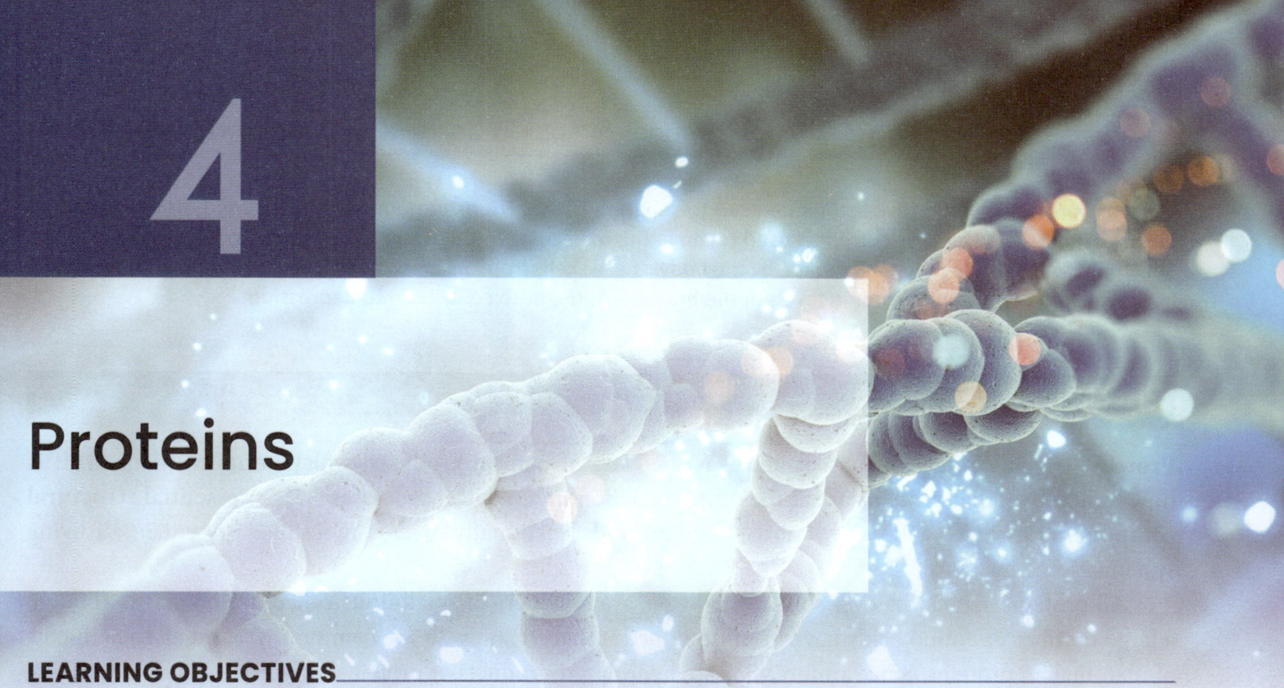

LEARNING OBJECTIVES

After the completion of the chapter, the readers will be able to:
- Explain the metabolism of proteins and amino acids and its alterations.
- Explain plasma proteins.
- Explain biologically important compounds synthesized from histidine.
- Explain metabolism of amino acids.
- Explain protein denaturation.

CHAPTER OUTLINE

KEY TERMS

Ampholytes: Compounds that when dissolved in water (which is itself an amphoteric compound) can act either as acid or as a base.

Catecholamines: A monoamine neurotransmitter, an organic compound that has a catechol and a side-chain amine; important in stress responses. High levels cause high blood pressure which can lead to headache, sweating, pounding of the heart, pain in the chest, and anxiety.

Denaturation: Process modifying the molecular structure of a protein; the proteins or nucleic acids lose folded structure present in their natural state.

Electrophoresis: A laboratory technique used to separate DNA, RNA or protein molecules based on their size and electrical charge. An electric current is used to move the molecules through a gel or other matrix.

Serotonin: A chemical messenger made by the body's nerve cells from an amino acid called tryptophan. It is involved in controlling mood. Low serotonin levels in the brain are thought to contribute to depression.

PROTEINS

Protein (Greek: *Proteios* means primary) is the class of natural products, which **contain nitrogen**. It is now well known that proteins are at the center of action in biological processes and are **essential structural components of a cell**. These are most abundant and functionally diverse molecules present in all living systems.

All proteins, from whatever source it may be, are polymers of small units called **amino acids**. Though, a large number of amino acids have been described in nature, only **20** are commonly found as constituents of mammalian proteins. Since amino acids are hydrolyzed products of proteins, they are also called building blocks of proteins.

AMINO ACIDS

Commonly occurring amino acids are designated as α-**amino acids** because both, the **primary amino group (–NH$_2$)** and a **distinctive side chain (R-group)**, are attached to the α-carbon atom, i.e., the carbon atom next to the **carboxyl group (–COOH)**.

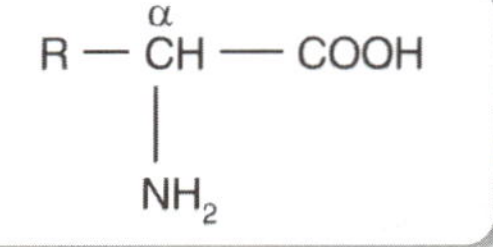

Fig. 4.1: General structure of an amino acid

General structure of an amino acid is shown in Figure 4.1.

Biological Significance of Amino Acids

- Amino acids are important **dietary source of nitrogen.**
- These are also used in protein biosynthesis.
- **Glucogenic amino acids**, e.g., alanine, serve **as a source of energy**.
- Some of the **amino acids are also used in the biosynthesis** of various **specialized products.**
  For example:
  - **Glycine** is a precursor of **creatine, glutathione, heme, bile acids** and **purines.**
  - **Sulfur-containing amino acids** are the **source of sulfur** for the body.
  - **Cysteine is also used in the biosynthesis of glutathione** while **methionine** is important in **one-carbon metabolism.**
  - **Aromatic amino acids** are the precursors **of thyroid hormones, catecholamines** (hormones of the adrenal medulla, i.e., dopamine, norepinephrine and epinephrine), and **melanin** (a brown-black pigment in skin).
  - **Aspartate** and **glutamate** participate in **transamination reactions.**
  - **Aspartate and glutamine** are used **in the biosynthesis of purines** and **pyrimidines.**

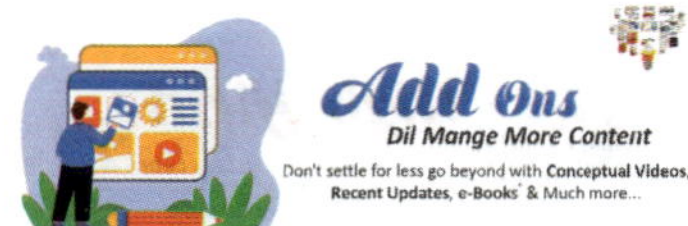

Classification of Amino Acids

Classification of Amino Acids Based on Nutritional Requirement

According to nutritional requirement, amino acids are divided into three groups, referred to as **essential amino acid, semi-essential amino acids** and **nonessential amino acids** (Table 4.1).

TABLE 4.1: Classification of amino acids according to nutritional requirement

Essential	Semi-essential	Nonessential
Methionine	Arginine	Glycine
Threonine	Histidine	Alanine
Tryptophan		Serine
Valine		Cysteine
Isoleucine		Tyrosine
Leucine		Aspartate
Phenylalanine		Glutamate
Lysine		Asparagine
		Glutamine
		Proline

Essential Amino Acids

As all amino acids cannot be synthesized in the body and are to be essentially included in the diet, hence those amino acids which are to be essentially included in the diet are called indispensable or **essential amino acids**.

There are eight amino acids which are essential for adult human beings. These are **methionine, threonine, tryptophan, valine, isoleucine, leucine, phenylalanine** and **lysine**.

Semi-Essential Amino Acids

Arginine and **histidine** are not essential for a normal adult human being. However, under certain conditions, e.g., growth, pregnancy and lactation (when their requirement is increased) or under conditions such as a high grade fever and chronic infections (when their catabolism is increased), arginine and histidine also become dietary essential. Hence, these two amino acids are called **semi-essential amino acids**.

Nonessential Amino Acids

Remaining all the amino acids, since can be synthesized by a normal human being and **are not dietary essential,** are called **nonessential amino acids**.

Classification of Amino Acids Based on Metabolic Fate

Carbon skeletons of amino acids, after the removal of α-amino group as ammonia, **form amphibolic intermediates, which** can be **converted to** either **glucose or ketone bodies**. Accordingly, based on their metabolic fates, amino acids are classified into three groups, as follows:

1. **Glucogenic amino acids:** These amino acids **serve as precursors of glucose**. For example, transamination of alanine, glutamate and valine forms pyruvate, α-ketoglutarate and succinyl CoA, respectively. As these

are **the intermediates of the citric acid cycle** and can be converted to glucose by gluconeogenesis, these amino acids are called glucogenic amino acids. These include **glycine, alanine, serine, aspartic acid, asparagine, glutamic acid, glutamine, proline, valine, methionine, cysteine, histidine** and **arginine**.

2. **Ketogenic amino acids:** These **amino acids** breakdown to **form ketone bodies**. These include **leucine** and **lysine**. The end products of the catabolism of leucine are acetyl CoA and acetoacetyl CoA, whereas the end product of the catabolism of lysine is acetoacetyl CoA.

3. **Both glucogenic and ketogenic amino acids:** These **amino acids** breakdown to **form** precursors for **both ketone bodies and glucose**. For example, **catabolism** of phenylalanine, **in addition to an intermediate of the citric acid cycle (i.e., formate)** also **forms acetoacetyl CoA**, which is the precursor of the ketone bodies. Therefore, **these amino acids are** referred to as **both, glucogenic and ketogenic**. These include **isoleucine, phenylalanine, tryptophan** and **tyrosine**.

Classification of amino acids based on metabolic fate is shown in Table 4.2.

TABLE 4.2: Classification of amino acids based on metabolic fate

Metabolic fate of amino acids	End products of their catabolism
Glucogenic	
Gly, Ala, Ser, Cys, HO-Pro	Pyruvate
Glu, Gln, Pro, Arg, His	α-Ketoglutarate
Val, Met	Succinyl CoA
Asp, Asn	Oxaloacetate
Glucogenic and Ketogenic	
Ile	Succinyl CoA and Acetyl CoA
Phe and Tyr	Fumarate and Acetoacetyl CoA
Trp	Pyruvate and Acetoacetyl CoA
Thr	Pyruvate and Acetyl CoA
Ketogenic	
Leu	Acetyl CoA and Acetoacetyl CoA
Lys	Acetoacetyl CoA

Properties of Amino Acids

Isomerism

All the naturally occurring **amino acids** except glycine, **have at least one asymmetric carbon atom and are optically active. These amino acids have L-configuration.**

Acid Base Properties

Amino acids exhibit acid base properties. An amino acid may have either a positive charge or a negative charge. **At low pH, an amino acid exists in the cationic form** as its amino group is protonated and is present as $-NH_3^+$. As the pH rises, carboxyl group loses its proton and the ampholyte form appears. With further increase in pH, the amino group is deprotonated and the anionic form is formed. At physiological pH

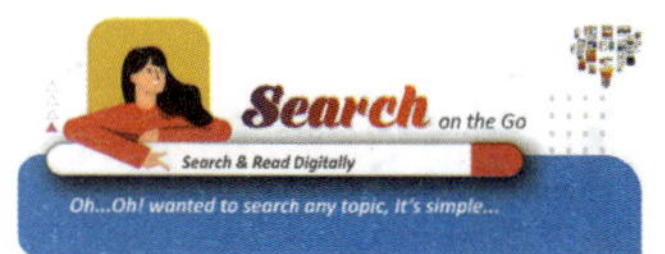

(pH 7.4), carboxyl group of the amino acids are dissociated (R–COO⁻) while their amino groups are protonated ($R–NH_3^+$).

Such ionized molecules, which have both negative as well as positive charges, are called **ampholytes**. **Molecules with equal number of ionizable groups**, i.e., when the number of cations is equal to the number of anions, **are called zwitterions**.

The pH at which a molecule exists as a zwitterion is called **isoelectric pH** or **isoelectric point (pI)**.

At pH more than its pI, an amino acid is negatively charged while at pH less than its pI, it is positively charged (Fig. 4.2).

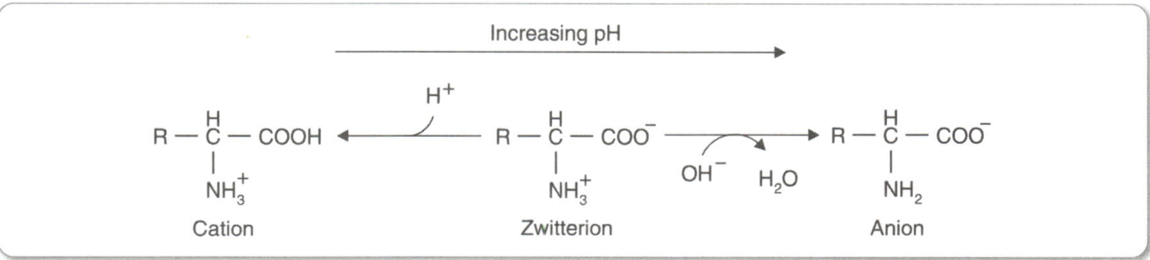

Fig. 4.2: Various ionic forms of an amino acid

Buffer Action

Amino acids in an aqueous solution contain weakly acidic α-carboxyl group and weakly basic α-amino group. In addition, acidic and basic amino acids also contain an ionizable group in its side chain. Hence, ***amino acids also act as buffers.***

FORMATION OF PEPTIDE BOND

Most important property of amino acids is the formation of a **peptide bond (–CO–NH–)**. During this process, the carboxyl group of an amino acid reacts with the amino group of the other amino acid. This is a condensation reaction and results in the formation of an **amide linkage**, called a peptide bond (Fig. 4.3).

Fig. 4.3: Formation of peptide bond

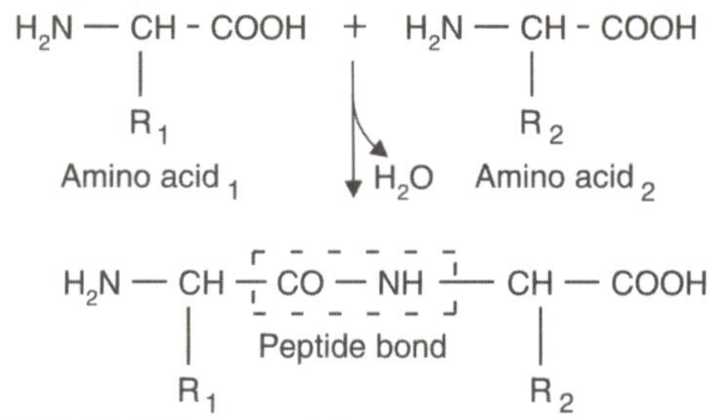

When several amino acids are linked together, they form **polypeptides and proteins**. Each polypeptide has a **free α-amino group** on the **left hand** side of the peptide chain. This end of the protein chain is referred to as **N-terminal (amino terminal) end**. The protein chain also has a free **α-carboxylic group** on the **right hand** side of the peptide chain. This end of the protein chain is referred to as **C-terminal (carboxyl terminal) end** (Fig. 4.4).

$$H_2NAA_1 - AA_2 - AA_3 \text{ -------------------- } AA_{n-1} - AA_nCOOH$$

N-Terminal end ... C-Terminal end

Fig. 4.4: A polypeptide

BIOLOGICAL SIGNIFICANCE OF PROTEINS

With respect to their biological importance, proteins are divided into several groups, as shown in Table 4.3.

- **Structural proteins:** Some of the proteins, e.g., **collagens** (found in bone and cartilage), **keratins** (found in hair and nail), etc., form an essential part of particular structures with in the body.
- **Enzymes:** Some of the proteins such as **pepsin**, catalyze biological reactions and act as enzymes.
- **Hormones:** Some of the proteins act as hormones, e.g., **insulin**, and regulate metabolic processes within the body.
- **Transporters:** Some of the proteins, e.g., **hemoglobin**, **ceruloplasmin**, etc., serve as carriers for the transport of certain substances with in the body and are called transport proteins.
- **Receptors:** Proteins such as **hormone receptors**, act as receptors for certain hormones and play an important role in signal transduction.
- **Storage proteins:** Some of the proteins bind to a substance for its storage in different tissues in the body, e.g., **ferritin** for the storage of Fe^{3+}.
- **Antibodies:** Proteins such as γ-**globulin**, act as antibodies and provide immunity.

TABLE 4.3: Biological importance of proteins

Biological role of protein	Examples
As structural proteins	Collagen, keratins, etc.
As enzymes	Pepsin, amylase, etc.
As hormones	Insulin
As transporters	Hemoglobin
As receptors	Hormone receptors
As storage molecules	Ferritin
In immune response	γ-Globulin

CLASSIFICATION OF PROTEINS

Depending upon their **solubility** and **physical properties**, proteins are classified into three classes (Table 4.4).

TABLE 4.4: Classification of proteins based on their solubility

Simple proteins	Conjugated proteins	Derived proteins
Albumins	Nucleoproteins	Primary derived proteins
Globulins	Glycoproteins	Secondary derived proteins
Prolamines	Phosphoproteins	
Glutelins	Metalloproteins	
Scleroproteins	Lipoproteins	
Histones		

Simple Proteins

Simple proteins are further subdivided into several groups, as follows:

- **Albumins:** These are found in serum, milk, egg, etc. These are soluble in water as well as salt solutions.
- **Globulins:** These are found in serum, milk and egg along with albumin. These are sparingly soluble in water but soluble in a neutral salt solution.
- **Prolamines:** These proteins, e.g., gliadin of wheat or zein of maize, are insoluble in water but soluble in 60–80% of alcohol.

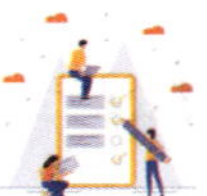
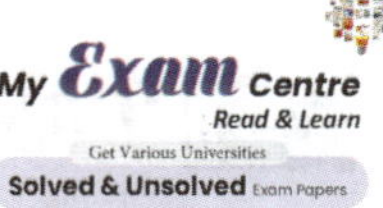

- **Glutelins:** These proteins, e.g., gluten of wheat or oryzenin of rice, are soluble in dilute acids and alkalies.
- **Scleroproteins:** These proteins are highly insoluble. These are present in supporting tissues such as bones, cartilages, etc. These are also found in protective tissues like skin, hair, nail, etc.
- **Histones:** These proteins, e.g., nucleohistones are rich in basic amino acids. These are soluble in water.

Conjugated Proteins

Proteins are conjugated **with** a **nonprotein substance**, called prosthetic group. Such proteins are referred to as conjugated proteins. For example, **nucleoproteins** (histones conjugated with nucleic acids), **glycoproteins** (proteins conjugated with carbohydrates), **phosphoproteins** (phosphoric acid attached through serine or threonine in the protein, such as casein in milk), **metalloproteins** (metal-containing proteins such as ceruloplasmin, a copper containing protein) and **lipoproteins** (lipid-associated proteins).

Derived Proteins

These are the derivatives of simple proteins such as denatured and coagulated proteins (**primary derived proteins**) or those produced by cleavage of the peptide bonds (**secondary derived proteins**).

STRUCTURAL ORGANIZATION OF PROTEINS

Variations in the number and order of amino acids, i.e., the manner in which various amino acids are arranged in a polypeptide chain, reflect structure of a protein. There are four levels of protein structure, referred to as primary, secondary, tertiary and quaternary levels of protein structure.

Primary Structure of Proteins

Primary structure of a protein refers to the **order and sequence of amino acids in a protein chain** (Fig. 4.5).

Some proteins such as insulin, are synthesized as a single polypeptide and are later cleaved into two or more chains. These proteins have intra-chain as well as interchain disulfide linkages.

$$H_2N - CH - CO - NH - CH - CO - NH - CH - CO \cdots \cdots NH - CH - COOH$$
$$\qquad\quad |\qquad\qquad\qquad |\qquad\qquad\qquad |\qquad\qquad\qquad\qquad\quad |$$
$$\qquad\quad R_1\qquad\qquad\qquad R_2\qquad\qquad\qquad R_3\qquad\qquad\qquad\qquad\quad R_n$$

Fig. 4.5: Primary structure of a protein

Secondary Structure of Proteins

Secondary structure of a protein **refers to folding and twisting patterns of a polypeptide chain,** i.e., the spatial arrangement of a polypeptide. Secondary structures include α-helix and β-sheet structures.

α-Helix

This refers to the twisting pattern of the backbone of a polypeptide which in turn forms coil or helix. As a result of its folding, hydrogen bonds may also be formed between the –CO and the –NH groups, with in the polypeptide chain. These types of linkages are called intra-chain peptide linkages.

The helix may be α-helix or β-helix.

α-Helix refers to **right handed folding** of the protein chain. It is the most stable conformation of the polypeptide chain, e.g., α-keratin. There are 3.6 amino acid residues per turn of the helix (Fig. 4.6).

Left-handed helix generally does not occur in proteins.

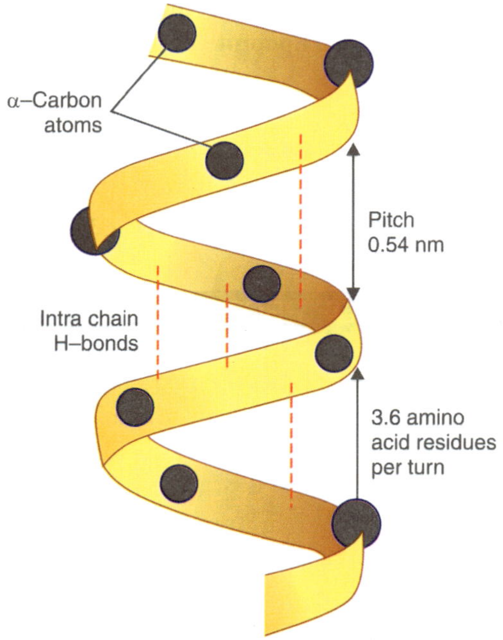

Fig. 4.6: Secondary structure of protein: α-helix (right-handed helix)

β-Pleated Sheet

The second regular conformation found in proteins is referred to as β-**sheet structure.** β-Denotes the second regular structure that was described after α-helix. The conformation, in which β-structure is optimally hydrogen bonded, has rippled or pleated-edge appearance. Therefore, this conformation is also called **pleated sheet-like** structure.

Such proteins, e.g., wool, may contain 2–12 polypeptides in β conformation. Each strand may contain up to 15 residues. β-Sheet orientation is formed due to **stretching of the polypeptide chain**, as a result of the formation of hydrogen bonds between –CO and –NH groups of the neighboring polypeptides. These types of linkages are called **intra chain peptide linkages** (Fig. 4.7).

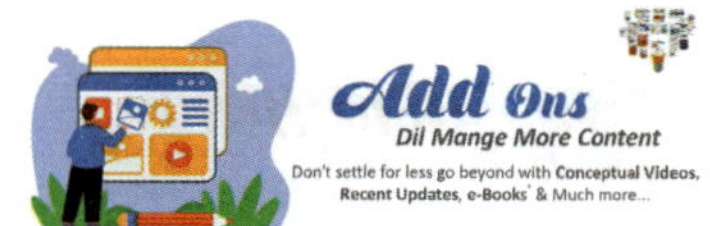

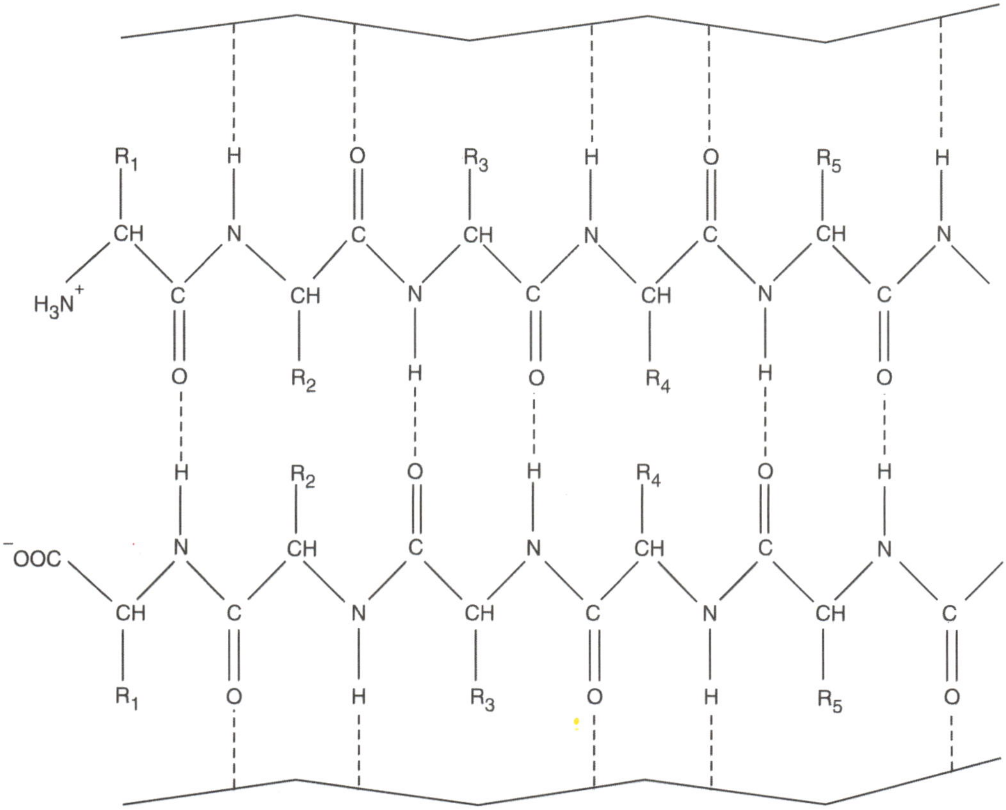

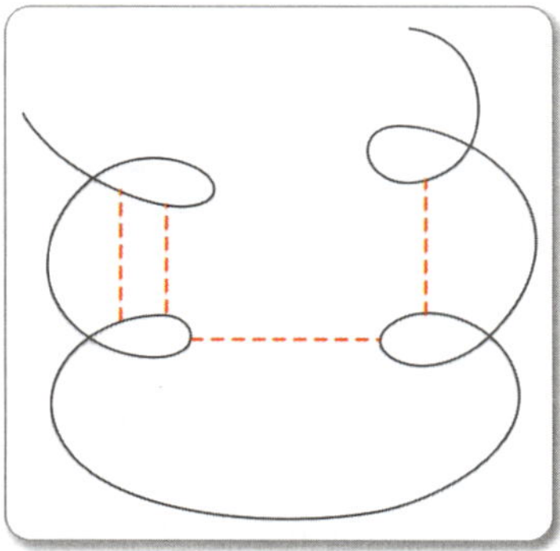

Fig. 4.7: Secondary structure of protein: β-pleated sheet

In these types of proteins, polypeptide chains may run either in antiparallel or parallel directions.

- **Antiparallel β-sheet:** It is formed when two polypeptide chains run in the **opposite directions**.
- **Parallel β-sheet:** It is formed when two chains run in the **same direction**.

Various **forces** which stabilize secondary structure of a protein, include **hydrogen bonds**, **hydrophobic interactions**, **electrostatic interactions** and **van der Waals forces**.

Tertiary Structure of Proteins

Tertiary structure involves **intramolecular folding** of the polypeptide chain thereby forming a compact three dimensional structure which has a specific shape.

Electrovalent linkages, hydrogen bonds, disulfide bridges, van der Waals forces and hydrophobic interactions maintain tertiary structure of proteins (Fig. 4.8).

Depending on their overall morphology, a protein may aquire either globular or fibrous structure.

Fig. 4.8: Tertiary level of protein structure

Globular Proteins

Globular proteins have a spheroidal shape and vary in size. They have relatively high water solubility and function as catalysts, transporters and regulators of metabolic pathways and gene expression. Their shapes are the result of complex interactions between secondary, tertiary and sometimes quaternary structural elements. Both types of the secondary structural elements, i.e., the α-helices and the β-sheets, occur in globular proteins in varying proportions and combinations. Certain groupings of the secondary structural elements, called **super-secondary structures** or **motifs**, also occur in many unrelated globular proteins. Some proteins such as cytochromes, consist of only α-helices spanned by short connecting links. Others, such as immunoglobulin folds, have a large proportion of β-sheets and are devoid of the α-helices. Most of the proteins, such as lactate dehydrogenase, however, have significant amounts of both types of the secondary structures. Most common globular proteins are hemoproteins, such as hemoglobin, myoglobin, cytochromes and catalase.

Fibrous Proteins

Fibrous proteins exhibit special mechanical properties. They characteristically, contain large amounts of the regular secondary structures and have long cylindrical (rod-like) shapes. They have low solubility in water. Fibrous proteins have a protective, connective or supportive role in living organisms, e.g., collagen, keratin and tropomyosin, etc. These are found as components of the skin, connective tissue, blood vessel walls, and sclera and cornea of the eye.

Quaternary Structure of Proteins

Multisubunit proteins contain several identical and/or different chains, where each one of the peptide chains is referred to as a **subunit**. These polypeptide subunits are associated with a specific geometry. Spatial arrangement of these subunits is referred to as the quaternary structure of proteins (Fig. 4.9).

Proteins with **more than one subunit** are called **oligomeric** proteins. For example **hemoglobin**, is an oligomeric protein with **four subunits** called $\alpha_2\beta_2$.

Disintegration of the monomeric subunits of a multimeric protein results **in the loss of its biological activity**.

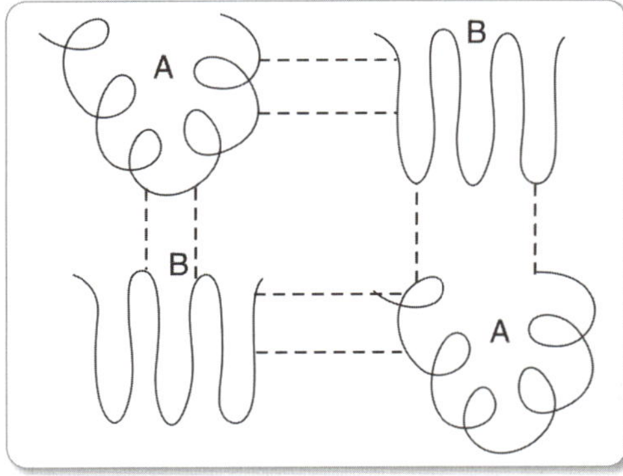

Fig. 4.9: Quaternary level of protein structure

PROTEIN DENATURATION

Usually, proteins are soluble in water due to their organized structures. On **heating** or adding a **strong acid**, protein loses its native structure and gets precipitated. This is referred to as **denaturation**. Usually, on denaturation, protein **loses** its **biological activity** since denaturation results in unfolding and disorganization of its secondary and tertiary structures.

Denaturing agents include **heat, mechanical force, detergents, strong acids** or **bases** and the **ions of heavy metals** such as lead and mercury. Under ideal conditions, denaturation may be reversible, however, most proteins, once denatured remain permanently disordered. Denatured proteins are often insoluble and therefore, precipitate from the solution.

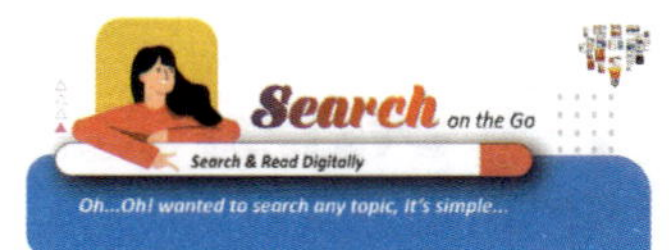

PRECIPITATION OF PROTEINS

Proteins are charged, high molecular weight, colloidal particles and can be precipitated from the solution by a number of compounds.

- **Salting out:** Proteins can be precipitated by the addition of a salt solution. This process is known as salting out. Highly soluble salts like $NaCl$ and $(NH_4)_2SO_4$ are generally, used for this purpose. Albumin is more soluble in water than globulins hence, **globulins get precipitated at half the saturation by ammonium sulphate while albumin precipitates only at full saturation.**

   Precipitation of protein by a salt solution is, apparently, due to neutralization of the charges as well as dehydration of the molecule. Protein, which has been precipitated by a salt solution, remains native and usually redissolve, when placed back in the solvent.

- **Precipitation by other reagents:** Since proteins are not soluble in organic solvents, they can also be precipitated with the addition of some nonaqueous solvents like alcohol, acetone, etc. Proteins get precipitated due to dehydration of the molecule.

- **By heavy metals:** Most commonly used metals as protein precipitants include metal salts such as lead acetate, mercuric chloride, barium chloride, zinc sulfate, etc. Proteins get precipitated due to adsorption of the metallic cations by the negatively charged colloidal particles of the protein.

- **By alkaloid reagents:** Proteins can also be precipitated by the addition of some alkaloid reagent. Precipitation by an alkaloid reagent is due to the formation of an insoluble salt between the anions of the reagent and the positively charged protein particles.

- **By heating:** By heating protein gets coagulated. This is referred to as **heat coagulation**. Coagulation is the maximum at isoelectric pH.

DIGESTION AND ABSORPTION OF PROTEINS

Proteins are degraded to amino acids, which contribute to the **amino acid pool**. Amino acids are used for protein biosynthesis. Excess of the amino acids are also used for energy. Amino acids are also important source of nitrogen for the body.

Digestion of Proteins

Digestion of proteins begins in the gastrointestinal tract and is carried out by proteases secreted by the stomach, the pancreas and the small intestine:

- Digestion of proteins starts in the stomach by the action of proteolytic enzyme **pepsin**, at pH of the gastric juice (1.5–2.5). Pepsin is secreted by the cells of the gastric mucosa in the form of a zymogen (proenzyme), called **pepsinogen**, which is activated by hydrogen ions of the gastric juice (HCl) and later autocatalytically by pepsin itself.

- Proteolytic products of pepsin pass into the small intestine where these are attacked by proteases which are secreted by the pancreas, i.e., trypsin, chymotrypsin and carboxypeptidases.

- **Trypsin** is secreted in the zymogen form as **trypsinogen**, which is converted to trypsin by another enzyme called enterokinase (enteropeptidase) that acts as an activator of trypsinogen and is secreted by the intestinal mucosa. Once trypsin is formed, it acts on trypsinogen and converts it to trypsin, autocatalytically.

- **Chymotrypsin** is also synthesized and secreted as a zymogen, designated as **chymotrypsinogen**. It is activated by trypsin.
- Pancreatic juice also contains **collagenase** and **elastase**, which specifically act on collagen and elastin, respectively.
- In addition to the above endopeptidases, some exopeptidases are also secreted by the pancreatic juice, in the zymogen forms. These include **procarboxypeptidase A** and **procarboxypeptidase B**. These are also activated by trypsin. These two enzymes attack peptide linkages, specifically those having a free carboxyl group. **Carboxypeptidase A** hydrolyzes the C-terminal amino acid in peptides, particularly of those where the terminal amino acid is an aromatic or aliphatic amino acid, while **carboxypeptidase B** hydrolyzes the terminal peptide bond between the basic amino acids (arginine and lysine).
- The digestion of proteins thereafter, is completed by the action of **aminopeptidases** and **dipeptidases** which are secreted by mucosa of the small intestine.

Any part of the protein that is not hydrolyzed in the small intestine enters the large intestine and excreted in the feces.

Absorption of Amino Acids

The end products of the digestion of proteins, i.e., amino acids, are absorbed from the small intestine into the portal blood. Absorption of L-amino acids is a Na^+-dependent active transport and requires ATP and specific transport proteins. Pyridoxal phosphate (vitamin B_6) is also required for the absorption of amino acids.

There are several transport systems for the uptake of different amino acids. These include:

- A transport system for **neutral amino acids with short or polar side chains** such as Ala, Ser and Thr
- For **neutral amino acids with an aromatic or hydrophobic side chain** such as Phe, Tyr, Met, Val, Leu, Ile
- For **imino acids**, i.e., Pro and hydroxyproline (HO-Pro)
- For **basic amino acids** such as, Arg and Cystine (Cys-Cys)
- For **acidic amino acids**, i.e., Asp and Glu
- For **β-amino acids**, e.g., β-Ala and taurine; and
- For **dipeptides**, e.g., peptide-1 (pep-1), glycyl-sarcosine, etc. These dipeptides are absorbed through the intestinal cells where they are hydrolyzed by dipeptidases to the constituent amino acids.

Besides, the small intestine of the fetus and the neonate can absorb intact proteins by endocytosis (pinocytosis).

Absorption of amino acids may be affected in specific transport disorders or other diseases involving the small intestine or the immune system, such as Hartnup's disease and cystinuria.

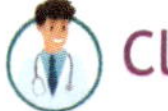 Clinical Correlation

Amino Acids Transport Disorders

Hartnup's disease: It is a genetic lesion in epithelial amino acid transport, named after the family in which the disease was first recognized. Transport and absorption of neutral amino acids including that of tryptophan, is decreased in the epithelial cells of the small intestine and proximal tubules of the kidney. The intestinal defect results in malabsorption of free amino acids from the diet. The inability to reabsorb amino acids by the kidney manifests in the excretion of neutral amino acids including tryptophan and other indole derivatives in the urine, resulting in **neutral aminoaciduria**. Symptoms of the disease are mainly those due to tryptophan amino acid and nicotinamide deficiencies. Due to tryptophan deficiency there are **pellagra like features**, such as dermatitis, diarrhea and dementia. Women are more susceptible to pellagra since kynurenine hydroxylase (an enzyme of the tryptophan niacin pathway) is inhibited by estrogen.

Cystinuria: It involves the carrier for sulfur-containing amino acid, cystine and the basic amino acids, i.e., lysine and arginine.

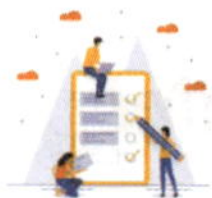
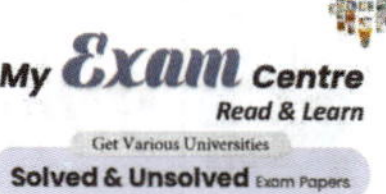

METABOLISM OF AMINO ACIDS

There are two processes by which the α-**amino group can be removed** from amino acids. These are referred to as **transamination** and **deamination.**

Transamination

Transamination is a process of **transfer of the α-amino group** from an **amino acid to a keto acid.** As a result of it, the **amino acid is converted to a keto acid** while the **keto acid is converted to an amino acid** (Fig. 4.10).

Enzymes, which catalyze transamination, are called **transaminases (aminotransferases)**. Although, liver contains transaminases for all the amino acids (except for threonine and lysine), most important of these transaminases are glutamate pyruvate transaminase (GPT, also called alanine **aminotransferase** or ALT) and glutamate oxaloacetate transaminase (GOT, also called **aspartate aminotransferase** or AST).

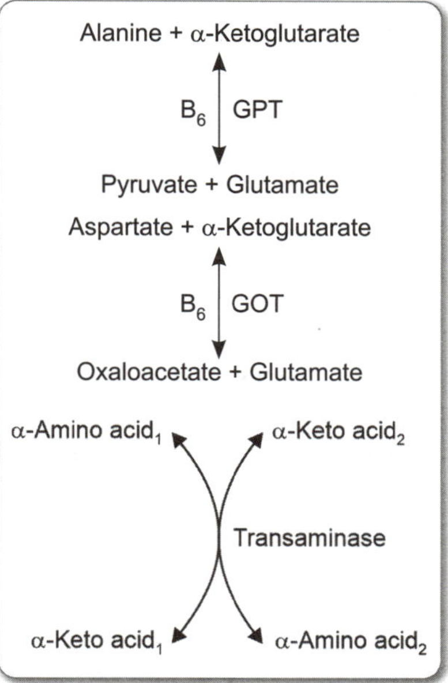

Fig. 4.10: Transamination reactions

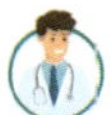

Clinical Correlation

Diagnostic Significance of Transaminases

*Serum GOT and GPT have diagnostic significance. These are present in large amounts in cardiac muscle and liver, respectively. Although serum levels of both the enzymes are raised in heart as well as liver diseases, **SGOT is markedly raised in myocardial infarction** while **SGPT is more increased in liver disorders** such as viral hepatitis or toxic liver necrosis (Table 4.5).*

TABLE 4.5: Diagnostic significance of transaminases

Enzyme	Comparatively more raised in
SGOT	Cardiac disorders, e.g., myocardial infarction
SGPT	Liver disorders, e.g., viral hepatitis

An obligate amino acid or the α-keto acid, which participates in these reactions, is glutamate or α-ketoglutarate.

During the process of transamination, the amino acid first reacts with the coenzyme pyridoxal-5-phosphate (PLP) and forms **Schiff's base**. Coenzyme in turn becomes protonated and is subsequently hydrolyzed to release the α-keto acid of the corresponding amino acid while retaining the α-amino group ($-NH_2$). Pyridoxal-5-phosphate thus, gets aminated and is converted to pyridoxamine-5-phosphate. Thereafter, α-keto acid combines with the coenzyme bound amino group (pyridoxamine-5-phosphate) which in turn releases the keto acid as a new amino acid and regenerates the coenzyme (Fig. 4.11).

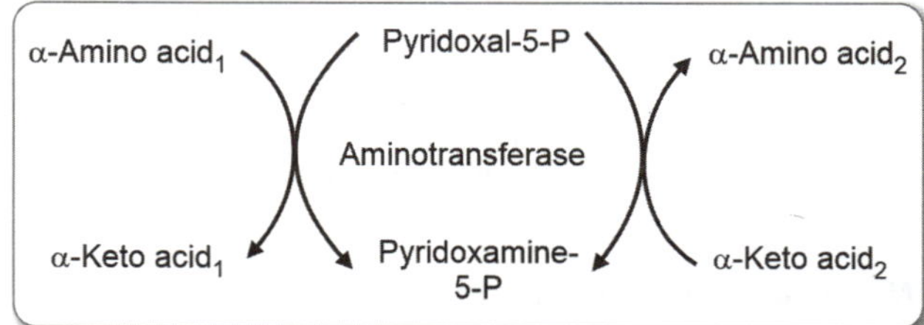

Fig. 4.11: Role of vitamin B6 in transamination

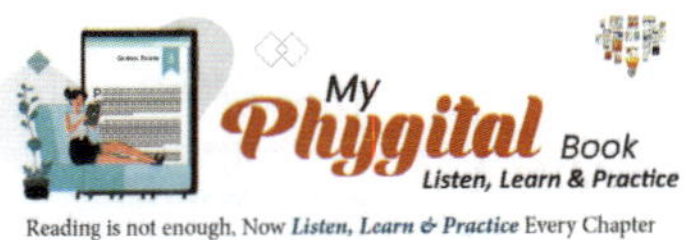

Deamination

Process of **removal of the α-amino group from amino acids** is referred to as deamination. Liver and kidney are the main organs, which are responsible for the deamination of amino acids. Deamination may take place either by oxidative or nonoxidative process.

Oxidative Deamination

As the name suggests, oxidative deamination refers to the process of the removal of ammonia from an amino acid in the presence of oxygen, through the transfer of reducing equivalents. This reaction is catalyzed by a group of enzymes referred to as amino acid oxidases.

Liver and kidney contain several **enzymes, which catalyze deamination** of amino acids, such as amino acid oxidases, glutamate dehydrogenase, etc.

- **Amino acid oxidases:** L-amino acid oxidase is linked to FMN (the prosthetic group) and catalyzes the oxidation of an L-amino acid producing α-keto acid, ammonia and water, as the final products (Fig. 4.12).

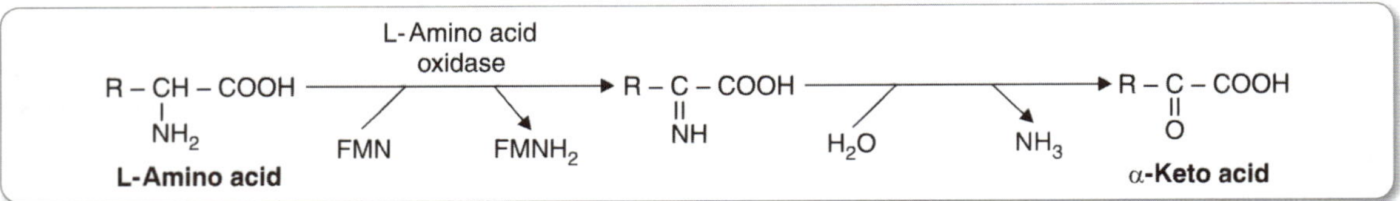

Fig. 4.12: Oxidative deamination

Some of the tissues also contain **FAD-linked D-amino acid oxidases**, which **catalyze oxidation of glycine and the D-amino acids.**

- **Glutamate dehydrogenase:** Glutamate **is produced from α-ketoglutarate** by the enzyme glutamate dehydrogenase (GDH). This enzyme is also important for the release of ammonia from glutamate, when glutamate is degraded and used for gluconeogenesis.

  Glutamate dehydrogenase thus, catalyzes reversible set of reactions. NADPH is used as coenzyme in the synthetic reaction while NAD^+ is used in the degradative reaction (Fig. 4.13).

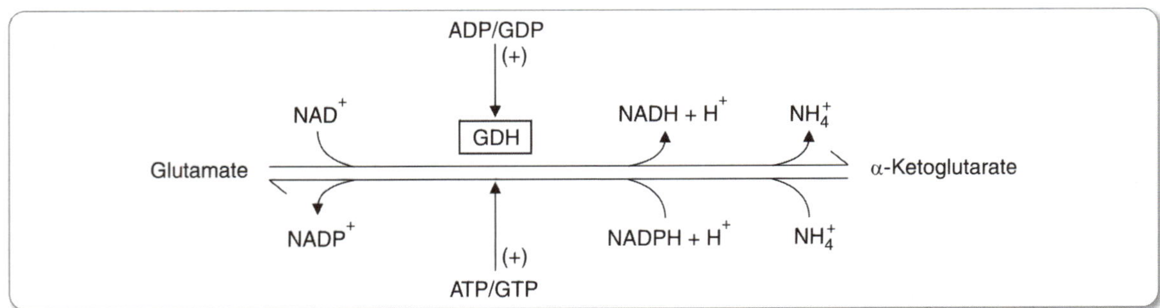

Fig. 4.13: Reactions catalyzed by glutamate dehydrogenase

Nonoxidative Deamination

In this process, ammonia is removed from some of the amino acids, such as serine, cysteine and histidine, in the absence of oxygen, without the use of reducing equivalents.

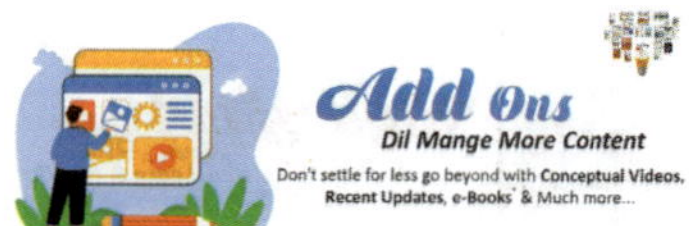

Dehydratase, desulfhydrase and histidase catalyze deamination of serine, cysteine and histidine, respectively. They catalyze dehydration followed by nonoxidative deamination of the amino acid, spontaneously (Fig. 4.14).

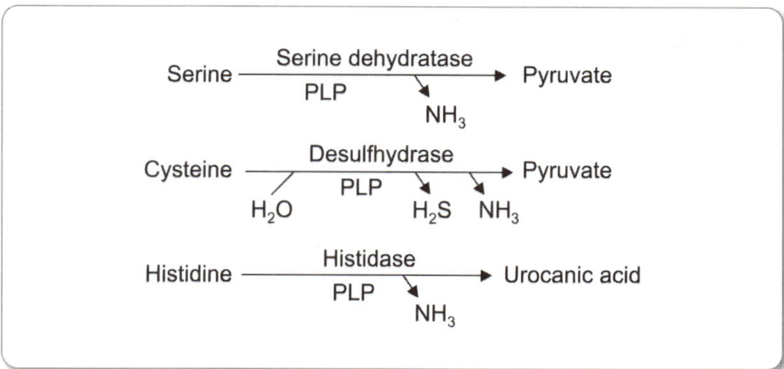

Fig. 4.14: Nonoxidative deamination reactions

METABOLIC FATES OF AMMONIA

Ammonia which is produced as a result of deamination of amino acids is removed as glutamine from the brain. It is also removed as urea, by urea cycle, from the liver.

Transport of Ammonia as Glutamine

From the brain, ammonia is removed as glutamine, which is synthesized by the enzyme **glutamine synthetase**. Glutamine is transported to the kidney, where **glutaminase** removes the amide group from glutamine as ammonia, which is excreted in the urine (Fig. 4.15).

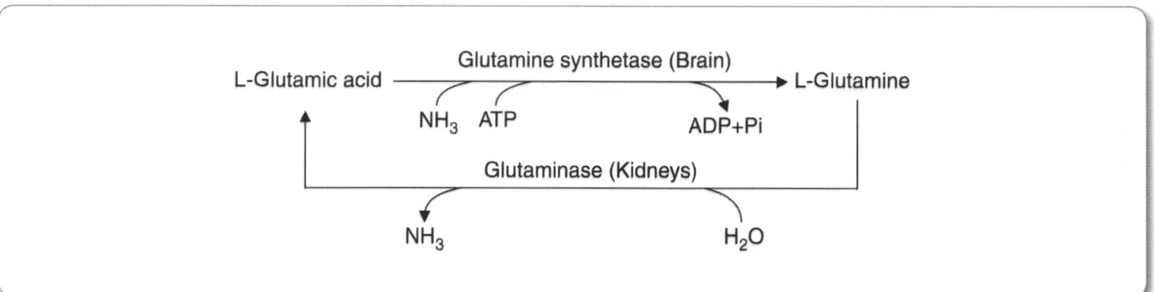

Fig. 4.15: Synthesis and degradation of glutamine

Transport of Ammonia as Urea

Urea cycle is the process by which ammonia that is a highly toxic substance, is converted to urea, which is a less toxic, water soluble, excretory waste product, in the liver (Fig. 4.16).

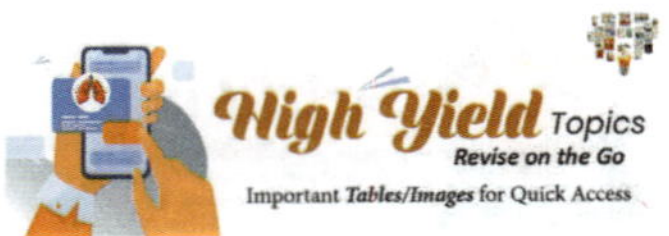

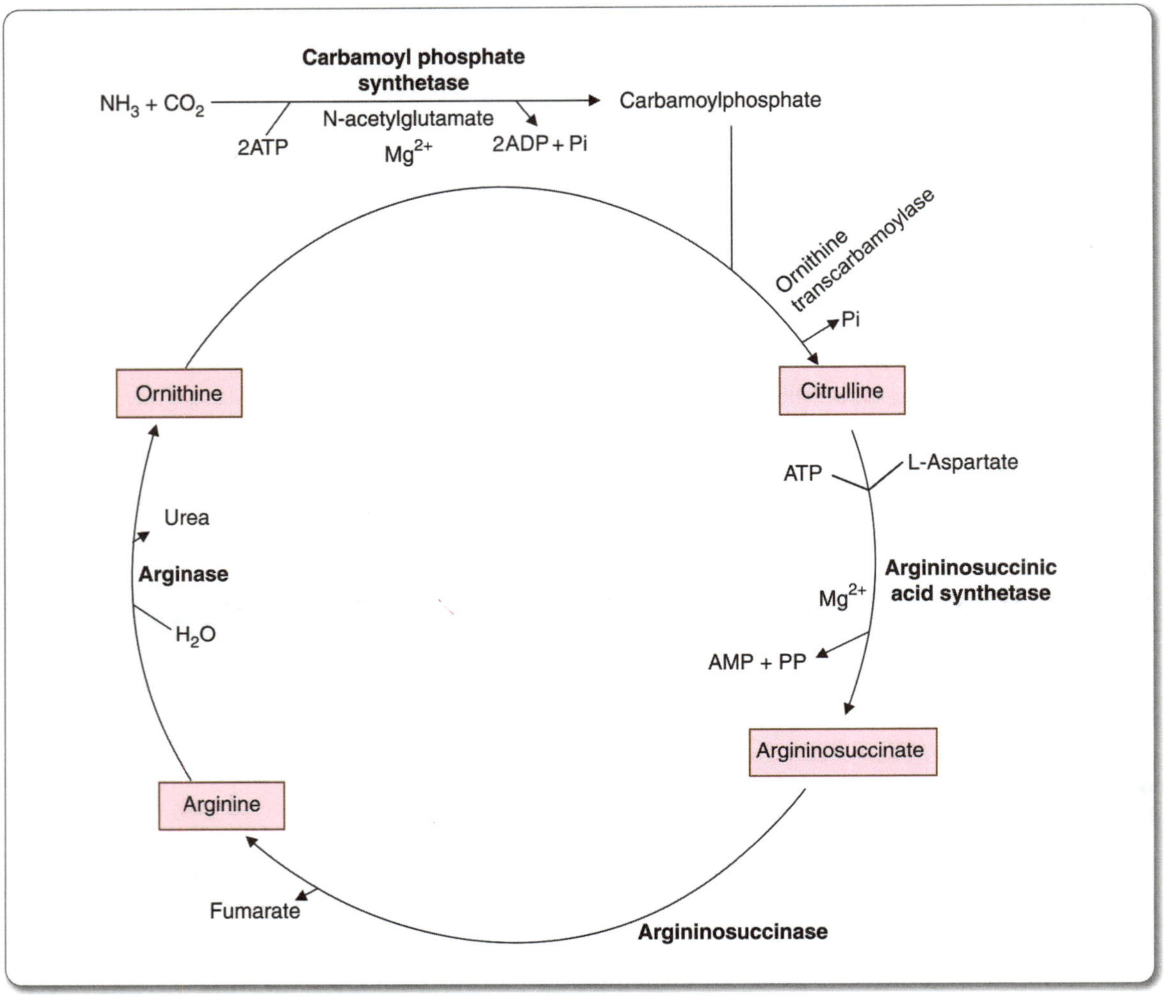

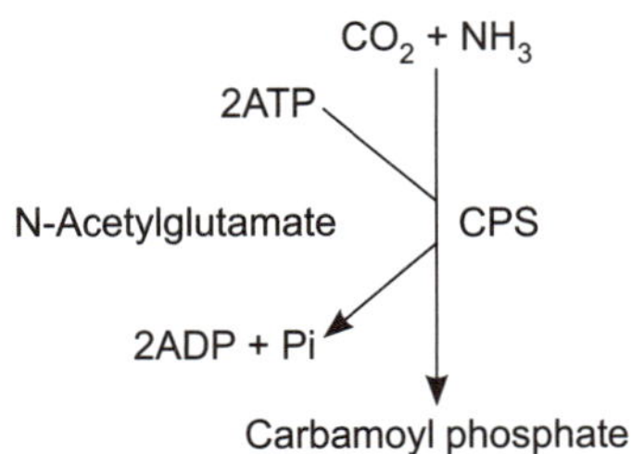

Fig. 4.16: Urea cycle

- In the first step, **ammonia reacts with carbon dioxide** and **forms carbamoyl phosphate,** in the mitochondria.

  This reaction is catalyzed by the enzyme **carbamoyl phosphate synthetase** (CPS), which requires N-acetylglutamate as coenzyme.

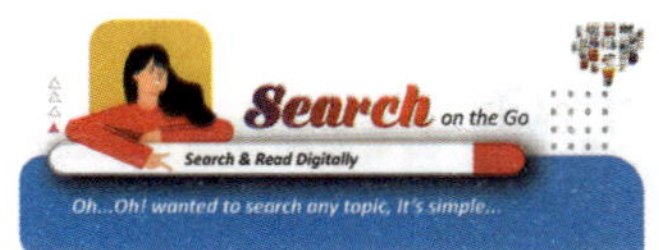

- **Thereafter, ornithine transcarbamylase transfers carbamoyl group from carbamoyl phosphate to ornithine** and forms **citrulline.**

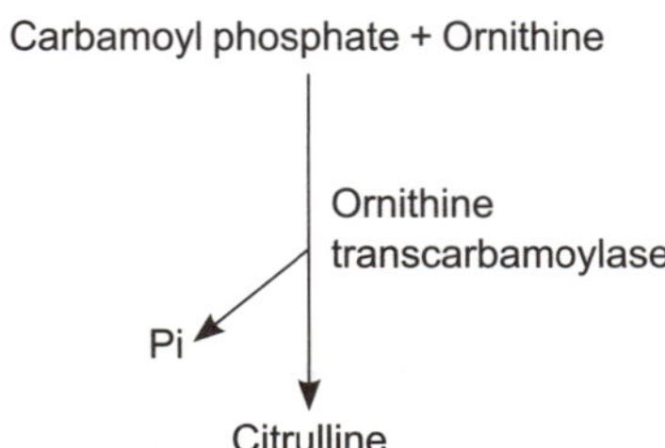

- In the presence of the enzyme **argininosuccinate synthetase, citrulline** combines with L-aspartate and **forms argininosuccinate**.

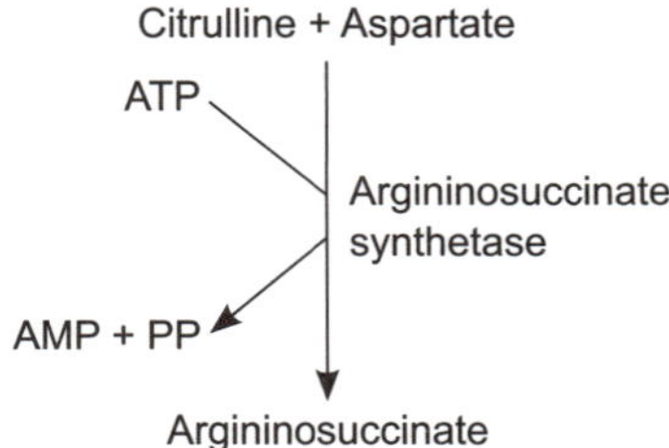

- Subsequently, **argininosuccinase** hydrolyzes **argininosuccinate** to **arginine and fumarate**.

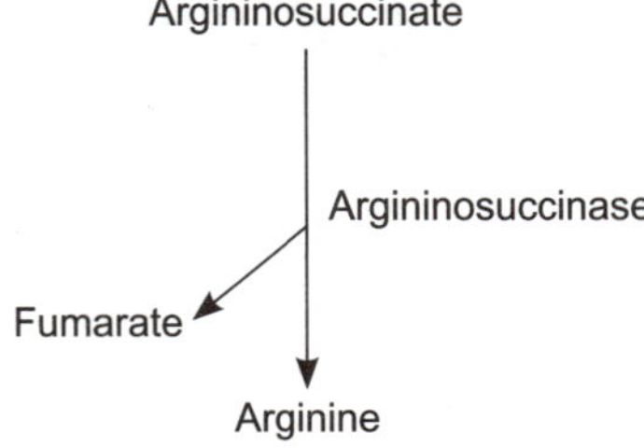

Fumarate, which is released in this reaction, enters mitochondria where it is converted to oxaloacetate via citric acid cycle.

Hence, urea cycle is coupled with the Krebs cycle, both of which were discovered by Sir Hans Krebs and Coworkers.

- In the last reaction, **arginine** is hydrolyzed, **by the enzyme arginase,** to **ornithine** and **urea**.

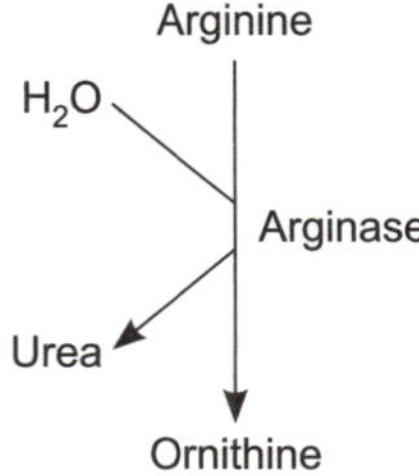

Ornithine is transported to mitochondria and re-enters the cycle.

This is the mechanism for the excretion of nitrogen in humans and other primates.

Two atoms of nitrogen, in urea, are derived from two different sources, i.e., from NH_3 and the amino group of aspartate.

Clinical Correlation

Defects in the Urea Cycle Enzymes

Since ammonia is very toxic, a metabolic disorder of urea cycle may result in coma and may be potentially fatal.

Defects in various enzymes of the urea cycle have been reported (Table 4.6).

TABLE 4.6: Disorders of urea cycle

Enzyme	Disorder
Carbamoyl phosphate synthetase	Hyperammonemia type I
Ornithine transcarbamoylase	Hyperammonemia type II
Argininosuccinate synthetase	Citrullinemia
Argininosuccinase	Argininosuccinic aciduria
Arginase	Hyperargininemia

Regulation of Urea Cycle

N-acetylglutamate acts as an allosteric activator for the enzyme **carbamoyl phosphate synthetase**.

Induction of the urea cycle enzymes occurs when either the delivery of ammonia or amino acids, to the liver, is increased. Thus, a high protein diet and starvation result in induction of enzymes of the urea cycle.

BIOLOGICALLY IMPORTANT COMPOUNDS SYNTHESIZED FROM VARIOUS AMINO ACIDS

Biologically Important Compounds Synthesized from Glycine

Biologically important compounds synthesized from glycine are shown in Figure 4.17.

- **Serine:** Glycine is converted to serine. Formation of serine from glycine is a reversible reaction. It is catalyzed by the enzyme **serine hydroxymethyltransferase**, which requires pyridoxal-5-phosphate and N^5, N^{10}-methylenetetrahydrofolate (N^5, N^{10}-methylene • FH_4; Fig. 4.18).

  The demand for glycine or serine and the availability of N^5, N^{10}-methylene • FH_4 determines the direction of the reaction.

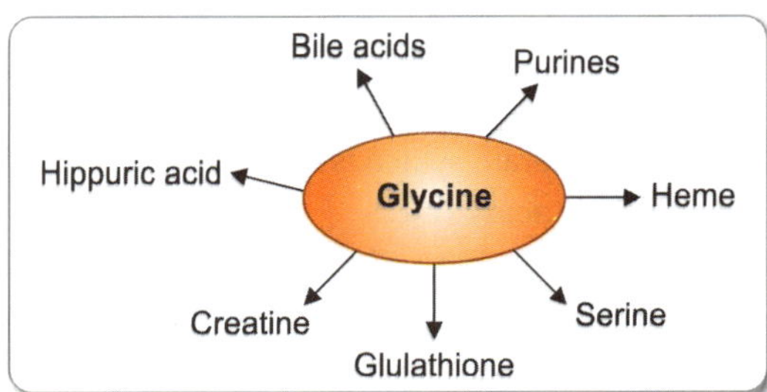

Fig. 4.17: Biologically important compounds synthesized from glycine

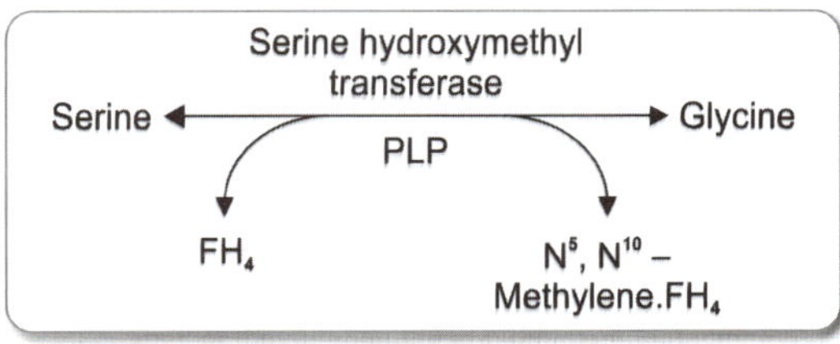

Fig. 4.18: Interconversion of glycine and serine

- **Purine ring:** Glycine is an important contributor in the biosynthesis of a purine ring. It contributes nitrogen and both the carbons, which form N_7, C_4 and C_5 of a purine ring (Fig. 4.19).
- **Heme:** Glycine joins with succinyl CoA and forms δ-aminolevulinic acid, a precursor of heme. This reaction is catalyzed by aminolevulinic acid (ALA) synthase (Fig. 4.20).
- **Creatine:** Glycine also contributes in the biosynthesis of creatine, a reservoir of energy in muscle (Fig. 4.21).
- **Glutathione:** Glycine is also a constituent of the tripeptide glutathione.
- **Bile acid:** Glycine conjugates with cholic acid and forms glycocholic acid (a bile acid).
- **Hippuric acid:** Glycine is also used in the detoxification of benzoic acid, which is excreted in urine as hippuric acid.

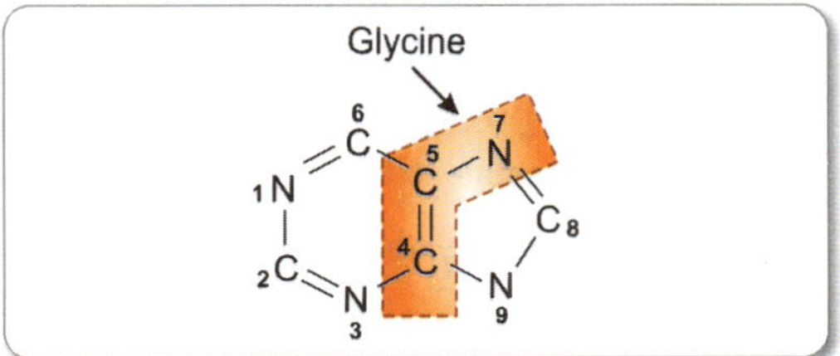

Fig. 4.19: Contribution of glycine in the synthesis of a purine ring

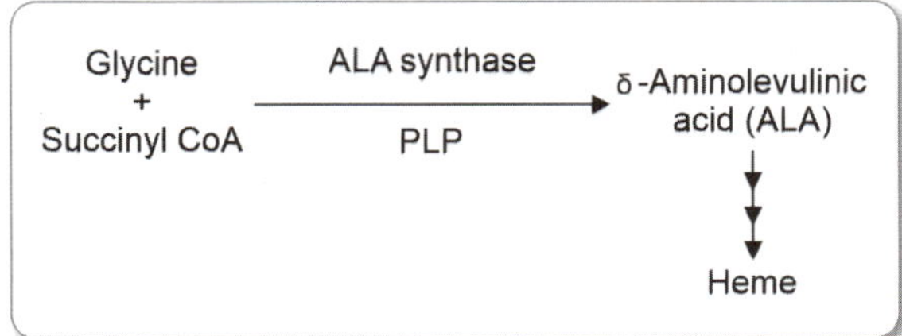

Fig. 4.20: Contribution of glycine in the synthesis of heme

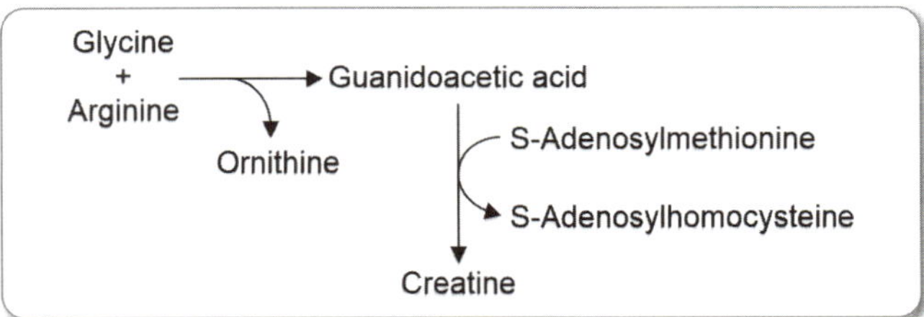

Fig. 4.21: Contribution of glycine in the synthesis of creatine

BIOLOGICALLY IMPORTANT COMPOUNDS SYNTHESIZED FROM AROMATIC AMINO ACIDS

Biologically Important Compounds Synthesized from Phenylalanine and Tyrosine

Biologically important compounds synthesized from phenylalanine and tyrosine are shown in Figure 4.22.

Synthesis of Norepinephrine and Epinephrine

In adrenal medulla, tyrosine is converted to norepinephrine (noradrenaline) and epinephrine (adrenaline), the two hyperglycemic hormones, secreted by the gland.

- First, tyrosine is converted to dihydroxyphenylalanine (**DOPA**) by the enzyme **tyrosine hydroxylase**.
- Thereafter, **DOPA-decarboxylase converts DOPA to dopamine**, which enters the storage granules as an active neurotransmitter.

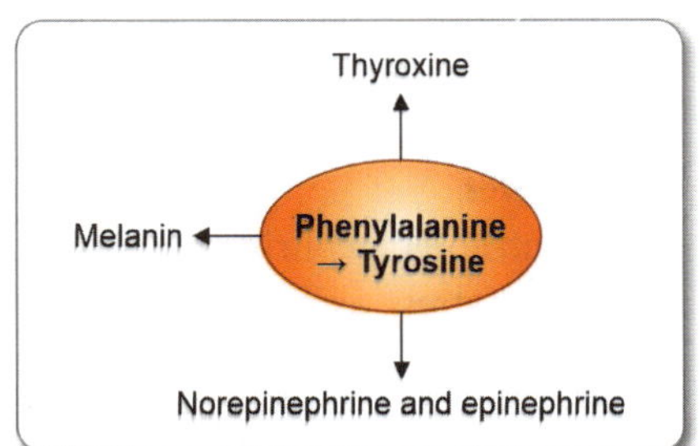

Fig. 4.22: Biologically important compounds synthesized from phenylalanine and tyrosine

- In the next step, **dopamine** is converted to **norepinephrine by dopamine-β-hydroxylase**.

  Norepinephrine is a hormone, present in sympathetic nerve endings. Its synthesis is regulated by plasma tyrosine in the brain.

- In the next step, methylation of **norepinephrine** by the enzyme **phenylethanolamine-N-methyltransferase** (PNMT), converts it to **epinephrine**. In this reaction active methionine (S-adenosylmethionine) is used as a methyl donor (Fig. 4.23).

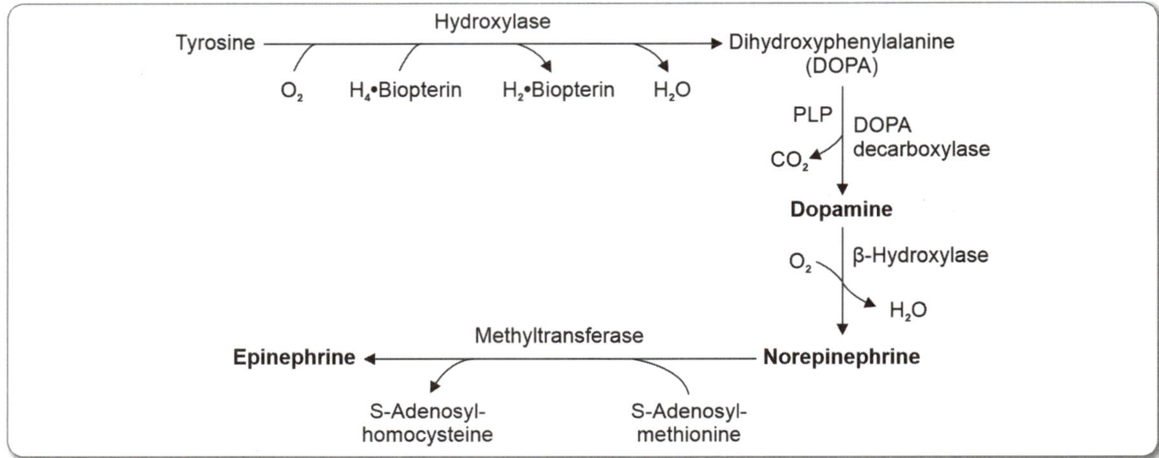

Fig. 4.23: Synthesis of norepinephrine and epinephrine from tyrosine in the adrenal medulla

Catecholamines

Aromatic amines with a catechol ring (3,4-dihydroxyphenyl ring), i.e., dopamine, norepinephrine and epinephrine, are collectively called catecholamines.

These have general modulatory effects on overall brain functions, such as mood and arousal.

- **Dopamine:** It is an intermediate in the synthesis of norepinephrine. It is a neurotransmitter in nerves, that interconnect nuclei of the basal ganglia in brain, and controls voluntary movement. Damage to these nerves causes Parkinson's disease, which is characterized by tremor and difficulties in initiating and controlling movement.

- **Norepinephrine:** It is a major transmitter in sympathetic nervous system. Stimulation of these nerves is responsible for various features of **fight or flight** response such as stimulation of heart rate, sweating and vasoconstriction in skin and bronchodilation.

- **Epinephrine:** It is produced by adrenal medulla under the influence of acetylcholine-containing nerves analogous to the sympathetic pre-ganglionic nerves. It has stimulatory effect on glycogen metabolism in the liver.

Both, norepinephrine and epinephrine are released from the storage vesicles in adrenal medulla, in response to stress, exercise, cold and hypoglycemia. They increase degradation of glycogen and triacylglycerols as well as increase blood pressure and output of the heart.

Synthesis of Thyroid Hormones

In the thyroid gland, iodination of tyrosyl residues of thyroglobulin results in the synthesis of thyroid hormones (Fig. 4.24).

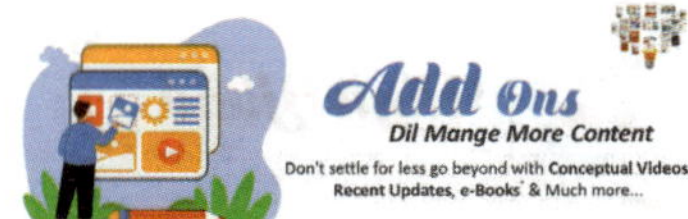

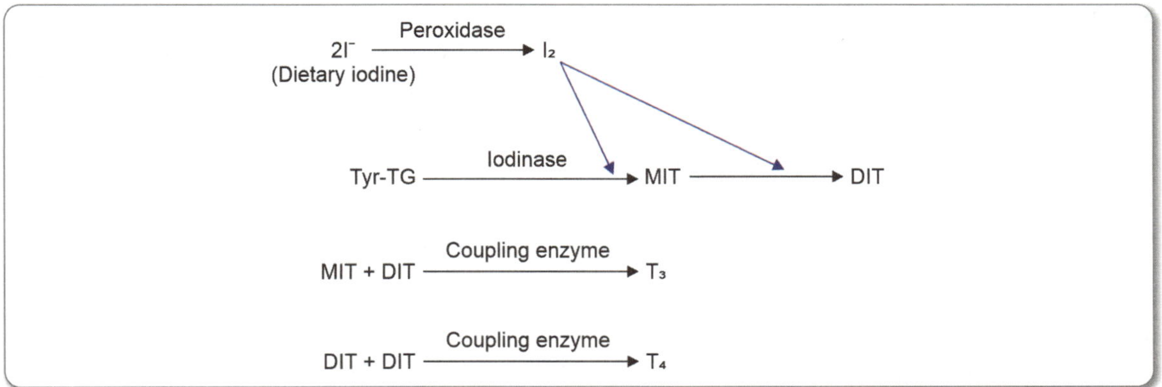

Fig. 4.24: Role of iodine in the synthesis of thyroid hormones (T_3 and T_4); (Tyr-TG = Tyrosine amino acids or tyrosyl-residues in a thyroglobulin molecule)

- In the first step of **iodination**, iodine is activated by peroxidase.
- Subsequently, iodinase catalyzes iodination of the tyrosyl residues of thyroglobulin and converts these tyrosine molecules to monoiodotyrosine (MIT) and diiodotyrosine (DIT).
- Thereafter, **coupling** of either a molecule of MIT with DIT or two molecules of DIT, forms triiodothyronine (T_3) and thyroxine (tetraiodothyronine or T_4), respectively. This is an intramolecular process and the two hormones are synthesized within the protein chain of the thyroglobulin molecule.

Synthesis of Melanin

In melanocytes, tyrosine is converted to melanin.

- In the first step, **tyrosine is converted to DOPA** and **then to dopaquinone** by the enzyme **tyrosinase** (a copper-containing protein).
- Subsequently, dopaquinone **forms melanin**, a brown-black pigment, found in skin, hair and retina (Fig. 4.25).

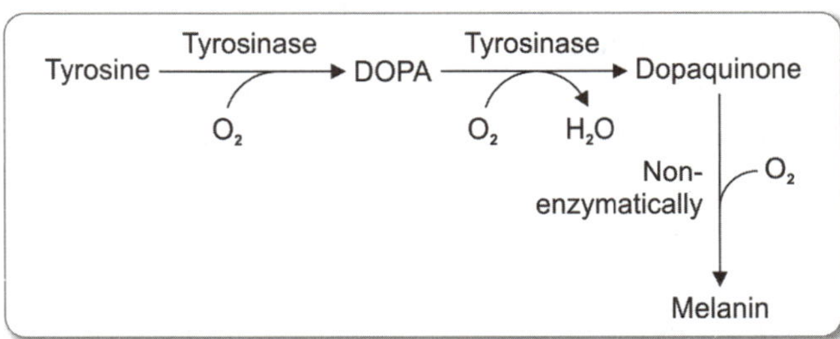

Fig. 4.25: Synthesis of melanin from tyrosine in melanocytes

Biologically Important Compounds Synthesized from Tryptophan

Various biologically important compounds synthesized from tryptophan are shown in Figure 4.26.

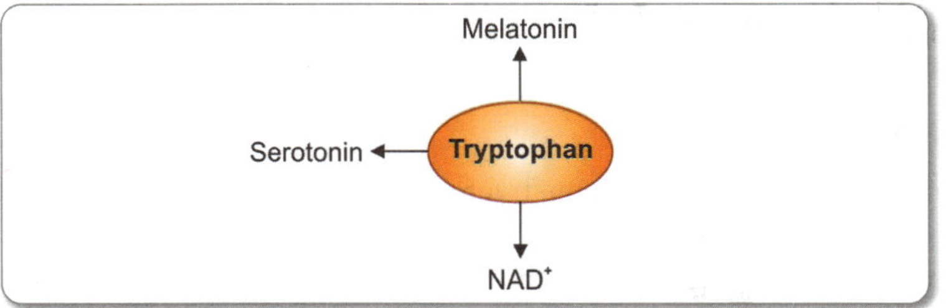

Fig. 4.26: Biologically important compounds synthesized from tryptophan

Synthesis of NAD

- Synthesis of NAD from tryptophan starts with the opening of the indole ring, leading to the formation of N-formylkynurenine. This reaction is catalyzed by a heme-containing enzyme, tryptophan dioxygenase, also called tryptophan pyrrolase, in the liver.
- In the next step, N-formylkynurenine is converted to kynurenine with the removal of formate by the enzyme formamidase (formylase).
- Thereafter, kynurenine is hydroxylated to produce 3-hydroxykynurenine by kynurenine hydroxylase.
- In the next step, with the cleavage of alanine from the side chain, by kynureninase, 3-hydroxykynurenine is converted to 3-hydroxyanthranilate. This enzyme requires pyridoxal-5-phosphate (vitamin B6) as a coenzyme.
- Subsequent oxidation of 3-hydroxyanthranilate, by 3-hydroxyanthranilate oxidase forms an unstable intermediate 2-amino-3-carboxymuconate-6- semialdehyde.
- Thereafter in the liver and some other tissues, nonenzymatic cyclization, of **aminocarboxymuconic semialdehyde**, converts it to **quinolinic acid**.
- Thereafter, **quinolate phosphoribosyltransferase** (QPRT) transfers a ribonucleotide moiety from phosphoribosylpyrophosphate (PRPP), subsequent decarboxylation of which leads to the synthesis of nicotinate mononucleotide (NMN, a derivative of niacin). NMN is finally converted to NAD (Fig. 4.27).

Sixty mg of tryptophan is converted to 1 mg of niacin. In B_6 deficiency quinolinic acid is not converted to niacin but to nicotinamide and its N^1-methyl derivative (N^1-methylnicotinamide). Vitamin B_6 deficiency, thus, results in urinary excretion of large quantities of these metabolites.

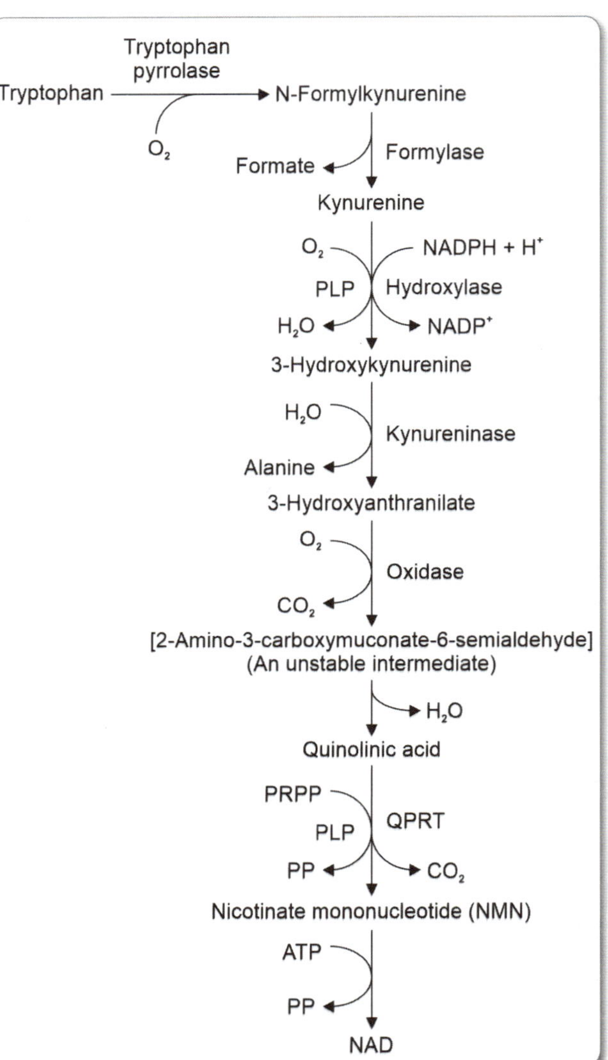

Fig. 4.27: Synthesis of NAD from tryptophan

Synthesis of Serotonin

- In platelets, brain and intestinal epithelium, tryptophan is hydroxylated by **tryptophan hydroxylase**, to form **5-hydroxytryptophan**.
- 5-hydroxytryptophan is subsequently decarboxylated to **5-hydroxytryptamine**, also called **serotonin**, by a **decarboxylase**, which also requires B_6 for its activity (Fig. 4.28).

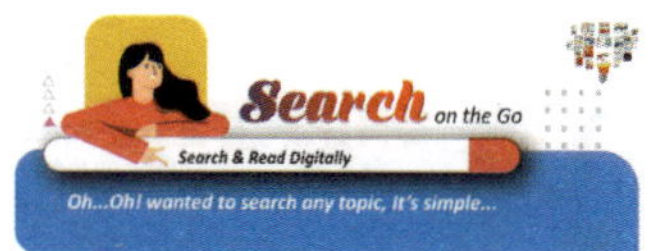

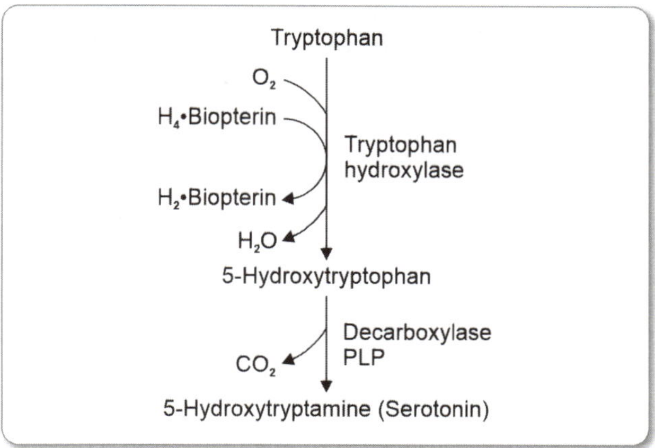

Fig. 4.28: Synthesis of serotonin from tryptophan

Serotonin is a neurotransmitter (in the brain), vasoconstrictor and bronchoconstrictor. Serotonin-producing tumor cells in the intestine results in a condition referred to as **malignant carcinoid syndrome**, also called **argentaffinoma**, because this tumor arises from the intestinal argentaffin cells, that normally secrete serotonin. There is an increased production of serotonin that causes flushing, anxiety and gastrointestinal upset.

Serotonin is normally catabolized to **5-hydroxy-indoleacetic acid** (**5-HIAA**). In this condition, urinary excretion of 5-HIAA is increased by >50 folds. Estimation of 5-HIAA is used to establish the diagnosis.

Synthesis of Melatonin

An **acetyltransferase**, present in the pineal gland and retina, converts **serotonin** into **N-acetyl-5-methoxytryptamine**, also called **melatonin** (Fig. 4.29).

Melatonin is a sleep-inducing substance and maintains circadian rhythm of sleep wake cycle. It also inhibits synthesis and secretion of other neurotransmitters, such as dopamine and GABA.

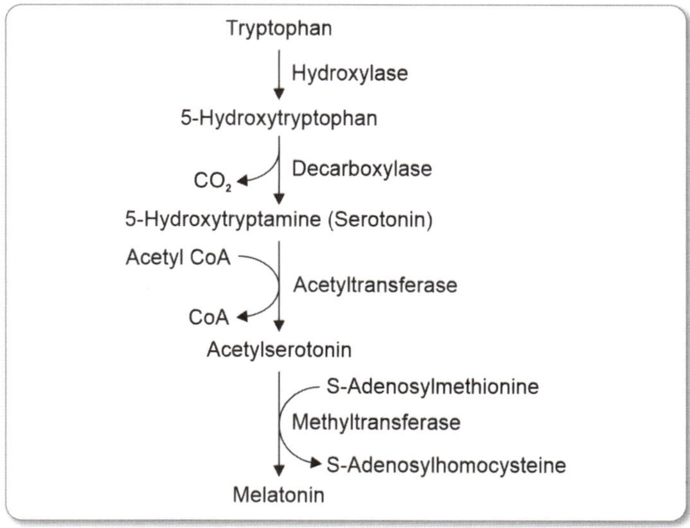

Fig. 4.29: Synthesis of melatonin from tryptophan

BIOLOGICALLY IMPORTANT COMPOUNDS SYNTHESIZED FROM SULFUR-CONTAINING AMINO ACIDS

Biologically Important Compounds Synthesized from Methionine

Methionine is a precursor of **cysteine**, which is synthesized as follows:

- After removal of the active methyl group, by a methyltransferase, **S-adenosylmethionine** is converted to **S-adenosylhomocysteine**.
- Thereafter, **adenosylhomocysteinase**, cleaves the adenosyl moiety (a molecule of adenosine) and forms **homocysteine**, which has one carbon more than cysteine.
- In the next step, **homocysteine** is coupled with **serine** and forms **cystathionine**. The reaction is catalyzed by the enzyme **cystathionine synthase**, which also requires pyridoxal phosphate as a coenzyme.
- In the next step, **cystathionine** is cleaved by a splitting enzyme, **cystathionine lyase**, also called **cystathionase**, and forms **cysteine** and α-**ketobutyrate** (Fig. 4.30).

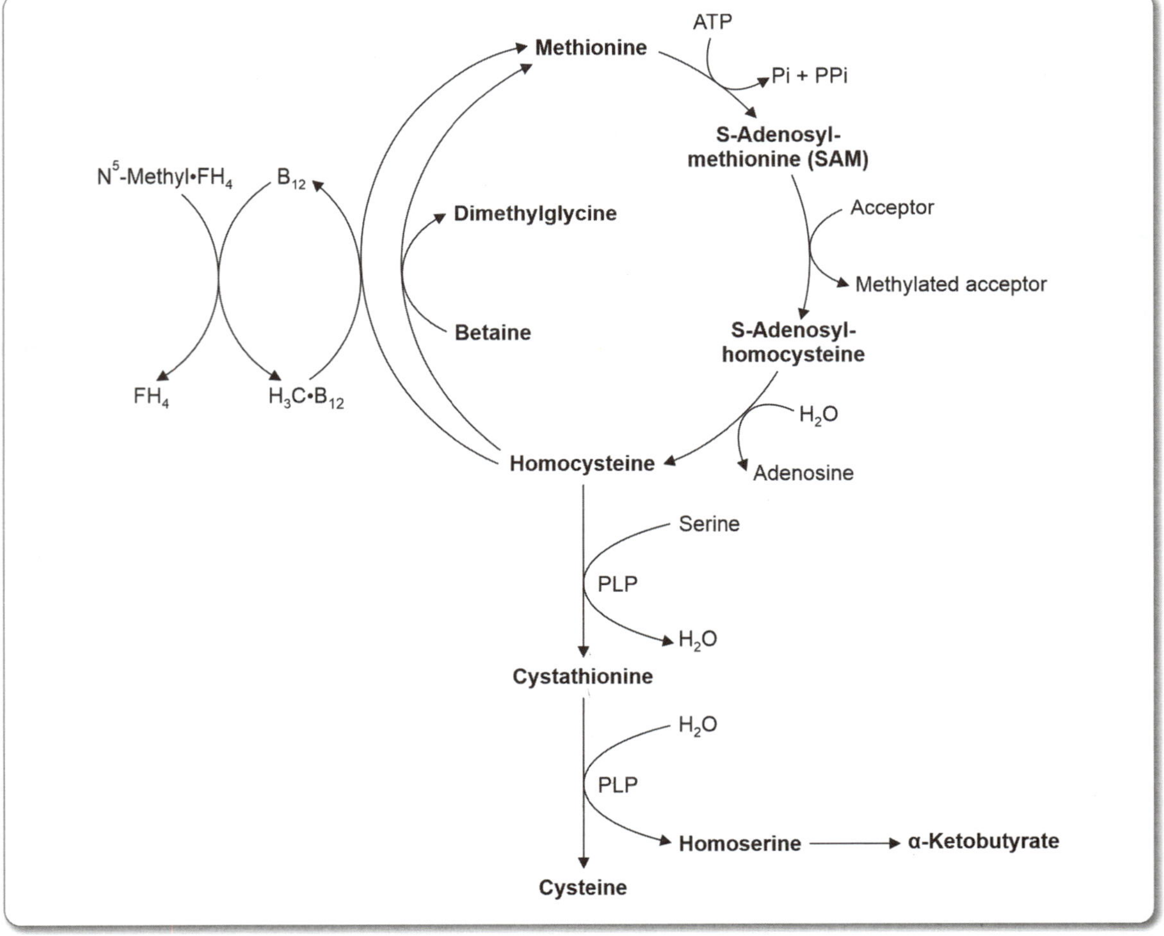

Fig. 4.30: Conversion of methionine to S-adenosylmethionine (active methionine), homocysteine and cysteine

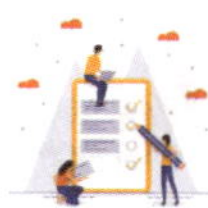
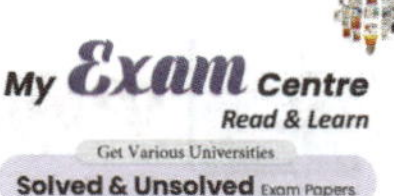

Biologically Important Compounds Synthesized from Cysteine

Synthesis of Taurine

- **Cysteine** is oxidized by the enzyme **cysteine dioxygenase** to form **cysteine sulfinate**.
- The latter is decarboxylated to **hypotaurine** (2-aminoethane sulfate), which is oxidized to form **taurine**.

Synthesis of Active Sulfate

- **Taurine**, as synthesized above, undergoes transamination with α-ketoglutaric acid and is converted to **bisulfite** and pyruvate.
- In the next step, **sulfite oxidase** oxidizes **bisulfate**, which is converted to **sulfate**.
- In the next step, **sulfate** in the presence of ATP and the enzyme **adenosine phosphosulfate pyrophosphorylase**, is converted to **3′-phosphoadenosine-5′-phosphosulfate** (PAPS), also called **active sulfate**.

Active sulfate is used as a source of sulfate for the formation of sulfate esters of steroids, alcohols and phenols.

Synthesis of SH-containing Peptides

Cysteine is also used in the synthesis of other sulfur-containing compounds of physiological importance such as insulin, CoA, glutathione and vasopressin.

BIOLOGICALLY IMPORTANT COMPOUNDS SYNTHESIZED FROM HISTIDINE

Histamine

Histidine is converted to histamine by a decarboxylase.

Histamine is a pharmacologically active compound. It is a vasodilator and reduces blood pressure. It is also a stimulant of gastric juice secretion. Allergic reactions increase liberation of histamine.

INBORN ERRORS OF AROMATIC AMINO ACIDS METABOLISM

Inborn errors of metabolism of phenylalanine and tyrosine are shown in Table 4.7.

TABLE 4.7: Inborn errors of aromatic amino acids metabolism

Inborn error	Deficient enzyme
Phenylketonuria	Phenylalanine hydroxylase
Tyrosinemia type I	Fumarylacetoacetate hydrolase
Tyrosinemia type II	Tyrosine transaminase
Alkaptonuria	Homogentisic acid oxidase
Albinism	Tyrosinase

Phenylketonuria

Autosomal recessive deficiency of hepatic **phenylalanine hydroxylase** results in a condition called **phenylketonuria.**

The alternative pathway catabolizes an excess of phenylalanine, which cannot be converted to tyrosine. It is transaminated to phenylpyruvic acid, which is subsequently reduced to phenyllactic acid as well as decarboxylated to phenylacetic acid (Fig. 4.31).

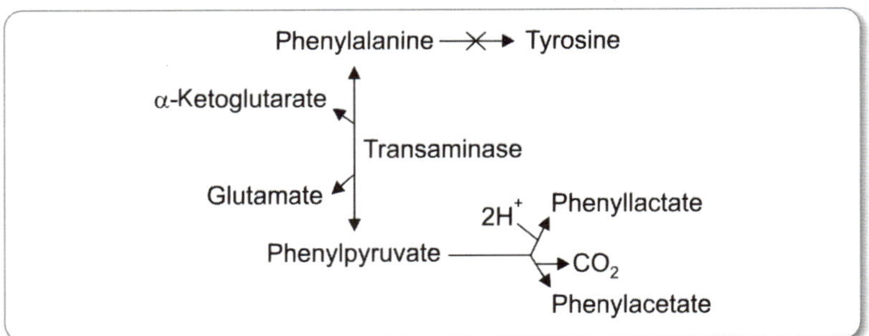

Fig. 4.31: Conversion of phenylalanine to phenyl-ketoacids in phenylketonuria

Due to increased urinary excretion of phenylpyruvic acid (a phenylketone), this disease is called phenylketonuria. Increased levels of phenyl keto acids in the blood cause mental retardation and convulsions.

Such infants are given low phenylalanine diet and under these conditions tyrosine becomes dietary essential.

Tyrosinemias

A complete or partial **deficiency of tyrosine aminotransferase** may result in **tyrosinemia**, which in turn leads to accumulation and excretion of tyrosine and its metabolites. Tyrosinemias are of two types:

Tyrosinemia Type I

It is also called **hepatorenal tyrosinemia**. It is caused by the **deficiency of fumarylacetoacetate hydrolase** and is characterized by liver failure, renal tubular dysfunction, rickets and polyneuropathy.

Tyrosinemia Type II

It is also called **oculocutaneous tyrosinemia**. It is due to the **deficiency of tyrosine transaminase**. It results in eye and skin lesions and mental retardation.

Alkaptonuria

Hereditary **deficiency of homogentisic acid oxidase** causes **alkaptonuria**. Such individuals excrete homogentisic acid in their urine. Homogentisic acid, in turn, gets auto-oxidized and is subsequently polymerized to form intensely dark substance, referred to as **alkapton.**

Dark urine is the only consequence of this condition in early life. Homogentisate is slowly oxidized and deposited in the bone, connective tissue and other organs. This condition is called **ochronosis** because of ochre color of the pigment.

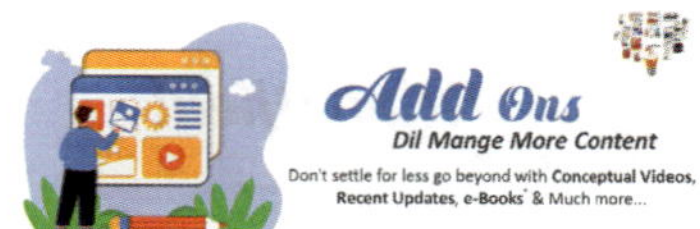

Albinism

Lack of tyrosinase, in the melanocytes, affects the synthesis of melanin and leads to the formation of white patches on the skin and iris in the eyes. This condition is referred to as **albinism**.

Lack of the pigment in the skin makes these albinos more sensitive to sunlight and increases the risk of carcinoma of skin. Lack of the pigment in the eyes contributes to photophobia.

PLASMA PROTEINS

Plasma contains over 300 proteins. Albumin, globulins and fibrinogen are the major plasma proteins, all of which are synthesized in the liver (except γ-globulins). Others include apolipoproteins (present in lipoproteins), protein hormones (such as insulin, prolactin, etc.), enzymes and coagulation proteins. Total plasma protein concentration varies from 6.3–8.0 g/dL, out of which albumin constitutes 3.7–5.3 g/dL while globulins constitute 1.8–3.7 g/dL. The range for various globulin fractions are - $\alpha_1 + \alpha_2 = 0.4$–$1.4$ g/dL, $\beta = 0.5$–1.3 g/dL and $\gamma = 0.6$–1.5 g/dL.

A/G Ratio

A/G ratio refers to plasma albumin: globulin ratio. The normal plasma A/G ratio is 1.2–2.0:1, which may be altered in a number of conditions. For example, an increase in total plasma proteins occurs in dehydration, due to prolonged diarrhea, vomiting and diabetes insipidus.

In hemoconcentration, both albumin and globulins are increased proportionately but A/G ratio remains unaltered.

A decrease in total plasma proteins is generally due to hypoalbuminemia as seen in liver cirrhosis, nephrotic syndrome, kwashiorkor, etc. It may be accompanied by either no increase in globulins or an increase in globulins that is proportionately less than the fall in albumin, resulting in a reversal of A/G ratio.

Functions of Plasma Albumin

Albumin performs several functions:
- Maintenance of **plasma colloidal osmotic pressure** and hence the regulation of blood volume.
- **Transport** of various molecules such as long chain fatty acids, unconjugated bilirubin, steroids, Cu^{2+} and drugs like salicylates, barbiturates, penicillin, sulfonamides and warfarin (Table 4.8).
- Makes plasma **antioxidant** because of the presence of sulfhydryl (–SH) groups.
- Acts as **protein reserve** in case of nutritional depletion.

Functions of Plasma Globulins

- α and β-globulins transport various molecules such as hormones, copper, iron, etc.
- γ-globulins constitute the defense proteins that combat antigenic challenge.

TABLE 4.8: Transport proteins

Proteins	Molecule transported
Albumin	Cu^{2+}, Fe^{3+}, bilirubin, free fatty acids, steroids, heme
Ceruloplasmin	Copper
Transferrin, ferritin, hemosiderin	Iron
Haptoglobin, hemopexin	Free hemoglobin
Thyroid binding globulin	Thyroid hormones
Cortisol binding globulin	Cortisol
Sex hormone binding globulin	Androgens, estrogens

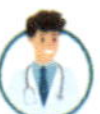 ## Clinical Correlation

Plasma Protein Disorders

Hypoproteinemia

*Causes of hypoproteinemia (**low total protein concentration**) are **overhydration**; **excessive loss** through the kidney (mainly albumin) such as in nephrotic syndrome, and from the skin after burns or loss through the intestine such as in protein losing enteropathy; **decreased synthesis** such as in a severe liver disease, or **reduced intake** either due to severe dietary protein deficiencies like kwashiorkor, or severe malabsorption.*

Hypoalbuminemia

It refers to low plasma albumin and may arise due to several reasons such as protein malnutrition (e.g., kwashiorkor and marasmus), malabsorption (e.g., inflammatory bowel disease), impaired synthesis in chronic liver diseases (e.g., cirrhosis), excessive losses in urine (e.g., nephrotic syndrome) or increased catabolism (e.g., major surgery, trauma, sepsis and malignancy).

Hyperglobulinemia

Increase in globulins occurs most commonly in advanced liver disease (e.g., cirrhosis), chronic infectious diseases (e.g., tuberculosis or viral hepatitis) or multiple myeloma.

ELECTROPHORESIS

The term electrophoresis means, Electro = electric field + Phoresis = migration. So, as the name indicates, electrophoresis is a **method of separation where charged molecules migrate in differential speeds in an applied electric field**.

- The charged molecules under the influence of electric field migrate toward oppositely charged electrodes. Molecules with positive (+ve) charge move towards cathode while negative (–ve) molecules move toward anode.
- The migration is due to charge on the molecules and potential applied across the electrodes.
- The sample, under test, is placed at one end, near one of electrodes. When current is applied, the molecules start moving to respective electrodes.
- The movement is influenced by molecular weight of the molecule. So, when a mixture is placed on the electrophoresis paper or agarose gel, different bands are seen along the paper after the process. This is due to differential rate of movement by molecules, based on their weight. Those with high molecular weight move slower while those with small weight move faster.

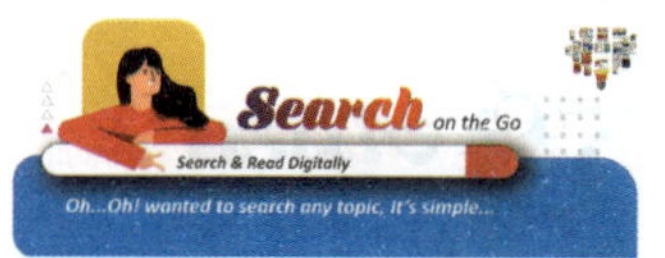

Electrophoresis is one of the **widely used techniques in molecular biochemistry, microbiology and biomedical research**. It is one of the highly efficient techniques of analysis and sole method for separation of proteins for western blot and RNA studies.

Electrophoresis Systems

There are two types of electrophoresis systems, referred to as **horizontal electrophoresis system** and the **vertical electrophoresis system**.

Each system requires the equipment, which consists, basically, of two items, i.e., **a power pack** and **an electrophoresis unit**.

- **Power pack:** It provides a stabilized direct current and controls both voltage (0–500 V) and current output (0–150 A). The power pack **supplies a direct current between the two electrodes** in the electrophoresis unit. Electrophoresis is carried out in an appropriate buffer, which is essential to maintain a constant state of ionization of the molecules being separated. Any variation in pH will alter the overall charge and hence, the mobilities (rate of migration in the applied field) of the molecules being separated.
- **Electrophoresis unit:** It **consists of electrodes, buffer reservoir, supporting medium and transparent insulating cover**. Electrodes are made of platinum or stainless steel.

Types of Electrophoresis Units

Electrophoresis units are available for running either **vertical or horizontal systems**.

Horizontal type: It consists of **two buffer reservoirs** (compartments), which are placed side by side to each other. Separate compartments are necessary because any change in pH occurring at electrodes, does not affect the buffer that is in contact with the supporting medium.

- It has a transparent insulating cover which provides electrical insulation and also prevents evaporation of buffer. The supporting medium is cast on a glass/plastic sheet and is placed on a cooling plate.
- Support for electrophoresis medium (supporting medium) may be paper, cellulose acetate or gel.
- Contact between the supporting medium and the buffer reservoir is through a wick.

Types of Electrophoresis

Electrophoresis can be broadly divided into two types, designated as **slab electrophoresis and capillary electrophoresis**.

Slab Electrophoresis

Slab electrophoresis is the classical method, which is widely used for industrial use. It is slow, time consuming and bulky. Yet, it is the sole method available for separation of proteins, enzymes, hormones, antibodies and nucleotides. Based on the principle used for separation, it is further divided into three types, as zone electrophoresis, isoelectric focusing and immunoelectrophoresis.

Zone Electrophoresis

In zone electrophoresis, the charged particles are separated into different zones or bands such as in paper electrophoresis.

Paper Electrophoresis

Paper electrophoresis employs a Whatman filter paper No. 1, which is moistened by a buffer and then connected at two ends, to the oppositely charged electrodes. The sample is applied on one end and let for separation of the components under electric gradient. After separation, paper is dried and stained to get colored bands, which are later recognized by comparing with the standard.

Principle and procedure of paper electrophoresis: In paper electrophoresis, a strip of filter paper is taken and about 10 µL of serum is applied along a thin line, near the cathode. The strip is dipped in a buffered solution (barbitone buffer, pH 8.6) and is laid on a platform. The apparatus is covered with a sheet, to minimize evaporation. Two electrodes are also dipped in the two compartments containing buffer. Current is supplied through a power supply, which either supplies constant current and/or voltage. The current is carried by the charged particles and depending upon the charge, proteins migrate towards either anode or cathode. At pH 8.6, all the proteins carry a net negative charge and tend to migrate towards anode. Thus, on passing a constant current (about 1–2 mA per strip), different proteins migrate at different rates. At the end, their positions are revealed by some dye such as bromophenol blue, which stains proteins. Different proteins form separate bands on the paper strip.

Normal Electrophoretic Pattern of Plasma Proteins

In the normal serum, five bands are observed. Since albumin carries the largest number of the negative charges, it moves farthest while γ-globulin has less negative charges, it moves least. Starting from anode, these bands are designated as albumin, α_1-globulin, α_2-globulin, β-globulin and γ-globulin (Figs 4.32A and B).

Abnormal Electrophoretic Patterns of Plasma Proteins

Abnormal electrophoretic patterns of plasma proteins in some disease conditions are shown in Figures 4.32C to J.

As shown in the Figures 4.32A to J, these patterns help in the diagnosis of several diseases.

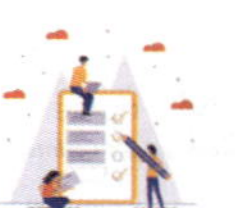
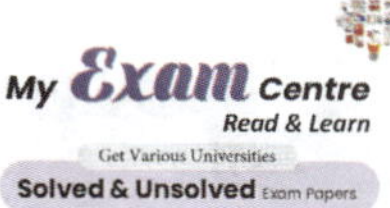

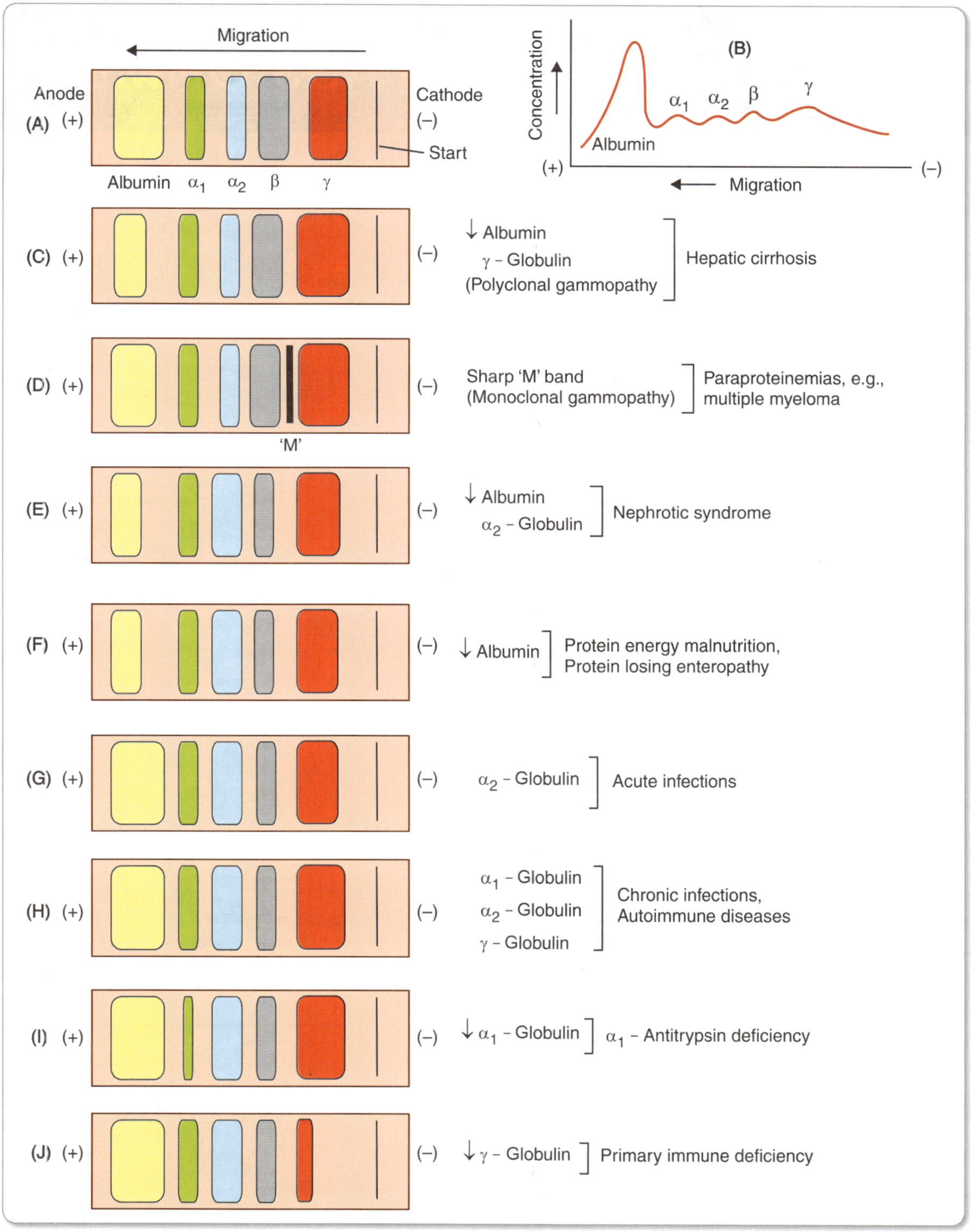

Figs 4.32A to J: Normal and abnormal electrophoretic patterns of plasma proteins

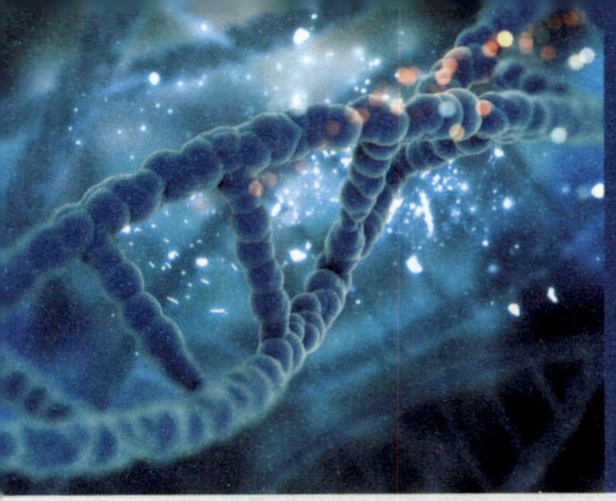

STUDENT ASSIGNMENT

LONG AND SHORT ANSWER QUESTIONS

1. What are proteins? Classify proteins based on their solubility.
2. What are amino acids? Classify them based on nutritional requirements.
3. Outline urea cycle. What is the site of urea synthesis? What is the need for urea synthesis in the body?
4. Describe various mechanisms of the removal of ammonia from amino acids.
5. How is ammonia removed from the body?
6. Explain how phenylalanine and tyrosine are metabolized. Describe biologically important compounds synthesized from these amino acids.
7. **Discuss briefly:**
   a. α-Helix
   b. β-Sheets
   c. Quaternary structure of proteins
   d. Biological significance of amino acids
   e. Essential amino acids
   f. Classification of amino acids according to nutritional requirement
   g. Classification of amino acids according to their metabolic fate
   h. Synthesis of urea and its abnormalities
   i. Transamination and its importance
   j. Metabolism of phenylalanine
   k. Processes of the removal of NH_3 from amino acids
8. **Write notes on:**

a. Fibrous proteins	b. Globular proteins
c. Protein denaturation	d. Alkaptonuria
e. Plasma proteins	f. Phenylketonuria
g. Disposal of ammonia from the body	h. Serum proteins electrophoresis

MULTIPLE CHOICE QUESTIONS

1. **Essential amino acids are named so:**
   a. Because these are produced in the body
   b. Because these are not synthesized in the body
   c. Because these are not important for life
   d. Because every foodstuff essentially contains them

2. **Nonessential amino acids are:**
   a. Not needed in the diet
   b. Not essential for growth
   c. Not required for protein synthesis
   d. Not synthesized in the body

3. **TRUE about denaturation of proteins:**
    a. Biological property is lost
    b. Primary structure is lost
    c. Always irreversible
    d. Proteins are soluble

4. **Transamination of aspartate forms:**
    a. Pyruvate
    b. Acetyl CoA
    c. Oxaloacetate
    d. Alanine

Notes

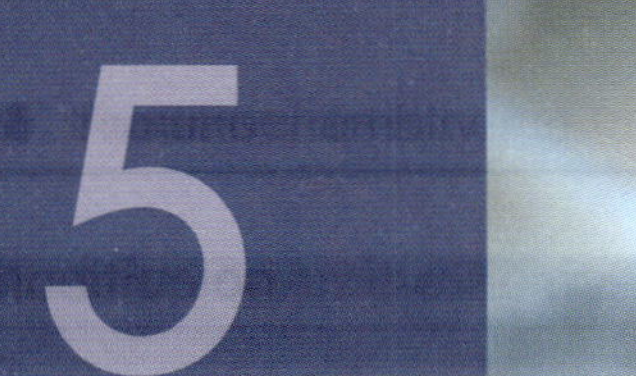

5

Clinical Enzymology

LEARNING OBJECTIVES

After the completion of the chapter, the readers will be able to:
- Explain enzymes, their chemical nature and classification.
- Understand the regulation of enzyme activity.
- Know the enzymes of diagnostic importance in various disease conditions.

CHAPTER OUTLINE

- Enzymes
- Enzyme Inhibition
- Regulation of Enzyme Activity
- Isoenzymes
- Enzymes of Diagnostic Importance

KEY TERMS

Alanine aminotransferase: An enzyme found primarily in the liver and kidney. High levels of alanine aminotransferase (ALT) in the blood may indicate damage or injury to the liver.

Allosteric regulation: A substance that binds to a site on an enzyme or receptor distinct from the active site, resulting in a conformational change that alters the protein's activity, either enhancing or inhibiting its function.

Aspartate transaminase: An enzyme found in the liver, heart, and other tissues. A high level of aspartate transaminase released into the blood may be a sign of liver or heart damage, cancer, or other diseases.

Cofactors: A nonprotein chemical compound or metallic ion that is required for an enzyme's role as a catalyst; these can be considered "helper molecules" that assist in biochemical transformations.

Creatine phosphokinase: An enzyme in the body, which is found mainly in the heart, brain, and skeletal muscle.

Isoenzymes: A group of enzymes that catalyzes the same reaction but have different enzyme forms and catalytic efficiencies.

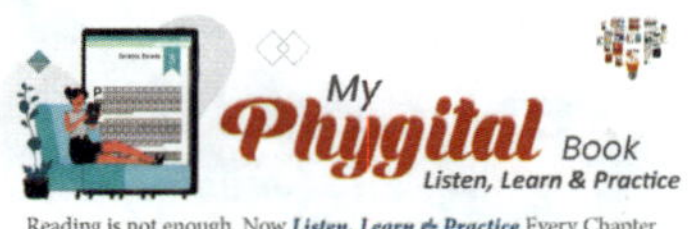

ENZYMES

Enzymes are **organic** molecules that are produced in the living organisms and increase the rate of a biochemical reaction without being utilized in the overall process. They are **nondialyzable, colloidal particles** which are **thermolabile proteins** with **highly specific catalytic activity**. An enzyme **increases rate of a chemical reaction** by lowering its free energy barrier that separates a substrate (reactant) from the product.

Most of the enzymes are produced within the cell of a particular tissue and function there only. Such enzymes are called **intracellular enzymes**, e.g., **enzymes of the glycolysis**, **citric acid cycle**, **fatty acid synthesis**, etc. On the other hand, there are certain enzymes, which are produced by the cells of a particular tissue from where they are liberated but function in some other tissues. Such enzymes are called **extracellular enzymes**, e.g., proteolytic enzymes **trypsin**, **chymotrypsin**, **etc**. They are secreted in the pancreatic juice for their action in the small intestine.

Proenzymes

Most of the intracellular enzymes are secreted in their active form called **zymase**. Some of the enzymes, however, are secreted in their **inactive** form called proenzyme or **zymogen**. After coming in contact with certain activating agent, the proenzyme undergoes some modifications and is converted to active enzyme (zymase).

The activating agent can be H^+, some other enzyme or the active form of the zymogen itself. For example, gastric juice contains **pepsin** which is secreted as **pepsinogen** (a zymogen). Pepsinogen is changed to its active form pepsin by the H^+ of the gastric juice. Once pepsin has been formed, it acts on pepsinogen and catalyzes its conversion to pepsin. This process is referred to as **autocatalysis** (Fig. 5.1).

Table 5.1 lists some of the proenzymes, their activators and the active enzymes.

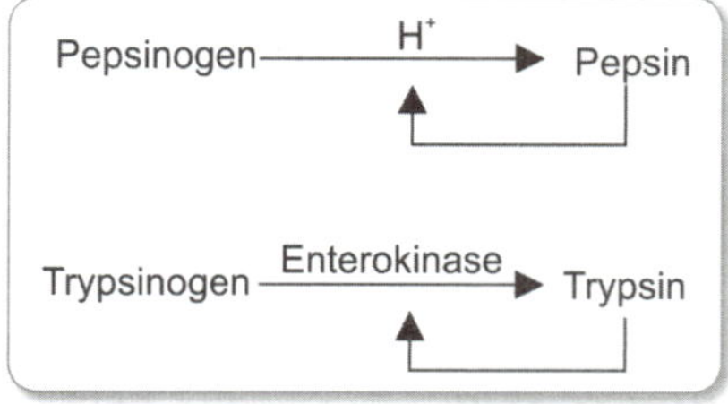

Fig. 5.1: Conversion of a proenzyme to active enzyme

TABLE 5.1: Some of the proenzymes, their activators and active enzymes

Proenzyme	Activator	Active enzyme
Pepsinogen	H^+, pepsin	Pepsin
Trypsinogen	Trypsin, enterokinase	Trypsin
Chymotrypsinogen	Trypsin	Chymotrypsin
Procarboxypeptidase	Trypsin	Carboxypeptidase
Proelastase	Trypsin	Elastase

Chemical Nature of Enzymes

All enzymes are **proteinaceous** in nature and have large molecular weights. Some RNA molecules called **ribozymes**, also have catalytic activity.

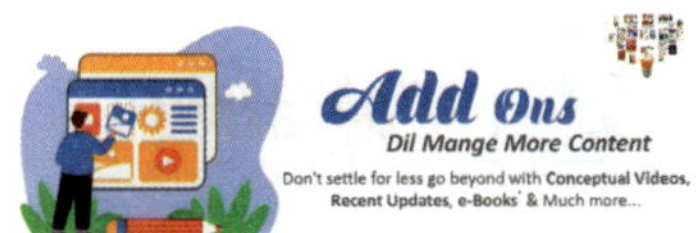

Ribozymes

A ribozyme is an RNA molecule, which exhibits highly substrate-specific catalytic activity. It catalyzes hydrolysis of phosphodiester bonds within the RNA molecules and plays a key role in intron splicing, in the conversion of pre-mRNA to mature mRNA, e.g., RNase P from *E. coli*.

Although, most of the enzymes are simple proteins and have a single polypeptide chain, there are various **enzymes** which have more than one catalytic activity and are called multimeric enzymes. They may be grouped as **oligomeric enzymes** or **multienzyme complexes**.

Oligomeric Enzymes

Oligomeric enzymes are the **multimeric proteins**, i.e., they have more than one protein subunits, **which have a catalytic activity only when associated with each other**. These multi-subunit enzymes are called **oligomeric enzymes**. For example, phosphorylase, hexokinase, and lactate dehydrogenase, each one is a tetramer, i.e., each one of these enzymes has four subunits. Phosphofructokinase, fructose-1,6-bisphosphatase, and creatine phosphokinase are dimers, i.e., each one of these enzymes has two protein subunits.

Multienzyme Complexes

Multienzyme complexes are single polypeptide chains with several catalytic sites. Due to multienzyme activities associated with a single protein, these enzymes are called **multienzyme complexes**. They act on a substrate and catalyze series of reactions, e.g., pyruvate dehydrogenase complex, α-ketoglutarate dehydrogenase complex, etc. Each of these enzymes is a complex having three different enzyme activities. Fatty acid synthetase is a multienzyme complex with seven enzyme activities.

Enzyme Specificity

Enzymes are highly specific, interacting with only one or a few substrates and catalyzing one type of a chemical reaction only. They exhibit several types of catalytic specificities such as stereospecificity, reaction specificity, etc.

Coenzymes and Cofactors

Several enzymes require the presence of some nonprotein organic substances or metal ions for their activity. These enzymes are referred to as holoenzymes (conjugated proteins). The protein part of such an enzyme is called **apoenzyme** (apo-protein) while the nonprotein component is called **prosthetic group.**

Proenzyme (protein) + prosthetic group (nonprotein component) = Holoenzyme

- If the prosthetic group is removed, enzyme loses its biological activity and becomes inactive.
- If the prosthetic group is an organic compound, it is called coenzyme while inorganic ions are called cofactors.

Coenzymes

A coenzyme is a **dialyzable, thermostable, low-molecular weight, organic substance**, which may be referred to as co-substrate or second substrate.

Generally, coenzymes are the **derivatives of the B complex** group of **vitamins,** e.g., **TPP** (coenzyme form of vitamin B_1), **FMN** and **FAD** (derivatives of B_2), **pyridoxal-5-phosphate** (coenzyme form of vitamin B_6), etc. (Table 5.2).

TABLE 5.2: Coenzymes, their precursor vitamins and some of the reactions catalyzed by them

Vitamin	Coenzyme form	Reaction catalyzed
Thiamine	TPP	Pyruvate → Acetyl CoA α-Ketoglutarate → Succinyl CoA
Riboflavin	FMN, FAD	α-Amino acids → α-Keto acids; Succinate → Fumarate
Niacin	NAD^+, $NADP^+$	Lactate → Pyruvate; Glucose-6-P → 6-P-Gluconolactone
Pyridoxine	Pyridoxal-5-P	Alanine + α-Ketoglutarate → Pyruvate + Glutamate; Tyrosine → Tyramine
Pantothenic acid	CoA	Pyruvate → Acetyl CoA; Fatty acid → Fatty acyl CoA
Biotin	Active biotin	Acetyl CoA → Malonyl CoA; Pyruvate → Oxaloacetate
Folate	Tetrahydrofolate	Glycine → Serine; Homocysteine → Methionine
B_{12}	Deoxyadenosylcobalamin/ Methylcobalamin	Methylmalonyl CoA → Succinyl CoA Homocysteine → Methionine
Lipoic acid	Lipoic acid	Pyruvate → Acetyl CoA; α-Ketoglutarate → Succinyl CoA

Cofactors

Several enzymes require certain **metal ions** called cofactors for their activity, e.g., Mg^{2+}, Zn^{2+} or Cl^-, etc.

A metal ion may be either tightly bound to the enzyme (**metalloenzymes**) or loosely associated with it (**metal-associated enzymes**).

Metalloenzymes: When a **metal ion forms an integral part of the enzyme,** such enzymes are referred to as **metalloenzymes.** For example, zinc is an essential component of superoxide dismutase. Some of the metalloenzymes and their cofactors are shown in Table 5.3.

TABLE 5.3: Some metalloenzymes and their cofactors

Metalloenzymes	Cofactor
Cytochromes, peroxidases, catalase	Fe
Ascorbic acid oxidase, cytochrome oxidase, tyrosinase	Cu
Aldehyde oxidase, xanthine oxidase, nitrate reductase	Mo
Carbonic anhydrase, lactate dehydrogenase, carboxypeptidase	Zn
Glutathione peroxidase	Se

Metal-associated enzymes: In certain enzymes, a **metal ion** may be **loosely associated** with it, forming a **metal-enzyme complex.** Such enzymes are called **metal-associated enzymes.** They require the presence of the particular ions for their activity, e.g., Cl^- (as NaCl) acts as an activator for salivary amylase. Table 5.4 lists metal-associated enzymes and the associated metal.

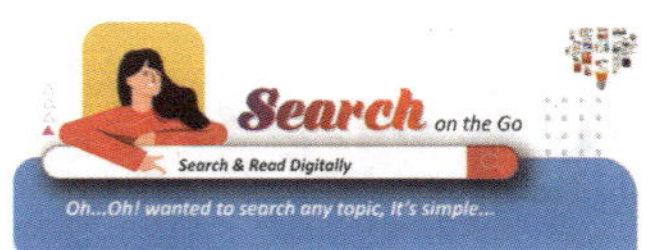

TABLE 5.4: Some metal-activated enzymes

Metal Ion	Associated enzymes
Ca	Lipase, ATPase, succinate dehydrogenase
Co	Lecithinase, peptidases
Mg	Phosphorylase, enolase, DNA polymerase
Mn	Arginase, phosphoglucomutase, cholinesterase
Cl	Salivary amylase
K	Pyruvate kinase

Nomenclature of Enzymes

Enzymes are usually named by **the suffix "-ase"** with the **name of the substrate** or the **catalytic action** of the enzyme, e.g., lipase catalyzes the hydrolysis of lipids, fatty acid synthase catalyzes the synthesis of fatty acids, etc. These names are called the **trivial names**. While assigning a trivial name to an enzyme, no systematic rules are followed.

Enzyme Commission Number

International Union of Biochemistry and Molecular Biology (IUBMB) adopted a scheme for the rational naming of each enzyme and suggested a **functional classification**. According to IUBMB, **each enzyme is assigned a four-digit systematic code**, commonly known as **Enzyme Commission number (EC number)**.

- The **first digit of the code denotes main class of the enzyme**, which is according to general type of the chemical reaction an enzyme catalyzes.
- Its **second digit** characterizes the **sub-class**, which may be based on the nature of the chemical group removed or transferred, or any bond spliced or formed.
- Its **third digit** indicates the **sub-sub-class** and describes detailed subdivision of each subclass.
- The **last digit** of the EC number indicates **serial number** of the particular enzyme in the sub-sub-class. For example, 1.1.1.1 is the enzyme code for alcohol dehydrogenase, which is the first enzyme of the sub-sub-class 1, of the sub-class 1, of the class 1.

Classification of Enzymes

According to the enzyme commission, enzymes are classified into six classes, as follows:

1. **Oxidoreductases:** These are involved in **oxidation and/or reduction of the substrate**, i.e., they catalyze addition of oxygen, or removal of hydrogen or electrons. Their sub-classes include dehydrogenase, oxidase, oxygenase, etc.
   Examples of the class oxidoreductase are alcohol dehydrogenase, xanthine oxidase, glutathione reductase, etc.
2. **Transferases:** These catalyze **transfer of a particular group from one substrate to another**. On the basis of the group transferred, transferases are sub-classified as aminotransferases, phosphotransferases, etc.
   Glutamate oxaloacetate transaminase, hexokinase, glucose-1-phosphate uridyltransferase, etc., are some of the examples of the class transferase.

3. **Hydrolases:** These bring about **hydrolysis of a substrate with the addition of a molecule of water**. According to the nature of the group or bond hydrolyzed, hydrolases are sub-classified as peptidases, glycosidases, etc.
   Examples of the class hydrolase include glucose-6-phosphatase, amylase, pepsin, etc.
4. **Lyases:** These catalyze **splitting of a substrate into two products without the addition of water**. They are sub-classified on the basis of the linkage splitted. Its various sub-classes include lyases catalyzing the breakdown of the C–C, C–N or C–S bond, etc.
   Examples of the class lyase include fumarase, pyruvate decarboxylase, histidase, etc.
5. **Isomerases:** These are involved in the conversion of one isomeric form of the substrate into another, i.e., in **isomerization of the substrate.** Racemases, epimerases and mutases, etc., are the sub-classes of the class isomerase.
   Examples of the class isomerase include phosphohexose isomerase, phosphoglucomutase, alanine racemase, etc.
6. **Ligases:** These are involved in the **synthesis of a product by linking two substrates together**. This joining of the two substrates requires energy which is coupled with the hydrolysis of some high-energy bond. Its various sub-classes include ligases that can form a C–C, C–N or C–S bond.
   Examples of the class ligase include glutamine synthetase, acetyl CoA carboxylase, glutathione synthetase, etc. (Table 5.5).

TABLE 5.5: Classification of enzymes with examples

Classes of enzymes	Examples
Oxidoreductases	Alcohol dehydrogenase, xanthine oxidase, catalase
Transferases	Glutamate pyruvate transaminase, serine hydroxymethyl transferase, hexokinase
Hydrolases	Glucose-6-phosphatase, carboxypeptidase, pepsin
Lyases	Pyruvate decarboxylase, aldolase, histidase
Isomerases	Phosphotriose isomerase, phosphoglucomutase, alanine racemase
Ligases	Glutamine synthetase, acetyl CoA carboxylase, glutathione synthetase

ENZYME INHIBITION

Phenomenon of decrease in the rate of the enzymatic reaction brought about by the addition of some substances is called enzyme inhibition. An inhibitor may affect enzyme activity either competitively or noncompetitively.

Competitive Inhibition

A competitive **inhibitor competes with the substrate** for binding at the active sites of the enzyme. **Chemical structure** of such an inhibitor closely **resembles the substrate**, e.g., malonate, which inhibits the action of succinate dehydrogenase, has structure similar to succinate.

The inhibitor forms the complex with the enzyme, which is called the **enzyme-inhibitor complex** (EI) and inhibits the action of the enzyme.

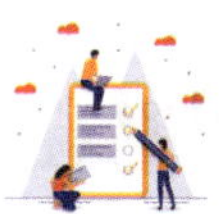
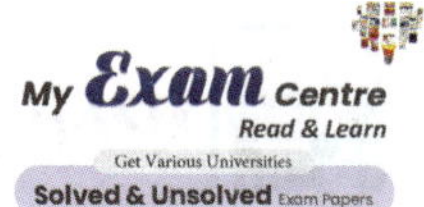

Binding of enzyme with the competitive inhibitor and the substrate depends upon the relative concentrations of the two and is usually a reversible process. By increasing the concentration of the substrate, degree of inhibition can be reduced. Presence of the competitive inhibitor increases the K_m without any change in V_{max} of the enzymatic reaction (Fig. 5.2).

Several drugs are used as competitive inhibitors.

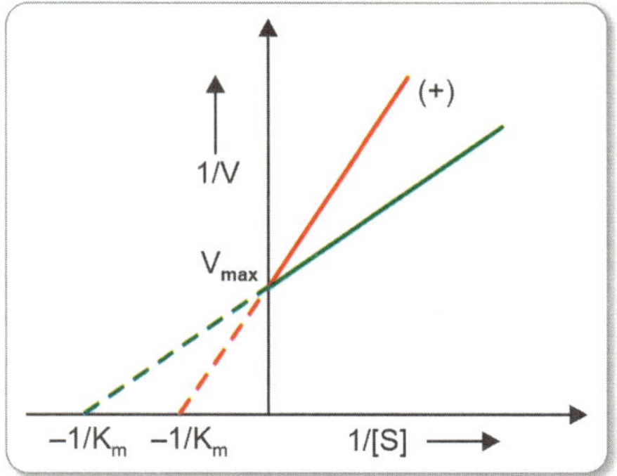

Fig. 5.2: Effect of a competitive inhibitor on enzyme activity (+ means with inhibitor)

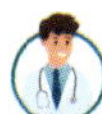
Clinical Correlation

Drugs as Competitive Inhibitors

*Due to their structural similarity with the substrate, several drugs are used as inhibitors of the enzyme in a particular metabolic pathway. For example, **sulfanilamide** (a sulfa drug) is an antibacterial agent and resembles **p-aminobenzoic acid**, structurally. It is used as a **competitive inhibitor of** the enzyme **dihydropteroic acid synthase** in bacteria. Similarly, **methotrexate**, a structural analog of folate, competitively inhibits **dihydrofolate reductase** and is used in the treatment of childhood leukemias (Fig. 5.3).*

Fig. 5.3: Substrates and their structural analogs used as competitive inhibitors

Table 5.6 lists some of the competitive inhibitors and the enzymes inhibited by them.

TABLE 5.6: Some enzymes, their substrates and competitive inhibitors

Enzyme	Substrate	Competitive inhibitor
Succinate dehydrogenase	Succinate	Malonate
Carbonic anhydrase	Carbonate	Acetazolamide
Dihydrofolate reductase	Dihydrofolate	Amethopterin (methotrexate)
L-histidase	L-Histidine	D-Histidine
Xanthine oxidase	Hypoxanthine	Allopurinol
HMG CoA reductase	HMG CoA	HMG

Noncompetitive Inhibition

Several **substances react covalently with the functional groups that** are present on the active site **of the enzyme** and thus inactivate the enzyme, non-competitively. For example, enzymes which have free SH-groups in their molecules are inhibited by substances like iodoacetate or *p*-chloromercuribenzoate that bind SH-groups and inactivate the enzyme. Heavy metals like Hg^{2+} and Ag^+ also inactivate some of the enzymes. This type of inhibition is usually irreversible and makes active sites of the enzyme ineffective.

A **noncompetitive inhibitor** may also **bind at a site other than the substrate-binding site**. In such cases, either the enzyme or the enzyme-substrate complex binds the inhibitor. As a result, both binary (EI) as well as ternary (ESI) complexes are formed. ESI may break down to form a product but at a slower rate, a reversible noncompetitive inhibitor thus **decreases V_{max}** but **does not change the K_m** (Fig. 5.4).

Some antimetabolites act as noncompetitive inhibitors.

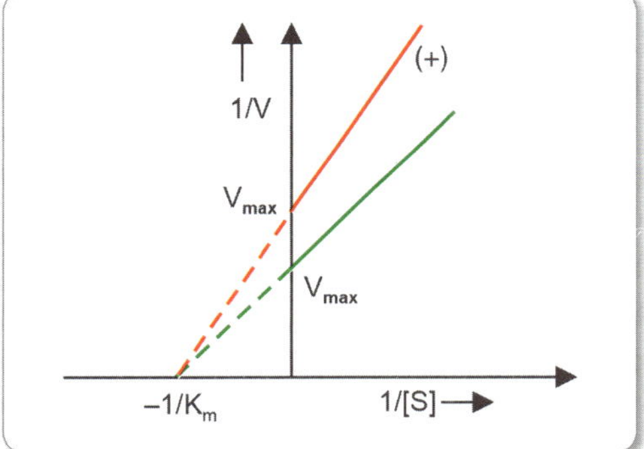

Fig. 5.4: Effect of a noncompetitive inhibitor on enzyme activity (+ means with inhibitor)

REGULATION OF ENZYME ACTIVITY

Regulation of the enzyme activity is essential for the coordination of numerous metabolic processes. Besides changes in the substrate concentration, enzyme activity is also regulated by modifying the activity of the existing enzyme molecules by a number of processes which include allosteric regulation, covalent modifications and induction/repression.

Allosteric Regulation

Oligomeric enzymes, having two or more subunits, have two different sites, which are called the **catalytic site** or regulatory site (also known as the **allosteric site)** and the **substrate-binding site** (active site). These two sites are **located apart from each other on two different subunits of the oligomeric enzymes**. Such enzymes are called **allosteric enzymes or regulatory enzymes**. Allosteric enzymes frequently catalyze the committed

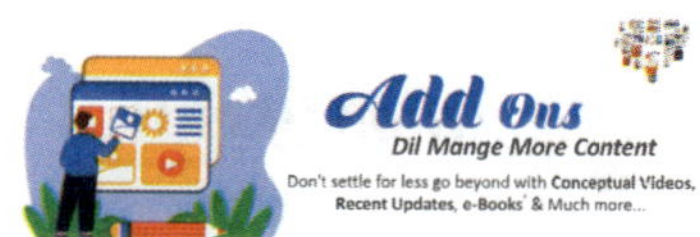

step that is generally present in the beginning of the pathway. For example, HMG CoA reductase (a regulatory enzyme of cholesterol biosynthesis), aspartate transcarbamoylase (of pyrimidine synthesis), etc.

Certain substances, called **allosteric modulators or effectors**, bind reversibly to such an enzyme at the allosteric site and regulate its activity. An interaction with the effector molecule brings about conformational changes at the catalytic site of the enzyme. An **effector molecule may** either **activate an enzymatic reaction (called positive effector or allosteric activator)** or **inhibit it (called allosteric inhibitor)**, and is referred to as allosteric regulator.

Due to interaction between the substrate and the activator/inhibitor, a characteristic **sigmoid curve** (S-shaped curve) is obtained. Presence of an **allosteric activator (+) shifts** the **curve to the right** whereas an allosteric inhibitor (–) **shifts the curve to the left** (Fig. 5.6).

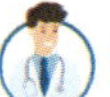 ## Clinical Correlation

Antimetabolites

Certain derivatives of purines and pyrimidines, called **antimetabolites,** *act as noncompetitive inhibitors and are used as chemotherapeutic agents, e.g.,* **5-fluorouracil.** *It is an analog of* **thymine** *but inhibits* **thymidylate synthetase, noncompetitively** *(Fig. 5.5).*

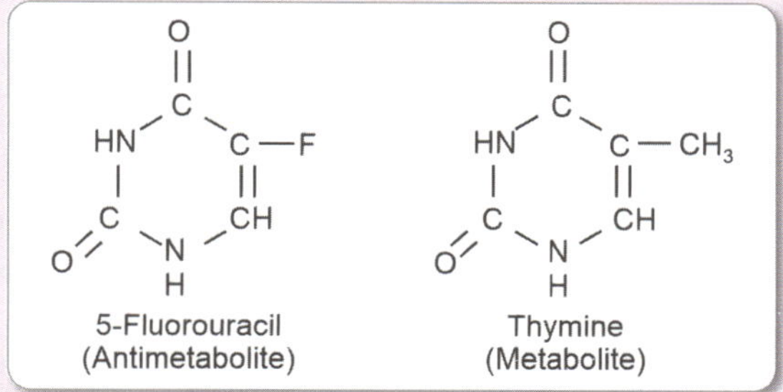

Fig. 5.5: Thymine and its analog 5-fluorouracil (an antimetabolite, which is used as a noncompetitive inhibitor)

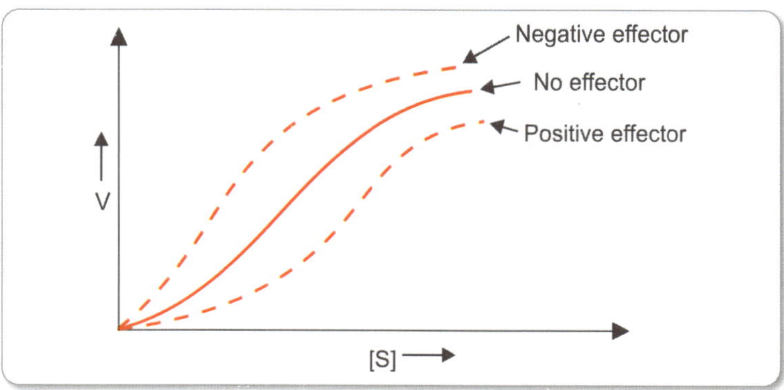

Fig. 5.6: Effect of an allosteric activator/inhibitor on enzyme activity

Table 5.7 lists some of the enzymes that are allosterically regulated along with their allosteric activators/inhibitors.

TABLE 5.7: Some allosteric enzymes with their allosteric activators/inhibitors

Enzyme	Allosteric activator	Allosteric inhibitor
Hexokinase	ADP	Glucose-6-P, ATP
Isocitrate dehydrogenase	ADP	Glucose-6-P, ATP
Glutamate dehydrogenase	ADP	ATP, NADH
Pyruvate carboxylase	Acetyl CoA	ADP

Covalent Modifications

Several enzymes are regulated by covalent modification, most frequently by the addition or removal of a phosphate group from serine, threonine or tyrosine residues of the enzyme. Protein kinases catalyze phosphorylation of enzymes while phosphoprotein phosphatases remove phosphate groups from the phosphorylated enzymes. Depending upon the specific enzyme, either the phosphorylated (such as for glycogen phosphorylase) or the dephosphorylated (e.g., glycogen synthase) enzyme is active.

Induction/Repression

Cells can also regulate the amount of an enzyme, usually by altering its rate of synthesis. Increased (**induction**) or decreased (**repression**) synthesis of the enzyme in turn regulates its activity. Enzymes that are required only at one stage of development or under selected physiological conditions are regulated in this way. For example, elevated levels of insulin, as a result of high blood glucose level, cause increased synthesis of the key enzymes that are involved in glucose utilization.

Units of Enzyme Activity

Amount of an enzyme in any sample of a biological fluid, such as serum, or tissue is measured in terms of the rate of reaction catalyzed and is directly proportional to quantity of the enzyme present in the sample. The result is expressed in terms of **enzyme units**. Thus, **unit of an enzyme activity** is a measure of the rate at which a reaction proceeds, e.g., quantity of the substrate consumed or product formed, in mg or micromoles, or change in absorbance, etc., in a unit time (second, minute or hour). In clinical chemistry, result of the enzyme activity is, generally, expressed in a fixed volume, such as per 100 mL (dL) or per liter (L) of serum.

Historically, different types of units have been introduced by different workers, e.g., King-Armstrong units (KA units) and Bodansky units for alkaline and acid phosphatases; Somogyi units for amylase, etc. These units, however, are still in use, in some labs.

International units

As per Enzyme Commission of the International Union of Biochemistry (IUB), enzyme activity is expressed in terms of **international units** (IU). An IU is defined as quantity of the enzyme which catalyzes reaction using 1 mmol of the substrate or formation of the product that is transformed per minute (1 mmol/min). This is expressed in terms of a fixed volume, e.g., IU/L.

SI units

To overcome the problem of different units being reported by different laboratories, in different countries, IUB suggested SI units (Systeme Internationale de units, i.e., International System of units). According to it, mole is a measure of the substrate transformed while second is the unit of time. Further, it has been recommended that enzyme activity should be expressed in terms of katal, which is defined as moles/second. It is further recommended that the enzyme concentration should be expressed in terms of katal per liter (kat/L).

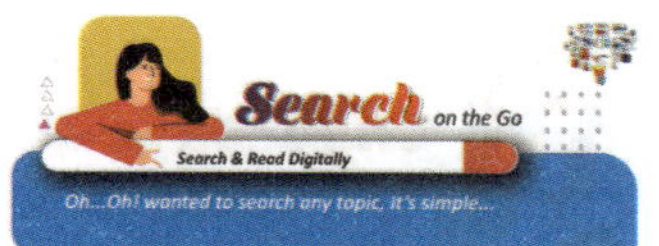

ISOENZYMES

The **enzymes that occur in a number of different forms** and **differ from each other chemically**, **immunologically** and **electrophoretically** are called isoenzymes or **isozymes** (or more generally as **multiple forms of an enzyme**). Isozymes are present in the serum and tissues of mammals, amphibians, birds, insects, plants and unicellular organisms.

Properties of Isoenzymes

- Isoenzymes are the **multiple forms of an enzyme** that **have different amino acid sequences** and, therefore, **different shapes**, **sizes** and **electrical charges**, but **perform the same function**. So, they catalyze the same reaction but can be distinguished by physical methods, such as electrophoresis, or by immunological methods.

- They display **different kinetic parameters** as well as **regulatory properties**. For example, isozymes have **different K_M** and **V_{max}** values, and can be distinguished from one another by biochemical properties such as electrophoretic mobility.

- The difference between some isozymes is **due to differences in the quaternary structure of the enzymes**, e.g., lactate dehydrogenase (LDH) exists in five isozymic forms. The isozymic forms of LDH are tetramers; each is made up from two types of units H and M. Only the tetrameric molecule possesses catalytic activity. The subunits are expressed in the following 5 ways, i.e., HHHH (H_4), HHHM (H_3M), HHMM (H_2M_2), HMMM (HM_3) and MMMM (M_4).

- Isozymes are **encoded by different genes** and **expressed in a distinct organelle**, or **at a distinct stage of development**. Different isozymes appear in specific regions of the body; differing in specifics organelles or tissues. The purpose of isozymes is to allow fine adjustment of metabolism to meet the need of different development stages and help the different tissues and organs function properly depending on their physiology make up and in what kind of environment which they function. For example, the isoenzymes of lactate dehydrogenase in animal organs are different in term of their amino acid sequences and the level of their expression. The level of the different isozymes in a certain organ is related to the level of oxygen supply.

- Isozymes in general can be used **to meet the metabolic needs of different tissues and developmental stages**, e.g., LDH. LDH is used to catalyze the synthesis of glucose in anaerobic metabolism of glucose. As discussed above, its isozymes are divided into two forms, i.e., the H isozyme and the M isozyme. The H isozyme is expressed more in the heart, whereas the M isozyme is expressed more frequently in the skeletal muscle. Both isozymes have two polypeptide chains, and each isozyme share 75% of the amino acid sequence for the chains. Both isozymes metabolize glucose, but the difference is that the H isozymes have a higher affinity for their substrates than the M isozyme. Another difference is that the H isozyme functions better in aerobic environments such as the heart, whereas the M isozyme functions better in anaerobic environments such as the muscle, where strenuous activity may deplete the oxygen supplies.

- Isozymes may also be **utilized to diagnose tissue damage** such as damaged heart muscle cells during a heart attack or myocardial infarction. When heart muscle cells are damaged, they release the cellular material such as the H isozyme. When taking blood samples, if the H isozymes appear in increased levels, then there is a possibility that the heart cells are damaged.

Some Isoenzymes of Clinical Significance

Lactate Dehydrogenase

Lactate dehydrogenase **is a tetramer**, i.e., it **has four polypeptide subunits**. Its each subunit may be one of the two types, known as the H (heart) type and the M (muscle) type. **LDH** thus exists in serum in **five distinct forms** (isoenzymes) with different proportions of the H and the M subunits. **LDH_1 has four polypeptide chains of the H type (H_4)** while **LDH_5 has four subunits of the M type (M_4)**. Other forms include LDH_2 (H_3M), LDH_3 (H_2M_2) and LDH_4 (HM_3).

LDH_1 and LDH_2 are **predominant in the myocardium** and erythrocytes while LDH_4 and LDH_5 are predominant in liver and skeletal muscle. LDH_1 **increases between 12 and 24 hours following myocardial infarction**. LDH_5 is diagnostic of secondary congestive liver involvement.

Creatine Phosphokinase

Creatine phosphokinase **(CPK)**, also referred to as **creatine kinase (CK)** has **three isoenzymes**. Each of its **isoenzyme** is a **dimer,** i.e., **composed of two subunits** which may either be of M (muscle) type or B (brain) type. Hence it has **three isoenzymes** which are called CPK_1 **(CK_1 or CK-BB)** that is mainly **found in the brain**; CPK_2 **(CK-MB) found in the myocardium**; and CPK_3 **(CK-MM) found in skeletal muscle**.

Normally, **CK-MB** is present in very small amount in serum. Its **level rises within 4 hours**, reaching a maximum value within 1 day, **of myocardial infarction**.

Alkaline Phosphatase

Alkaline phosphatase **exists in three forms.** Different tissues contain a distinct form of the enzyme. **Major portion** of the enzyme in serum is **from liver** whose level **rises in post-hepatic jaundice**.

In **growing children**, the serum enzyme is **mainly from bone** and is related to **increased osteoblastic activity**.

During the last trimester of **pregnancy**, there is an increase in serum alkaline phosphatase, which is primarily of the **placental origin**. This form of the enzyme is heat-stable; hence, placental enzyme is also called **heat-stable alkaline phosphatase**.

ENZYMES OF DIAGNOSTIC IMPORTANCE

Measurement of certain enzymes in serum is helpful in the diagnosis of various diseases. The level of a particular enzyme increases in serum when it is released in large amounts due to the damage to the tissue. Several of these enzymes also have a prognostic significance. Some of the enzymes, which have diagnostic importance, include transaminases, alkaline phosphatase, etc.

Some enzymes of diagnostic importance along with their principal tissue of origin and clinical applications are listed in Table 5.8.

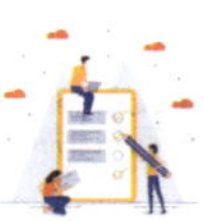
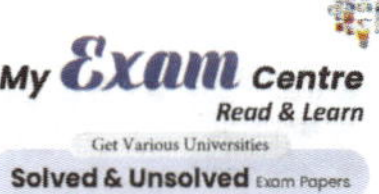

TABLE 5.8: Some enzymes of diagnostic importance

Enzyme	Principal source	Clinical situation in which altered
Acid phosphatase	Prostate and RBC	**Increases** in carcinoma of prostate
Alkaline phosphatase	Liver, bone, placenta and kidney	**Increases** in obstructive jaundice, rickets, Paget's disease and hyperparathyroidism
Aldolase	Skeletal muscle and heart	**Increases** in muscular dystrophies and acute liver diseases
Amylase	Salivary glands, pancreas and ovaries	**Increases** in acute pancreatitis, intestinal obstruction and acute parotitis. **Decreases** in acute liver diseases
Ceruloplasmin	Liver	**Increases** in cirrhosis. **Decreases** in Wilson's disease
Choline esterase	Liver	**Increases** in nephrotic syndrome and organophosphorus poisoning. **Decreases** in acute liver diseases
Creatine phosphokinase	Skeletal muscle, brain and heart	**Increases** in myocardial infarction and muscular dystrophies
Glutamate oxaloacetate transaminase (GPT)	Liver, skeletal muscle, heart, kidney and RBCs	**Increases** in myocardial infarction, toxic liver cell necrosis, acute liver diseases, and muscle diseases
γ-glutamyl transferase	Liver and kidney	**Increases** in alcoholism and hepatobiliary diseases
Lactate dehydrogenase	Heart, liver, skeletal muscle, RBCs and platelets	**Increases** in acute myocardial infarction, acute hepatitis, and muscle disorders
Lipase	Pancreas	**Increases** in acute pancreatitis and pancreatic carcinoma. **Decreases** in liver diseases and diabetes mellitus
5'-nucleotidase	Hepatobiliary tract	**Increases** in liver diseases, obstructive jaundice and hepatic carcinoma
Trypsin	Pancreas	**Increases** in acute pancreatic diseases

Enzymes of Diagnostic Importance in Liver Diseases

Alanine Transaminase and Aspartate Transaminase

Alanine Transaminase (**ALT**; also called alanine aminotransferase; glutamic pyruvic transaminase or GPT; serum glutamic pyruvic transaminase or SGPT) and aspartate transaminase (**AST**; also known as aspartate aminotransferase; glutamic oxaloacetic transaminase or GOT; serum glutamic oxaloacetic transaminase or SGOT), are pyridoxal phosphate (PLP)-dependent transaminases. While **ALT catalyzes** the reversible transfer of an α-amino group between **alanine** and **glutamate**, **AST** catalyzes the reversible transfer of an α-amino group between **aspartate** and **glutamate** and, as such, both the enzymes are important in amino acid metabolism.

In healthy individuals, **ALT** is found **predominantly in the liver** with clinically negligible quantities found in the kidneys, heart and skeletal muscle. On the other hand, **AST** is found **in the** liver, **heart (cardiac muscle), skeletal muscle**, kidneys, brain and red blood cells. Thus, ALT is similar to AST in the way that both the enzymes are associated with liver parenchymal cells.

The difference, however, is that **ALT is a more specific indicator of liver inflammation** than AST, as **AST** may also be **elevated in diseases** affecting other organs, **such as** myocardial infarction, acute pancreatitis, acute hemolytic anemia, severe burns, acute renal disease, musculoskeletal diseases and trauma.

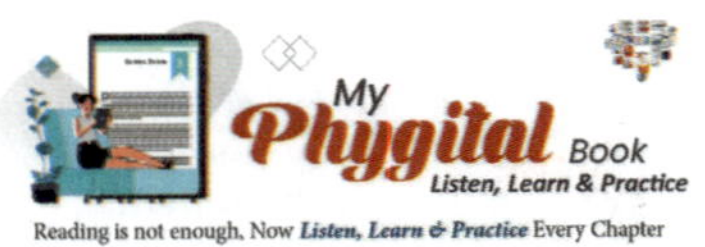

Normally, levels of AST in the blood are low, however, when liver or muscle cells are injured, they release AST into the blood. This makes AST also a useful test for detecting or monitoring liver damage. Therefore, **AST** is usually measured together **with ALT** to check **for liver problems**. Thus, **serum ALT** and **AST levels** as well as their ratio (**AST/ALT ratio**) are commonly measured as **biomarkers** for liver health.

Both, the enzymes (**ALT** and **AST**) are **raised** when there is a **liver injury** or **inflammation**. These enzymes may also be raised in, both, **alcoholic** and **nonalcoholic fatty liver diseases.** Their levels are also elevated in **viral hepatitis** and other forms of a liver disease that may be associated with **hepatic necrosis**, even before the clinical signs and symptoms of the disease appear. Under these conditions, levels of both the enzymes may reach the values as high as 100 times of the upper normal limits. Peak values are observed between day seven and day twelve in viral hepatitis. Thereafter, their activities gradually decrease and reach towards normal by third to fifth week of recovery. Five to ten-fold increase in both the enzymes occur in patients with primary metastatic carcinoma of the liver.

Reference range	
ALT (SGPT)	8–56 IU/L
AST (SGOT)	8–40 IU/L

Alkaline Phosphatase

Alkaline phosphatase (**ALP**) or **basic phosphatase** is **optimally active at alkaline pH** (pH 9–10).

ALP is found in many tissues, with the **highest concentration** in the **liver, biliary tract** and **bone**. This test may be performed to **assess liver functioning and to detect liver lesions that may cause biliary obstruction such as tumor or abscess. As biliary obstruction results in induction of the enzyme, rise is more** marked in extrahepatic obstruction than in intrahepatic obstruction. In intrahepatic obstruction of the bile, flow increase in serum ALP is nearly 2–3 times of the upper normal limit.

High levels of ALP may indicate **liver inflammation, blockage of the bile duct** or a **bone disease**. **Children** and **adolescents** may have elevated levels of ALP because their bones are growing. ALP level is also increased in **pregnancy**.

Reference range
Up to 120 U/L in adults

Gamma-glutamyltransferase

Gamma-glutamyltransferase, also referred to as γ-**glutamyltranspeptidase (γ-GT or GGT)** is an enzyme that catalyses the **transfer of γ-glutamyl group from peptides**, and compounds, **to some acceptor** that may be the substrate itself, some amino acid or peptide, or even water.

GGT is **present in proximal renal tubules, liver, pancreas** and **intestine**. GGT, although, primarily, originates from the hepatobiliary system, its activity in serum comes from the liver. So, its activity is increased in all types of liver diseases. However, it is present in high concentration in the serum in intrahepatic or posthepatic biliary obstruction. Accordingly, it is a sensitive indicator of the presence of hepatobiliary disease and the test is, often, performed to assess liver function, to provide information about the liver diseases and to detect alcohol ingestion.

High elevations are observed in primary and metastatic liver neoplasms, whereas moderate elevation (2–5 times the normal value) is seen in infectious hepatitis.

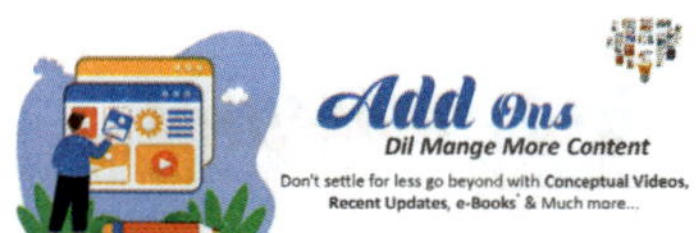

GGT is of special significance in detecting an **alcohol-induced liver disease**, since its levels are significantly increased in patients with **alcoholic cirrhosis** as well as in people who are **heavy drinkers**.

> **Reference range**
>
> 5–35 U/L

Enzymes of Diagnostic Importance in Myocardial Infarction

Most of the early markers of myocardial infarction include CPK (and its isoenzyme CPK-MB), AST and LDH. Besides, cardiac troponins (troponin I and T), though not enzymes, are also important markers of myocardial infarction.

Creatine Phosphokinase

Creatine phosphokinase **(CPK)** or **creatine kinase (CK)**, also known as **phosphocreatine kinase**, is an enzyme expressed by various tissues and cell types. It catalyzes the conversion of creatine, and utilizes ATP to form phosphocreatine and ADP. This reaction is reversible and, thus, ATP can be generated from phosphocreatine and ADP. In tissues and cells that consume ATP rapidly, especially, skeletal muscle and smooth muscle, phosphocreatine serves as an energy reservoir for the rapid buffering and regeneration of ATP *in situ*, as well as for intracellular energy transport by the phosphocreatine shuttle. Thus, CK is an important enzyme in such tissues.

The CK is assayed in blood tests as a marker of the damage of the CK-rich tissues, such as in **myocardial infarction** and **muscular dystrophies**. Increased levels are also seen in polymyositis, motor neuron disease and in acute cerebrovascular accidents.

As discussed above, CK has 3 isoenzymes, out of which CPK-MB (CK_2 or CK-MB) is predominant in cardiac muscle. **Measurement of CK-MB, in serum, is used in the diagnosis of acute MI**, where initial rise occurs within 4–6 hours. Peak levels are observed after approximately 24 hours and return towards normal within 48–72 hours. The areas under the peak and the slope of the initial rise are proportional to the size of the infarct. In such patients, CK-MB isoenzyme, usually, exceeds 6% of the total activity. In patients of MI, though, first rise is seen within 6 hours after the onset of symptoms but for diagnosis with high specificity and sensitivity, serial sampling, over a period of 8–12 hours is required.

> **Reference range for creatine kinase**
>
> - **Men:** 20–50 IU
> - **Women:** 10–37 IU

> **Reference range for CK-MB**
>
> 0–24 IU

Aspartate Aminotransferase

After **myocardial infarction** (MI), **increased AST** (and also ALT) activity appears **in serum**, as its concentration is highest in the cardiac muscle. Since ALT concentration is less than that of AST in the cardiac muscle, there is comparatively lesser rise in ALT.

Peak level of AST is reached after 18–24 hours and returns towards normal by fourth or fifth day.

Lactate Dehydrogenase

Lactate dehydrogenase (**LDH** or **LD**) is an enzyme involved in energy production and catalyzes the conversion of lactate to pyruvate and back. It is found in almost all the body's cells, with the highest level found in cells of the heart, liver, muscles, kidneys, lungs and blood cells.

Elevated levels of LDH in blood, usually, **indicate some type of tissue damage**. LDH levels are elevated in a wide variety of conditions, reflecting its widespread tissue distribution. An elevated level of LDH may be seen in patients with hemolytic anemia, pernicious anemia (megaloblastic anemia), infections such as infectious mononucleosis, meningitis, encephalitis and HIV; sepsis, intestinal and lung (pulmonary) infarction, acute kidney disease, acute liver disease, acute muscle injury, pancreatitis, bone fractures, testicular cancer, lymphoma and other cancers.

LDH also has a **diagnostic significance in MI**. Rise in serum LDH starts 12–18 hours after the onset of acute MI with a peak after 48–72 hours. Levels return towards normal after 6–10 days.

As discussed above, LDH has 5 isoenzymes, out of which LDH_1 or **LD_1 is predominant in myocardium**. Rise in total LDH, in patients with MI, parallels a rise in LDH_1. **Total LDH** as well as **LDH_1** (H4) levels are significantly increased in patients with MI. LDH_1 becomes greater than LDH_2 between 12–24 hours following myocardial infarction with peak after 48–72 hours. The levels return towards normal after 6–10 days.

Low levels are, sometimes, seen when someone ingests **large amount of ascorbic acid** (vitamin C).

Reference range for CK-MB

70–240 IU

Cardiac Troponins

Troponin (or the **troponin complex**) is a component of the thin filaments (along with actin and tropomyosin) and is the protein complex to which calcium binds to trigger the production of muscular force. It is integral to muscle contraction in skeletal muscle and cardiac muscle, but not smooth muscle. Troponin has three subunits, i.e., troponin-C (TnC), troponin-I (TnI) and troponin-T (TnT), each play a role in force regulation. Individual subunits serve different functions:

- **TnT is a tropomyosin-binding subunit**. It regulates the interaction of troponin complex with thin filaments, interlocking them to form a troponin-tropomyosin complex.
- **TnI inhibits ATPase activity of actomyosin**. It binds to actin in thin myofilaments, to hold the troponin-tropomyosin complex in place.
- **TnC is a Ca^{2+}-binding subunit**. It binds to calcium ions, to produce a conformational change in TnI, thereby, playing a main role in Ca^{2+}-dependent regulation of muscle contraction.

Troponin-I and **troponin-T** are found in the **heart muscle** and are released into blood when there is damage to the heart. Though, troponin tests are, generally, ordered along with other cardiac markers, such as CK-MB, however, troponin is the preferred test for a suspected heart attack, because it is more specific for heart injury than other tests (which may also be elevated in patients with skeletal muscle injury) and remain elevated for a longer period. So, troponin tests are, primarily, done to help diagnose a heart attack and rule out other conditions with similar signs and symptoms, such as chest pain that may be due to other causes. Either a troponin-I or troponin-T test can be performed. The concentrations are different but they, basically, provide the same information.

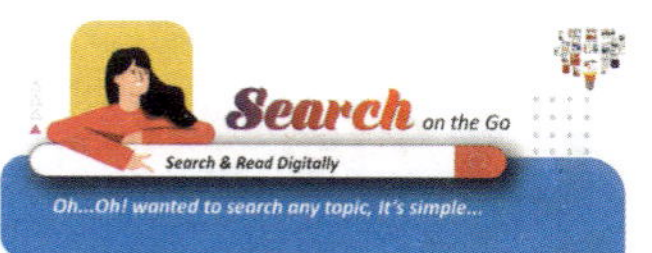

Troponin proteins are released when the heart muscle has been damaged, such as occurs with a heart attack. The more damage there is to the heart, the greater the amount of troponin-T and troponin-I will be in the blood. So, serial sampling is required. Test may also be done to evaluate people with angina, if their signs and symptoms worsen. Both the proteins are now widely used to diagnose acute myocardial infarction (AMI), unstable angina, postsurgery myocardium trauma and some other diseases related with cardiac muscle injury.

Cardiac troponins (troponin-I and troponin-T) levels **rise within 4–6 hours of MI**, reaching peak level within 16–30 hours. Elevated concentration of TnI and TnT in blood samples can be detected even 5–8 days after onset of the symptoms, making both the proteins useful for the late diagnosis of AMI.

> **Reference range of TnI**
> 0–1.5 ng/mL

Enzymes of Diagnostic Importance in Muscle Diseases

Creatine Kinase

As discussed above, CK catalyzes the production of high-energy adenosine triphosphate (ATP) *via* transfer of a phosphate from creatine phosphate, which is the major storage reservoir of energy during muscle rest, to adenosine diphosphate (ADP). The enzyme is located on the inner mitochondrial membrane on myofibrils and in the muscle cytoplasm.

Creatine kinase (CK) is the most widely used enzyme to diagnose and follow muscle disease. It is present in the highest concentrations in serum in response to muscle injury. It is the most sensitive indicator of muscle injury, and is the best measure of the course of muscle injury.

Measurement of the serum CK level is traditionally the first step in the assessment of patients with a muscle disease. In comparison with other serum muscle enzymes, CK appears to be a relatively specific and sensitive indicator of the degree of muscle fiber injury. **In skeletal muscle, the CK_3** (MM form) **predominates** (90–95%), whereas immature muscle may have increased concentrations of the MB form (20–30% in children younger than 1 year of age). It is the CK_3 activity, which is **markedly elevated in a muscle disease**.

Aldolase

Aldolase is a key enzyme of glycolysis, as well as in the reverse pathway (gluconeogenesis). It catalyzes the reversible conversion of fructose-1,6-bisphosphate to glyceraldehydes-3-phosphate and dihydroxyacetone phosphate. As a result, it is a crucial player in ATP biosynthesis. Aldolase A also contributes to other functions such as muscle maintenance, regulation of cell shape and motility, striated muscle contraction, actin cytoskeleton organization and regulation of cell proliferation. It is ubiquitously expressed in most tissues, though it is predominantly expressed in developing embryo and adult muscle.

Elevated serum aldolase levels may indicate damage to different organ systems.

Elevated aldolase is usually a **sign of muscle** or **liver damage**. Aldolase level is an early, but nonspecific, marker of a muscle disease, e.g., muscle damage from a heart attack releases aldolase in large quantities. Liver damage, such as hepatitis or cirrhosis, raises aldolase levels as well. It can also be used to assess rare genetic disorders of the skeletal muscles, such as dermatomyositis and polymyositis. Exercise can also affect aldolase test results.

Higher or abnormal levels may be due to health conditions, including muscle damage, dermatomyositis, viral hepatitis, cancers of the liver, pancreas or prostate, muscular dystrophy, heart attack, polymyositis, leukemia and gangrene. At first, muscle destruction causes higher aldolase levels. However, aldolase levels actually decline as the amount of muscle in the body decreases.

Low aldolase levels can be seen in people with fructose intolerance, muscle-wasting disease and late stage muscular dystrophy.

> **Reference range**
>
> For people up to 16 years age—14.5 U/L
> For people 17 years old and up—1.0–7.5 U/L

Enzymes of Diagnostic Importance in Bone Diseases

Alkaline Phosphatase

As discussed above, alkaline phosphatase (**ALP**) is **found in many tissues**, with the highest concentrations in the **liver, biliary tract** and **bone. High levels of ALP may indicate** liver inflammation, blockage of the bile ducts, or **a bone disease. Children and adolescents may have elevated levels of ALP because their bones are growing.**

Condition of abnormal ALP levels may indicate less regularly include rickets (a weakening of the bones in children, usually as a result of a vitamin D or calcium deficiency), osteomalacia (a weakening of the bones in adults, usually relating to vitamin D deficiency) and Paget's disease (a condition that causes significant bone deformity and problems with bone regeneration).

> **Reference range**
>
> **Up to 120 U/L** in adults

Enzymes of Diagnostic Importance in Prostate Cancer

Prostate-specific Antigen

Prostate-specific antigen (PSA) is a protein produced by normal, as well as malignant cells of the prostate gland. The prostate is a small gland that is part of a man's reproductive system. It is located below the bladder and makes a fluid that is part of semen. PSA is a substance made by the prostate.

Men normally have low PSA levels in their blood. The blood level of PSA is often **elevated in men with prostate cancer**. In addition to prostate cancer, a number of benign (noncancerous) conditions can cause a man's PSA level to rise. The most frequent benign prostate conditions that cause an elevation in PSA level are prostatitis (inflammation of the prostate) and benign prostatic hyperplasia (BPH, i.e., enlargement of the prostate). Also, PSA levels normally increase with age.

Free versus total PSA—The amount of PSA in the blood that is free (not bound to other proteins) divided by the total amount of PSA (free plus bound) is denoted as the proportion of free PSA. Some evidence suggests that a lower proportion of free PSA may be associated with more aggressive cancer.

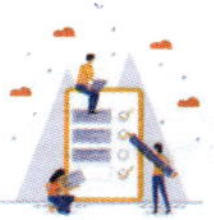
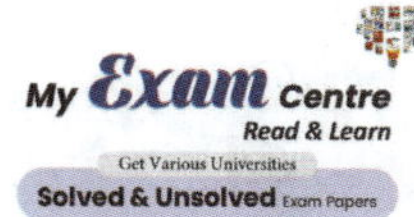

Certain drugs used to treat BPH or urinary conditions, and large doses of certain chemotherapy medications, may lower PSA levels. Obesity can also lower PSA levels.

> **Reference range**
> <4.0 ng/mL

Acid Phosphatase

Acid phosphatase **(ACP)** is an enzyme that liberates phosphate under acidic conditions **(optimum pH of 4.9)**. It is made in the liver, spleen, bone marrow and prostate gland.

Abnormally **high serum levels of acid phosphatase** may indicate infection, injury, or **cancer of the prostate**. It is released into the circulation in metastatic cancer of the prostate and that prostate acid phosphatase has been used extensively as a serum marker for cancer of the prostate.

> **Reference range**
> Up to 3 U/L

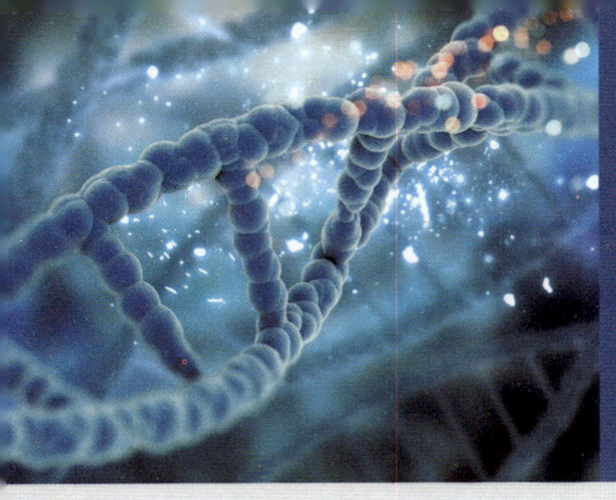

LONG AND SHORT ANSWER QUESTIONS

1. What are enzymes? Classify them. Discuss factors affecting enzyme activity.
2. Define enzyme, coenzyme and cofactor. Discuss role of B complex vitamins as coenzymes.
3. Define an enzyme. What are isoenzymes? Discuss importance of enzymes in clinical diagnosis.
4. What are allosteric enzymes? How their activity is modulated? Give examples.
5. Give brief account of factors affecting enzyme activity.
6. **Discuss briefly:**
   a. Various types of enzyme inhibition, giving examples.
   b. Apoenzyme, holoenzyme and coenzyme with examples.
   c. Classify enzymes giving examples.
7. **Write notes on:**
   a. Diagnostic significance of enzymes
   b. Noncompetitive inhibition of enzyme activity
   c. Isoenzymes and their importance
   d. Proenzymes
   e. Competitive inhibitors
   f. Enzyme specificity
   g. Coenzymes
   h. Classification of enzymes
   i. Ribozymes
   j. Allosteric regulation
   k. Covalent modification of enzyme activity
   l. Induction and repression of enzyme activity

MULTIPLE CHOICE QUESTIONS

1. **Hexokinase is a:**
   a. Ligase
   b. Transferase
   c. Oxidoreductase
   d. Lyase

2. **Tyrosinase is a:**
   a. Oxidase
   b. Transferase
   c. Lyase
   d. Isomerase

3. **Coenzymes are _____________ organic compounds:**
   a. Lipoprotein
   b. Proteinaceous
   c. Non proteinaceous
   d. None of these

4. **All are true regarding competitive inhibition, except:**
    a. Inhibitor molecules compete with normal substrate
    b. Is usually irreversible
    c. Inhibitor is a structural analogue of substrate
    d. K_m increase in presence of competitive inhibitor

Notes

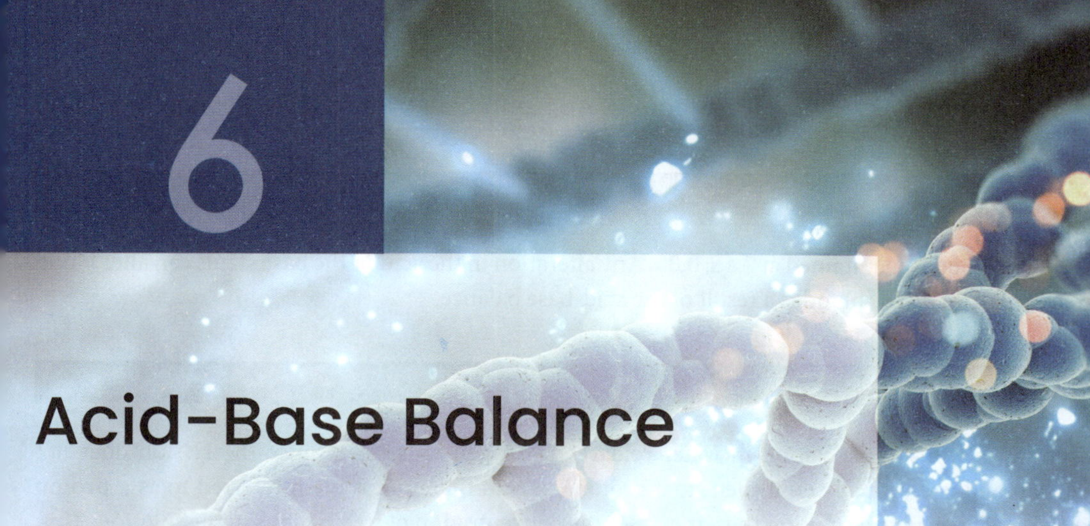

6

Acid-Base Balance

LEARNING OBJECTIVES

After the completion of the chapter, the readers will be able to:
- Explain acid-base balance, imbalance and its clinical significance.
- Explain pH, buffers and regulation of blood pH.
- Name the components of arterial blood gases.
- Explain the acid-base disorders.

CHAPTER OUTLINE

- Introduction
- Acids
- Bases
- Amphoteric Substances
- pH
- Buffers
- Regulation of Blood pH
- Arterial Blood Gases
- Acid-base Disorders

KEY TERMS

Amphipathic: A chemical compound containing both polar (water-soluble) and nonpolar (not water-soluble) portions in its structure, such as a phospholipid.

Amphoteric substances: A molecule or ion that can act both as an acid and as a base such as an amino acid.

INTRODUCTION

Normal pH of the blood is maintained at 7.4 ± 0.05. Any alteration in the acid or the base status can alter blood pH. Maintenance of the pH of blood is a result of the acid-base balance.

ACIDS

Acid is a substance whose dissociation in water **releases hydrogen ions** (H^+). Since the H^+ ion does not contain neutron and is essentially equivalent to a proton, an acid therefore is often referred to as a **proton donor**. Addition of an acid to a solution thus, increases the concentration of free H^+ ions in the solution. This, in turn, produces a more acidic solution and results in a **decrease in pH**.

An acid, e.g., HA, in aqueous solution reversibly dissociates into **H^+ ion** and a **conjugate base (A^-)**. This dissociation of HA thus can be represented symbolically by the following equation:

$$HA \longrightarrow H^+ + A^-$$

where A^- represents an anion (a conjugate base) that remains when H^+ (a cation) is released. This tendency of an acid to give up H^+ ions depends upon its strength.

- A **strong acid** such as HCl completely dissociates in an aqueous solution as follows:

$$HCl \longrightarrow H^+ + Cl^-$$

- On the other hand, a **weak acid** gives up H^+ ions less rapidly and does not dissociate completely. A solution of a weak acid thus, contains both dissociated ions as well as undissociated molecule. Most of the acids produced in the living systems are weak acids.

BASES

A base **releases hydroxyl ions** (OH^-) in an aqueous solution and **decreases its H^+ ions concentration** by accepting or binding with the free H^+ ions. This in turn results in **increase in pH** of the solution.

A strong base such as sodium hydroxide (NaOH) dissociates completely as follows:

$$NaOH \longrightarrow Na^+ + OH^-$$

The OH^- ions, so produced, accept H^+ ions and result in the formation of water. This in turn, lowers the concentration of the H^+ ions in the solution.

$$OH^- + H^+ \rightleftharpoons H_2O$$

A weak base such as bicarbonate (HCO_3^-) can also utilize H^+ ions and thus lowers H^+ ions concentration of the solution.

$$HCO_3^- + H^+ \rightleftharpoons H_2CO_3$$

Amount of an acid or a base is expressed in terms of **equivalents.** One mole of HCl contains one equivalent of acid and neutralizes one equivalent of base. On the other hand, one mole of sulfuric acid (H_2SO_4) contains two equivalents of acid since sulfuric acid can donate two H^+ ions and requires two moles of NaOH to neutralize it.

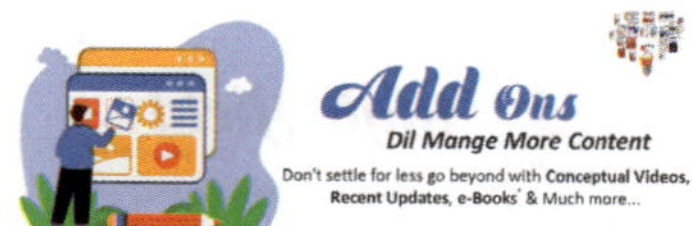

AMPHOTERIC SUBSTANCES

Some substances such as amino acids and proteins can act as **acid** as well as **base**. These substances are referred to as amphoteric substances, e.g., glycine.

$$H_2N - CH_2 - COOH \rightleftharpoons H_3N^+ - CH_2 - COO^-$$

- **It acts as an acid** when its ammonium group donates the H^+ ion:

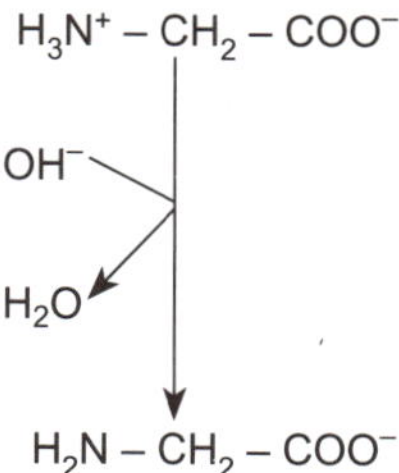

- On the other hand, glycine **acts as a base** when its carboxylate group accepts H^+ ion:

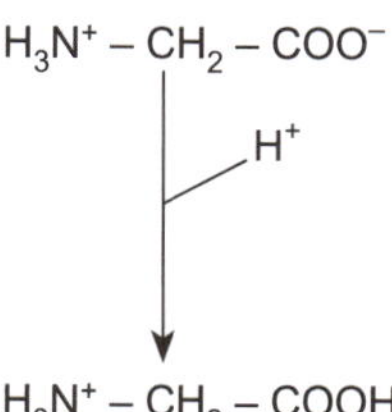

pH

pH is defined as the **negative logarithm to the base 10 of the molar concentration of the hydrogen ions (H^+) in a solution**.

$$pH = - \log [H^+]$$
$$= \log (1/[H^+])$$

The pH of the solution is inversely related to **free H^+ ions concentration**, i.e., $[H^+]$. Low pH indicates high H^+ concentration while high pH indicates low H^+ concentration.

If we add a strong base such as NaOH to water, the OH^- ions from NaOH will combine with the H^+ ions supplied by water. This in turn will shift the equilibrium towards the undissociated water and lower its free H^+ ions concentration thereby resulting in increase in pH.

The **scale of pH measurement** varies from 0 to 14.

If pH of a solution is **below 7**, the solution is said to be **acidic**; if it is equal to **7** it is referred to as **neutral**, and if its pH is **greater than 7** the solution is said to be **alkaline** or basic in nature.

BUFFERS

A buffer is a solution, which **resists change in pH**; i.e., it minimizes the change in the H^+ ions concentration following the addition of an acid or a base.

A buffer can be prepared by mixing **a weak acid**, e.g., HA, **with its conjugate base** (A^-). When a strong acid such as HCl is added to it, the conjugate base A^- reacts with the H^+ ion, neutralizes it and forms HA. On the other hand, if a base is added, HA gets dissociated to give H^+ ions and the conjugate base A^-, as follows:

$$HA \rightleftharpoons H^+ + A^-$$

(Weak acid)   (Proton)   (Salt or conjugate base)

- **Dissociation constant** (Ka) of the weak acid can be expressed as follows:

$$Ka = \frac{[H^+]\,[A^-]}{[HA]}$$

Larger the value of Ka, stronger the acid is, because most of the acid gets dissociated and converted to H^+ and A^-. On the other hand, if the Ka value is small, less acid is dissociated, being a weak acid.

A buffer has maximum **buffering capacity** at its pKa (–log Ka), i.e., when its acidic and basic forms are present in equal concentrations. Its acid (protonated) form reacts with the added base while the basic (unprotonated) form neutralizes the added acid.

The quantitative relationship between the concentration of a weak acid, e.g., HA, and its conjugate base, i.e., A^-, is described by an equation, referred to as **Henderson-Hasselbalch equation.**

Henderson-Hasselbalch Equation

The general dissociation of a weak acid such as a carboxylic acid is given by the equation (1):

$$HA \rightleftharpoons H^+ + A^- \tag{1}$$

where HA is the protonated form or the conjugate acid (associated form) and A^- is the unprotonated form or the conjugate base (the dissociated form).

The dissociation constant (Ka) for such a weak acid is defined as the equilibrium constant for the dissociation reaction of the acid, by equation (2):

$$Ka = \frac{[H^+]\,[A^-]}{[HA]} \tag{2}$$

The hydrogen ion concentration [H^+] of a solution of a weak acid then can be calculated by rearranging this equation, to equation (3):

$$[H^+] = Ka \times \frac{[HA]}{[A^-]} \tag{3}$$

A negative logarithm of the above can be expressed, as equation (4):

$$-\log\,[H^+] = -\log Ka - \log \frac{[HA]}{[A^-]} \tag{4}$$

Since pH is the negative logarithm of [H^+], multiplying the equation (4) by –1, arrives at the equation (5) which is referred to as the Henderson-Hasselbalch equation:

$$pH = pKa + \log \frac{[A^-]}{[HA]} \tag{5}$$

where pH is the negative logarithm of [H^+], i.e., – log [H^+], pKa is equal to the negative logarithm of dissociation constant (Ka), i.e., as – log Ka.

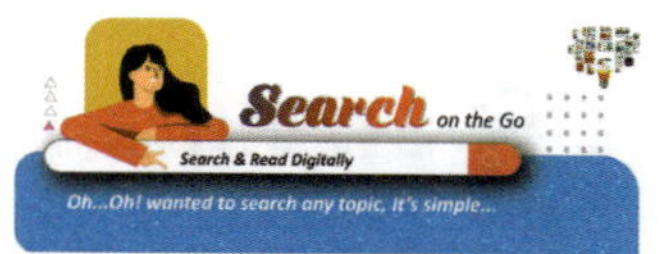

Henderson-Hasselbalch equation can be used for the analysis of acid-base equilibrium systems. The extent of protonation of acidic and basic functional groups and therefore the net charge will vary with the pKa of the functional group and the pH of the solution. For example, for alanine, which has two functional groups with pKa_1 of 2.4 and pKa_2 of 9.8, the net charge varies with pH from −1 to +1. At a point intermediate between the two pKa values (6.2), it has a net zero charge. This pH is called its **isoelectric point** (pI).

The effectiveness of a buffer, in minimizing changes in pH, **depends upon** two factors:

1. **The pK′a of the buffer** in relation to the desired pH, e.g., pK′a of the imidazole group of histidine in hemoglobin is close to 7.4 and thus, it is an ideal buffer in the blood.

2. The **concentration of the buffer:** Greater the concentration of the buffer more is its ability to bind or release H^+.

REGULATION OF BLOOD pH

Metabolism of food consumed in our diet results in the production of CO_2 as well as acids, in the body. For example, most carbohydrates and fats are normally, completely oxidized to CO_2 and water. Metabolism of dietary protein results in the production of strong acids, etc. In the pulmonary capillary blood, CO_2 reacts with water and forms carbonic acid (H_2CO_3). A zinc containing enzyme carbonic anhydrase, which also catalyzes the dissociation of carbonic acid to H^+ and HCO_3^-, catalyzes this reaction. Dissociation of H_2CO_3 or association of H^+ and HCO_3^- to form H_2CO_3 occurs, instantaneously.

$$H_2O + CO_2 \rightleftharpoons H_2CO_3 \rightleftharpoons H^+ + HCO_3^-$$

Despite metabolic production of acids in the body, blood and intestinal fluid pH is maintained within the normal limits in a healthy person. Here, **first line of defense** of pH **consists of chemical buffers that are present in the extracellular and the intracellular fluids,** and the bone while the **second line of defense are the lungs** that maintain blood pH by disposing of CO_2.

Regulation of Blood pH by Buffers

Blood plasma is a mixed buffer system and has **three major buffers,** i.e., HCO_3^-/CO_2, $HPO_4^{2-}/H_2PO_4^-$ and **protein⁻/H. protein.**

- **Phosphate buffer:** Phosphate buffer has a pK of 6.8. It is a good buffer for stabilizing the pH of the blood. It is also an important buffer in the urine.

- **Protein buffer:** A protein contains many different ionizable groups, each one of which can donate or accept H^+. Protein comprises of the largest amount of buffer in the body. For example, albumin acts as a buffer in the blood plasma. An important example of the intracellular protein buffer is hemoglobin (Hb).

- **Bicarbonate/CO₂ buffer:** Bicarbonate/CO_2 buffer **has special importance in buffering pH in the extracellular fluid,** due to the reason that:

  - **The components of this buffer system,** i.e., HCO_3^- and CO_2, **are present in large quantities.** In the course of metabolism, a normal adult produces about 300 L of CO_2 every day. Further, there is also an appreciable concentration of HCO_3^- in the extracellular fluid.

  - This buffer pair is quite effective since **it operates as an open system,** i.e., **either of its components can be removed or added.** Although CO_2, truly, is not an acid but is an acid anhydride, since it readily reacts with water and forms H_2CO_3, which ionizes to H^+ and HCO_3^-.

The sum of the two equations is:

$$CO_2 + H_2O \rightleftharpoons H^+ + HCO_3^-$$

As concentration of water, generally, does not alter much, equilibrium expression for the above reaction can be represented as:

$$K' eq = ([H^+] [HCO_3^-]/[CO_2]),$$

where $[CO_2]$ represents concentration of dissolved CO_2. Since concentration of a gas, in a solution, is directly proportional to its partial pressure, therefore, concentration of the dissolved CO_2 in the blood is proportional to pCO_2.

Two components of the buffer can be easily regulated. Whereas lungs control arterial blood pH by regulating pCO_2, the kidney controls plasma HCO_3^-.

Respiratory Regulation of Blood pH

The respiratory system controls partial pressure of CO_2 and thus minimizes pH changes in the arterial blood.

- **Normally,** CO_2 is expired at the same rate at which it is produced and thus pCO_2 is maintained.
- **If blood becomes acidic** by the addition of the fixed acids, pulmonary ventilation is increased. **In the state of hyperventilation, CO_2 is flushed-out at a rate greater than the rate at which it is produced and** consequently pCO_2 falls. This reduction in arterial blood pCO_2, in turn, results in fall in H^+ concentration of the blood. The reactions are pulled to the left, which in turn lowers HCO_3^- concentration and reduces acidic shift in the blood.

$$CO_2 + H_2O \rightleftharpoons H_2CO_3 \rightleftharpoons H^+ + HCO_3^-$$

On the other hand, **if blood becomes more alkaline, changes occur in the opposite direction.** Accordingly, hypoventilation takes place, blood pCO_2 rises, and these reactions are pushed to the right, which in turn **results in a high carbonic acid concentration in the blood** and a less alkaline shift in blood pH. Hypoventilation, however, is limited because it causes retention of CO_2, which further stimulates ventilation.

$$CO_2 + H_2O \rightleftharpoons H_2CO_3 \rightleftharpoons H^+ + HCO_3^-$$

Buffering of acid-base disturbances by the respiratory response although is rapid but is relatively coarse. It brings blood pH close to normal but cannot eliminate a fixed acid or base from the body. Therefore, it cannot restore the pH to normal.

Renal Regulation of Blood pH

Kidneys regulate acid-base balance by controlling bicarbonate (HCO_3^-) reabsorption and secreting acid (H^+). In addition, kidneys also excrete anions, such as phosphate, chloride, sulfate, etc., which are liberated from the strong acids.

Secretion of H⁺ Ions

In a basic ion exchange mechanism, carbonic anhydrase-catalyzed reaction in the tubule cells generates bicarbonate (HCO_3^-) and hydrogen ions (H^+). The H^+ are actively secreted into the tubular fluid (lumen) in exchange for Na^+ (*via* Na^+/H^+-antiport system). Within the tubule cell, Na^+ combines with HCO_3^- and generates sodium bicarbonate ($Na^+ + HCO_3^-$), that is pumped out of the cell into the blood (interstitial fluid) and equilibrates with the plasma (Fig. 6.1).

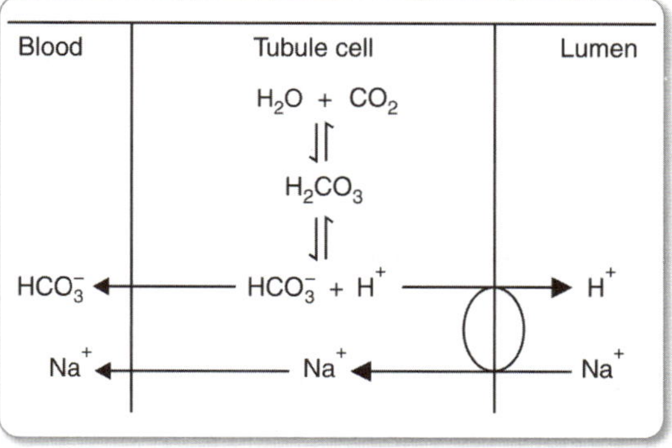

Fig. 6.1: Secretion of H^+

Mechanisms of the Removal of the Secreted H⁺ Ions

H^+ ions that are secreted into the tubular fluid can be removed by any of the three mechanisms, suggesting that three processes are involved in the acidification of urine.

1. By reabsorption of the filtered bicarbonate
2. By excretion of titratable acids, and
3. Excretion of ammonium ions.

All the three mechanisms involve H^+ secretion and are associated with the addition of bicarbonate to the peritubular capillary blood by the kidney tubules.

Reabsorption of the Filtered Bicarbonate

H^+ ions that are secreted into the tubules (in exchange for Na^+) combine with bicarbonate that has been filtered by the glomeruli. This, in turn, leads to the formation of carbonic acid in the tubular fluid. Dissociation of this acid to CO_2 and water is catalyzed in the lumen by carbonic anhydrase. The CO_2 rapidly diffuses through the cell membrane. **The secretion of H^+, thus, reabsorbs the filtered HCO_3^-, indirectly** (Fig. 6.2).

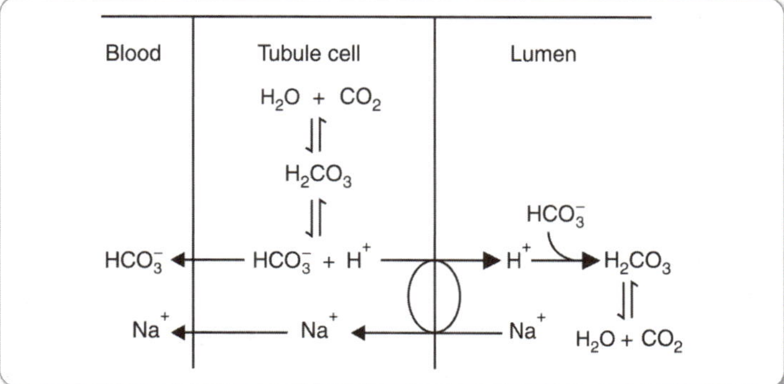

Fig. 6.2: By the reabsorption of the filtered bicarbonate

Excretion of Titratable Acid

As reabsorption of sodium bicarbonate proceeds, the tubular fluid becomes depleted of HCO_3^- and the pH drops. Following this, **H^+ ions are taken up by the phosphate buffer**. At this stage, hydrogen ions that are secreted into the tubular fluid (in exchange for Na^+) react with the phosphate buffer:

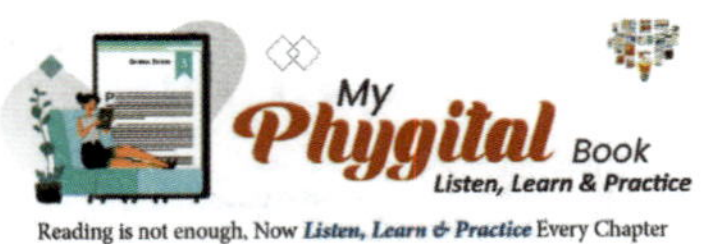

$$HPO_4^{2-} + H^+ \longrightarrow H_2PO_4^-$$

As a result of it, basic form of phosphate (HPO_4^{2-}) is converted to acidic form ($H_2PO_4^-$). Besides phosphate, which is the most important buffer in the urine, other ions are also important in the excretion of H^+. For example, **in diabetic ketoacidosis** when pH of the urine reaches at its minimum (about 4.4), **acetoacetate and β-hydroxybutyrate** pass through the glomerular filtrate and appear in the tubular fluid. Under these conditions these ions **also serve as buffer**.

Excretion of titratable acids thus, not only eliminates H^+ from the body but also restores depleted plasma bicarbonate reserve since for each mEq of H^+ excreted as titratable acid, a new HCO_3^- ion is added to the blood (Fig. 6.3).

The amount of the acid excreted (as the acid component of a urinary buffer) can be measured by the titration of the urine back to the normal pH of the plasma (to pH 7.4). The quantity of the base so required is equivalent to the quantity of the acid excreted and is referred to as **titratable acidity of urine**.

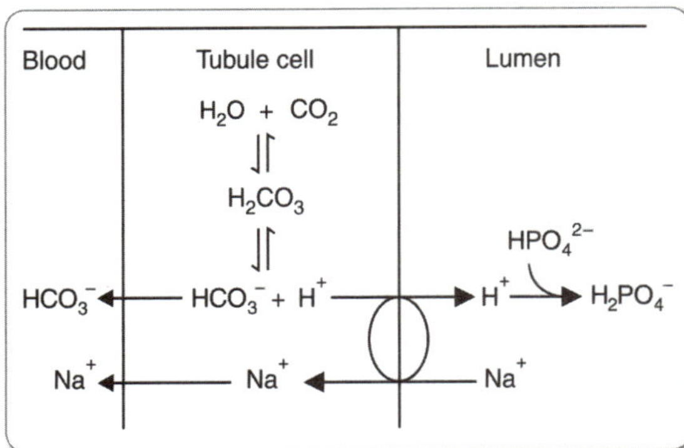

Fig. 6.3: By the excretion of the titrable acids

Excretion of Ammonia

The third fate of H^+ in the tubular fluid is neutralization by NH_3. Ammonia is mainly synthesized in the proximal tubule from amino acids, predominantly glutamine. It readily gets diffused through the cell membrane and combines with the secreted H^+ and forms NH_4^+. NH_4^+ is usually accompanied by an anion, e.g., chloride, in the urine. For **each H^+ excreted in the urine as NH_4^+, an equivalent quantity of HCO_3^- is added to the blood** (Fig. 6.4).

Elimination of NH_4^+ in the urine contributes to net acid excretion, as NH_4^+ is normally a major urinary acid. Nearly, one-half to two-thirds of our daily acid load is excreted as NH_4^+.

Ability of the kidney to synthesize NH_3, from glutamine, is increased under conditions of excess acid in the body.

The sum of the titrable acidity and NH_4^+ comprises **total acidity of urine** (total acid excretion).

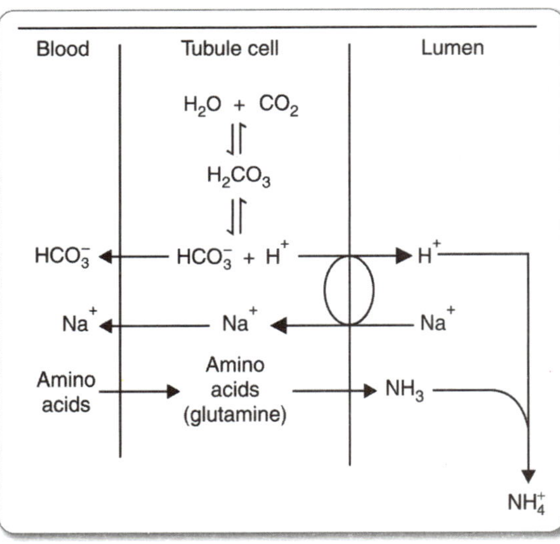

Fig. 6.4: Excretion as ammonium ion

ARTERIAL BLOOD GASES

Arterial Blood Gases (ABG) is one of the most commonly used tests that measures the acidity, or pH, and the levels of oxygen (O_2) and carbon dioxide (CO_2) from an artery. The test is used to check the function of the

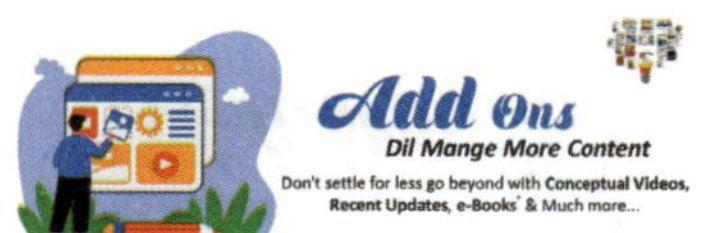

patient's lungs, and how well they are able to move oxygen into the blood and remove carbon dioxide. There are six key components to an ABG. These include:

1.   pH
2.   Partial pressure of oxygen
3.   Partial pressure of carbon dioxide
4.   Bicarbonate (HCO_3^-)
5.   Oxygen saturation
6.   Oxygen content

When interpreting ABG results, it is essential to know what ABG values are considered normal. From this baseline, one can then begin to recognize significant variations in a patient's results, which could indicate clinical deterioration:

- The first value is the **pH**, which measures how many **hydrogen ions** (H^+) are in the sample. This determines if the blood is acidotic or alkalotic. **Normal values for pH range from 7.35 to 7.45**.
- The next value is the **carbon dioxide level**, and this tells us, if the problem is **respiratory, in origin**, as CO_2 is **regulated by the lungs. The normal range for PaCO$_2$** is 35–45 mm Hg.
- Finally, **bicarbonate ions (HCO_3^-)** tell us, if the problem is related to **metabolic changes** in patient and refers **to the renal system. Normal is considered to be from 22 mmol/L to 26 mmol/L.**

Besides the above parameters, **calculated values** of **base excess** and **anion gap** may also be helpful in the interpretation of acid-base disturbances.

Base Excess

Base excess is defined as the amount of acid, which is required to titrate the blood to the pH value of 7.4 at pCO_2 of 40 mm Hg (at 37°C). If pH of the blood is low, base excess will be negative. Normally, the base excess value may be in the range of –2.0 to +3.0 mmol/L.

Anion Gap

Anion gap is a difference between the sum of Na^+ and K^+ (cations) from the sum of Cl^- and HCO_3^- (anions).

Anion gap thus, represents plasma anions other than Cl^- and HCO_3^-, which are not routinely measured.

$$\text{Anion gap} = (Na^+ + K^+) - (Cl^- + HCO_3^-)$$

Normal value for the anion gap is in the range of 12–16 mEq/L. This is the most commonly used parameter to establish differential diagnosis for metabolic acidosis.

Results of ABG are considered in the light of the clinical findings as well as other types of investigations such as plasma creatinine, urea, Na^+ and K^+. Normal values for various parameters related to ABG are shown in Table 6.1.

TABLE 6.1: Normal blood values for some of the parameters related to ABG

Parameter	Normal value
pH	7.35–7.45
pCO_2	35–45 mm Hg
HCO_3^-	22–26 mEq/L
Base excess	–2.0–3.0 mmol/L
Anion gap	10–20 mmol/L
Serum creatinine	0.8–1.3 mg/dL
Blood urea	15–40 mg/dL
Serum electrolytes	
Na^+	136–145 mEq/L
K^+	3.5–5.0 mEq/L
Cl^-	98–107 mEq/L

ACID-BASE DISORDERS

Acidosis or Alkalosis

If the ABG results reveal pH numbers are not within the normal range, the patient's pH level is either acidotic or alkalotic.

Acidosis

The lower the number, the more acidotic the patient is. For instance, a pH of 4 refers to severe acidosis and requires emergency intervention.

Alkalosis

Alkalosis is the opposite. The higher the pH, the more base is in the blood sample, which can disrupt the normal functioning of the body.

Once we have determined whether there is too much acid or too much base, one can move on to determine the cause of it.

HCO_3^-: Respiratory or Metabolic?

After we know whether the sample is acidic or alkaline, we need to work out if the cause is respiratory or metabolic:

- If the cause is **respiratory in nature**, the **$PaCO_2$** will be out of the normal range, whereas for **metabolic problems the HCO_3^-** will be abnormal.
  - It means that **low $PaCO_2$** points to respiratory alkalosis and that
- **High HCO_3^-** indicates **metabolic alkalosis**.

  Accordingly, there are four types of acid-base disturbances. The changes in arterial blood values and compensatory responses in different types of acid-base disorders have been given in Table 6.2.
  - Respiratory acidosis
  - Respiratory alkalosis
  - Metabolic acidosis, and
  - Metabolic alkalosis

TABLE 6.2: Changes in arterial blood values and compensatory responses in different types of acid-base disorders

Compensated or Uncompensated?	Respiratory or Metabolic?	Acidic or Alkalotic?	pH	$PaCO_2$	HCO_3^-
Uncompensated	Respiratory	Acidosis	Low	High	
Uncompensated	Respiratory	Alkalosis	High	Low	
Uncompensated	Metabolic	Acidosis	Low		Low
Uncompensated	Metabolic	Alkalosis	High		Low
Compensated	Respiratory	Acidosis	Normal	High	
Compensated	Respiratory	Alkalosis	Normal	Low	
Compensated	Metabolic	Acidosis	Normal		Low
Compensated	Metabolic	Alkalosis	Normal		High

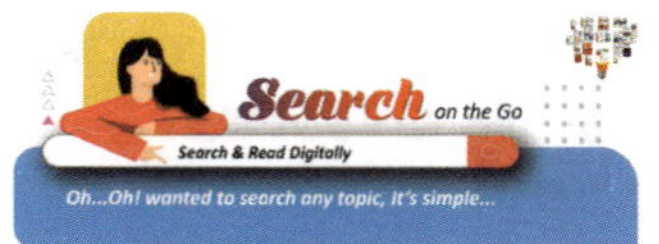

PaCO$_2$: Compensated or Uncompensated?

Compensation is the body's attempt to correct the imbalance, i.e., it is the system in the body, which it is trying to compensate for an abnormality in another system. This can be investigated by looking at the opposing component of the problem. For example:

- **In acidosis**, we look at the **level of HCO$_3^-$**. Whereas, **in alkalosis**, to determine if the body is compensating, we look at the **level of PaCO$_2$**.
- **If the other component is within normal range**, then **the problem is** noncompensated or **uncompensated**. Ultimately, the body is yet to fix the problem or has been unable to fix the problem.
- However, **if the other component has gone outside its normal reference range**, we can think of it as **compensation occurring** and that the body is trying to fix the problem. To assess how well it has been able to do this, we need to **look back to the pH**.
  - If the **pH is not** within or **close to the normal range**, then **a partial-compensation exists**.
  - If the **pH is back within normal ranges** then **a full-compensation has occurred**.
  - A **noncompensated** or **uncompensated abnormality** usually represents an **acute change occurring in the body**.

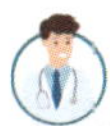 ## Clinical Correlation

Acidosis

Acidosis refers to a decrease in pH of the blood. It includes respiratory acidosis and metabolic acidosis.

Respiratory acidosis

Respiratory acidosis is due to inadequate ventilation *(hypoventilation)* **by the alveoli. This in turn results in the retention of CO$_2$ and fall in blood pH.**

Alveolar hypoventilation occurs when depth or rate of respiration is diminished such as in airways obstruction or a pulmonary disease. It results in a rise in pCO$_2$. As pCO$_2$ rises, plasma pH drops and HCO$_3^-$ concentration rises.

Kidney compensates for the respiratory acidosis by increasing the output of H$^+$ in the urine. The filtered HCO$_3^-$ in turn is reabsorbed and the increased amounts of H+ combine with the urinary buffers and are excreted in the urine.

Metabolic acidosis

Metabolic acidosis is characterized by the accumulation of nonvolatile acids *(gain of fixed acids other than H$_2$CO$_3$)* **and loss of HCO$_3^-$.**

The gain of metabolically produced acid may be due to several reasons such as:

- *Renal failure, due to reduced excretion of metabolically produced acids.*
- *Uncontrolled diabetes mellitus, due to the production of large quantities of ketone bodies.*
- *Inadequate circulation, due to cardiogenic or hemorrhagic shock, which in turn promotes anaerobic glycolysis and increases production of lactic acid.*
- *Heavy exercise, resulting in the production of lactic acid, or*
- *Ingestion of certain acidifying agents such as ammonium chloride.*

Metabolic acidosis may also be due to the loss of HCO$_3^-$ from the body such as due to diarrhea, or abnormal excretion of HCO$_3^-$ in the urine.

Two **compensatory mechanisms** *are usually available to deal with:*

1. *Due to the acidic pH, respiratory system is stimulated. This in turn lowers pCO$_2$ and hence carbonic acid concentration in the blood.* **Respiratory compensation** *although is prompt but usually does not restore the blood pH to normal.*
2. *The other mechanism, which begins almost instantly, is the* **renal compensation**. *The kidney increases H$^+$ excretion. This, however, takes time and alone is not adequate to return HCO$_3^-$ concentration (and the pH) to normal.*

Contd...

Alkalosis

Alkalosis refers to an increase in pH of the blood. It includes respiratory alkalosis and metabolic alkalosis.

Respiratory alkalosis

Respiratory alkalosis is a result of hyperventilation, *which may be caused by anxiety, central nervous system injury involving the respiratory center, salicylate poisoning or fever. This in turn causes* **a fall in arterial blood pCO$_2$.** *At high altitude also, due to decrease in total atmospheric pressure, alveolar pCO$_2$ falls and there is chronic respiratory alkalosis.*

The **kidney compensates for respiratory alkalosis, by excreting HCO$_3^-$ in the urine.** *Low pCO$_2$ leads to decreased H$^+$ secretion by the tubular epithelium. This in turn results in reduced reabsorption of the filtered bicarbonate and increases its excretion in the urine. This loss of HCO$_3^-$ in the urine results in further decrease in plasma HCO$_3^-$ and brings plasma pH towards normal.*

Metabolic alkalosis

Metabolic alkalosis is characterized by the intake of excess alkali, *i.e., by the gain of strong base or HCO$_3^-$, or* **abnormal loss of acid** *other than H$_2$CO$_3$. For example, ingestion of excess sodium bicarbonate used in treating gastric ulcer or oxidation of organic anion such as citrate, lactate and acetate.*

A common cause of abnormal loss of acid causing metabolic alkalosis is prolonged vomiting or gastric lavage since loss of gastric contents results in net addition of HCO$_3^-$ to the blood. It may also be a result of rapid loss of body water, e.g., in diuresis which in turn may result in temporary rise in HCO$_3^-$ in the plasma and the extracellular fluid.

Characteristic **arterial blood changes include a primary increase in plasma HCO$_3^-$ concentration, a rise in pH and a compensatory rise in pCO$_2$.** *Metabolic alkalosis is seldom long lasting.*

In metabolic alkalosis, as a primary defect is increase in plasma HCO$_3^-$ concentration, immediate **physiological compensation** *is* **hypoventilation, followed by increased renal excretion of HCO$_3^-$.**

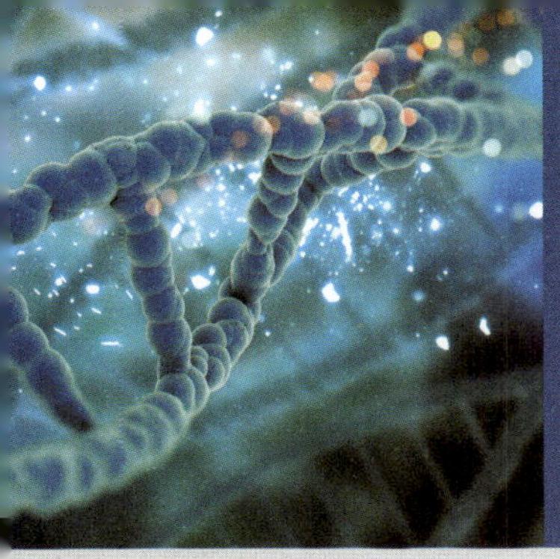

STUDENT ASSIGNMENT

LONG AND SHORT ANSWER QUESTIONS

1. Define buffer. What are the important buffers present in the body? Explain the role of various body buffers in the regulation of blood pH.
2. Define pH. How pH of blood is regulated?
3. **Explain:**
   a. Renal regulation of blood pH.
   b. Various mechanisms of H^+ secretion.
   c. Disorders of the acid-base balance.
   d. Biochemical assessment of acid-base balance.
   e. Respiratory regulation of blood pH.
4. **Write notes on:**

   a. pH
   b. Chemical buffers found in the body
   c. Respiratory acidosis
   d. Respiratory alkalosis
   e. Metabolic acidosis
   f. Metabolic alkalosis
   g. Base excess
   h. Anion gap

MULTIPLE CHOICE QUESTIONS

1. **Proteins act as buffer due to which property:**
   a. Colloid
   b. Basic
   c. Acidic
   d. Amphipathic (amphoteric) in nature

2. **Most important buffer in extracellular fluid is:**
   a. Acetate buffer
   b. Bicarbonate buffer
   c. Phosphate buffer
   d. Glycine buffer

3. **Anion gap represents:**
   a. Gap in anion molecule
   b. Difference between high and normal anion gap acidosis
   c. Unmeasured anions present in plasma
   d. Primary deficit of anions

4. **The following is a correct representation of pH:**
   a. $\log_{10}[H^+]$
   b. $\log_{10}[1/H^+]$
   c. $\log_e[H^+]$
   d. $\log_e[1/H^+]$

ANSWER KEY

1. d   2. b   3. c   4. b

Notes

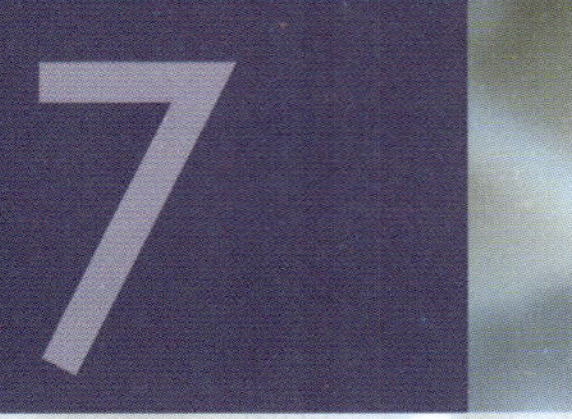

Heme Catabolism

LEARNING OBJECTIVES

After the completion of the chapter, the readers will be able to:
- Describe the metabolism of hemoglobin and its clinical significance.
- Describe bilirubin, its metabolism and the disorders.

CHAPTER OUTLINE

- Hemoglobin
- Heme Degradation Pathway
- Bilirubin

KEY TERMS

Enterohepatic circulation: The circulation of bilirubin, biliary acids, drugs or other substances from the liver to the bile, followed by entry into the small intestine, absorption by the enterocyte and transport back to the liver.
Neonatal jaundice: A condition in which an infant's skin appears yellow and the whites of the eyes, within the first few days of life.
Unconjugated bilirubin: Indirect bilirubin, formed by the breakdown of hemoglobin in the red blood cells.

HEMOGLOBIN

Hemoglobin is a globular protein, which is present in high concentration in red blood cells. It binds oxygen in the lungs and transports it to different cells in the body. A molecule of hemoglobin consists of four heme groups along with the four polypeptide chains, which are synthesized separately and subsequently, bind to four heme groups.

HEME DEGRADATION PATHWAY

Red blood cells have limited lifespan of approximately 100–120 days. These senescent cells are recognized by their membrane changes, removed and engulfed by the reticuloendothelial system, at the extravascular site. Degradation of red blood cell occurs in spleen, bone marrow, liver and lymph glands.

Degradation of heme occurs mainly, in the liver. If degradation of red blood cells occurs in the tissues other than the liver, hemoglobin is transported to the liver by means of haptoglobulin.

After the aged red blood cells are recognized by macrophages, they are rapidly engulfed by the phagocytes and form phagosomes. They fuse with the primary lysosomes and form secondary lysosomes. Lysosomal cathepsin results in complete degradation of the cellular proteins, including globin of hemoglobin, to the constituent amino acids, which are utilized for general metabolic needs.

Heme is degraded in the reticuloendothelial cells, to a linear tetrapyrrole (biliverdin IXa), by the microsomal enzyme system, which is designated as **heme oxygenase.** This enzyme requires molecular oxygen and NADPH, and is induced by heme. Heme oxygenase catalyzes the cleavage of α-**methenyl bridge** which **is quantitatively converted to carbon monoxide** (CO) that is trapped by the hemoglobin and eventually exhaled.

Biliverdin is reduced to bilirubin by the enzyme biliverdin reductase (Fig. 7.1).

One gram of hemoglobin yields about 35 mg of bilirubin.

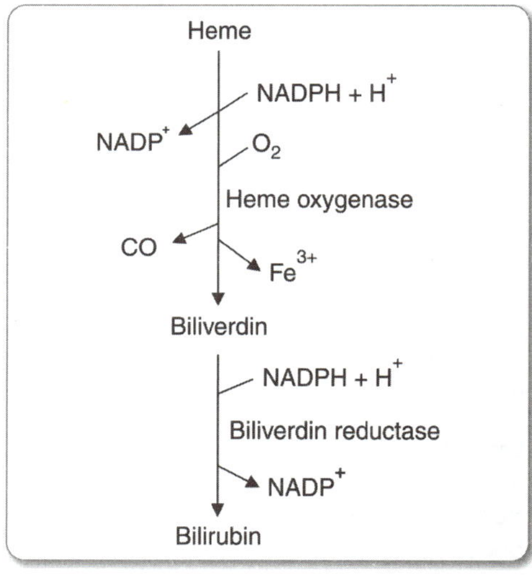

Fig. 7.1: Degradation of heme to bilirubin

BILIRUBIN

Bilirubin is an orange-yellow pigment, derived from the breakdown of red blood cells in the liver, spleen and bone marrow. Its daily production, in men, averages from 250 mg to 300 mg. Approximately, 85% of this is derived from the heme moiety of hemoglobin, which is released from the erythrocytes that are destroyed in the reticuloendothelial cells while rest of it is formed from catabolism of other heme containing proteins, such as myoglobin, cytochromes and other heme containing enzymes.

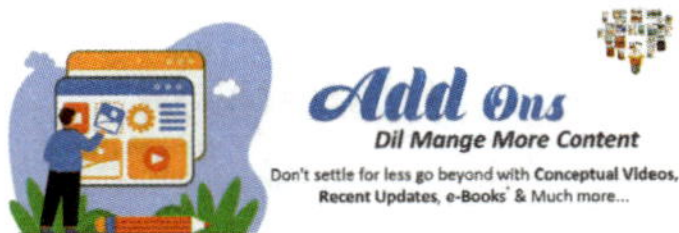

Metabolism of Bilirubin

Bilirubin, normally present in the blood, is bound to albumin and is transported to the liver.

Hepatocytes trap bilirubin by means of a specific binding protein, called **ligandin. In the hepatocytes, bilirubin** gets **conjugated with UDP-glucuronate,** which is derived from the oxidation of UDP-glucose. **This reaction is catalyzed by UDP-glucuronyltransferase** (Fig. 7.2).

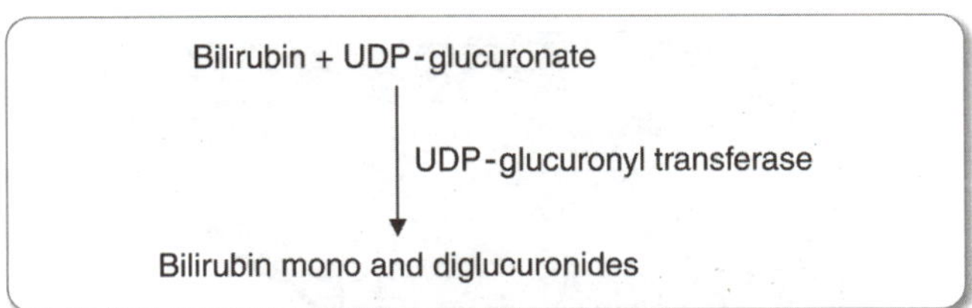

Fig. 7.2: Conversion of bilirubin to bilirubin glucuronides

Clinical Correlation

Thalassemias

Thalassemia is a family of related genetic disorders that arise due to the deletion of one or more globin-like genes in either the globin gene cluster or a defect in transcription, and/or processing of mRNA of the globin gene. If there is reduced synthesis or total lack of synthesis of α-globin mRNA, the disease is classified as α-thalassemia. On the other hand, if β-globin mRNA level is affected, it is called β-thalassemia.

One to four α-globin genes may be missing in the patients with α-Thalassemia. If one α-globin gene is missing, the condition is called α-thalassemia 1 (α-thal 1). When two α-globin genes are missing, it is called α-thal 2. Both the conditions are associated with mild to moderate anemia. On the other hand, if three α-globin genes are missing it results in the synthesis of more β-globin molecules, forming a tetramer containing four β-globin subunits. This condition is called HbH disease. When all the four α-globin genes are absent, it results in a fatal condition called hydrops fetalis.

β-thalassemias also exhibit different degrees of severity and can be caused by a variety of defects or deletions.

In the normal bile, bilirubin diglucuronide is the major form of excreted bilirubin with only a small amount of the bilirubin monoglucuronide. As bilirubin diglucuronide is much more water soluble than free bilirubin, transferase thus facilitates the excretion of bilirubin, via bile duct, into the intestine.

Enterohepatic Circulation of Bilirubin

As **bilirubin diglucuronide** is poorly absorbed by the intestinal mucosa, glucuronide residues are **released in the terminal ileum and large intestine, by intestinal β-glucuronidases and by the enzymes produced by anaerobic bacteria. It is reduced to** colorless linear tetrapyrroles, called stercobilinogen, mesobilinogen and urobilinogen. These compounds are collectively referred to as urobilinogens.

A large portion of **urobilinogens are excreted in the feces.**

Majority of these recirculating pigments are taken up by the liver and re-excreted in the bile. Some of the urobilinogens (only up to 2%) are also reabsorbed passively from the colon and return to the liver via the portal venous blood. This is referred to as **enterohepatic circulation of urobilinogen** (Fig. 7.3).

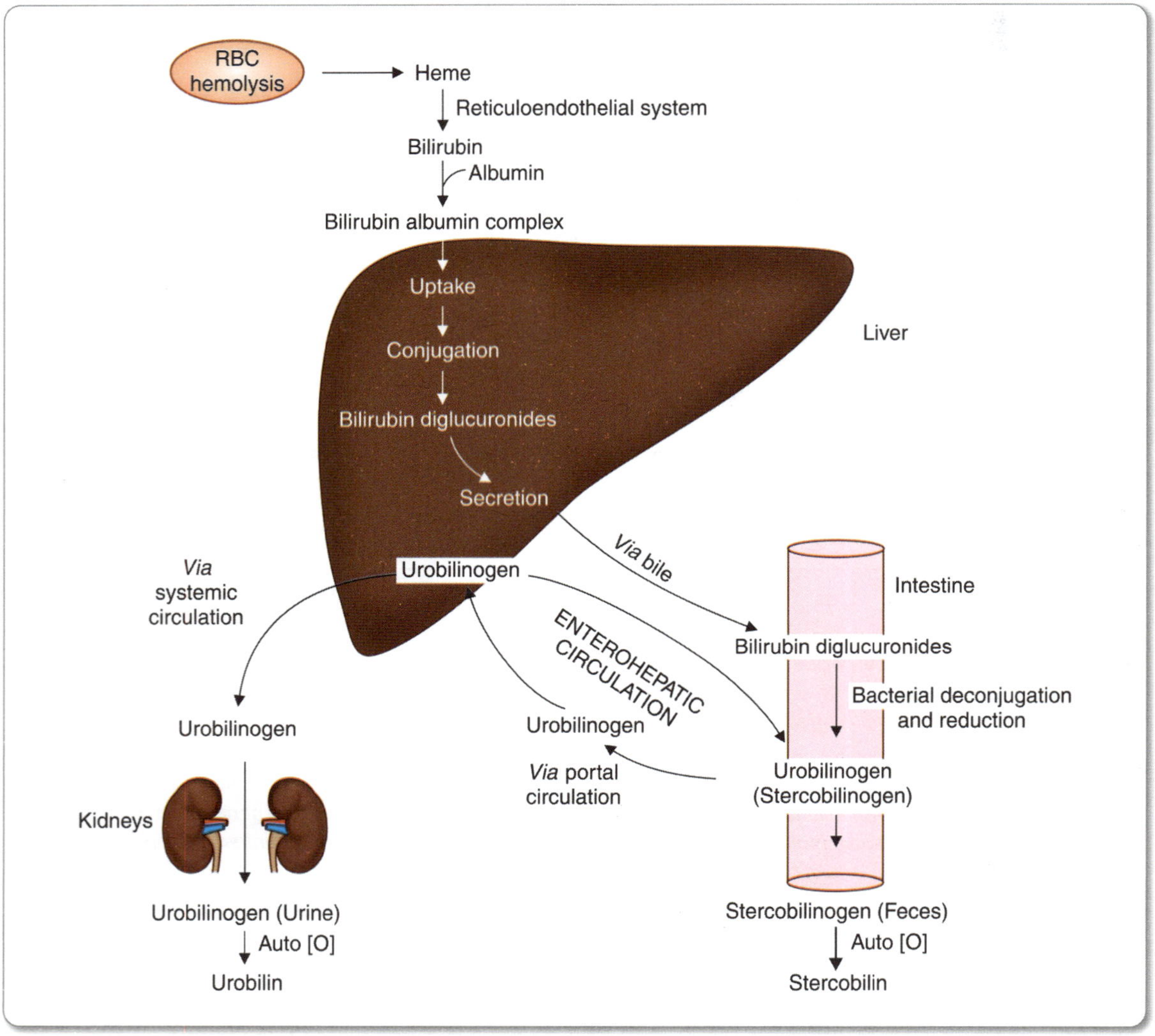

Fig. 7.3: Formation, conjugation and enterohepatic circulation of bilirubin

Most of the reabsorbed urobilinogen is taken up by the liver and is re-excreted in the bile. **A small portion of urobilinogen (2–5%),** however, escapes hepatic extraction, **reaches the peripheral circulation and is excreted in the urine**.

Serum thus contains two different forms of bilirubin, which are referred to as:

- **Unconjugated** (lipid soluble) form that is bound to albumin and is transported from the reticuloendothelial system to the liver, and
- **Conjugated** (water soluble) form that is regurgitated from the liver into the plasma

> Normal value, for the sum of the unconjugated and conjugated bilirubin, is 0.1–1.0 mg/100 mL of serum or plasma.

Normally, almost all the bilirubin in plasma is unconjugated.

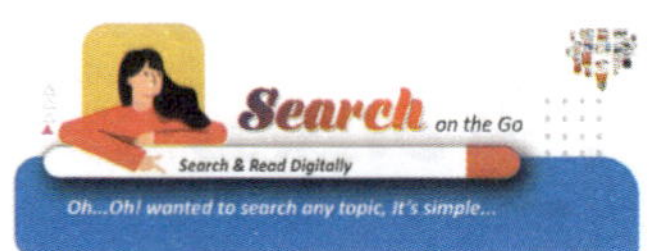

Disorders of Bilirubin Metabolism

Disorders of bilirubin metabolism lead to **hyperbilirubinemia** where serial measurement of bilirubin is helpful in knowing the severity of a liver disease.

Bilirubin fractionation is also helpful in differential diagnosis of **jaundice**.

Jaundice

Jaundice is a physical sign characterized by yellow appearance of the patient and is the most characteristic clinical manifestation of hyperbilirubinemia. It results from the deposition of bilirubin (bile pigment) in the skin, mucous membrane and sclera of the patient (Fig. 7.4).

Jaundice is apparent clinically, when serum bilirubin level is >2 mg/dL. If serum bilirubin is below 2 mg/dL, it is called **latent jaundice** (subclinical jaundice) since it is not detectable at this stage, clinically.

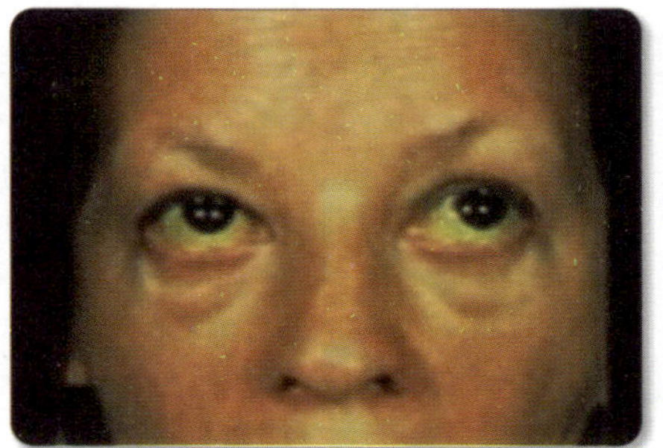

Fig. 7.4: Clinical manifestation of hyperbilirubinemia (Jaundice)

Types and Causes of Jaundice

There are three types of jaundice, referred to as prehepatic, hepatic and posthepatic jaundice.

1. **Prehepatic jaundice:** Prehepatic jaundice is also called **hemolytic jaundice**. It is characterized by the excessive presence of **unconjugated bilirubin**. It may be a result of increased production of unconjugated bilirubin such as in hemolysis, decreased uptake of unconjugated bilirubin across the hepatocyte membrane as in Gilbert's syndrome, or decreased biotransformation such as in neonatal jaundice, Crigler-Najjar syndrome, etc.

   - **Hemolysis:** In disorders associated with hemolysis (hemolytic anemia), rate of bilirubin production is increased, which may exceed the amount that cannot be removed by the liver.
   - **Gilbert's syndrome:** This is a heterogeneous group of disorders inherited as autosomal recessive trait. Several defects include deficiency of the enzyme bilirubin-glucuronyl transferase, a defect in hepatic uptake of bilirubin, or a decrease in red cell survival.
   - **Neonatal jaundice:** Neonatal jaundice is also called physiological jaundice of the newborn. Every infant exhibits some transient unconjugated hyperbilirubinemia (about 5 mg/dL) between the second and the fifth day of life, as at this stage hepatic glucuronyltransferase activity is not fully developed. Activity of the enzyme increases within 2 weeks after birth when serum bilirubin returns to normal. Neonatal jaundice is more pronounced in a premature infant.

   > Unconjugated bilirubin levels above 18 mg/dL lead to deposition of bilirubin in the lipid-rich basal ganglia. This is referred to as kernicterus.

   - **Crigler-Najjar syndrome:** This disorder is known to exist in two forms:
     Type I: It is clinically more severe form of the disease. It is due to complete absence of glucuronyltransferase.
     Type II: It has moderate clinical findings and is due to partial deficiency of the enzyme. In both the conditions, unconjugated bilirubin is significantly raised.

2. **Hepatic jaundice:** Plasma, usually, shows elevated levels of **both conjugated as well as unconjugated bilirubin**.

- **Some primary diseases**: Hepatic jaundice is due to a primary disease, e.g., in **viral hepatitis, liver cirrhosis,** etc. In these conditions, there is also an increase in ALT and AST levels.
- **Dubin-Johnson syndrome:** Elevated levels of conjugated as well as unconjugated bilirubin along with the dark-brown pigmentation, in the liver cells, are also observed in a benign, autosomal recessive condition known as Dubin-Johnson syndrome.
- **Liver injury due to some chemicals:** Inhalation, ingestion or parenteral **administrations of** several **pharmacological** and **chemical agents**, such as **carbon tetrachloride, acetaminophen, isoniazid** or **chlorpromazine**, which result in **liver injury**, also lead to hepatic jaundice.

3. **Posthepatic jaundice:** Posthepatic jaundice is also referred to as **obstructive jaundice** or **posthepatic cholestasis**. It is caused by obstruction of the bile duct, may be due to gallstones, carcinoma of the head of pancreas or carcinoma of the bile duct. Serum of such a patient shows excessive amount of conjugated bilirubin. It is also characterized by the presence of the excessive amount of bilirubin (bile pigment) in the urine.

Blood and Urine Investigations for Jaundice

Blood Investigations

- **Serum Bilirubin:** It refers to the estimation of the levels of total bilirubin, direct bilirubin and indirect bilirubin.
  - **Indirect bilirubin** refers to the bilirubin formed by the breakdown of red blood cells which travels from the blood to the liver. It is the **lipid soluble** form and is bound to albumin. It is also referred to as **unconjugated bilirubin**. Majority of the bilirubin in plasma is unconjugated. Its serum level is increased in conditions associated with prehepatic jaundice.
  - **Direct bilirubin** refers to the bilirubin which undergoes chemical change (conjugation) in the liver. It is the **water soluble** form which has been regurgitated from the liver into the plasma. It moves to the intestine and is then removed through stools. Its serum level is increased in conditions associated with posthepatic jaundice.
  - Serum levels of both, i.e., unconjugated as well as conjugated bilirubins are increased in conditions associated with hepatic jaundice.
- **Serum enzymes and proteins:** If elevated levels of bilirubin are found, various liver function tests can be performed to determine the underlying cause of jaundice, by estimating serum **ALT, AST** and **ALP**, and **albumin** and **total proteins**. None of these parameters are altered in prehepatic jaundice. Serum ALT and AST levels are increased while serum albumin and total protein concentrations are decreased in conditions associated with hepatic jaundice. On the other hand, serum ALP levels are significantly increased in posthepatic jaundice.

Urine Investigations

- **Bilirubin: Unconjugated bilirubin** is hydrophobic and, therefore, **cannot be excreted in urine.** Conversely, **conjugated bilirubin** is hydrophilic and, thus, can be **excreted in the urine**, i.e., as bile pigment. Presence of bilirubin in urine indicates liver dysfunction.
- **Urobilinogen:** Normally, 0.5–4.0 mg of urobilinogen is excreted in the urine in 24 hours. Increased excretion of urobilinogen occurs when hepatocellular function is impaired. Urobilinogen may also increase in the urine if there is an excess of urobilinogen in the gastrointestinal tract that exceeds the capacity of the liver to re-excrete it, e.g., in hemolysis, viral hepatitis and cirrhosis. In contrast, when

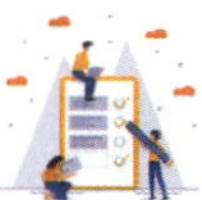
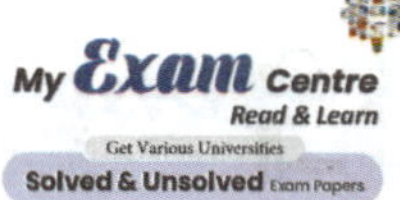

biliary excretion of bilirubin is impaired, e.g., in cholestasis, urinary excretion of urobilinogen is decreased due to limited delivery of bilirubin to the gut and due to low rate of urobilinogen production. This also results in clay-colored or chalky white, stool of patients with cholestatic jaundice.

Blood and urine investigations for biochemical differentiation of the three types of jaundice are shown in Table 7.1.

TABLE 7.1: Blood and urine investigations for biochemical differentiation of the three types of jaundice

Investigation	Prehepatic jaundice	Hepatic jaundice	Posthepatic jaundice
Total serum bilirubin	Normal/increased	Increased	Increased
Conjugated bilirubin	Normal	Increased	Increased
Unconjugated bilirubin	Normal/increased	Increased	Normal
Urine Urobilinogen	Normal/increased	Decreased	Decreased/negative
Urine color	Normal	Dark (urobilinogen, conjugated bilirubin)	Dark (conjugated bilirubin)
Stool color	Brown	Slightly pale	Pale, white
Alkaline phosphatase level	Normal	Increased	Highly Increased
ALT and AST levels	Normal	Highly Increased	Increased
Conjugated bilirubin in urine	Not present	Present	Present

Van den Bergh Test

Van den Bergh test is a chemical reaction used to measure bilirubin levels in blood. This test helps to identify the type of jaundice; **more specifically**, it determines the amount of **conjugated bilirubin in the blood**.

In the normal state, plasma bilirubin concentration is 0.3–1.0 mg/dL. Almost all of this is **unconjugated** (bound noncovalently to albumin) and does not react, until it is released by the addition of an organic solvent such as methanol. **Unconjugated bilirubin** binds so tightly to serum albumin and lipid that it does not diffuse freely in plasma, and, therefore, does not lead to an elevation of bilirubin in the urine. The reaction with diazonium salt yields azo dye after the addition of methanol and is called **indirect Van den Bergh reaction**.

Conjugated bilirubin is relatively water soluble and elevation of conjugated bilirubin leads to its high urinary excretion with the characteristic deep yellow-brown color to the urine. The conjugated bilirubin is also referred to as **direct bilirubin**, because it can be coupled readily with diazonium salt to yield azo dye. This is called **direct Van den Bergh reaction**.

In **Van den Bergh** test, bilirubin reacts with diazotised sulfanilic acid to produce purple colored azobilirubin. The serum of patient is mixed with diazo reagent:

- If red colour develops immediately, it is called **direct positive**. It happens if **conjugated bilirubin** is present.
- In **indirect positive** test, patient's serum is first treated with alcohol and later mixed with diazo reagent. This causes development of red color. It is seen if **unconjugated bilirubin** is present.
- If **both, conjugated and unconjugated bilirubin** are present, the reaction is termed **biphasic reaction**.

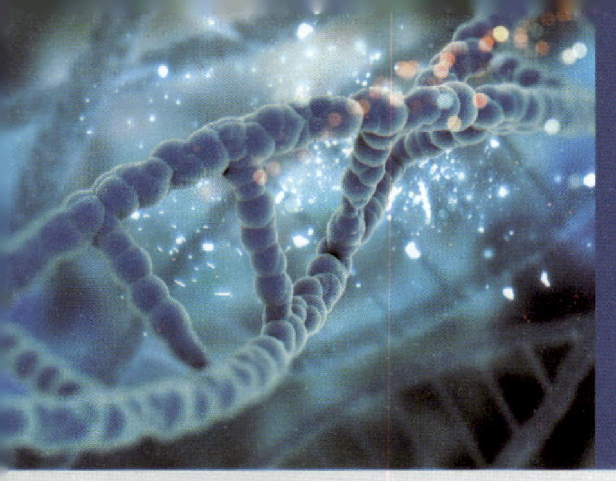

LONG AND SHORT ANSWER QUESTIONS

1. Describe the process of heme degradation.
2. Describe types and causes of jaundice.
3. **Write notes on:**
   a. Conjugated bilirubin
   b. Unconjugated bilirubin
   c. Van den Bergh test
   d. Thalassemias
   e. Jaundice

MULTIPLE CHOICE QUESTIONS

1. **Conjugated bilirubin in urine in the absence of urobilinogen suggests:**
   a. Hemolytic jaundice
   b. Hepatocellular jaundice
   c. Obstructive jaundice
   d. None of these

2. **Which of the following is correct about breakdown of hemoglobin (Hb)?**
   a. Hb-Heme-bilirubin-urobilinogen
   b. Heme-Hb-biliverdin-bilirubin-urobilinogen
   c. Hb-Heme-biliverdin-bilirubin-urobilinogen
   d. Hb-Heme-bilirubin-urobilinogen-biliverdin

3. **In the plasma, conjugated bilirubin is bound to:**
   a. α_2-Globulin
   b. α_1-Globulin
   c. β-Globulin
   d. None of these

4. **The following is not true for heme oxygenase system:**
   a. Requires oxygen
   b. Requires NADPH
   c. Produces CO
   d. Repressed by heme

ANSWER KEY

1. c   **2.** c   **3.** d   **4.** d

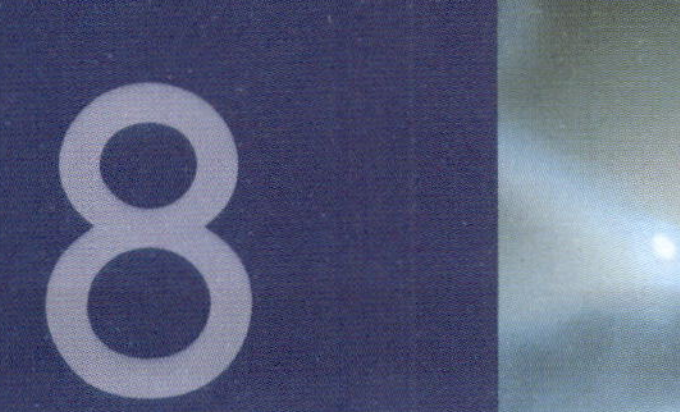

8

Organ Function Tests

LEARNING OBJECTIVES

After the completion of the chapter, the readers will be able to:
- Explain renal, liver and thyroid function tests.
- Describe the biochemical parameters of renal, liver and thyroid functions.

CHAPTER OUTLINE

Renal Function Tests
- Functions of the Kidneys
- Biochemical Parameters for the Evaluation of Kidney Functions

Liver Function Tests
- Commonly Used Biochemical Parameters for the Evaluation of Liver Functions
- Normal Values of Some Biochemical Parameters of Liver

Thyroid Function Tests
- Thyroid Hormones
- Commonly Used Biochemical Parameters for the Evaluation of Thyroid Functions
- Normal Values of Some Biochemical Parameters of Thyroid Function

KEY TERMS

Glomerular filtration rate: The volume of plasma that is filtered by the glomeruli per unit of time, and is usually measured by estimating the rate of clearance of a substance from the plasma.

Renal clearance: Renal clearance is a measure of the rate at which a substance is cleared from the blood by the kidneys through urine production. It is used to estimate the kidney's ability to remove that specific substance from the bloodstream.

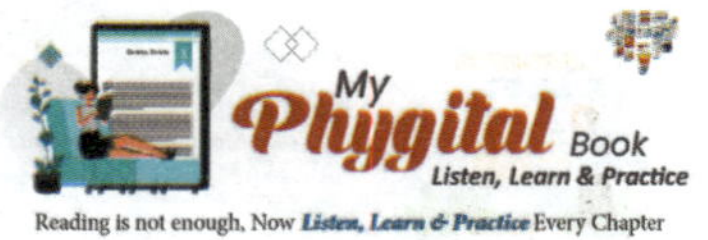

RENAL FUNCTION TESTS

Various metabolic processes occurring in the body produce a number of substances, many of which, such as CO_2, water, nitrogenous compounds and inorganic salts, are waste products. If not regularly removed from the body, these toxic metabolites may severely affect normal health. The kidneys excrete most of the water, and organic and inorganic substances, whereas CO_2 is expired through lungs.

FUNCTIONS OF THE KIDNEYS

Kidneys perform several biochemical functions (Table 8.1).

TABLE 8.1: Important functions of the kidney

- Filtration of blood and preparation of ultrafiltrate fluid as urine.
- Reabsorption of useful substances such as glucose, amino acids, electrolytes, etc.
- Homeostasis of the extracellular volume.
- Maintenance of the acid-base status, water and electrolytes
- Endocrine functions and activation of hormones such as synthesis of erythropoietin, activation of vitamin D, etc.

Excretion of Waste Products

Urine is an ultrafiltrate of plasma. It is formed in the kidney, a paired organ, which is meant for filtration, concentration and reabsorption of various constituents. Each kidney has nearly one million basic filtration units called nephrons.

Filtration of Blood

Filtration is carried out in the nephron through glomeruli. As blood passes through the glomeruli, non-colloidal substances (usually of low molecular weight), filter through capillaries, with the retention of protein (not normally found in the urine).

Total amount of the filtrate formed per minute, by all the nephrons of both the kidneys, is known as **glomerular filtration rate** (GFR). Under normal physiological conditions, **GFR is 125 mL/min**.

Reabsorption of Useful Substances

About 150–200 L of the ultrafiltrate passes through the glomeruli in 24 hours. Reabsorption of water and solutes in various regions of the tubule reduces its volumes to nearly 500–1800 mL/day, as urine.

In the proximal tubule, nearly 60–80% of the ultrafiltrate is absorbed in an obligatory fashion, along with Na^+, Cl^-, HCO_3^-, Ca^{2+}, HPO_4^{2-} and other ions. **Glucose** is reabsorbed almost completely, predominantly in the proximal tubule by a Na^+-dependent active transport process. **Uric acid** is also reabsorbed in the proximal tubule. When blood level of creatinine increases above normal, creatinine is secreted in this region.

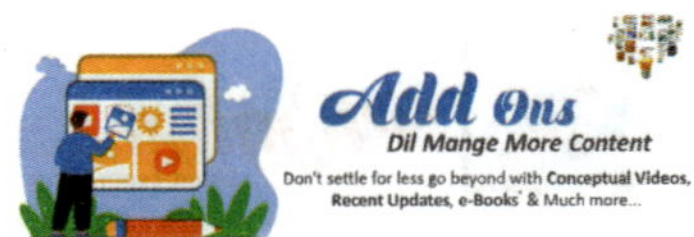

- **In the loop of Henle**, Cl^- and more of the Na^+ but without water are reabsorbed, resulting in diluted urine. Water reabsorption is then regulated in the distal tubule and collecting duct by antidiuretic hormone (ADH or vasopressin).
- **In the distal tubule**, **secretion** is the prominent activity as organic ions; K^+ and H^+ are transported from the blood in the efferent arteriole into the tubular fluid. This region also secretes H^+ and reabsorbs Na^+ and HCO_3^-.

At the same time, certain solutes are added to the fluid by an excretory function of the tubule. These include hippuric acid and other organic waste products.

Substances, which are reabsorbed by the renal tubules, are divided into two groups, according to their threshold value:

1. **High threshold substances:** These compounds are vital for life and body cannot afford to lose them. Such substances are completely reabsorbed by the renal tubule, e.g., glucose, amino acids, etc.
   - **Glucose** is reabsorbed in the tubular epithelial cells.
   - **Sodium, potassium, amino acids** and other substances are reabsorbed, apparently by specific transport mechanisms.
   - Transfer of **carbon dioxide and bicarbonate** is controlled by carbonic anhydrase.
2. **Low threshold substances:** These compounds are not required by the body and are reabsorbed to a very small extent only, e.g., urea, creatinine, etc.
   Urine thus, carries off:
   - Water and salts in such amount so as to maintain normal equilibrium between extracellular and intracellular fluids,
   - Acids or bases, to maintain a normal acid-base balance,
   - Waste products
   - Toxic and detoxified substances, and
   - Other substances, those are present in the blood in excessive amount.

Regulation of Water and Electrolytes

Regulatory functions of the kidney have a major role in homeostasis, by maintaining constant optimal chemical composition of the blood as well as interstitial and intracellular fluids.

Regulation of Water

The kidney plays an important part in regulating water balance. If excessive amount of water (fluid) is ingested, kidney excretes the same. On the other hand, if intake is low, kidney excretes more concentrated urine.

- Water homeostasis is intrinsically linked to renal urea handling. Only 40–50% of the filtered load of urea is reabsorbed.
- Most of the glomerular filtrate is reabsorbed through tubule cells.
   About 90% of water is reabsorbed as a result of the difference in pressure. The remaining 10% of water is reabsorbed actively, by tubular cells, as a result of the action of ADH.
- In the absence of ADH, little water and urea are reabsorbed, and a large amount of water is excreted. On the other hand, in the presence of ADH only 1.0–1.5 L of the filtrate is excreted as urine.
   Regulation of ADH excretion is thus of vital importance to fluid homeostasis.

Regulation of Electrolytes

The kidney plays an important role in the maintenance of electrolyte balance. Salts are either excreted or conserved by the kidney by tubular reabsorption, depending upon dietary intake and physiological need.

Plasma electrolytes pass through the glomerulus but some potassium leaves the blood by way of tubules, by active secretion.

Sodium and Chloride

Sodium and chloride ions predominate in the glomerular filtrate, as in plasma. As the glomerular filtrate flows through tubule, these electrolytes are absorbed into the blood.

Reabsorption of Na^+ is required for the reabsorption of water, Cl^-, glucose, HCO_3^-, urea and amino acids.

The proximal tubule is highly permeable to Na^+. Approximately 80% of the Na^+ entering tubular cells do so in exchange for H^+ secretion, which, in turn, leads to the entry of both Cl^- and HCO_3^- into the cells.

Sodium transport is regulated by many factors:
- Protein kinase-dependent phosphorylation
- Aldosterone
- Na^+, K^+-ATPase
- Na^+-H^+ exchanger
- H^+-ATPase

Calcium and Phosphorus

Approximately 98% of filtered Ca^{2+} is reabsorbed. Out of which 65–75% in the proximal tubule, 20–25% in the thick ascending limb of the loop of Henle, 10% in the distal tubule and a small amount in the collecting duct.

A passive process that is linked to active Na^+ reabsorption predominantly absorbs calcium. However, in the distal tubule, Ca^{2+} reabsorption is an active process catalyzed by Ca^{2+}-ATPase.

Reabsorption of Ca^{2+} is increased by the action of PTH and calcitonin.

Normally, less than 20% of the filtered load of phosphorus is excreted in the urine. Its excretion is directly related to the filtered load when plasma phosphorus concentration is above normal. Reabsorption of phosphorus, though dependent on Na^+ reabsorption, is regulated by:
- Protein kinase C-dependent phosphorylation
- PTH
- Active vitamin D
- Calcitonin, and
- Dopamine and serotonin

Maintenance of Acid-Base Balance

Oxidation of various metabolites in the living organism results in the formation of a variety of acids as well as bases. For example, protons are generated from ionization of various substances such as organic acids (produced during metabolism of glucose, fatty acids and amino acids), uric acid (from purines), sulfates (from sulfur-containing amino acids) and carbonic acid (from CO_2).

Similarly, bases arise during catabolism of various metabolites such as ammonia (from amino acids), bicarbonate, phosphates, acetate and citrates.

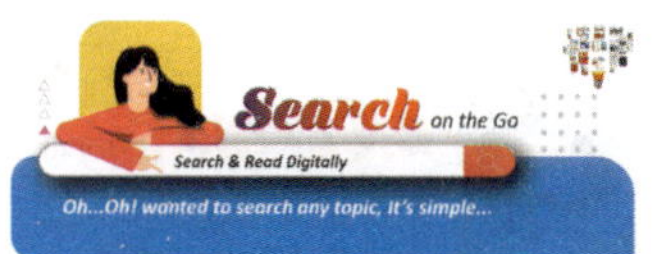

All these substances enter blood plasma and other extracellular fluids for disposal. In spite of the entry of these acids and bases, pH of the blood does not alter much and remains within the normal limit of 7.35–7.45. This is due to the presence of various defense mechanisms, which include:

- Buffer systems of the blood, tissue fluids and cells
- Excretion or retention of CO_2 by lungs
- Excretion of an acid or alkaline urine
- Formation and excretion of ammonia as well as organic acids

Regulation of Acid-Base Balance

Four reactions are mainly involved in the regulation of acid-base balance by the kidneys:

1. ***Exchange of H^+ for Na^+***
   - Na^+ that is present in the lumen of the renal tubule, i.e., in the ultrafiltrate of plasma, is exchanged for H^+, which is formed in the tubular epithelial cells from CO_2 and H_2O. Na^+ is transported from the epithelial cells into the blood plasma for recycling. This transport of Na^+ is mediated by sodium pump.
   - In the presence of carbonic anhydrase, CO_2 and H_2O form carbonic acid, which is dissociated into H^+ and HCO_3^-. HCO_3^- diffuses from the epithelial cells into the blood plasma as the accompanying ion to Na^+, and thus, HCO_3^- is conserved.

2. ***Reabsorption of HCO_3^- from the tubular urine***
   - The H^+ that is exchanged into the tubular urine reacts with HCO_3^- in the plasma ultrafiltrate and forms H_2CO_3.
   - This is dissociated to CO_2 and H_2O from where CO_2 diffuses back into the epithelial cells.

3. ***Formation and excretion of NH_3***
   - Glutamine is extracted from the renal blood plasma of the peritubular capillaries and is deaminated by glutaminase in the tubular epithelial cells, to release NH_3 and glutamate.
   NH_3 so formed is diffused into the tubular urine and binds with H^+ to form NH_4^+.

4. ***Excretion of H^+***
   - The H^+ ions that are exchanged for Na^+ bind to HPO_4^{2-} to form $H_2PO_4^-$ (titratable acid). Both $H_2PO_4^-$ and NH_4^+ are then excreted in the urine.
   - The accompanying ions are predominantly, Na^+ and Cl^-, respectively.
   - Kidney, thus, participates in the regulation of acid-base balance, primarily, by maintaining the HCO_3^- concentration in the plasma.
   - In the event of acidosis, excretion of both $H_2PO_4^-$ and NH_4^+ are increased in the urine while the reverse occurs in alkalosis, until acid-base balance is restored (Chapter 6).

Synthesis and Activation of Hormones

Kidney synthesizes some hormones such as erythropoietin, renin and prostaglandins. It is also the site for the activation of vitamin D.

BIOCHEMICAL PARAMETERS FOR THE EVALUATION OF KIDNEY FUNCTIONS

Commonly used biochemical parameters for the assessment of the functions of kidney are shown in Table 8.2.

TABLE 8.2: Commonly used biochemical tests for the assessment of the kidney functions

Routine laboratory tests	Tests for glomerular functions	Tests for tubular functions
Urine • Volume • pH • Normal constituents • Abnormal constituents **Blood** • Urea • Creatinine • pH, gases and electrolytes	**Renal clearance test** • Insulin clearance • Urea clearance • Creatinine clearance **Renal plasma flow**	• Urine concentration test • Urine dilution test • Urine acidification test

Examination of Urine

Physical Examination of Urine

Volume

Volume of the urine varies from person to person and time to time.

- Average volume of urine, excreted by a normal individual, over a period of 24 hours, is **1000–1500 mL**. It is influenced by diet, particularly, ingestion of fluids. Strenuous physical exercise, hot weather and fever diminish urine output.
- Certain pathological conditions alter urine output. If 24 hours volume is increased, the condition is called **polyuria**, such as seen in diabetes and early renal failure.
- When urine output is decreased, it is termed **oliguria** such as seen in acute renal failure, dehydration (diarrhea and vomiting), edema and urinary obstruction.
- In acute renal failure or shock, urine is usually not formed. This condition is called **anuria**.

Color

Normal urine is usually pale, straw-yellow colored, due to the presence of urochrome, uroerythrin and urobilin.

- Change in color may be due to some pathology, secondary to the intake of some drug or a particular type of food.
- In fever it is usually dark in color, if there is blood in the urine (due to hemorrhage in the kidney or the urinary tract), urine becomes red in color. In jaundice urine may be dark-yellow or green due to the oxidation of bilirubin to biliverdin.

General Appearance and Odor

Freshly excreted urine is normally clear and transparent, as all the substances are present in the soluble form. On standing, it becomes turbid due to precipitation of phosphates.

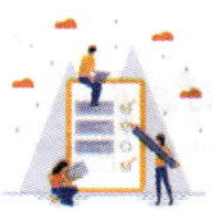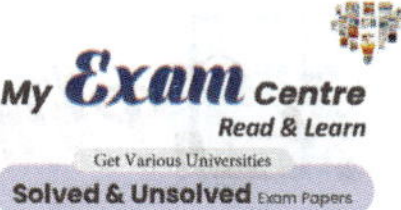

Pathological urine may be turbid due to the presence of fat globules or pus cells.

- **Odor of the urine is usually aromatic,** due to the presence of volatile acids. On standing, urine may develop pungent odor due to formation of ammonia from urea because of its decomposition by bacteria.
- In acidosis and diabetes mellitus, urine has a peculiar sweet smell due to the presence of ketone bodies.

Specific Gravity

Specific gravity of urine normally varies between 1.010 and 1.030. Volume has a great influence on specific gravity of urine.

- Low values (up to 1.003) are observed after large water intake, on diuretic therapy or excretion of large amount of ketone bodies.
- High values (up to 1.040) are seen in dehydration or due to the presence of large amount of glucose.

Specific gravity of urine is measured by means of hydrometer, known as urinometer. Mark on the urinometer, in contact with surface of urine, indicates specific gravity of the sample.

pH (Reaction)

Under normal circumstances urine is slightly acidic in reaction, with a **mean pH of about 6.0 (ranging from 4.8 to 8.0)**

The pH of urine varies widely depending upon the nature of the food taken. High protein diet leads to acidic urine while alkaline urine is excreted after a vegetarian diet, particularly after large intake of vegetables and fruits.

Following meal, pH of the urine becomes alkaline due to the production and secretion of HCl by the stomach.

- Alkaline urine is seen in patients with systemic alkalosis since body attempts to conserve H^+ ions and remove fixed bases.
- Strongly acidic urine is seen in patients with systemic acidosis, e.g., diabetes mellitus, due to the excretion of large amount of ketone bodies.
- An increase in pH, greater than 8.0, indicates urinary tract infection by an organism that splits urea to ammonia.

The pH of urine is routinely checked with the help of pH paper. Its reaction can be tested with the help of litmus paper.

Chemical Examination of Urine

Normal Constituents

Major constituents of normal urine are shown in Table 8.3.

Normally, 50–60 g of solids are excreted in the urine over a period of 24 hours. About half of the total solids are urea. It comprises of nearly 80–90% of total organic substances. Other organic constituents of normal urine include creatinine, uric acid, hippuric acid and ethereal sulfates.

Major inorganic substance excreted is chloride (as sodium chloride). It constitutes about 25% of the total solids excreted in 24 hours. Other inorganic constituents normally excreted in the urine include ammonia, phosphates and sulfates.

In certain pathological conditions these constituents may be excreted in abnormal amounts.

TABLE 8.3: Normal constituents of urine

Constituent	Daily excretion (g/24 hours)
Water	1000–1500 mL
Total solids	50–60
Organic substances	30–35
Urea	25–30
Uric acid	0.5–1.0
Creatinine	1.0–2.0
Free amino acids (as amino acid N)	0.15–0.20
Inorganic substances	20–25
Chloride (as NaCl)	10–15
Total sulfates (as sulfur)	0.7–1.0
Total phosphates (as inorganic phosphorus)	0.8–1.1
Ammonia	0.5–0.7

Organic Substances

- **Urea:** Urea is a principal end product of protein catabolism in mammals. An adult man excretes 25–30 g of urea under normal conditions, in 24 hours.
  - Urea excretion is increased on high protein diet or in protein catabolic states such as fever.
  - On low protein diet, urea excretion is reduced. Decrease in urea excretion is also observed in disorders which are associated with impaired liver function, such as cirrhosis as well as in a kidney disease, such as nephritis.
- **Uric acid:** Uric acid is derived from nucleic acids by the oxidation of purine bases. It is found in urine to the extent of 0.5–1.0 g/24 hrs. Its daily excretion, however, varies, depending upon the diet and several other factors.
  - On a purine-free diet, uric acid output may be reduced up to 0.1 g/24 hrs.
  - On a high purine diet, uric acid excretion may be increased up to 2.0 g/24 hrs.
  Pathologically, uric acid excretion is increased in gout and leukemia.
- **Creatinine:** Creatinine (a waste product) is anhydride of creatine. Creatinine is present in considerable amount in muscle, in the form of creatine phosphate. Very little of creatine is found in the urine.
  On the other hand, about 1.0–1.8 g of creatinine is excreted by an adult in 24 hours. Excretion of creatinine is related to the amount of body creatine, i.e., muscle mass. Daily excretion of creatinine is, therefore, fairly constant and is used to check the accuracy of 24 hours urine collection.
  - Creatinine content of urine is increased in conditions associated with increased muscular activity.
  - A decrease in creatinine excretion may be observed in disorders, which are associated with muscular weakness as well as in a kidney disease.
- **Amino acids:** Due to high thresh-hold, normally only small amount of free amino acids are found in the urine. Their daily excretion (as amino acid nitrogen) is about 150–200 mg. Infants excrete more amino acids as compared to adults. During pregnancy excretion of amino acids is increased.

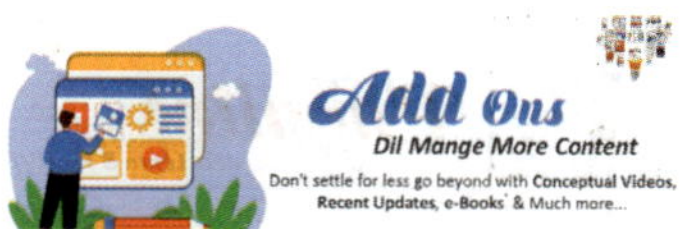

Aminoaciduria may be prominent in certain liver diseases and after poisoning by chloroform or carbon tetrachloride.

In certain metabolic diseases increased excretion of some of the amino acids may be observed, such as arginine, cystine, lysine and ornithine in cystinuria.

Inorganic Substances

- **Chloride:** It is a major inorganic constituent of the normal urine. Its excretion is dependent upon chloride content of the food. On an average daily output of chloride (expressed as sodium chloride) varies between 10 and 15 g. Fasting and excessive perspiration decreases its urinary output.

  Pathologically, its excretion may be decreased in chronic nephritis, fever, burn, diarrhea and vomiting.
- **Phosphates:** These are present in the urine in various forms, e.g., alkaline phosphates, such as sodium, potassium and ammonium phosphates, which are derived from the ingested inorganic phosphate or earthy phosphates such as phosphates of calcium and magnesium. These are insoluble phosphates and get precipitated in alkaline urine.
  - Excretion of phosphorus is dependent upon diet but on an average nearly 1 g of phosphates (as inorganic phosphorus) is excreted in 24 hours.
  - Urinary phosphorus is increased in acidosis and certain bone diseases, e.g., rickets and osteomalacia.
  - Phosphorus excretion is reduced in pregnancy, renal and infectious diseases as well as in hyperparathyroidism.
- **Sulfates:** These arise in the urine from the oxidation of sulphur, which is obtained from the sulphur-containing amino acids. Only a small amount of the ingested sulphur is excreted.
  - Sulfates are present in the urine in various forms, e.g., **inorganic sulfates** such as sodium, calcium and magnesium sulphates; **ethereal sulfates** which are mostly the detoxification products, and **neutral sulfates**, e.g., cystine, taurine, etc.
  - Under normal conditions about 1 g of sulfates (as sulfur) are excreted in the urine daily.
- **Ammonia:** Tubular cells of the kidney form ammonia. Precursor for ammonia is the amide nitrogen of glutamine. A decrease in blood pH speeds up ammonia production.
  - Normally, about 0.5–0.7 g of ammonia is excreted in 24 hours. Although very little of it is present in a fresh sample of the urine, its level increases on standing, due to bacterial decomposition of urea.
  - Ammonia excretion is decreased in a kidney disease while its excretion is increased in acidosis such as in diabetic ketoacidosis.

Abnormal Constituents of Urine

In the process of filtration of plasma through glomeruli, large molecular weight substances such as proteins are retained while small molecular weight substances, which are useful for the body, are reabsorbed. Normally, their amount is so low that it is not detectable, by the routine laboratory tests.

Under certain pathological conditions, when either their metabolism is disturbed or a tubular damage occurs, large quantities of these substances are excreted in the urine. Hence, these substances are called **abnormal constituents of urine.** These include sugar (glucose), ketone bodies, protein (albumin), blood, bile salts and bile pigments (Table 8.4).

TABLE 8.4: Abnormal constituents or urine

Constituent	Conditions in which excreted
Sugar (glucose)	Diabetes mellitus, renal glycosuria
Ketone bodies	Prolonged starvation, low-carbohydrate high-fat diet, diabetic ketoacidosis
Protein (albumin)	Nephrotic syndrome, glomerulonephritis
Blood	Hematuria, hemoglobinuria
Bile salts/pigments	Different types of jaundice

Sugar

Excretion of, readily detectable amount of sugar in the urine is known as mellituria or glycosuria whereas **excretion of glucose** is referred to as **glucosuria**.

When blood glucose concentration exceeds 180 mg/100 mL such as in diabetes mellitus, reabsorptive capacity of the tubule is reduced and glucose appears in the urine. Glucose may also be found in the urine in hyperthyroidism, hyperpituitarism, hyperadrenalism or I-cell disease of the pancreas.

- Glucosuria may also be observed in a proximal tubular disease that impairs re-absorptive mechanism. This is known as **renal glucosuria**. In this condition, glucose utilization as well as blood glucose level may be normal.

Besides glucose, other sugars that may be excreted in the urine include lactose, galactose, fructose or pentoses.

- **Lactosuria** may be observed in lactating women.
- **Fructose** may be present in the urine after ingestion of large quantity of honey. Essential fructosuria is an inborn error of metabolism due to the deficiency of the enzyme fructokinase.
- **Pentoses** may be found after ingestion of large quantities of fruits like plums and cherries. Pentosuria, referred to as L-xylulosuria, is an inborn error of metabolism due to the deficiency of xylitol dehydrogenase.
- **Galactosuria** may be observed in infants suffering from congenital galactosemia. Galactosuria may also be seen in infants as well as adults with a liver disease.

Ketone Bodies

Ketone bodies (acetoacetate, β-hydroxybutyrate and acetone) are formed in considerable amounts when fat is metabolized, excessively.

- Their accumulation in the blood is called ketonemia while their excretion in the urine is referred to as ketonuria.
- Ketonemia and ketonuria occur in a condition, which is referred to as ketosis.
- Ketosis may occur during prolonged fasting or carbohydrate deprivation. Pathologically, ketone bodies appear in the urine in diabetic ketoacidosis.

Proteins

Normal urine contains only traces of protein, which cannot be detected by routine procedures. When readily detectable amount of protein is seen in urine, this condition is called proteinuria. Since it is mainly the albumin that is detected abnormally, hence, proteinuria may also be referred to as albuminuria.

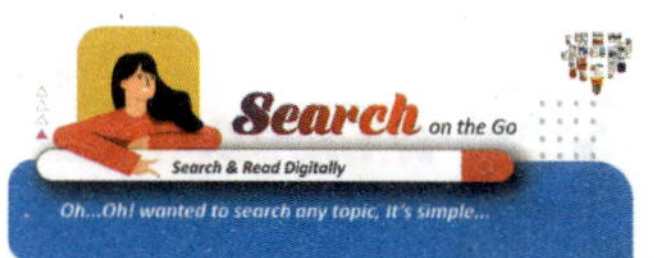

- Proteinuria or albuminuria may be physiological (benign albuminuria) or pathological (renal albuminuria).
- **Physiological proteinuria** is usually transitory. There is no evidence of kidney damage but proteinuria may be observed after severe exercise, high protein diet, pregnancy or postural effect (when an individual assumes an upright position for a long period). The latter is called **orthostatic** or **postural proteinuria**.
- **Pathological proteinuria** may be classified as:
  - *Prerenal proteinuria:* Pre-renal proteinuria may be observed in conditions that are primarily not related to the kidney, e.g., a cardiac disease, by affecting the circulation of the kidney, may lead to proteinuria. Besides, fever, convulsions, anemia and liver diseases may also result in proteinuria.
  - *Renal proteinuria:* Renal proteinuria may be observed due to inflammation of the kidney (nephritis) or kidney damage (nephrosis). Proteinuria due to a glomerular disease can lead to nephrotic syndrome where large amount of protein is excreted.
    Acute tubular necrosis and pyelonephritis also lead to proteinuria, which is generally mild.
  - *Postrenal proteinuria:* Post-renal proteinuria may occur due to some inflammatory, degenerative or traumatic lesions of the pelvis of the kidney, ureter, bladder, prostate or urethra.

Blood

Either intact red blood cells or hemoglobin may be present in the urine.

Presence of red blood cells in the urine is referred to as **hematuria**. It can be confirmed by the presence of red blood cells by microscopic examination of the urine. RBCs may be seen in acute glomerulonephritis or trauma to the urinary tract.

Hemoglobinuria may be observed due to intravascular hemolysis. This, in turn, results in the liberation of the hemoglobin which is filtered in the glomerulus and appears in the urine. Hemoglobinuria may occur under various pathological conditions such as mismatched transfusion of blood, hemolytic jaundice, typhoid or malaria.

Bile

Bile is produced in the liver. It is secreted through biliary tract and enters duodenum. It is alkaline in reaction and bitter in taste. Its color varies from yellowish-brown to dark green. Important constituents of the bile are bile salts, bile pigments, lipids particularly phospholipids and cholesterol, proteins like mucin, urea and certain inorganic salts such as sodium chloride and bicarbonate.

- **Bile salts** are the sodium and potassium salts of glycocholic and taurocholic acids. Cholic acid has the basic ring structure of cyclopentanoperhydrophenanthrene, like cholesterol. In glycocholic acid, glycine is conjugated with cholic acid through a peptide linkage. Similarly, in taurocholic acid, taurine is conjugated with cholic acid. Bile salts are essential for the digestion of fat. Since fat is insoluble in water, it is not digested in the absence of bile salts. Bile salts emulsify fat by lowering surface tension of water and help to bring fat in intimate contact with the lipase.
- **Bile pigments** are the degradation products of hemoglobin. When hemolysis of red blood cells takes place, hemoglobin is dissociated into heme and globin. Globin is hydrolyzed to amino acids by the proteolytic enzymes, while heme loses its iron, which is reutilized for heme synthesis. The tetrapyrrole ring (protoporphyrin) is broken down to biliverdin, which is further oxidized to bilirubin. Bilirubin is predominant in human bile. When it enters the intestine, further changes take place due to bacterial action and a number of pigments are formed. Some of these are reabsorbed into blood through the intestine, modified and excreted through urine.

Urobilinogen

Urobilinogen is an important constituent of the freshly voided normal urine. Following its oxidative degradation, it disappears quickly. Increased amount of urobilinogen may be seen in the urine of patients with hemolytic jaundice.

Estimation of Some Biochemical Parameters of Blood

Blood Urea

Urea is a major nitrogenous metabolic product of protein catabolism in man, accounting for more than 75% of the nonprotein nitrogen which is eventually excreted. Urea is freely filtered by the glomeruli. In a normal kidney, 40–70% urea moves passively out of the renal tubule into the interstitium.

> Blood urea level, in a normal individual, may vary between 15 and 40 mg/dL. In patients with untreated chronic renal failure, blood urea level may be increased to 100–150 mg/dL.

Measurement of blood urea is widely used as a test of renal function. However, a number of non-renal factors influence circulating urea concentration. For example, urea production and consequently blood urea concentration are increased on a high protein diet, in protein catabolic states, gastrointestinal hemorrhage and treatment with cortisol in some cases of chronic liver disease and with decreased perfusion of the kidney. Blood urea also depends upon the state of hydration of the patient.

Estimation of plasma urea concentration, however, is a less valuable test of renal function than plasma creatinine concentration. This is due to the reason that nearly 50% of the urea, filtered at the glomerulus, is passively reabsorbed through the tubules and this fraction increases if urine flow rate increases, such as in dehydration. Plasma urea concentration is also more affected by diet than plasma creatinine.

- **Low blood urea** concentration may be observed in several situations, such as reduced synthesis, e.g., on a low protein diet or in an acute liver disease. Blood urea level may also fall as a result of water retention.
- **High blood urea** concentration may be due to several causes, which may be subdivided into pre-renal, renal and post-renal:
  - *Pre-renal causes* of increase in blood urea concentration include increased production by the liver (such as on a high protein diet), hemorrhage in the upper gastrointestinal tract, or in protein catabolic states (e.g., due to trauma, major surgery, or starvation). It may also be due to impaired renal perfusion (e.g., extracellular fluid loss, cardiac failure, hypoproteinemia, etc.).
  - *Renal causes* of increase in blood urea concentration include acute or chronic renal failure with reduction in glomerular filtration.
  - *Post-renal causes* include obstruction to urine flow, such as stone, benign prostatic hypertrophy, malignant stricture, or obstruction.

Serum Creatinine

Creatinine is a waste product of creatine. Its daily excretion is related to muscle mass and does not vary greatly from day to day. Hence, its level in the blood remains fairly constant. Creatinine is freely filtered at the glomerulus. Although it is not reabsorbed to any great extent by renal tubules but a small amount of it is secreted. Its secretion is increased with the increasing level of plasma creatinine.

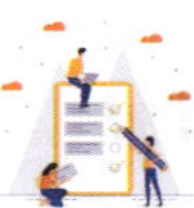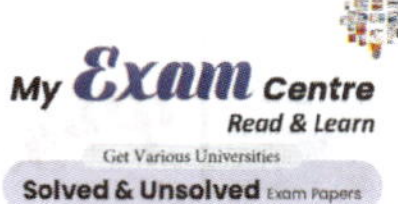

> Normal serum creatinine concentration varies between 0.8 and 1.5 mg/dL.
>
> Meal, containing meat may increase serum creatinine concentration. Certain drugs, e.g., salicylates, cimetidine, etc., also increase serum creatinine level.
>
> Serum creatinine values are lower in children than in adults, in women than in men, and during pregnancy. Determination of serum creatinine gives a useful indication of the degree of renal failure.

An increase in serum creatinine, due to fall in GFR is observed when:

- There is decreased renal perfusion, e.g., reduced blood pressure, fluid deprivation or renal arterial stenosis.
- There is a loss of functional nephrons, e.g., in acute and chronic glomerulonephritis, and
- Pressure is increased on the tubular side of the nephron, e.g., in urinary tract obstruction due to prostate enlargement.

Serum creatinine concentration is a more precise measurement than creatinine clearance and is usually sufficient for following the progress of patients with renal disease. Because:

- Plasma creatinine concentration normally remains fairly constant throughout adult life whereas creatinine clearance declines with advancing age.
- Plasma creatinine concentration correlates well with GFR as does creatinine clearance in patients with renal disease.
- Measurements of plasma creatinine concentration are as effective in detecting early renal disease as creatinine clearance, and
- Sequential plasma creatinine concentration measurements enable the progress of renal disease to be followed with better precision than creatinine clearance.
- **Reduced plasma creatinine** concentration is found in subjects with a small total muscle mass. Thus, a lower value is found in children. Values are, on average, normally lower in women than in men. Abnormally low values may be found in wasting diseases (reduced muscle bulk) and starvation, and in patients on steroid therapy, due to their protein catabolic effect. Plasma creatinine concentration is also usually low in pregnancy.
- **Increased plasma creatinine** concentration may be observed in several non-renal situations. For example:
    - High meat intake can cause temporary rise in plasma creatinine level.
    - Transient small increase in plasma creatinine level may occur after vigorous exercise.
    - Some drugs, e.g., salicylates, cimetidine, etc., reduce tubular secretion of creatinine hence, exhibit elevated plasma creatinine concentration.
    - High concentration of certain compounds, such as acetoacetate or cephalosporin antibiotic exhibit analytical interference and result in its overestimation.

An increased plasma creatinine concentration indicates a fall in GFR. Renal causes of increased plasma creatinine level include:

- A disease, in which there is impaired renal perfusion, e.g., reduced blood pressure, fluid depletion, renal artery stenosis, etc.
- Diseases in which there is loss of functioning nephrons, e.g., glomerulonephritis
- Urinary tract obstruction due to prostatic enlargement.

Blood pH and Gases

Diminished capacity of the kidney to excrete H^+ results in metabolic acidosis, the severity of which may be assessed by measuring arterial pH (H^+), HCO_3^- and pCO_2 concentrations.

Serum Electrolytes

Estimation of serum electrolytes, i.e., sodium and potassium are also of value in certain kidney conditions, e.g., chronic renal failure or metabolic acidosis accompanied by hyponatremia or hyperkalemia.

Renal Clearance Tests

Clearance is defined as the volume of plasma that is cleared-off a particular substance by the two kidneys in one minute. It is calculated by the following mathematical relationship:

$$C = \frac{U \times V}{P}$$

where:

C = Clearance of the substance (mL/min)

U = Concentration of the substance (mg/dL) in urine

V = Rate of flow of urine (mL/min)

P = Concentration of the substance (mg/dL) in plasma, blood or serum

Inulin Clearance Test

Inulin is a polymer of fructose. It is filtered by the glomeruli, but is neither reabsorbed nor secreted by the tubule. Inulin clearance, therefore, is nearly equal to glomerular filtration rate (GFR).

> Normal value for GFR, as per inulin clearance, found in adults, is about 125 mL/min.

Although inulin meets most of the criteria for measuring GFR, it is not suitable for routine use, because it is an exogenous substance and has to be administered intravenously.

Urea Clearance Test

Urea is an end product of protein catabolism. Its concentration varies depending on dietary protein intake. Further, after filtration from the glomeruli, it is both, secreted from as well as reabsorbed by the tubules, thus, its excretion is affected by the rate of flow of urine.

As both, blood urea as well as urine urea concentrations are variable; accordingly, urea clearance is calculated in two different ways, depending upon the rate of flow of urine, i.e., as standard urea clearance and maximum urea clearance.

Standard Urea Clearance

Standard urea clearance is calculated with standard rate of urine flow (approximately 1 mL/min), i.e., when the value of urine volume is below 2 mL/min:

$$\text{Standard urea clearance (mL/min)} = \frac{U}{B} \times \sqrt{B}$$

where U and B are concentrations of urea (mg/100 mL) in urine and blood, respectively, while B square root is the volume of urine excreted (mL/min). Mean value for standard urea clearance is 54 mL/min.

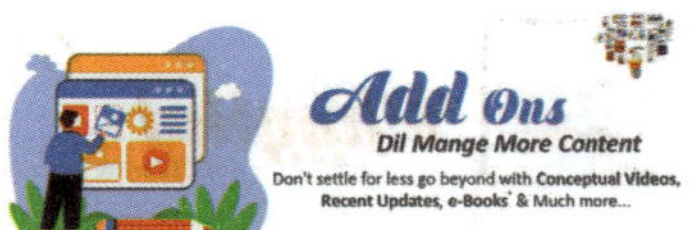

Maximum Urea Clearance

Maximum urea clearance is calculated when volume of urine excreted is 2 mL/min or more. It is calculated by putting the actual value of V in the above equation, instead of $\sqrt{V}$.

$$\text{Maximum urea clearance} = \frac{U}{B} \times V$$

Mean value for maximum urea clearance is 75 mL/min.

As discussed above, urea clearance depends upon the rate of urine flow and that blood urea concentration is affected by dietary protein, urea clearance test is not preferred to determine GFR.

Creatinine Clearance Test

Creatinine is produced endogenously from creatine and gains access to the urine by glomerular filtration. Its clearance is not affected by the volume of urine flow. Also, serum creatinine concentration is not affected by diet. Thus, creatinine clearance is preferred as a measure of GFR. Normal value for creatinine clearance is 95–105 mL/min.

> Creatinine clearance (per 1.73 m^2 surface area) is low at birth (35–40 mL/min) and reaches the normal adult value (80–120 mL/min) by 6 months of age. It further declines with age. Creatinine clearance is increased by 20% during pregnancy.

Normal Values of Some Biochemical Parameters of Renal Function

Normal values of biochemical parameters of significance in renal function tests are shown in Table 8.5.

TABLE 8.5: Normal values of some biochemical parameters related to renal function tests

Biochemical parameter	Normal value
Blood urea	15–40 mg/dL
Serum creatinine	0.8–1.3 mg/dL
pH	7.35–7.45
pCO_2	35–45 mm Hg
HCO_3^-	22–26 mEq/L
Na^+	136–145 mEq/L
K^+	3.5–5.0 mEq/L

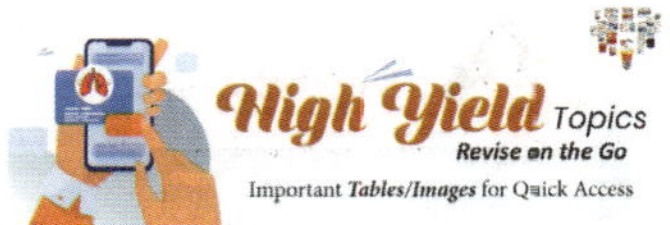

LIVER FUNCTION TESTS

The liver is a multifunctional organ that is involved in a number of excretory, synthetic and metabolic functions (Table 8.6).

- The liver has a major influence on the flow of nutrients to the rest of the body. It controls the release of absorbed material into the systemic circulation and has a central role in carbohydrate, protein and fat metabolism.
- The liver is an important site for the storage of glycogen and for gluconeogenesis.
- Most proteins in plasma including albumin, α- and β-globulins, clotting factors and transport proteins are synthesized by the liver.
- This is also the site for urea synthesis.
- Fatty acids and phospholipids are also taken up from circulation by the liver and are metabolized there.
- Cholesterol is also synthesized and esterified in the liver.
- Liver is also a site for the detoxification of exogenous compounds (such as alcohol, drugs and toxins) as well as endogenous materials (such as bilirubin and hormones) which are excreted via the kidney or the biliary system.
- Bile salts are synthesized in the liver.
- Liver stores various substances, such as vitamins and minerals, and releases them as and when required.
- Liver is also one of the biggest reticuloendothelial organ and has important immune functions.

TABLE 8.6: Important biochemical functions of the liver

Metabolism of nutrients
- Carbohydrates
- Proteins
- Fats

Synthesis of proteins
- Albumin
- α- and β-globulins
- Clotting factors
- Transport proteins

Metabolism and excretion of exogenous substances
- Alcohol
- Drugs
- Toxins

Metabolism and excretion of endogenous substances
- Bilirubin
- Hormones

Storage of vitamins
- Vitamin A
- Vitamin B_{12}

Storage of Mineral
- Iron

COMMONLY USED BIOCHEMICAL PARAMETERS FOR THE EVALUATION OF LIVER FUNCTIONS

Various liver functions tests that are useful in the assessment of a liver disease include the estimation of serum proteins, serum bilirubin, various enzymes and prothrombin time (Table 8.7).

TABLE 8.7: Commonly used biochemical tests for the assessment of liver functions in serum

Total proteins
Albumin
Bilirubin
Prothrombin time
Enzymes • GPT and GOT • Alkaline phosphatase • γ-Glutamyl transpeptidase (γ-GT) • 5′-Nucleotidase • Glutamate dehydrogenase

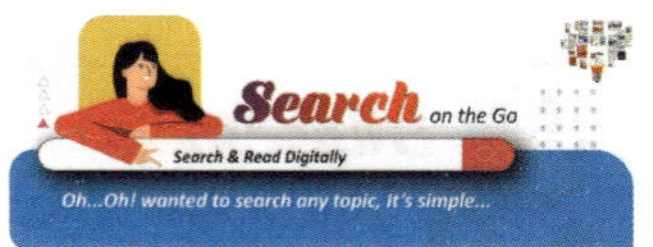

Serum Bilirubin

Bilirubin is an orange-yellow pigment, derived from the breakdown of red blood cells in the liver, spleen and bone marrow (Chapter 7).

Normal value for the sum of the unconjugated and conjugated forms is 0.1–1.0 mg/100 mL of serum. Normally, almost all the bilirubin in plasma is unconjugated. Bilirubin fractionation is also helpful in differential diagnosis of **jaundice**.

Plasma Proteins

As liver is the primary site of the synthesis of plasma proteins, a disturbance in protein synthesis occurs as a consequence of impaired hepatic function. Decreased synthesis of protein leads to a decrease in their plasma concentration. Pattern of alteration in plasma proteins, however, depends upon the type, severity and duration of the liver injury.

In a severe liver disease, hepatic synthesis of albumin is decreased. In chronic hepatocellular damage also, serum albumin concentration falls.

Serum protein electrophoresis, to determine the proportion of different serum proteins, is also helpful in the diagnosis of a liver disease, e.g., α_2- and β-globulins are increased in cirrhosis due to their increased production and decreased clearance. In cholestasis, there is a small increase in serum γ-globulin with a more increase in α- and β-globulins due, in part, to increase serum lipoproteins.

Serum Enzymes

Serum levels of several enzymes are elevated in liver diseases.

ALT and AST

In viral hepatitis and other forms of a liver disease, which may be associated with hepatic necrosis, serum ALT and AST levels are elevated even before clinical signs and symptoms of the disease appear. Levels of both the enzymes may reach values as high as 100 times the upper normal limit. Peak values occur between day seven and day twelve. Thereafter, their activities gradually decrease and reach toward normal by third to fifth week of recovery.

Five to ten-fold increase in both the enzymes occur in patients with primary metastatic carcinoma of the liver. Although serum levels of both ALT and AST are elevated in a liver disease, however, ALT is more liver specific.

Alkaline Phosphatase

Serum alkaline phosphatase (ALP) levels are important in a hepatobiliary disease as well as in bone diseases that are associated with increased osteoblastic activity.

As biliary obstruction results in induction of the enzyme, rise is more marked in extrahepatic obstruction than in intrahepatic obstruction.

Glutamate Dehydrogenase

Glutamate dehydrogenase (GDH) is found in the liver, heart, muscle and kidney. It is present only in traces in normal serum but increased activity is observed in a liver disease with hepatocellular damage.

5′-nucleotidase

5′-nucleotidase (5′-NT) activity is increased by two to six folds, in some of the hepatobiliary diseases. It may be due to extrahepatic causes such as stone or tumor, obstructing the bile duct or in intrahepatic conditions, e.g., cholestasis that may be caused by chlorpromazine, malignant infiltration of the liver or biliary cirrhosis.

γ-glutamyltransferase

γ-glutamyltransferase is also referred to as γ-glutamyltranspeptidase or γ-GT. It is present in high concentration in the serum in intra-hepatic or post-hepatic biliary obstruction.

Elevated levels of γ-GT are also observed in the sera of people who are heavy drinkers. Accordingly, this enzyme has been shown to be of significance in the detection of an alcohol-induced liver disease.

NORMAL VALUES OF SOME BIOCHEMICAL PARAMETERS OF LIVER

Normal values of biochemical parameters of significance in liver function tests are shown in Table 8.8.

TABLE 8.8: Normal values of some biochemical parameters related to liver function tests

Biochemical parameter	Normal value
Bilirubin	
Total Bilirubin	0.2–0.8 mg/dL
Conjugated Bilirubin	0.0–0.3 mg/dL
Unconjugated Bilirubin	0.2–0.8 mg/dL
Proteins	
Total proteins	6.3–8.0 g/dL
Albumin	3.7–5.3 g/dL
Globulins	1.8–3.7 g/dL
$\alpha_1 + \alpha_2$-Globulins	0.4–1.4 g/dL
β-Globulin	0.5–1.3 g/dL
ϒ-Globulin	0.6–1.5 g/dL
Enzymes	
ALT	8–56 IU/L
AST	8–40 IU/L
ALP	39–117 U/L
GDH	<7.0 U/L
5′-NT	2–15 U/L
ϒ-GT	5–35 U/L

THYROID FUNCTION TESTS

The thyroid is a gland found in the neck. Its **main function is to make thyroid hormones**, the chemicals which are released into the bloodstream.

THYROID HORMONES

Thyroid makes three hormones that it secretes into the bloodstream. Two of these hormones called **thyroxine** (T_4) and **triiodothyronine** (T_3), increase body's metabolic rate. The third hormone calcitonin, helps to control the amount of calcium in the blood.

In order to make T_3 and T_4, the thyroid gland needs iodine, a substance found in the food. It is taken up from bloodstream into the thyroid gland. In the thyroid gland, it undergoes a number of different chemical reactions which result in the production of T_3 and T_4. T_4 is so called because it contains four atoms of iodine. T_3 contains three atoms of iodine. In the cells and tissues of the body most T_4 is converted to T_3. T_3 is the more active hormone; it influences the activity of all the cells and tissues of the body.

Thyroid function tests (TFTs) is a collective term for **blood tests** used to check the function of the thyroid. These tests are requested if a patient is thought to suffer from **hyperthyroidism** (overactive thyroid) or **hypothyroidism** (underactive thyroid), or to monitor the effectiveness of either thyroid-suppression or hormone replacement therapy. It is also requested routinely in conditions linked to thyroid disease, such as atrial fibrillation and anxiety disorder.

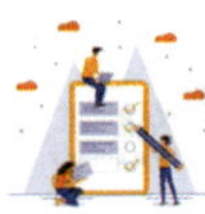
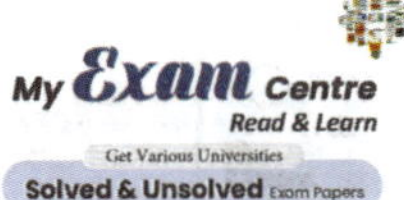

Hyperthyroidism

Hyperthyroidism, often called **overactive thyroid** and sometimes **hyperthyreosis**, is a condition in which the thyroid gland produces and secretes excessive amounts of the free (not protein bound circulating in the blood) thyroid hormones, T_3 and/or T_4.

A variety of conditions can cause hyperthyroidism. Graves' disease (an autoimmune disorder) is the most common. Other causes of hyperthyroidism include excess iodine (iodine is needed to make T_4 and T_3), inflammation of the thyroid gland (thyroiditis causes T_4 and T_3 to leak out of the gland), tumors of the ovaries or testes, benign tumors of the thyroid or pituitary gland or taking large amount of thyroxine (through dietary supplements or medication).

Graves' Disease

Graves' disease is the most common form or cause of hyperthyroidism. In this condition antibodies stimulate the thyroid to secrete too much hormone, the eyes may look enlarged because the eye muscles swell and push the eye forward. This symptom is called exophthalmos.

Some patients have swelling of the front of the neck from an enlarged thyroid gland. It occurs more often in women and tends to run in families. Other symptoms include weakness, irregular heartbeat, difficulty in sleeping, itching, hair loss, nausea and vomiting, and breast development in men.

Thyrotoxicosis

Hyperthyroidism is one cause of thyrotoxicosis, the hypermetabolic clinical syndrome, which occurs when there are elevated serum levels of T_3 and/or T_4. Thyrotoxicosis can also occur without hyperthyroidism. Some people develop thyrotoxicosis due to inflammation of the thyroid gland (thyroiditis) which can lead to excessive release of thyroid hormone already stored in the gland (without the accelerated hormone production that characterizes hyperthyroidism). Thyrotoxicosis can also occur after ingestion of excessive amounts of exogenous thyroid hormone in the form of thyroid hormone supplements.

Thyrotoxicosis or hyperthyroidism may be asymptomatic but when it is not, symptoms are due to an excess of thyroid hormone. If there is too much thyroid hormone, every function of the body tends to speed up.

- Some of the **symptoms of hyperthyroidism** may be nervousness, irritability, increased perspiration, heart racing, hand tremors, anxiety, difficulty sleeping, thinning of the skin, fine brittle hair and muscular weakness, especially in the upper arms and thighs, unintended weight loss and low serum cholesterol. For women, menstrual flow may lighten and menstrual periods may occur less often.
- **Major clinical signs** include weight loss (often accompanied by an increased appetite), anxiety and intolerance to heat, hair loss (especially of the outer side of the eyebrows), muscle ache, weakness, fatigue, hyperactivity, irritability, hyperglycemia, polyuria, polydipsia, delirium, tremor and sweating.
- The first step to **diagnose hyperthyroidism** is a complete history and physical examination, which can reveal common symptoms such as weight loss, rapid pulse, elevated blood pressure, protruding eyes and/or an enlarged thyroid gland (which can appear either symmetrical or one-sided).
- Other tests may be performed to further evaluate the diagnosis. These include **serum cholesterol** (cholesterol levels vary with the metabolic rate, the rate at which cells use energy. In hyperthyroidism, cholesterol can be low due to the elevated metabolic rate), **T_4 and T_3**, **TSH** (a hormone produced by the hypothalamus that stimulates the thyroid gland to produce thyroid hormones. When thyroid hormones levels are normal or high, TSH should not be elevated).

Hypothyroidism

Hypothyroidism, often called **underactive thyroid** or **low thyroid** and sometimes **hypothyreosis**, is a common endocrine disorder in which the thyroid gland does not produce enough thyroid hormone.

- **Iodine deficiency** is the most common cause of primary hypothyroidism and endemic goiter worldwide.
- In areas of the world with sufficient dietary iodine, hypothyroidism is most commonly caused by the autoimmune disease, **Hashimoto's thyroiditis** (chronic autoimmune thyroiditis). Hashimoto's disease may be associated with a goiter. It is characterized by infiltration of the thyroid gland with T lymphocytes and autoantibodies against specific thyroid antigens such as thyroid peroxidase, thyroglobulin and the TSH receptor. Autoimmune thyroiditis is associated with other immune-mediated diseases such as diabetes mellitus type I, pernicious anemia, myasthenia gravis, rheumatoid arthritis, etc.
- Hyperthyroidism due to certain types of **thyroiditis** can eventually lead to hypothyroidism (lack of thyroid hormone), as the thyroid gland is damaged.
- Also, **radioiodine treatment of Graves' disease** often eventually leads to hypothyroidism. Such hypothyroidism may be treated by regular thyroid hormone testing and oral thyroid hormone supplementation.
- Hypothyroidism can cause a number of symptoms such as tiredness, poor ability to tolerate cold and weight gain. In children, hypothyroidism leads to delays in growth and intellectual development, called **cretinism** in severe cases. Cretin children are dwarf and mentally retarded.
- The diagnosis of hypothyroidism, when suspected, can be confirmed with blood tests measuring TSH and thyroxine levels.

COMMONLY USED BIOCHEMICAL PARAMETERS FOR THE EVALUATION OF THYROID FUNCTIONS

Biochemical tests to establish if there is any thyroid dysfunction, include measurement of thyroid hormones (T_3 and T_4) and TSH in serum. Other tests include radioactive iodine uptake, protein bound iodine, serum cholesterol, etc.

Thyroid Hormones

The thyroid function test panel typically includes thyroid hormones such as thyroid-stimulating hormone (TSH, thyrotropin), and thyroxine (T_4) and triiodothyronine (T_3). Measurement of the concentration of T_4 and T_3 in the serum is used in confirming the diagnosis of hyperthyroidism or hypothyroidism.

Thyroxine

Total thyroxine is rarely measured, having been largely superseded by free thyroxine test. It is generally elevated in hyperthyroidism and decreased in hypothyroidism. It is usually slightly elevated in pregnancy, secondary to increased levels of thyroid binding globulin (TBG). Serum T_4 value in a normal person ranges from 4.5–12.5 mg/dL. In hyperthyroidism, serum T_4 concentration is increased to >12 mg/dL whereas in hypothyroidism the value is <5 mg/dL. Estimation of free thyroxine (FT_4), however, provides more reliable information than does total T_4. Free T_4 is generally elevated in hyperthyroidism and decreased in hypothyroidism.

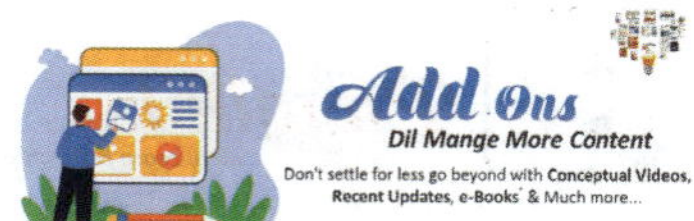

Triiodothyronine

Total triiodothyronine (Total T_3) is rarely measured, having been largely superseded by free T_3 test. Total T_3 is generally elevated in hyperthyroidism and decreased in hypothyroidism. Normal value for serum T_3 varies between 86 and 187 ng/dL. Serum T_3 concentration is low at birth. The value rises to near adult level in early childhood and then is maintained up to 30 years of age, after which it again falls.

Measurement of reverse T_3 (rT_3, a catabolic product of T_4) may also be helpful in some cases, e.g., in low T_3 syndrome where rT_3 concentration is increased. Free T_3 is generally elevated in hyperthyroidism and decreased in hypothyroidism.

Thyroid-Stimulating hormone

Thyroid-stimulating hormone (TSH) is the most sensitive test for thyroid hormone function. TSH is produced in the pituitary gland. The production of TSH is controlled by TRH, which is produced in the hypothalamus. TSH levels may be suppressed by excess free T_3 or free T_4 in the blood.

> Reference value for serum TSH concentration is in the range of 0.3–5.0 µIU/mL.

Measurement of TSH is most useful and sensitive for primary hypothyroidism.

Thyroxine-Binding Globulin

An increased thyroxine-binding globulin results in an increased total thyroxine and total triiodothyronine without an actual increase in hormonal activity of thyroid hormones. Reference range is 12–30 mg/L.

Serum Cholesterol

Increase in serum cholesterol is observed in hypothyroidism whereas it is decreased in hyperthyroidism or thyrotoxicosis.

Serum Calcium

Hyperthyroidism may result in increased plasma calcium along with increased plasma alkaline phosphatase activity.

NORMAL VALUES OF SOME BIOCHEMICAL PARAMETERS OF THYROID FUNCTION

Normal values of biochemical parameters of significance in thyroid function tests are shown in Table 8.9.

TABLE 8.9: Normal values of some biochemical parameters related to thyroid function tests

Biochemical parameter	Normal value
Thyroxine (T_4)	
Total T_4 (T_4)	4.5–12.5 µg/dL
Free T_4 (FT_4)	0.89–1.76 ng/dL
Triiodothyronine (T_3)	
Total T_3 (T_3)	86–187 ng/dL
Free T_3 (FT_3)	2.3–4.2 pg/dL
Thyroid stimulating hormone (TSH)	0.3–5.0 mIU/L (µIU/mL)
Thyroxine-binding globulin (TBG)	1.3–2.0 mg/dL
Serum cholesterol	120–200 mg/dL
Serum calcium	8.5–10.5 mg/dL

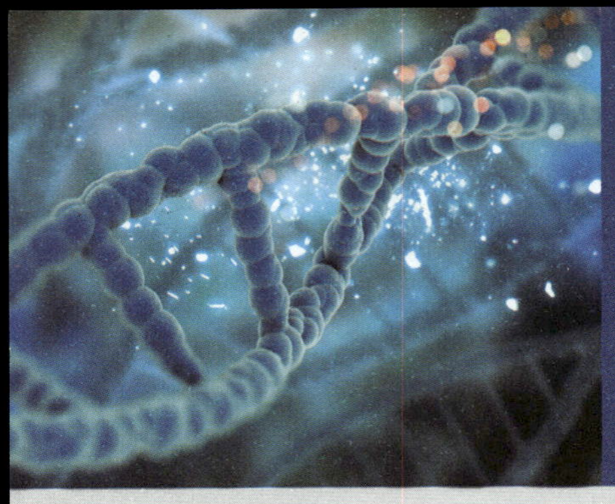

LONG AND SHORT ANSWER QUESTIONS

1. Explain biochemical parameters for the evaluation of thyroid functions.
2. **Write notes on:**
   a. Thyroid function tests
   b. Renal function tests
   c. Differential biochemical diagnosis of jaundice
   d. Clearance tests
   e. Tubular function tests

MULTIPLE CHOICE QUESTIONS

1. **The following proteins are not synthesized in the liver:**
   a. α_1-Globulins
   b. α_2-Globulins
   c. γ-Globulins
   d. β-Globulins

2. **Highest concentration of γ-GT normally occurs in:**
   a. Liver
   b. Kidneys
   c. Small intestine
   d. Lungs

3. **The maximum urea clearance is:**
   a. 54 mL/min
   b. 75 mL/min
   c. 100 mL/min
   d. 125 mL/min

4. **A useful index of renal plasma flow is:**
   a. Inulin clearance
   b. PAH clearance
   c. Creatinine clearance
   d. Urea clearance

ANSWER KEY

1. c   2. a   3. b   4. b

9

Immunochemistry

LEARNING OBJECTIVES

After the completion of the chapter, the readers will be able to:
- Explain about antigen.
- Explain about immune system.
- Understand the complement system.
- Illustrate the structure of Immunoglobulin.
- Understand antibody production.

CHAPTER OUTLINE

- Introduction
- Antigen
- Immune System
- The Complement System
- Molecules of Immune Response
- Immunoglobulins
- Degradation of Immunoglobulin
- Classification and Functions of Immunoglobulins
- Antibody Production
- Investigations and Interpretation

KEY TERMS

Complement system: Made up of a large number of distinct plasma proteins that react with one another to opsonize pathogens and induce a series of inflammatory responses that help to fight infection.

Immunoelectrophoresis: The separation and identification of proteins based on differences in electrical charge and reactivity with antibodies.

Interleukins: A class of cytokines that are secreted by different cells of the immune system and their main function is the regulation of immunity.

Lymphopoietic stem cells: Stem cells in bone marrow, from which lymphocytes generate.

Opsonization: A process that helps immune system identify and destroy old cells and germs (pathogens).

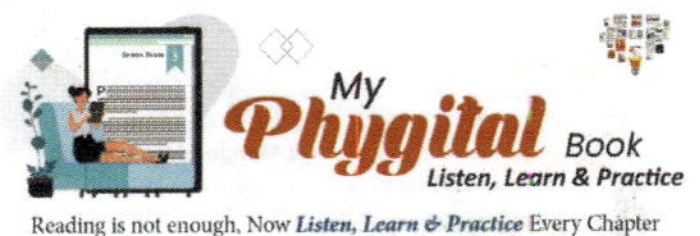

INTRODUCTION

Immunochemistry is the study of biochemical and molecular aspects of immunology, especially the nature of antibodies (immunoglobulins), antigens, their interactions, and determination of immune materials by immunochemical techniques such as enzyme-linked immunosorbent assay (ELISA), immunoblotting, and precipitation and agglutination reactions.

The immune system is a complex system; consisting of the tissues, cells, and molecules and genes involved in the recognition, reaction with, and elimination of foreign and non-self-substances called **antigens** that may disturb the homeostasis of the body.

ANTIGEN

Substances that interact with the immune system and elicit an immune response are referred to as immunogens or antigens. Any substance that is capable of stimulating an immune response is referred to as **immunogen**. In contrast, those substances that are capable of stimulating specific immune responses by binding with specific lymphocytes or antibodies are defined as **antigens**. The features of an antigen that make it immunogenic include foreignness, high molecular weight and chemical complexity. A wide variety of macromolecules, such as proteins, lipoproteins, peptides, glycoproteins, many polysaccharides and some nucleic acids that are foreign to the individual, can act as antigens.

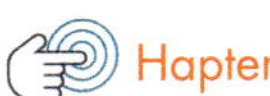 Hapten

Low molecular weight substances, such as amino acids, sugars and small polymers that by themselves are not able to initiate antibody formation but can combine with specific carrier molecules (e.g., a protein) and induce a specific antibody response, are called **haptens**.

IMMUNE SYSTEM

The immune system consists of a complex network of different cells and their products that interact in the immune response. The components, comprising the immune system, arise in the fetal bone marrow between the third and sixth month of fetal life.

Stem cells give rise to **lymphopoietic stem cells**, which **differentiate into T and B lymphocytes** after processing in the thymus and bursa equivalent (bursa, bone marrow or fetal liver), respectively.

T Lymphocytes

T Lymphocytes (T for thymus) or T cells comprise about 75% of lymphocytes in blood. They are the main components of cell-mediated immunity and (like B cells) they are derived from precursor lymphoid stem cells in the bone marrow. The T cells have surface antigens that make possible their identification. The **T cells further differentiate** in the thymus, as follows:

Cytotoxic T Cells

Cytotoxic T cells (Tc cells) are involved in killing foreign cells. They recognize foreign antigens, imbedded in MHC class I molecules. They possess the surface antigen CD8 and produce the cytokine γ-interferon.

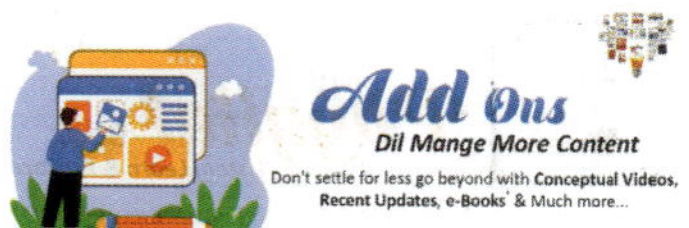

Helper T Cells

These cells have a surface antigen called CD4. Helper T cells (Th cells) are required for the production of normal levels of antibody by B cells and aid in development of cell-mediated immunity. The various functions of the Th cells are due to cytokines, interleukin-2 (IL-2), IL-4, IL-6, IL-10 and γ-interferon. There are two subsets of Th cells, referred to as Th1 (for macrophage activation) and Th2 (for antibody production).

Delayed Hypersensitivity Cells

Delayed hypersensitivity cells (Td cells) have the surface antigen CD4. They produce several cytokines whose functions include attracting macrophages and other defensive cells. Td cells are also involved in the rejection of transplant tissue, some allergic reaction and immunity to neoplasms.

Suppressor T Cells

Suppressor T cells (Ts cells) produce cytokines and other effects that suppress the immune response.

Besides these T cells, natural killer cells and macrophages also play an important role in cell mediated immunity.

Natural Killer Cells

Natural killer cells (Nk cells) are the cytotoxic lymphocytes, which are neither T cells nor B cells but are of lymphoid lineage. They are able to kill tumor and virus infected cells without specific antigen stimulation. They attack those cells that have reduced or altered major histocompatability complex expression and their mechanism of killing is similar to that of cytotoxic T cells.

Macrophages

Macrophage is the main phagocyte of tissues, organs and such serous membranes as the pleura and peritoneum. Macrophages have a role in all phases of the immune response. They are involved in the initial defense of the host by engulfing microbes and in response to the later, secreting cytokines that attract more phagocytes to the area.

Macrophages function as antigen presenting cells (APC), which determine the epitopes available to T cells that ultimately decide the immune response toward a particular antigen. Macrophages are effector cells in cell-mediated immunity and once activated by cytokines present in the area, they serve to produce additional cytokines, in addition to antitumor and antimicrobial activities. Macrophages play crucial role in inflammation, tissue reorganization and tissue repair.

B Lymphocytes

Most B lymphocytes (B for bursa) or B cells migrate from the bone marrow and liver to secondary lymphoid organs and tissues throughout the body. Roughly 20% remain in the circulation. B lymphocytes can transform into plasma cells, which produce antibodies and thus are responsible for humoral immunity. Plasma cells are found mainly in the spleen and lymphoid tissue, and only rarely in the blood, however, antibodies readily enter the circulation.

THE COMPLEMENT SYSTEM

The complement system consists of at least twenty proteins that interact in a complex reaction sequence, referred to as the complement cascade. The proteins of the system are referred to collectively as complement (C) because their action complements certain antibody-mediated reactions. Proteins of the complement system make up about 5% of the serum proteins and are designated by numbers following C, ranging from C1 through C9.

The various proteins act in a sequence or cascade in numerical order where each protein activates the next one in the series, often by cleaving it. The resulting components have new functions. The complement system employs two pathways to achieve its ends, called the classical pathway and the alternative pathway (Fig. 9.1).

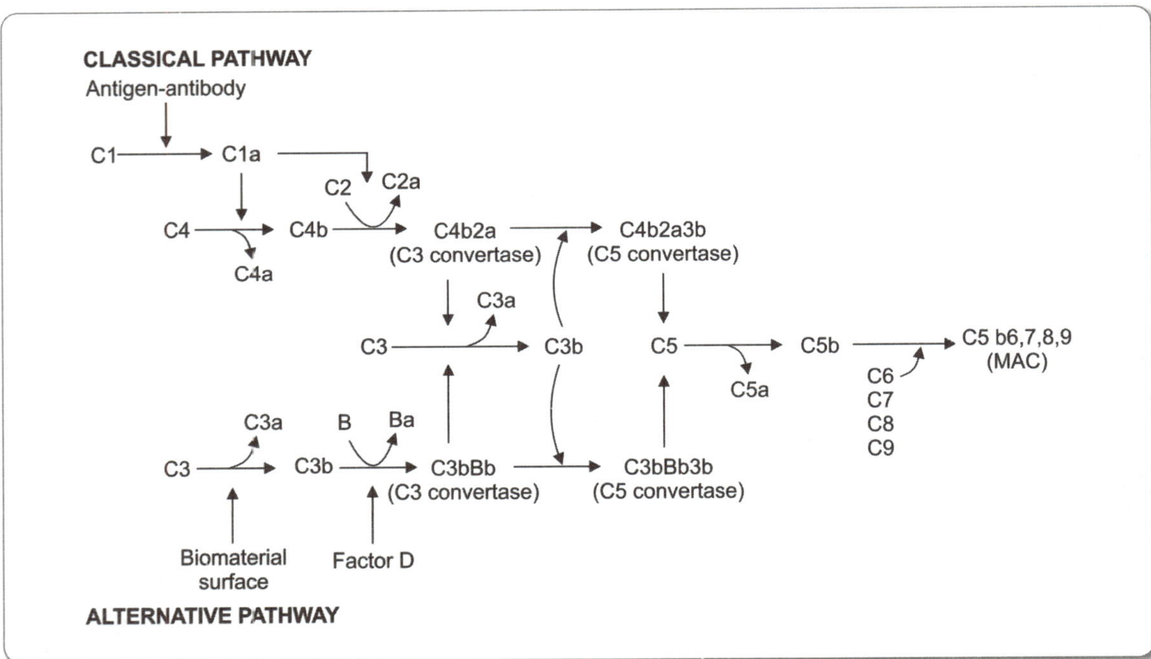

Fig. 9.1: The complement system

The classical pathway is initiated by the binding of antibodies to antigen, while **the alternative pathway** is initiated by cell-wall polysaccharides of the kind found in bacteria and fungi. Both the classical and alternative pathways lead to the cleavage of C3 into fragments C3a and C3b. These initiate cytolysis, inflammation and opsonization.

Cytolysis

The most important function of the complement cascade is to destroy foreign cells. This is accomplished by damaging the cell membrane to the point that the cellular contents leak out. This process is called cytolysis.

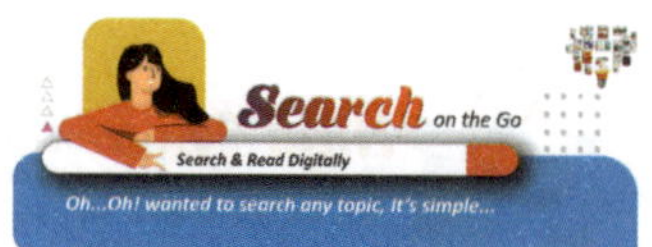

Inflammation

Inflammation is the localized tissue reaction to injury, caused by physical and chemical agents, and by introduction of foreign substances to tissues, including microorganisms. Components C3a to C5a contribute to acute inflammation. Their binding to mast cells, basophils and blood platelets results in the release of histamine, which increases the permeability of blood vessels.

Inflammation is characterized by redness, pain, heat and swelling. The functions of inflammation are:

- To destroy and remove a deleterious agent, if possible;
- If it cannot be removed, to sequester the injury to a localized area within the body; and
- To repair any damage that may have resulted from the injury.

Inflammation is the body's response to injury or tissue damage. It involves the interaction of the microvasculature, circulating blood cells, cells in the tissues and their secreted products. Cells involved in inflammation include those that usually circulate in the blood and are involved in phagocytic and secretory responses, such as polymorphonuclear leukocytes (neutrophil, eosinophil and basophil), mononuclear phagocytes (monocytes), lymphocytes, platelets and endothelial cells as well as those that are tissue-based, which include mast cells and macrophages.

All the cells involved in inflammatory response synthesize and secrete a wide variety of soluble chemical substances termed inflammatory mediators, such as acute-phase reactants like C-reactive protein (CRP) and components of the complement system, etc.

Opsonization

It is the promotion of phagocytosis by specific antibody in conjunction with complement. Component C3b coats foreign cells and interact with special receptors on phagocytes, to promote phagocytosis.

MOLECULES OF IMMUNE RESPONSE

Cytokines

Cytokines are soluble molecules that mediate interactions between cells. These are a diverse group of small, soluble proteins produced by leukocytes that mediate a variety of immune functions. Those cytokines produced by lymphocytes are sometimes called **lymphokines**.

Generally, they are secreted by one cell and bind to specific receptors on the corresponding target cells. Cytokines may also bind to the cells that produce them and have self-stimulation (autocrine) functions that result in such processes as cell division and protein synthesis, and ultimately differentiation and clonal proliferation.

Those cytokines that mediate interactions between leukocytes are called **interleukins** (ILs). Cytokines other than interleukins include interferon (IFN), granulocyte-monocyte colony stimulating factor (GM-CSF) and tumor necrosis factor (TNF).

Cytokines are antigen nonspecific glycoproteins that are rapidly secreted by the cells that produce them, rather than stored. Thus, they are very short-lived and are typically in minute quantities. These compounds are responsible for delayed type hypersensitivity responses and the recruitment of large number of monocytes to a site of infection. Each cell is capable of producing multiple cytokines while each cytokine also has a unique function. Each cytokine can affect many different types of cells, depending upon the cytokine receptors, present on a particular cell.

Over-expression of cytokines can have a devastating effect on the immune response. For example, overproduction of TNF by macrophages can lead to septic shock.

Cytokines are soluble mediators of the inflammatory and immune response. They are produced by a variety of cells and tissues, are peptides or glycoprotein in nature and are active at concentration between 10^{-9} and 10^{-15} molar. They act by interacting with receptors on the surface of their target cells.

Cytokines may be grouped as interferons, interleukins and chemokines.

Besides the prostaglandins and leukotrienes, cytokines form another group of inflammatory mediators.

Major Histocompatibility Complex

The collection of genes coding for the self-marking proteins or **major histocompatibility antigens** is referred to as major histocompatibility complex **(MHC)**. These antigens occur on the surface of all the body's cells and identify them as belonging to the body and not foreign. Some MHC antigens appear on the surface of cells of the immune system.

- The **human MHC region** is known as the *human leucocyte antigen (HLA)* **region** and the corresponding genes are located on chromosome 6. Although HLA complex pertains to the humans, sometimes MHC and HLA antigens are the terms that are used interchangeably.
- The **MHC** is subdivided into three regions, known as **Class I, Class II and Class III**. MHC Class I and Class II are associated with the stimulation of T cells. Class III MHC contains an assemblage of twenty different genes, some cytokines, heat-shock proteins and complement factors.

MHC Class I Antigens

In humans, the Class I genes contain three loci, i.e., A, B and C. These genes encode a transmembrane protein that possesses three extracellular domains, designated as α_1, α_2 and α_3. Chemically, class I antigens are glycoproteins composed of a heavy chain and a light chain, known as β_2-microglobulin.

MHC class I molecules are transplantation antigens and are expressed on most of the nucleated cells in mammals. These include HLA-A, HLA-B and HLA-C antigens. The β-microglobulin is essential for the expression of the MHC Class I molecules on the surface of the cell. Expression of the MHC Class I molecule on the cell surface can be either up-regulated (increased expression) or down-regulated (decreased expression) by a variety of stimuli.

When interacting with the T cell receptors, the CD8 molecule interacts with the invariant region of the MHC class I molecule. These transplantation antigens are the main determinants, which would decide whether a graft is to be accepted or rejected. If the transplantation antigens of a donor match the antigens found on the recipient, the transplant is successful.

MHC Class II Molecules

These are also known as immune responsiveness antigens. In humans, the MHC class II region includes three genes that are referred to as DP, DQ and DR. Each of these encodes an α chain and a β chain. MHC class II

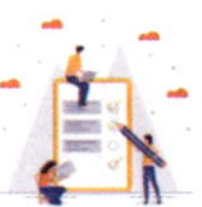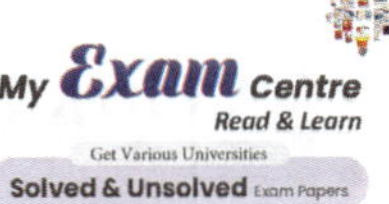

molecules are expressed constitutively on the surface of macrophages, monocytes, B cells, dendritic cells and thymic epithelial cells. The expression of MHC class II can be induced on other cells by IFNγ.

The CD4 molecule of the T cell receptors interacts with the invariant region of the MHC class II molecule.

HLA Typing

The HLA compatibility has to be determined prior to transplantation, paternity testing and any HLA associated diseases. This is referred to as HLA typing and is done with the help of serological tests, such as **lymphocyte cytotoxicity tests and mixed lymphocyte culture**.

IMMUNOGLOBULINS

Immunoglobulins form a related but enormously **diverse group of proteins** called **globulins**, which have **antibody activity.** They are **synthesized and secreted** by plasma cells, **in response** to invasion by **an antigen**, hence called **antibodies**. They are **glycoprotein** in nature and are present in the serum and some tissue fluids of all the mammals.

Immunoglobulins constitute approximately 20% of the total plasma proteins.

Some of them are carried to surface of the B cells where they act as receptors for the specific antigens while others are found in free form in blood or lymph. Contact between B cells and the antigen is needed to convert B cells into the antibody forming cells, also called plasma cells, which secrete large amount of antibodies.

Antibodies are highly specific for the three-dimensional conformation of the epitope.

Structure of an Immunoglobulin

- A molecule of immunoglobulin has **Y-shaped structure** with two arms and a stem.
- It has **four polypeptide chains**, which are bound by –S–S–linkages. They comprise of **two small subunits** called **L chains** and **two large subunits** called **H chains**.
- Each subunit has a **variable region**, which is located towards the **N-terminal end** and **constant region(s)** that are located towards the **C-terminal end**.
- Its two arms are called the **Fab fragments** whereas the stem is called **Fc fragment**.
- Both the **arms are linked** to the stem **by a flexible region**, called hinge region.

An Immunoglobulin has Four Polypeptide Chains

An immunoglobulin is a basic unit comprising of **four polypeptide chains**. Out of these, there are **two** identical **small polypeptides**, called L-chains **(light chains)** and **two** identical **large polypeptides**, which are designated as **H-chains (heavy chains)**. They occur in light-heavy-heavy-light arrangement. Its four chains are **joined** with each other **by disulfide bonds** (–S–S–) and form, roughly, a Y-shaped molecule, which has two arms and a stem (Fig. 9.2).

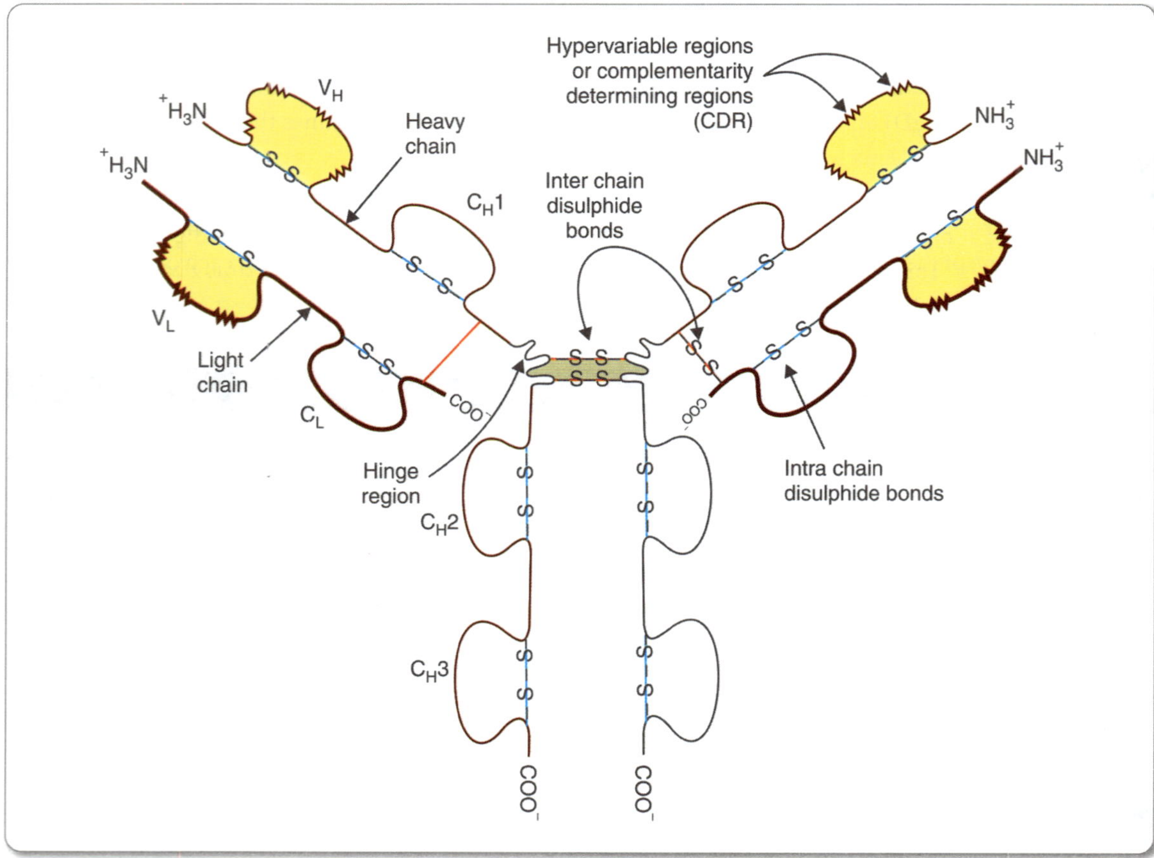

Fig. 9.2: Structure of an immunoglobulin

Light Chains

The **smaller polypeptides** (about 25 kD each) are designated as the **light chains (L-chains)**. Each L chain has approximately **220 amino acids**.

Two types of the **L chains** may occur in immunoglobulins. They are designated as **kappa** (κ-chain) and **lambda** (λ-chain).

Though any type of the L-chain may be found in an immunoglobulin molecule but, generally, an immunoglobulin has two identical chains, i.e., it has either two κ-chains (κ_2) or two λ-chains (λ_2) but never one κ-chain and one λ-chain (κλ).

These are referred to as the isotypes and are found in all the individuals. In human immunoglobulins, κ-chains are more prevalent than the λ-chains.

Heavy Chains

The **larger subunits** that are found in the immunoglobulins are called **heavy chains (H-chains)**.

Five different types of the **H chains**, each containing **440–450 amino acids**, are found in immunoglobulins, in human beings. Molecular mass of an H-chain may vary from 50 kD to 75 kD.

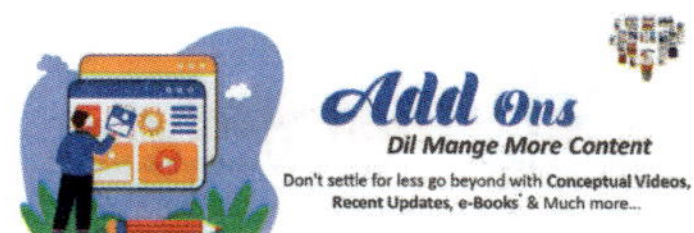

Various types of the H chains are designated as **gamma (γ)**, **alpha (α)**, **mue (μ)**, **delta (δ) and epsilon (ε)**. Each one of the H-chain is specific to a class of the immunoglobulin. Thus, depending upon the type of the **H-chain**, they are called **immunoglobulin G (IgG)**, **immunoglobulin A (IgA)**, **immunoglobulin M (IgM)**, **immunoglobulin D (IgD)** and **immunoglobulin E (IgE)**. The H-chain determines the class and subclass of the immunoglobulin molecule.

Both types of the chains, i.e., the L-chain and the H-chain, are synthesized **separately** and are subsequently **assembled** to form a mature immunoglobulin tetramer molecule (L_2H_2), within the plasma cells. During assembly, each one of the two-H chains is associated with the two-L chains as well as with each other **by –S–S– linkages**.

An L-chain is joined to the H-chain in such a way that they run parallel to each other. Since L-chain is only about half the size of the H-chain (as an L-chain contains nearly 220 amino acids as compared to 440–450 present in the H-chain), **L chain** is therefore, **associated with only NH_2-terminal half of the H-chain**.

Various chains in an immunoglobulin molecule are folded into discrete regions, called domains. There are two domains in the light chain while depending on their class, four or five domains are found in a heavy chain.

Each Polypeptide has Two Regions

Each chain has two regions called variable region and constant region.

1. **Variable regions: Amino acid sequences** that are found in the **NH_2-terminal half** of the **L chains** and **one-fourth** of the **H chains** are highly variable between the different immunoglobulin molecules. Therefore, these NH_2-terminal regions are **called variable regions (V regions)**. They are highly **heterogeneous** and vary to the extent that no two V regions, from different persons, have identical amino acid sequences. The V regions of the L-chains and the H-chains are designated as the V_L region and the V_H region, respectively.

2. **Constant regions:** Half of the **L-chain** towards the **COOH-terminal end** and **three-fourths** of the **H-chain** towards the **COOH-terminal end** has **homologous amino acid sequences**, i.e., these segments are homologous with the same segments of the other L or H-chains found in the same class of immuno-globulin. These regions, with a homologous primary structure, are called **constant regions (C region)**. The C regions of the L-chains and the H-chains are designated as the C_L region and **the C_H region**, respectively. C_H **region** is further **subdivided** into **three parts,** each comprising about 110 amino acids. These are designated as $C_H^{\,1}$, $C_H^{\,2}$ and $C_H^{\,3}$, respectively. Each such segment of the C_H region is **homologous to each other as well as to the C_L region**. Each of these segments (sequence repeats) contains an intrachain disulfide bond.

The μ type and ε type of the H chains have four C_H regions instead of three found in others.

V regions of the immunoglobulin is involved in **recognition and binding of the antigen with the antibody**. This ability of the antibody **resides in several short sequences**, which are located in small loops **within the V region**. These short loops are termed *hypervariable regions (hypervariable sequences)*.

Characteristics of the C_H Region

- C_H region **determines the antibody class** *of an immunoglobulin.*
- *This region of the immunoglobulin molecule provides a* **site for the binding of the complement protein.**
- *These are also the* **sites** *for the antibodies* **to cross the placental membrane.**
- *Depending upon the class of an immunoglobulin,* **variable amounts of carbohydrates** *(2–15%)* **are attached to the C_H^2 region.**
- *Amino acid sequences in C_H region, in some cases, also promote* **polymerization of the basic molecular structure** *of the* **immunoglobulin molecule.**

Only 5–10 amino acids in each of the hyper-variable sequence **contribute to the antigen-binding site** (ab site). These hypervariable sequences (the antigen-binding sites) are **complementary to the topology of the antigen** and are **designated as complementary-determining regions. Three hypervariable sequences** are commonly found in the V_L **region. A V_H region may have three or four hypervariable sequences**, depending upon the type of the antibody.

Amino acid segments separating different hypervariable sequences from each other are referred to as the **framework regions**.

In a polymeric structure, basic molecular structures are covalently linked to each other around a peptide, called joining subunit or J chain.

Immunoglobulins of the IgA class generally occur as dimmers while IgM occur as pentamers (Fig. 9.3).

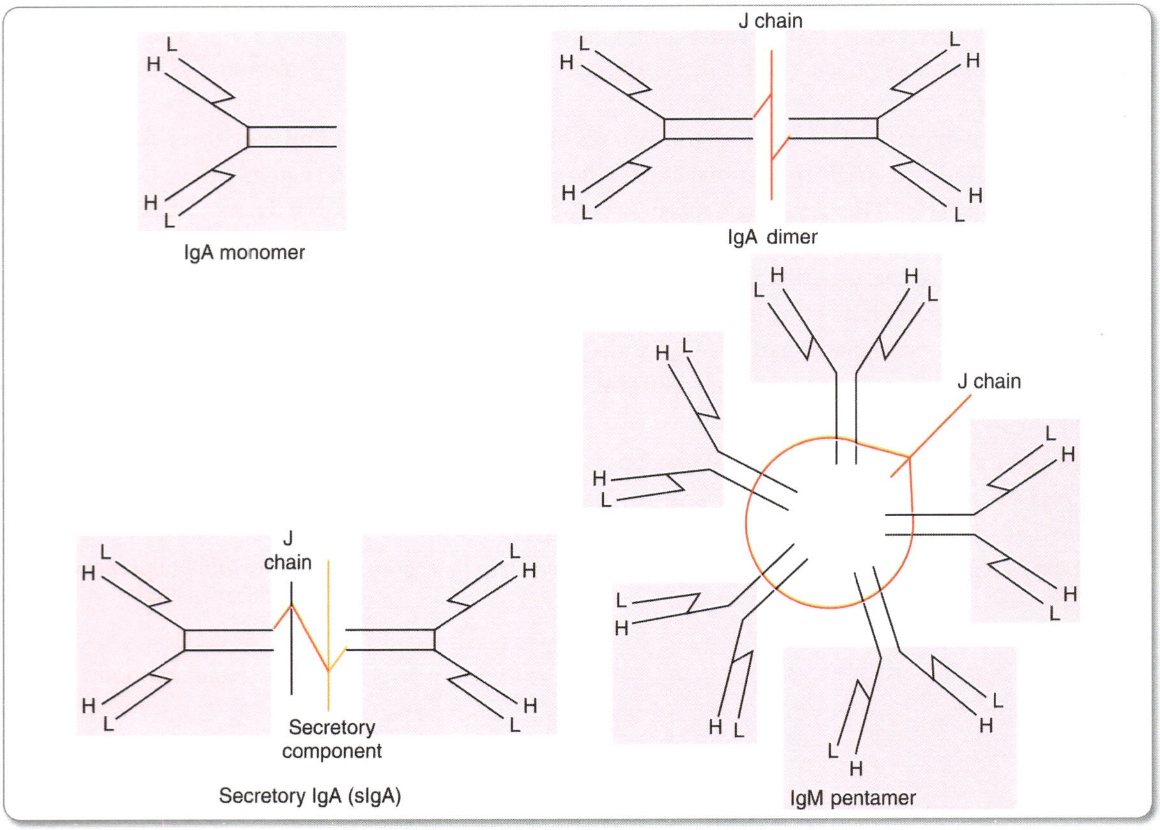

Fig. 9.3: Structures of IgA and IgM molecules

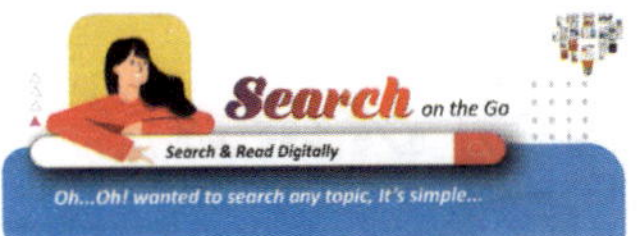

DEGRADATION OF IMMUNOGLOBULIN

An **immunoglobulin** molecule, such as IgG, can be **cleaved with** the enzyme **papain**, which hydrolyzes it **into three fragments** of approximately 50 kD each. **Two** of these fragments are identical and represents two arms. These are the fragments where an antigen binds and are called **Fab fragments**. The **third fragment represents the stem**. Since this fragment can be easily crystallized, it is called **Fc fragment** (Fig. 9.4).

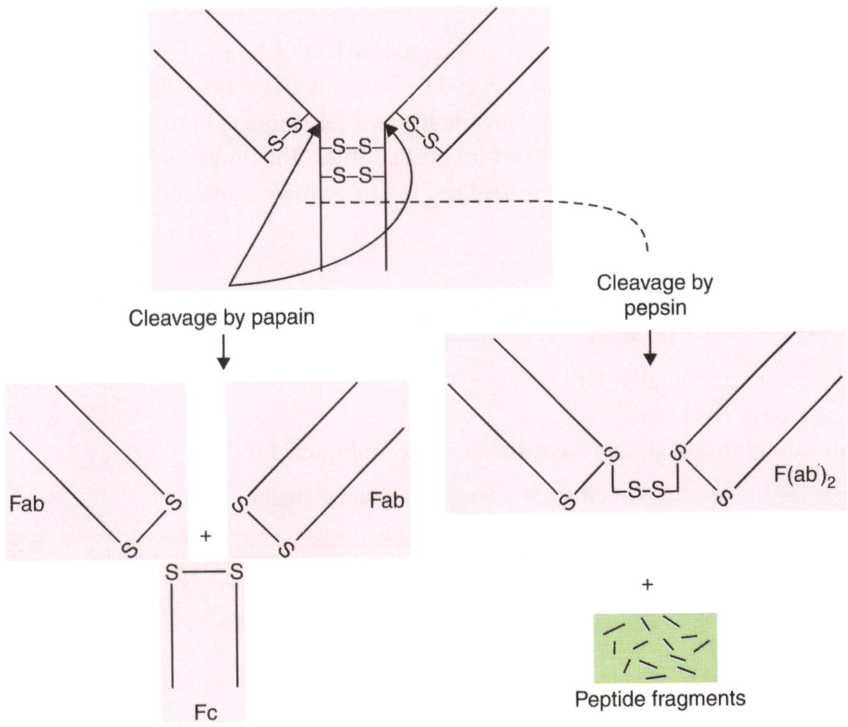

Fig. 9.4: Proteolytic degradation of an immunoglobulin molecule by papain and pepsin

Proteolytic cleavage by pepsin: Action of pepsin on an immunoglobulin molecule results in a fragment that has 2 Fab regions only, i.e., F(ab)$_2$ while the Fc fraction is hydrolyzed to oligopeptides and amino acids (Fig. 9.4).

Fab Fragment

Fab fragment has **entire L-chain** and **half of the H chain** (comprising of the V_H and the C_H^1 regions). Each of the Fab fragments can bind to an antigen with the affinity similar to that of the intact antibody. Because there are two Fab domains, a molecule of an immunoglobulin can bind two molecules of the antigen, simultaneously. Thus, an **antibody** is said to be **divalent**.

Fc Fragment

The **Fc fragment** consists of the **C-terminal halves of the two-H chains**, i.e., the C_H2 and C_H3 regions, which are joined together by disulfide bridges.

All antibodies thus are bifunctional, i.e., in addition to the antigen binding, they also exhibit one or more effector functions, such as complement activation and cell binding (in the Fc region).

Hinge Region

Two **Fab fragments** of the immunoglobulin are **connected to** the **Fc fragment by a flexible region,** referred to as the *hinge region*. It is present between the C_H1 and C_H2 regions and confers flexibility to the molecule. This in turn allows two Fab fragments to move independently and help them to bind two antigens, simultaneously, that may be present at different distances, apart from each other. The hinge region has one or more cysteine residues, which provide **interchain disulfide bridges**. It also controls interactions between different parts of an immunoglobulin.

CLASSIFICATION AND FUNCTIONS OF IMMUNOGLOBULINS

There are five classes of immunoglobulins called IgG, IgA, IgM, IgD and IgE. Each one differs from other with respect due to the type of its H chain.

Various immunoglobulin classes have different physiological functions (Table 9.1).

TABLE 9.1: Properties and functions of different classes of immunoglobulins

Ig class	Approximate molecular weight (kD)	H chain	Carbohydrate content (%)	Serum concentration (mg/dL)	Major physiological function
IgG	146	γ	2–4	800–1500	• Placental transfer • Provides immunity to neonates
IgA	160–380	α	5–9	150–250	• Protects outer surfaces • sIgA is present in mucous secretions
IgM	970	μ	8–12	70–150	• First line of defense, synthesized in neonates
IgD	160	δ	8–12	3–5	• Primary function unknown, acts as B cell receptor
IgE	190	ε	10–15	0.01–0.05	• Reaginic antibodies, implicated in allergic reactions • Release of histamine and other vasoactive amines

Immunoglobulin G

Immunoglobulin G (IgG) is a major immunoglobulin produced by the plasma cells. It accounts for **70–75% of the total** immunoglobulins found in serum.

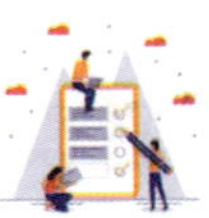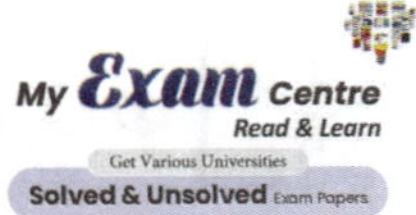

The IgG is the most important class of immunoglobulins that occurs in secondary immune response and is distributed evenly between the intravascular and the extra vascular pools.

Antibodies of the IgG class are **produced in response to most bacteria and viruses**. These antibodies **bind to macrophages and neutrophils**, and **promote phagocytosis**.

The IgG has four subclasses, which are referred to as IgG_1, IgG_2, IgG_3 and IgG_4. Structurally, these **subclasses differ,** primarily, **in the hinge region**. It is the IgG_1 and IgG_3 both of which bind firmly to Fc receptors of phagocytic cells and activate K cells (killer monocytes).

In human beings, IgG molecules of all the subclasses cross placenta and confer high degree of passive immunity to the newborn.

The major effector mechanism of the human IgG_1 and IgG_3 subclasses is the activation of the classical pathway of a complement.

Immunoglobulin A

Immunoglobulin A (IgA) accounts for about **15–20% of the total** serum immunoglobulins.

In human beings, >80% of the IgA occurs as a monomer but in most other mammals, serum IgA is mainly dimeric.

The IgA has two subclasses, designated as IgA_1 and IgA_2. In human serum, IgA_1 is the predominant subclass. It accounts for 75–90% of total IgA in many secretions, such as nasal secretion, tear, saliva and milk. In the colon IgA_2 predominates.

Secretory IgA

Secretory IgA (sIgA) is the most important form of IgA. It is called secretory IgA since it is the predominant immunoglobulin in seromucous secretions, such as saliva, colostrums, milk and tracheobronchial and genito-urinary secretions. It exists, mainly in the dimeric form, in association with another protein that is known as a secretory component. sIgA may be of either of the two subclasses, i.e., it may be IgA_1 or IgA_2.

The sIgA is assembled during an active transport process, as the locally produced dimeric IgA passes across the mucosal epithelium. It is the sIgA, which is found in the bronchial, nasal and intestinal mucous **secretions**, tear, milk and colostrum.

The sIgA provides initial defense against invading viral and bacterial pathogens, prior to their entry into the internal spaces. Its deficiency is the commonest disorder, which results in recurrent infections of the sinus and respiratory tract.

Immunoglobulin M

Immunoglobulin M (IgM) accounts for nearly **5–10% of the total** circulating immunoglobulins. Most of the IgM in serum is **a pentamer** consisting of five Y-shaped monomeric molecules, which are **arranged around the J chain**.

Two other features characterize an IgM molecule, i.e., an abundance of oligosaccharide units, which are associated with the μ chain and an additional peptide chain called joining chain (J-chain) that assist the process of polymerization, prior to its secretion.

The IgM is the **first** immunoglobulin, which is synthesized by the cell, on introduction of an antigen into the host. IgM thus, is called the **first line of defense**. It is the only immunoglobulin that **a neonate** normally synthesizes.

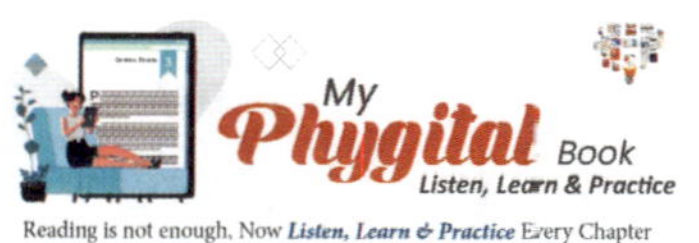

The IgM is the predominant antibody in primary immune response. It is largely confined to the intravascular pool and is frequently associated with the immune response to antigenically complex blood-borne infectious organisms.

Once bound to its target, IgM is a potent activator of the classical pathway of a complement.

Immunoglobulin D

Immunoglobulin D (IgD) accounts for **<1% of the total** serum immunoglobulins. It is the major component of the surface membrane of many B cells and may play a role in antigen-triggered lymphocyte differentiation though its primary function is unknown.

Immunoglobulin E

Immunoglobulin E (IgE) is normally present in blood in **minute concentrations**. It is found on the surface membrane of basophils and mast cells, in all individuals.

It also sensitizes cells on the mucosal surfaces, such as conjunctival, nasal and bronchial mucosa. It **protects** the host **against parasites** and has been **implicated in allergic reactions**. When antigen cross-links some of the attached IgE molecules, **mast cells** are stimulated to **release histamine** and other vasoactive amines, which, in turn, are responsible for vascular permeability and smooth muscle contraction.

The **IgE** is commonly associated with the **allergic diseases**, such as hay fever and asthma.

ANTIBODY PRODUCTION

Both, **L chains** and **H chains** are synthesized independently and form an immunoglobulin molecule.

The immune system has a potential to produce large number of different antibodies, which can react with almost every antigen that an organism encounters. A human, however, does not contain as many numbers of genes so that each one of it can code for an individual immunoglobulin. This is achieved by generating great diversity in the antibodies that are produced by the B cells.

Generation of such immense **antibody diversity** is achieved by recombination of a limited number of gene segments, to produce vast number of variable domains.

INVESTIGATIONS AND INTERPRETATION

Immune materials may be analyzed by various immunochemical techniques such as agglutination reactions, immunodiffusion, immunoelectrophoresis and enzyme-linked immunosorbent assay (ELISA).

Agglutination Reaction

This is the **binding of particulate antigen by antibody**, resulting in an observable **clumping** or aggregation. Antigens, both soluble and particulate, can be adsorbed to carrier red cells. When these coated red cells are mixed with specific antibody, hemagglutination takes place. This test is used for the diagnosis of a number of diseases.

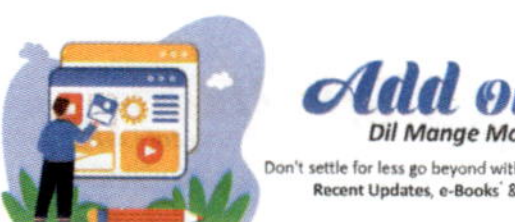

Immunodiffusion

It is based on the principal that when an **antigen is mixed with a specific antiserum,** they form an **antigen-antibody complex** which precipitates out. The amount of the precipitate depends on the relative concentration of the antigen and the antibody.

This is a precipitin test in which soluble antigen is placed in a well, in an agar gel containing antibody. The antigen and antibody diffuse towards one another and a specific reaction results in a visible precipitate within 48 hours. A **precipitin ring** is formed, the diameter of which is proportional to the concentration of the antigen.

Immunoelectrophoresis

In this technique, a sample containing mixture of proteins (antibodies) is subjected to electrophoresis in agar gel, which contains an antigen. Proteins migrate to various positions in the gel by an electric current. Thereafter, antiserum to a specific immunoglobulin is added into a horizontal trough, in agar gel. Development of the **precipitin arc** identifies the presence of the protein of interest.

Rocket immunoelectrophoresis is used to quantify antigen. In this technique, an agarose gel is prepared containing a predetermined concentration of antibody. Wells are cut into the agarose, once it has solidified, and are filled with antigen. An electric current is then passed through the gel. Antigen-antibody complexes are formed in the shape of rockets. The height of the rocket is proportional to the amount of antigen in the well.

Enzyme-Linked Immunosorbent Assay

Enzyme-linked immunosorbent assay (**ELISA**) is an antibody test, a test for immune response to immunogen which attack the body, such as virus, bacteria and allergens that may be related to certain infectious conditions, e.g., to diagnose HIV which causes AIDS. ELISA is a test where an **enzyme is linked to an antibody or antigen** for the qualitative detection and quantification of a specific substance.

Applications of ELISA

The ELISA tests are used as *in vitro* diagnostics in medical laboratories, such as for the:

- Estimation of hormones and tumor markers
- Detection of *Mycobacterium* antibodies in tuberculosis, hepatitis B markers and HIV antibodies in blood samples
- Detection of rotavirus in feces, etc.
- Besides, these are widely used in research, drug discovery, bioassay validation, quality control and manufacturing processes in the pharmaceutical and biotechnological industry and academic organizations.

General Principle of ELISA

The ELISA is a very sensitive immunochemical technique which is used to access the presence of specific protein (antigen or antibody) in the given sample. It requires at least one antibody with specificity for the particular antigen. An enzyme conjugated with an antibody reacts with a colorless substrate to generate a colored reaction product (Fig. 9.5).

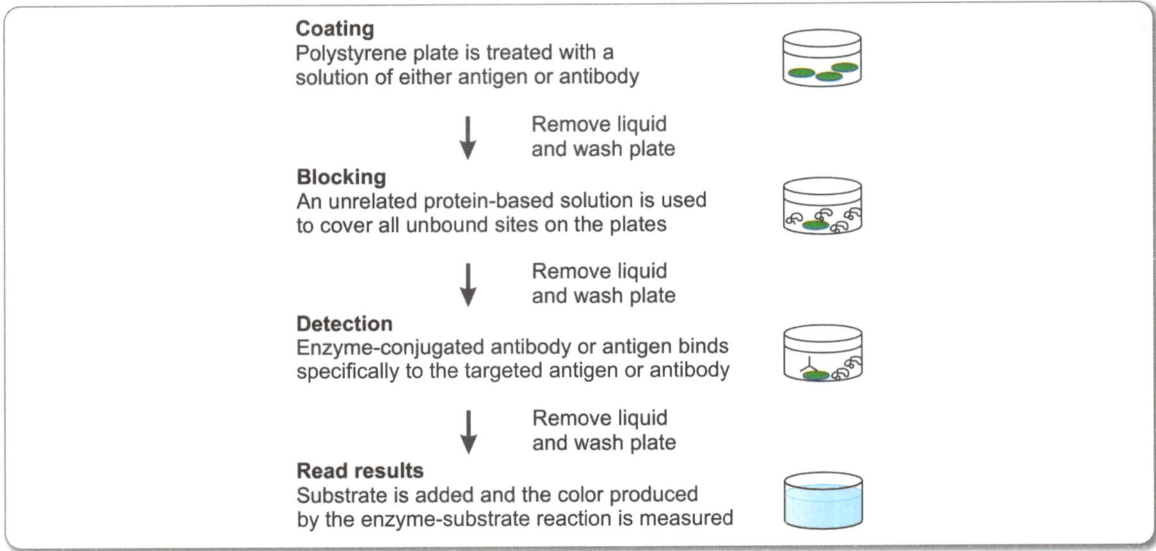

Fig. 9.5: General principle of ELISA

Enzyme Labels Used

Some of the commonly used enzymes and their substrates are shown in Table 9.2.

TABLE 9.2: Commonly used enzyme labels

Enzyme label	Substrate
Horse radish peroxidase	Tetramethylbenzidine (TMB)
Alkaline phosphatase	BCIP (5-bromo-4-chloro-3-indolyl-phosphate) with NBT (nitro blue tetrazolium)

General Procedure

- The sample with an unknown amount of antigen is immobilized on a solid support (usually a polystyrene microtiter plate) either non-specifically (via adsorption to the surface) or specifically (via capture by another antibody specific to the same antigen, in a sandwich ELISA).
- After the antigen is immobilized, the detection antibody is added, forming a complex with the antigen. The detection antibody can be covalently linked to an enzyme or can itself be detected by a secondary antibody that is linked to an enzyme through bioconjugation.
- Between each step, the plate is typically washed with a mild detergent solution to remove any proteins or antibodies that are non-specifically bound.
- After the final wash step, the plate is developed by adding an enzymatic substrate to produce a visible signal, a color change in the substrate, which indicates the quantity of antigen in the sample.

Types of ELISA

Indirect ELISA

The indirect ELISA detects the presence of **antibody** in a sample (Fig. 9.6):

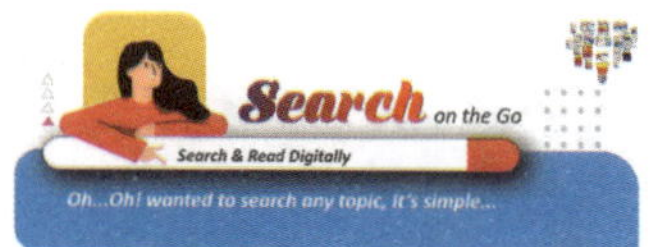

- The antigen, for which the sample is to be analyzed, is adhered to the wells of the microtiter plate.
- The primary antibody, present in the sample, binds specifically to the antigen after addition of the sample.
- The solution is washed to remove unbound antibodies and then enzyme conjugated secondary antibodies are added.
- The substrate for enzyme is added to quantify the primary antibody through a color change.
- The concentration of primary antibody present in the serum directly correlates with the intensity of the color.

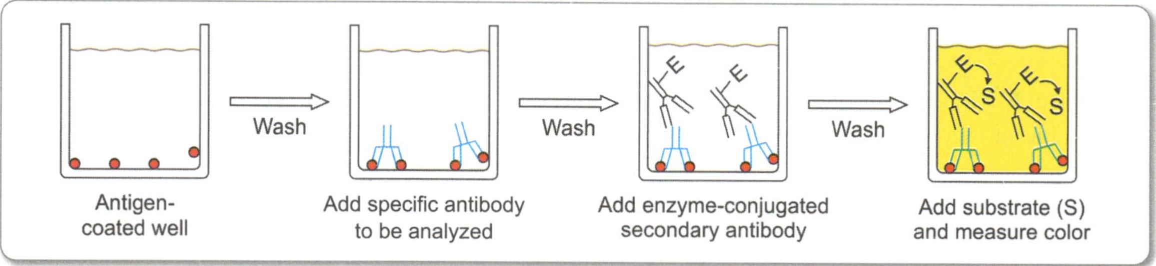

Fig. 9.6: Principle and procedure of indirect ELISA

Advantages of indirect ELISA

- A wide variety of labeled secondary antibodies are available, commercially. Further, it is a versatile procedure because many primary antibodies can be made in one species and the same labeled secondary antibody can be used for detection. As a result of it, maximum immunoreactivity of the primary antibody is retained since it is not labeled.
- Sensitivity is increased because each primary antibody contains several epitopes that can be bound by the labeled secondary antibody, allowing for signal amplification.

  This, however, requires an extra incubation step, as a result of which cross-reactivity might occur with the secondary antibody, thereby resulting in nonspecific signal.

Sandwich ELISA

The sandwich ELISA is used to detect a specific sample antigen (Fig. 9.7).

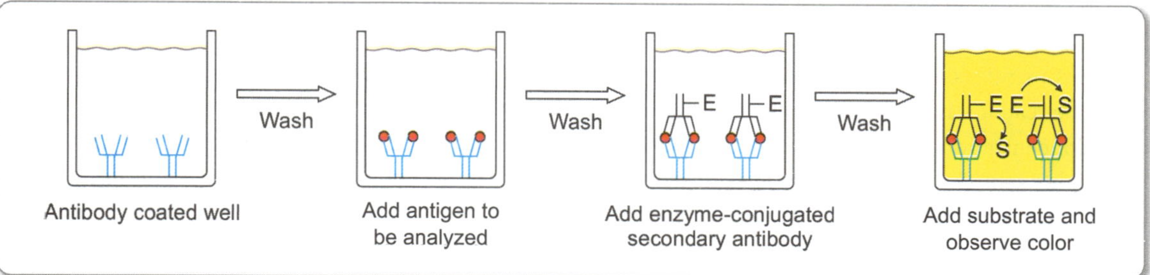

Fig. 9.7: Principle and procedure of sandwich ELISA

Various steps of the sandwich ELISA include:

- The wells of microtiter plate are coated with the antibodies.
- Nonspecific binding sites are blocked using bovine serum albumin.

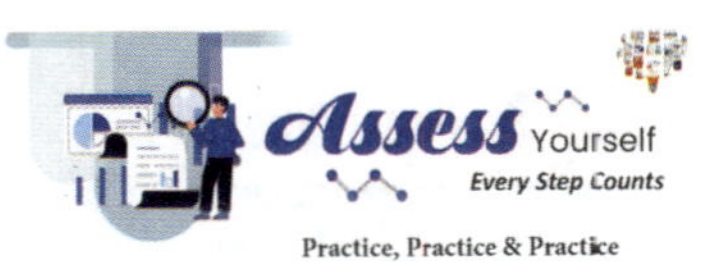

- The antigen-containing sample is applied to the wells and captured by antibody.
- The plate is washed to remove unbound antigen.
- Enzyme linked secondary antibody is added, which, in turn, binds to antigen (**sandwich**, i.e., the antigen is stuck between the two antibodies).
- The plate is washed to remove the unbound antibody-enzyme conjugates.
- The substrate for enzyme is added to quantify the antigen.
- The absorbance of the chromogen is measured to determine the presence and quantity of antigen.
  It has high specificity because the antigen is specifically captured and detected.

Competitive ELISA

This type of ELISA depends on the competitive reaction between the sample antigen and antigen bound to the wells of microtiter plate with the primary antibody (Fig. 9.8).

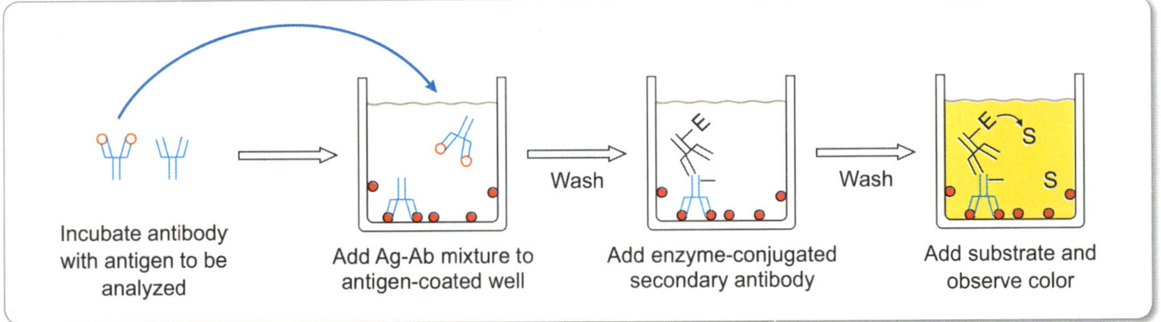

Fig. 9.8: Principle and procedure of competitive ELISA

Various steps of the competitive ELISA include:

- Unlabeled antibody is incubated in the presence of its antigen (sample).
- These bound antibody/antigen complexes are then added to an antigen-coated well.
- After the incubation, unbound antibodies are washed off, so unbound antibodies are removed. (The more the antigen in the sample, the more the Ag-Ab complexes is formed and so, there are less unbound antibodies available to bind to the antigen in the well, hence **competition**).
- Secondary antibody, specific to the primary antibody, is added. This second antibody is coupled to the enzyme.
- A substrate is added, and remaining enzymes elicit a chromogenic signal.
- The reaction is stopped to prevent eventual saturation of the signal.
- Concentration of color is inversely proportional to the amount of antigen present in the sample.

It is highly sensitive even when the specific detecting antibody is present in relatively small amounts.

Some competitive ELISA kits include enzyme-linked antigen rather than enzyme-linked antibody. The labeled antigen competes for primary antibody binding sites with the sample antigen (unlabeled). The less antigen in the sample, the more labeled antigen is retained in the well and the stronger are the signals.

High density microplates are, typically, used for screening applications, when throughput (number of samples processed per day) and assay cost per sample become critical parameters, with a typical assay volume between 5 and 50 µL per well.

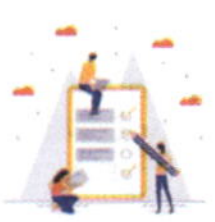
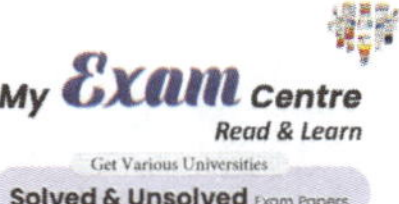

ELISA Readers

The ELISA reader is an instrument used for ELISA technique.

Types of ELISA readers

- Microplate ELISA readers
- Automated ELISA readers

Microplate ELISA readers

Microplate ELISA reader, also known as **microplate readers** or **microplate photometers**, are instruments which are used to detect biological, chemical or physical events of samples in microtiter plates. Common detection modes for microplate assays are absorbance, fluorescence intensity, luminescence, time-resolved fluorescence or fluorescence polarization.

A light source illuminates the sample using a specific wavelength (selected by an optical filter or a monochromator) and a light detector, located on the other side of the well, measures how much of the light is transmitted through the sample. The amount of transmitted light is related to the concentration of the molecule of interest (Fig. 9.9).

ELISA plate: The test is done in an **ELISA plate**, also known as a **96-well plate** or **microplate** (8 × 12 matrix), with a typical reaction volume between 100 and 200 μL per well. It is the most common microplate format used in academic research laboratories or clinical diagnostic laboratories (Fig. 9.10).

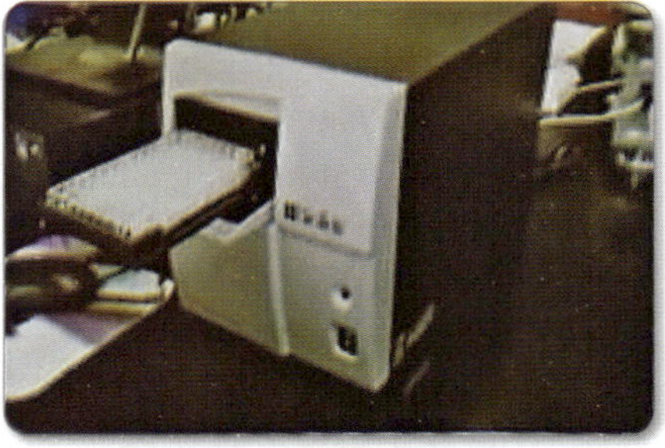

Fig. 9.9: A microplate reader with a 96-well microplate in the sample drawer

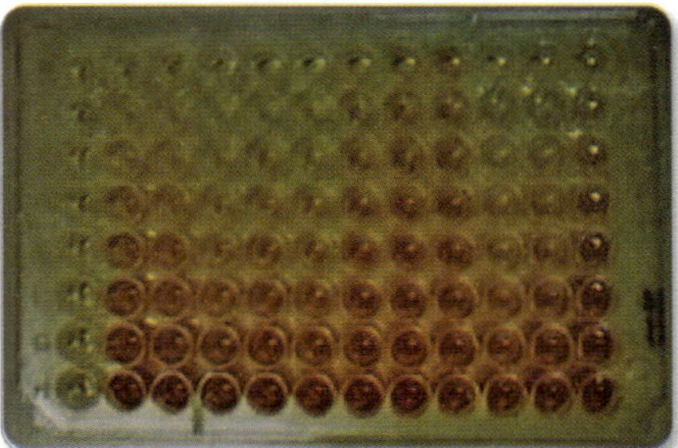

Fig. 9.10: ELISA plate

Automated ELISA readers

These are used for:

- **Microparticle enzyme immunoassay (MEIA):** It uses a solution of suspended submicron latex particles to measure analytes. The particles are coated with the capture molecule, specific for the analyte being measured. MEIA is less time consuming since the effective surface area of microparticles increases assay kinetics and decreases assay incubation time. This is the automated methodology.
- **Fluorescence polarization immunoassay (FPIA):** It combines two technologies to determine analyte concentration, i.e.,
  1. Competitive protein binding, and
  2. Fluorescence polarization
- **Radioactive energy attenuation assays (REA):** It involves color development reactions. The presence of the analyte converts chromogen (unreacted dye) to a chromophore (colored dye). A stable fluorescent substance (fluorophore) is also added in the reaction mixture. The light absorbing property of chromophore produced, causes a decrease of measured fluorescent light intensity from the fluorophore, which is measured by FPIA optics assembly. Change in radiant energy intensity follows Beer's law. Production of chromophore is linked by the reaction system to the consumption of analyte, hence, development of fluorescence attenuation can be calibrated to measure the concentration of analyte in the sample.

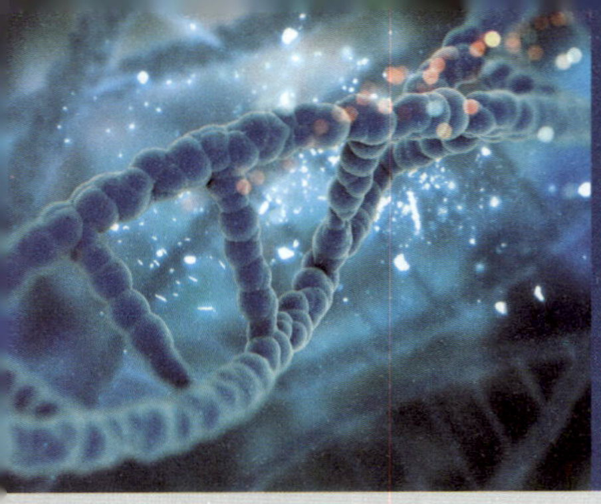

STUDENT ASSIGNMENT

LONG AND SHORT ANSWER QUESTIONS

1. What are immunoglobulins? Describe the structure of an immunoglobulin.
2. Classify immunoglobulins. Describe the function of each class of immunoglobulin.
3. **Write notes on:**
   a. Hinge region of an immunoglobulin
   b. Secretory IgA
   c. ELISA

MULTIPLE CHOICE QUESTIONS

1. **The earliest immunoglobulin to be synthesized by the fetus is:**
   a. IgD
   b. IgM
   c. IgA
   d. IgE

2. **Which antibody first appears following stimulation by an antigen?**
   a. IgG
   b. IgM
   c. IgE
   d. IgD

3. **IgM molecule consists of:**
   a. 2 subunits
   b. 3 subunits
   c. 4 subunits
   d. 5 subunits

4. **Which immunoglobulin (Ig) is found in highest concentration in serum of a normal person?**
   a. IgE
   b. IgD
   c. IgA
   d. IgG

10

Sample Collection and Normal Values

LEARNING OBJECTIVES

After the completion of the chapter, the readers will be able to:
- Explain about Sample collection understand.
- Explain about values of biochemical parameters.

CHAPTER OUTLINE

Sample Collection
- Collection of Blood Sample
- Use of Vacutainers
- Order of Blood Sample Collection
- Technique of Withdrawal of Blood
- Blood Collection of Babies
- Sequence of Filling the Sample Tubes after Withdrawal of Blood
- Collection and Handling of Urine Sample

Normal Values of Biochemical Parameters
- Normal Values of Common Biochemical Parameters in Blood
- Normal Values of Arterial Blood Gas Parameters
- Normal Values of Some Hormones in Blood
- Normal Values of Some Biochemical Parameters in Urine

KEY TERMS

Anticoagulant: A chemical substance which is added to in the tube during blood collection to prevent it from clotting.
Biochemical parameters: Estimated values, obtained by laboratory tests, of the concentration of various substances present in blood such as blood glucose, blood urea, total protein, etc.
Thromboplastin: A complex enzyme that is found in brain, lung, and other tissues and especially in blood platelets; functions in the conversion of prothrombin to thrombin in the clotting of blood, also called thrombokinase.
Venipuncture: A procedure in which a needle is used to take blood from a vein, usually for laboratory testing.

Note: This chapter does form a part of the syllabus but forms an essential part of the clinical chemistry. In my opinion every medical, paramedical as well as nursing student should know details of blood and urine sample collection and the normal range of some common biochemical parameters in these fluids.

SAMPLE COLLECTION

COLLECTION OF BLOOD SAMPLE

Biochemical tests are performed on all kinds of body fluid but mostly on **blood**, **plasma** or **serum**. The type of test required dictates what type of sample is required. Historically, serum is preferred for determining extracellular concentration of blood constituents. These days, however, even plasma is used for many, but not all, laboratory investigations.

Whole Blood, Serum or Plasma

- **Whole blood:** Whole blood is a body fluid that delivers necessary substances, such as nutrients and oxygen to the cells and transports metabolic waste products away from the cell.
  - Blood is composed of various types of cells suspended in plasma. These include red blood cells (also called RBCs or erythrocytes) and white blood cells, including leukocytes and platelets.
  - In a venous, arterial or capillary blood sample, concentration and properties of the various cellular and extracellular constituents remain relatively unaltered, when compared with their *in vivo* state.
  - Addition of anticoagulant, *in vitro*, stabilizes the constituents in the whole blood sample, for a certain period of time.
- **Serum:** Serum is undiluted **yellow watery part of blood**, which is left after blood has been allowed to clot and all the blood cells have been removed. This is, generally, done by centrifugation, which packs blood cells and platelets to the bottom of the centrifuge tube, leaving liquid (serum) fraction, resting above the packed cells. For this purpose:
  - Blood is collected in a tube **without any anticoagulant** and **allowed to clot**.
  - Thereafter, leave the tube at room temperature for at least 30 minutes, for the separation of the serum.
  - Serum is obtained after a clot is formed.
  - Centrifuge the sample to obtain a clear supernatant (serum).
- **Plasma:** Plasma is **cell free supernatant of blood containing an anticoagulant**. It is obtained after centrifugation of the blood.
  - Plasma constitutes about 55% of blood fluid. It is mostly water (92% by volume) and contains dissipated proteins, glucose, mineral ions, hormones and carbon dioxide.
  - From the same volume of blood, about 15–20% more volume of plasma is obtained than serum. For this purpose, blood is collected **in anticoagulant tubes** and **mixed**, by gently inverting the tube, several times. This, in turn, ensures even distribution of anticoagulant with the specimen.

However, it is essential that only a recommended quantity of the desired anticoagulant should be added to avoid any error in results.

Use of Anticoagulants

Anticoagulants are the additives, which inhibit blood and/or plasma from clotting, ensuring that the constituents to be measured are not significantly altered prior to the analytical process. Anticoagulation occurs by binding of the calcium ions (such as by EDTA or citrate) or by inhibiting the thrombin activity (such as by heparin).

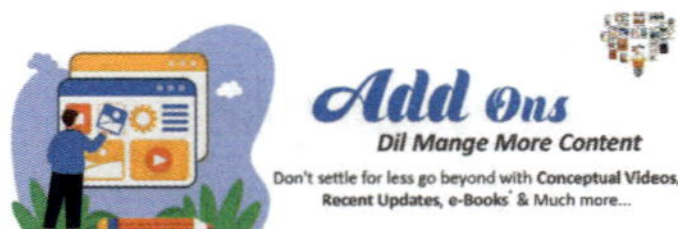

Commonly used Anticoagulants

Commonly used anticoagulants, which may be used in sample collection, include:

EDTA

- Ethylenediaminetetraacetic acid dipotassium (EDTA.K_2), tripotassium (EDTA.K_3) or disodium (EDTA.Na_2) salt, available in the powder form, may be used in a concentration of 1.2–2.0 mg/mL of blood.
- It strongly and irreversibly chelates calcium ions and prevents blood from clotting.
- EDTA (especially, dipotassium salt) interferes in some of the tests. Under these situations, heparin should be used as an alternative.
- Tubes with liquid EDTA reduce risk of hemolysis, which, sometimes, may be seen by using EDTA powder.

Citrate

- Trisodium citrate or acid-citrate-dextrose, with 0.10–0.136 mol/L (3–4%) citric acid (as buffered-citrate, pH 5.5–5.6) is used in the liquid form, in tubes for coagulation tests as well as in blood transfusion bags.
- Correct proportion of the anticoagulant is important to avoid dilution of the blood. Generally, a mixture of one part of citrate with nine parts of the blood is recommended for coagulation tests while one part of the citrate is mixed with four parts of the blood to determine erythrocyte sedimentation rate (ESR).
- Citrate binds calcium but not as strongly as EDTA.

Oxalate

Its mechanism is similar to that of citrate. It is used in fluoride-oxalate tubes, for use in blood collection for glucose and lactate determinations.

Heparin

About 12–30 IU/mL of the unfractionated sodium, lithium or ammonium salt of heparin is recommended. Calcium-titrated heparin, at a concentration of 8–12 IU/mL of blood, is recommended for the determination of ionized calcium.

Fluoride

For blood glucose determination fluoride is used as anticoagulant.

USE OF VACUTAINERS

A vacutainer, **blood collection tube**, is a sterile glass or plastic test tube with a colored rubber stopper creating a vacuum seal inside of the tube, thereby, facilitating the draw of a predetermined volume of blood. They are available with a safety engineered stopper and a variety of labeling options, and volumes. Each tube is topped with a color coded plastic or rubber cap. Tubes often include additives that mix with the blood when collected and the color of each tube's plastic cap indicates which additive it contains.

Principle of Working of a Vacutainer

Vacutainer needles are double ended, with one side being encased in a thin rubber coating for safety. When the needle is screwed into the translucent plastic needle holder, the rubber needle (inside the holder) and the exposed needle will be inserted into the vein. When a vacutainer tube is inserted into the holder, its rubber cap is punctured by the inner needle and the vacuum in the tube pulls blood through the needle into the tube. The filled tube is then removed and another can be inserted and filled the same way. The amount of air evacuated from the tube predetermines how much blood will fill the tube before blood stops flowing.

After the tube has been filled with blood, immediately invert the tube, containing additive, several times to prevent coagulation.

These tubes have an expiry, because over time, the vacuum is lost and blood will not be drawn into the tube when the needle punctures the cap.

Types of Vacutainer

- **Red-top tube (Plain tube):** This tube is a plain vacutainer containing no anticoagulant and is used for collection of serum for selected chemistry tests as well as clotted blood for immunohematology.
- **Gold-top tube (Serum gel tube):** This tube contains a clot activator and serum gel separator, and is used for various laboratory tests. Invert the tube to activate clotting, let it stand for 20–30 minutes before centrifuging for 10 minutes. If frozen serum is required, pour off serum into plastic vial and freeze. Do not freeze the vacutainer.
- **Green-top tube (Sodium heparin tube):** This tube contains sodium heparin or lithium heparin and is used for collection of heparinized plasma or whole blood in clinical chemistry, e.g., urea and electrolyte determination. Sodium heparin collection tubes are preferred for peripheral blood or bone marrow for cytogenetic studies. Lithium heparin is considered suboptimal for cytogenetics.
- **Purple or lavender-top tube (K_2.EDTA tube):** EDTA is a strong anticoagulant and these tubes are used for most hematological procedures, such as complete blood counts (CBC). These can also be used for some blood bank procedures, such as blood type and screening. EDTA tubes are also preferred by most molecular laboratories for genetic (DNA or RNA) studies.
- **Yellow-top tube (ACD tube):** This tube contains sodium polyanethol sulfonate (SPS) used for blood culture specimens, or acid-citrate-dextrose (ACD) for drawing whole blood required for special tests for blood bank studies, HLA phenotyping and paternity testing.
- **Grey-top tube (Potassium oxalate/Sodium fluoride tube):** This tube contains potassium oxalate as an anticoagulant and sodium fluoride as a preservative. Fluoride prevents enzymes in the blood from working, by preventing glycolysis and is used to preserve glucose in whole blood (Fig. 10.1).

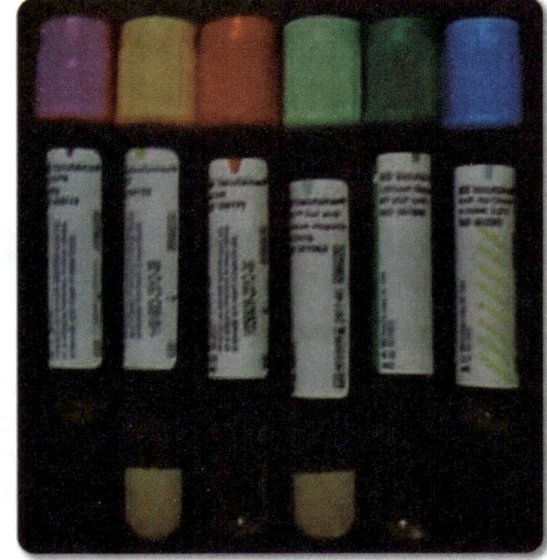

Fig. 10.1: Different types of vacutainers

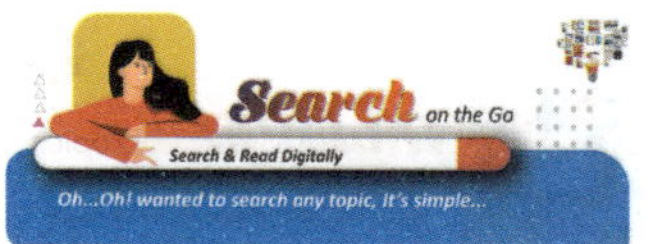

ORDER OF BLOOD SAMPLE COLLECTION

The term order of draw refers to the sequence in which tubes should be filled. Since the needle, which pierces the tubes, can carry additives from one tube to the next, the sequence is standardized to avoid any cross contamination of additives, so that the laboratory results are not affected.

If using vacutainer, the order of collecting the blood should be:

- Blood culture tube (yellow or yellow-black top).
- Coagulation tube (light blue top).

  If just a routine coagulation assay is the only ordered test, then a single light blue top tube may be used. If there is a concern regarding contamination by tissue fluids or thromboplastin, one may draw a non-additive tube first and then the light blue top tube.

- Non-additive tube (red top).
- Lastly, draw the tubes with different additives in the following order:
  - SST (red-gray or gold top), which contains a clot activator.
  - Sodium heparin (dark green top).
  - PST (light green top), which contains lithium heparin.
  - EDTA (lavender top).
  - ACDA or ACDB (pale yellow top), which contains acid citrate-dextrose.
  - Oxalate/fluoride (light gray top).

Timing of Blood Collection

As we know, blood composition of various analytes is significantly altered after consuming food, thus, it is necessary to provide the patient, in advance, with the appropriate collection instructions, information on fasting or diet and medication restrictions, if required.

- In routine, **overnight fasting sample** (early morning, approximately 12 hours after the last ingestion of food) is recommended for determining concentration of common blood constituents, such as glucose, triglycerides, lipoprotein fractions, electrolytes and proteins, etc.
- For glucose alone, **fasting of four hours** is sufficient.
- Blood can be taken at **any time of the day** for some of the tests, such as for total cholesterol.

Preparation of the Subject

- Exercise (muscular activity) has both, transient as well as long lasting effects. Thus, creatine kinase (CK), aspartate aminotransferase (AST), lactate dehydrogenase (LDH) and platelet counts may increase.
- Stress may cause transient elevation in elevated adrenal hormone values (cortisol and catecholamines). Anxiety results in hyperventilation. It may cause acid base imbalance and increase lactate concentration.
- Diurnal rhythms are body fluid and analyte fluctuations, during the day. For example, serum cortisol level is highest in early morning but is reduced in the afternoon. Serum iron levels tend to drop during the day. One must check timing of these variations for the desired collection point.
- Postural changes, supine to sitting, etc., are known to vary lab results of some of the analytes. Certain large molecules are not filtered into the tissue; therefore, they are more concentrated in the blood.

Levels of several enzymes, proteins, lipids, iron and calcium are significantly increased with a change in position.

- Age, gender and pregnancy also have influence on laboratory results. Normal reference range is often noted according to age.

Position of the Subject

Position of the subject can also influence results of some of the analytes, thus, standardization of the position is necessary.

- It is, generally, recommended that blood sample should be drawn in a sitting position.
- The subject should remain in the sitting position for about 15 minutes, prior to blood collection. This (waiting period) will allow equilibration of concentration of most of the blood components.

TECHNIQUE OF WITHDRAWAL OF BLOOD

There are many ways in which blood can be drawn from the vein. The method, however, may vary with age of the patient, equipment available and the tests required.

Various techniques of blood collection include:
- **Venipuncture:** Venipuncture using a needle and tube is the most common method for blood collection.
- **Vacutainer:** Blood collection can also be done with an evacuated tube system called vacutainer, which consists of a plastic hub, a hypodermic needle and a vacuum tube.
- **Lancet:** Blood may also be collected by puncturing the skin with a retractable lancet device.

Venipuncture

Venipuncture, **venopuncture** or **venepuncture** is a process of obtaining intravenous access for blood sampling of venous blood. This procedure is performed by a **phlebotomist** (professional who draws blood), nursing staff, medical laboratory technologists or medical practitioners. Though it is a complex procedure, requiring both knowledge and skill to perform, it is one of the most routinely performed invasive procedures carried out to obtain blood for diagnostic purposes as well as to monitor levels of blood components.

Requirements for Venipuncture

- **Vacutainers:** The tubes are designed to fill with a predetermined volume of blood, by vacuum. These are available in various sizes. Their rubber stoppers are color-coded, according to the additive, which the tube contains. Since these tubes have different additives or coatings, blood should never be poured from one tube to another.
- **Needles:** Needles are available for evacuated systems and for use with a syringe, single draw or butterfly system. The gauge number indicates the bore size. Larger the gauge number, smaller is the needle bore.
- **Holder/adapter:** It is used with the evacuated collection system.
- **Tourniquet**
- **Alcohol wipes:** 70% isopropyl alcohol.
- **Povidone-iodine wipes/swabs:** These are used if blood is to be drawn for culture.

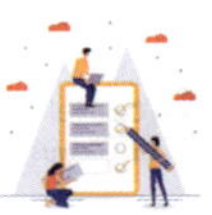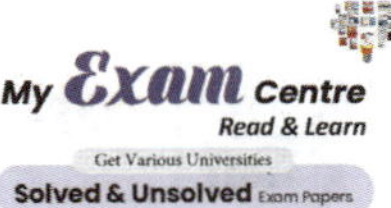

- **Gauze sponge:** It is required for application on the site from which the needle is withdrawn.
- **Adhesive bandage/tape:** It protects the venipuncture site after collection.
- **Needle disposal unit:** Needle should never be broken, bent, or recapped. It should be placed in a proper disposal unit, immediately after use.
- **Gloves:** Gloves made of latex, rubber, vinyl, etc., are worn to protect the patient and the phlebotomist.
- **Syringe:** It may be used in place of the evacuated collection tube, for special circumstances.

Use of Tourniquet

- Prolonged venous occlusion can cause change in the concentration of blood constituents. Therefore, use of tourniquet should be minimized. If a tourniquet is used to search for a vein, it should be released before withdrawal of blood begins. In any case, use of a tourniquet should be limited to <1 minute.
- Select a suitable site for venipuncture, by placing tourniquet 3–4 inches above the selected puncture site, on the patient.
- Do not put tourniquet too tight and do not leave it on the patient for longer than 1 minute.
- It should be wiped-off with alcohol and replaced frequently, because:

Prolonged use of tourniquet may have some undesirable effects, viz:

- Primary effect is hemoconcentration of non-filterable elements (i.e., proteins). The hydrostatic pressure causes some water and filterable elements to leave the extracellular space.
- Significant increase can be found in total protein, aspartate aminotransferase (AST), total lipids, cholesterol and iron.
- Affects packed cell volume (PCV) and other cellular elements.
- Hemolysis may occur, with pseudohyperkalemia.

Site of Venipuncture

- Preferably blood should not be collected from the arm that is used for blood pressure measurement, i.e., blood should usually be drawn from the **left arm**.
- Blood sample should be taken from vein in the **antecubital fossa**.
- Before blood collection, the subject should **remove tight clothes**, which may constrict the upper arm.
- During blood collection, the **arm should rest on some supportive prop**.
- Though **large median cubital** and cephalic **veins** are the usual choice but basilic vein on the dorsum of the arm or dorsal hand veins are also acceptable.
- **Foot veins** are the last resort because of the higher probability of complications.
- Palpate and trace path of veins with the index finger. Arteries pulsate, are most elastic and have a thick wall. Thrombosed veins lack resilience, feel cord-like and roll easily.
- If superficial veins are not readily apparent, you can force blood into the vein by massaging the arm from wrist to elbow, tap the site with index and second finger, apply a warm, damp washcloth to the site for 5 minutes, or lower the extremity over the bedside, to allow the vein to fill.

Areas to Avoid when Choosing a Site for Withdrawal of Blood

Certain areas should be avoided when choosing a site for blood withdrawal:
- **Extensive scars from burns and surgery**, since it is difficult to puncture the scar tissue and obtain a specimen from there.

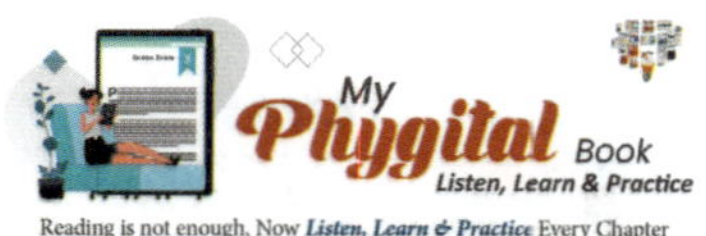

- **The upper extremity on the side of a previous mastectomy**, because test results may be affected due to lymphedema.
- **Hematoma**, since it may cause erroneous test results. If another site is not available, collect specimen distal to the hematoma.
- **Intravenous therapy (IV)/blood transfusion**, since fluid may dilute the specimen. If possible, collect from the opposite arm. Otherwise, a sample may be drawn below the IV, by following these procedures:
  - Turn off the IV set for at least 2 minutes before venipuncture.
  - Apply tourniquet below the IV site.
  - Select a vein other than the one with the IV set.
  - Perform venipuncture, draw 5 mL of blood and discard it, before drawing specimen, in tubes, for testing.
- **Intravenous line**, since drawing blood from an intravenous line may introduce problem, the line must be flushed, first. When using a syringe inserted into the line, blood must be withdrawn slowly to avoid hemolysis.
- **Fistula or cannula** blood should not be drawn from an arm with a fistula or cannula without consulting the attending physician.
- Edematous extremities should be avoided, as tissue fluid accumulation alters test results.

Venipuncture Procedure

Several essential steps are required for successful blood collection:
- A phlebotomist (professional who draws blood) must be a professional, who should be courteous and have understanding with the patient.
- First step to blood collection is to positively identify the patient by two forms of identification, i.e., ask the patient to state and spell his/her name, and give his/her age. Check these against the requisition form.
- Check the requisition form for requested tests, patient's information and special requirement, if any.
- Gather the tubes and supplies that will be required for the withdrawal of blood.
- Position the patient in a chair, or sitting or lying on a bed.
- Wash hands.
- Select a suitable site for venipuncture, by placing tourniquet 3–4 inches above the selected puncture site, on the patient. Do not put the tourniquet too tightly or leave it on the patient for longer than 1 minute.
- Put on non-latex gloves and palpate for the vein.
- After the vein has been selected, clean the area in a circular motion, beginning at the site and working outwards. Allow the area to air dry. After the area is cleansed, it should not be touched or palpated again. If it is necessary to re-evaluate the site by palpation, the area should be re-cleansed before the venipuncture is performed.
- Grasp patient's arm firmly, using thumb, to draw the skin taut and anchor the vein.
- Swiftly insert the needle, through the skin, into lumen of vein. The needle should form 15°–30° angle with the arm surface and avoid excess probing (Fig. 10.2).
- When the last tube is being filled, remove tourniquet.
- Remove needle from patient's arm, using a swift backward motion.

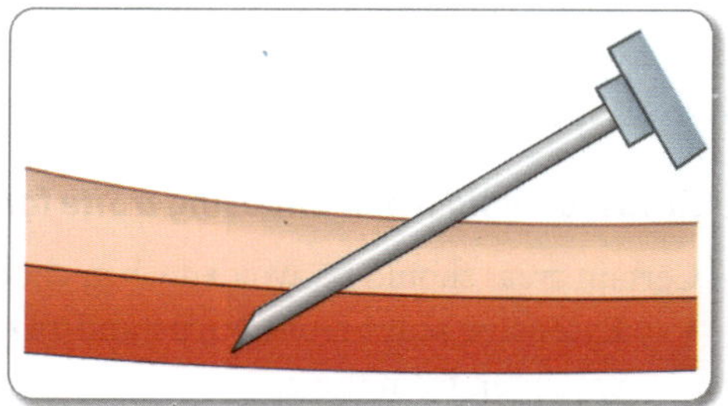

Fig. 10.2: Venipuncture

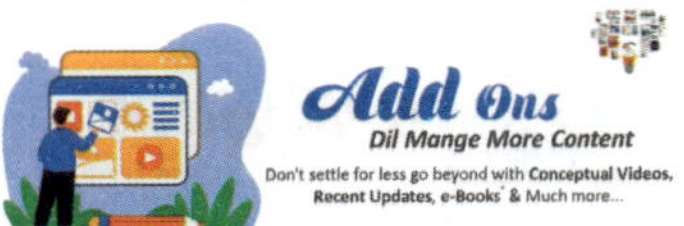

- Immediately place gauze on the puncture site.
- Apply and hold adequate pressure to avoid formation of hematoma.
- After holding pressure for 1–2 minutes, tape a fresh piece of gauze to the puncture site.
- Dispose-off the contaminated materials/supplies, in the designated containers.
- Mix and label all appropriate tubes at the patient's bedside.
- Deliver specimens promptly to the laboratory.

Trouble Shooting

If an Incomplete Collection or no Blood is Obtained

- Change the position of the needle. Move it forward (it may not be in the lumen) or move it backward (it may have penetrated too far; Fig. 10.3).
- Adjust the angle (the bevel may be against the vein wall).
- Loosen the tourniquet. It may be obstructing blood flow.
- Try another tube. Use a smaller tube with less vacuum. There may be no vacuum in the tube being used.
- Re-anchor the vein. Veins sometimes roll away from the point of needle or puncture site.
- Ask the patient to make a fist and flex the arm, which helps engorge muscles to fill veins.
- Pre-warm region of the vein to reduce vasoconstriction and increase blood flow.
- Ask the patient to drink fluid, if dehydrated.

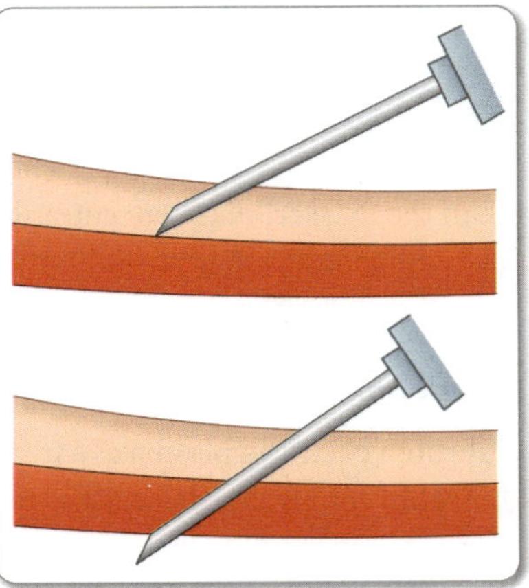

Fig. 10.3: Adjustment of position of the needle by moving it forward or backward

If Blood Stops Flowing

- The vein may have collapsed. Re-secure tourniquet to increase venous filling. If this is not successful, remove the needle, take care of the puncture site and redraw.
- The needle might have pulled out of the vein when switching tubes. Hold equipment firmly and place fingers against patient's arm, using the flange for leverage when withdrawing and inserting tubes.

Problems Other than an Incomplete Collection

- A hematoma may form under the skin adjacent to the puncture site. If so, release tourniquet immediately and withdraw the needle. Hematoma formation is a common problem in older patients.
- Apply firm pressure (Fig. 10.4).

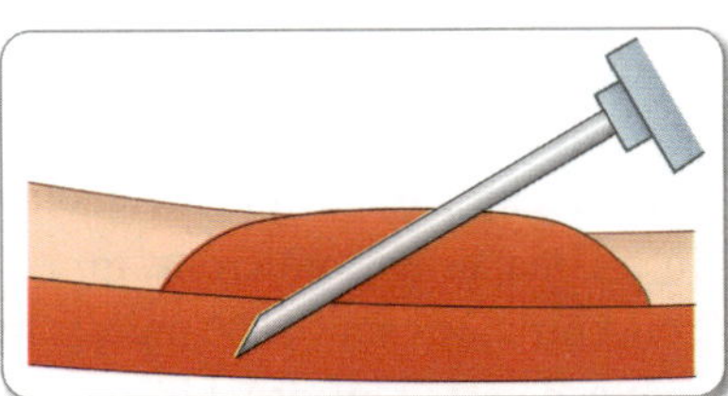

Fig. 10.4: Hematoma

Hemoconcentration

Hemoconcentration (an increased concentration of large molecules and formed elements in the blood) may be due to several factors:

- Prolonged tourniquet application (it should not be for >1 minute).
- Massaging, squeezing or probing a site.

- Long-term IV therapy.
- Sclerosis or occluded vein.

Hemolytic, Icteric or Lipemic Sample

Laboratory tests are affected by several endogenous and exogenous factors in the sample matrix. The relevant observation should be coined for each sample, e.g., **hemolytic**, **icteric**, **opalescent** and **turbid** or **lipemic**, if a relevant color or turbidity is seen.

Hemolytic Sample

Hemolysis is defined as release of the intracellular components of erythrocytes and other blood cells into the extracellular fluid of blood. After separation of the blood cells, hemolysis may be visible by the red color of serum or plasma. Cell constituents, particularly those with an intracellular concentration of 10 times higher than the extracellular concentration, will increase in plasma/serum during hemolysis, e.g., potassium, lactate dehydrogenase, aspartate aminotransferase, etc. Sample associated with greater degree of hemolysis may also interfere with other laboratory tests.

Icteric Sample

Bilirubin occurs in plasma as a free molecule as well as covalently bound to albumin. In addition, water-soluble bilirubin conjugates also exist as mono and di-glucuronides. Conjugated bilirubin also appears in urine, when present at increased concentration in blood. In patients with proteinuria, bilirubin bound to albumin can also appear in urine.

Bilirubin interferes in oxidase/peroxidase based test systems. Proportionally to its concentration, bilirubin reacts with H_2O_2 which is formed in the test system. This in turn causes systematically lower results in enzymatic procedures that are used for the measurement of glucose, cholesterol, triglycerides, uric acid and creatinine.

Bilirubin also competitively interferes with dyes binding to albumin.

Lipemic Sample

Lipemia is a turbidity of serum or plasma, which is caused by the elevated lipoprotein concentrations and is visible by the eye. A sufficiently transparent sample container must be used to detect lipemia. Post-centrifugal coagulation of serum samples of heparinized patients can also be the cause of turbidity.

Most often, lipemia results from increased triglyceride concentration in plasma/serum. This can be due to food intake, altered lipid metabolism or infusion of lipids. After intestinal absorption, triglycerides are present in plasma, as chylomicrons, for 6–12 hours. Lipemia in plasma or serum is visually observed at triglyceride concentrations above 300 mg/dL. In whole blood triglyceride concentrations above 1000 mg/dL cause turbidity that is detected by visual inspection. Centrifugation for 10 minutes at 1000 g is effective when chylomicrons cause turbidity.

Fingerstick Procedure of Blood Collection

- Follow the procedure as outlined above, i.e., identify the patient and the requisition form indicating the ordered test(s).

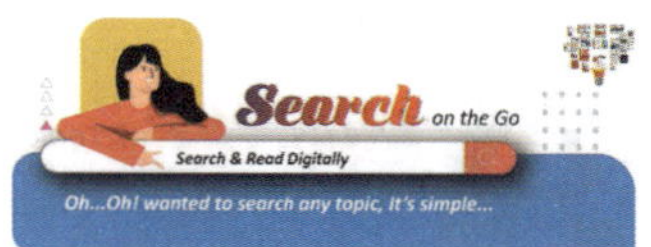

- Verify patient's condition, such as fasting, dietary restrictions, medications, timing and medical treatment, etc., since all the information is of concern and should be noted on the lab requisition slip.
- Position the patient who should either sit in a chair or lie down/sit in bed. Hyperextend the patient's arm.
- Best location for finger sticks is the 3rd (middle) and the 4th (ring) fingers of the non-dominant hand (Fig. 10.5).
- Do not use tip of the finger, or center of the finger. Avoid side of the finger, where there is less soft tissue, since vessels and nerves are located and the bone is closer to the surface.

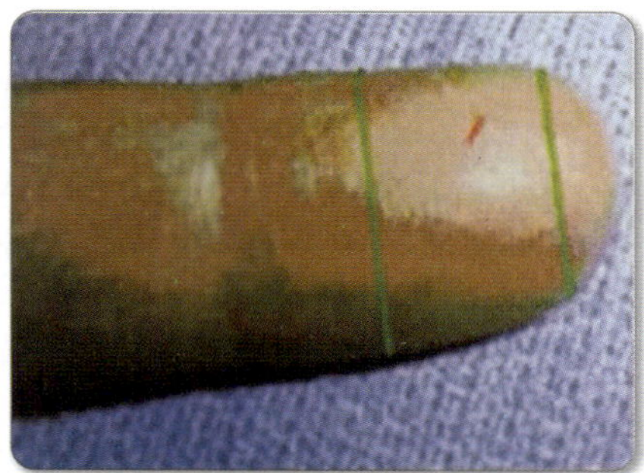

Fig. 10.5: Fingerstick procedure

The 2nd (index) finger tends to have thicker, calloused skin. The fifth finger tends to have less soft tissue overlying the bone. Avoid puncturing a finger that is cold or cyanotic, swollen, scarred or covered with a rash.

- Using a sterile lancet, make a skin puncture, just off the center of the finger pad. The puncture should be made perpendicular to the ridge of the fingerprint, so that the drop of blood does not run down the ridges.
- Wipe away the first drop of blood, which tends to contain excess tissue fluid.
- Collect drops of blood into the collection device, by gently massaging the finger. Avoid excessive pressure that may squeeze tissue fluid into the drop of blood.
- Cap, rotate and invert the collection device to mix the collected blood.
- Patient should hold a small gauze pad over the puncture site for a couple of minutes, to stop bleeding.
- Dispose of the contaminated materials/supplies in the designated containers.
- Label all appropriate tubes at the patient's bedside.
- Deliver specimen promptly to the laboratory.

BLOOD COLLECTION OF BABIES

Recommended location for blood collection on a newborn baby or an infant is the heel. To draw blood from a baby:

- Prewarm infant's heel (42°C for 3–5 minutes) to increase the flow of blood, for collection.
- Wash your hands and put gloves on.
- Clean the site, to be punctured, with an alcohol sponge.
- Dry the cleaned area with a dry gauze pad.
- Hold baby's foot firmly, to avoid sudden movement.
- Using a sterile blood safety lancet, puncture the side of the heel in the appropriate region (Fig. 10.6).
- Make a cut across the heel print lines, so that a drop of blood can well up and not run down along the lines.

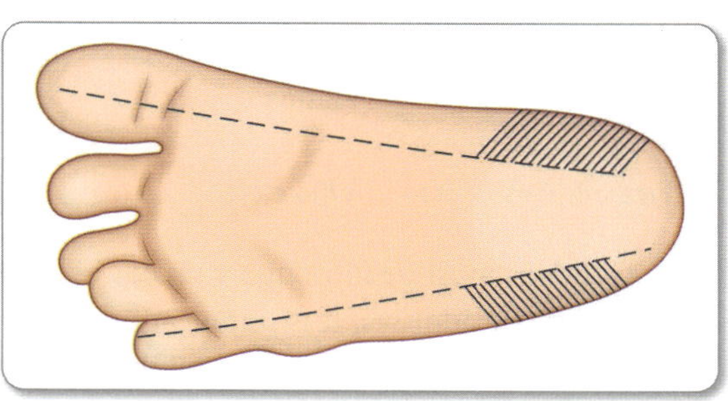

Fig. 10.6: Blood collection of babies

- Wipe away the first drop of blood with a piece of clean, dry cotton gauze.
- Since newborns do not, often, bleed immediately, use gentle pressure to produce a rounded drop of blood. Do not use excessive pressure because blood may become diluted with the tissue fluid.
- Fill the required microtainer(s), as needed. When finished, elevate the heel, place a piece of clean, dry cotton on the puncture site and hold it in place until bleeding has stopped. Apply tape or Band-Aid to area, if needed.
- Be sure to dispose of the lancet, in the appropriate container. Dispose of contaminated materials in appropriate waste receptacles.
- Remove gloves and wash your hands.

SEQUENCE OF FILLING THE SAMPLE TUBES AFTER WITHDRAWAL OF BLOOD

As mentioned above, tubes in which blood is to be transported to the laboratory may contain a variety of additives (anticoagulants). Accordingly, it is important to know that which tube the individual laboratory requires for the desired test, as the type of reagents used and accordingly the anticoagulant, may vary between different laboratories.

The order, in which various tubes should be filled, is determined by the risk of contamination and coagulation. The following sequence, for filling tubes with blood from a patient, is recommended to avoid contamination:

- Vial for blood culture
- Plain tubes (without any coagulant), for serum. Avoid serum as the first tube when electrolytes are to be measured.
- Citrate containing tubes
- Heparin containing tubes
- EDTA containing tubes
- Tubes containing additional anticoagulant, e.g., fluoride as glycolytic inhibitor.

Though, priority of the assay may affect order of filling of a particular tube but in general, specimen should be collected in the sequence, as shown in Table 10.1.

TABLE 10.1: Sequence of filling the tubes for various biochemical tests

Type of analysis	Specimen type	Type of tube
Lipids	Serum	10 mL, plain tube
Glucose	Plasma	4 mL, tube filled with glycolytic inhibitors, i.e., potassium oxalate and sodium fluoride
Glycated-hemoglobin	Whole blood	3 mL, tube with anticoagulant K_2 EDTA

Additives must be thoroughly mixed. Erroneous test results may be obtained, if blood is not thoroughly mixed with the additive. It is important that before the subject leaves the collection site and that before the specimen rack is moved anywhere, all the tubes should be labeled with the individual's identifications.

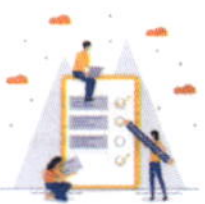
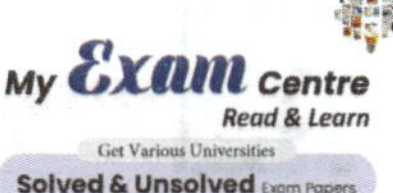

Disposal of the Syringe, Needle and Other Material

- Needle disposal box should be available for all personals, drawing blood samples.
- Needle should be released from the adapter directly to the needle disposal box.
- Needle should never be re-sheathed after use.
- The disposal box should not be allowed to become overfull, to avoid potential hazards.

Labeling of the Sample

A properly labeled sample is essential so that the results of the test match the patient. The key elements in labeling include:

- Patient's surname, first and middle name.
- Patient's OPD/CR number.
- Date and time.

Automated systems may include labels with bar codes (Fig. 10.7).

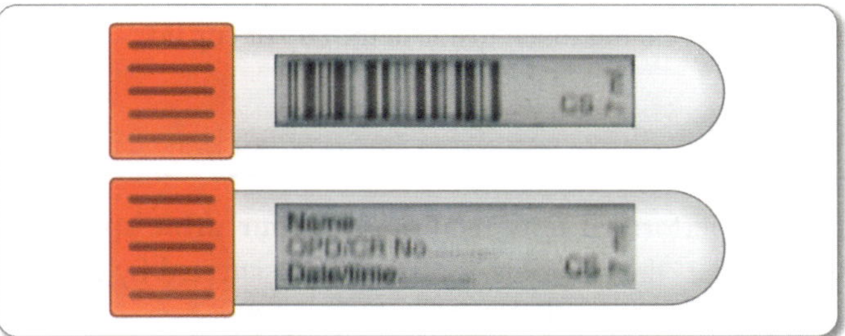

Fig. 10.7: Labeling of the sample

COLLECTION AND HANDLING OF URINE SAMPLE

Urine is an important tool for clinical diagnosis. The clinical information to be obtained from a urine specimen may be influenced by the collection method, timing and handling. A vast assortment of collection and transport containers for urine specimens are available. Determining which urine collection method and container should be used, depends upon the type of laboratory test ordered.

Types of Urine Specimen Collection

Laboratory urine specimens are classified by the type of collection or collection procedure used to obtain the specimen.

First-Morning Specimen

This is the specimen of choice for urinalysis and microscopic analysis, since the urine is generally more concentrated (due to length of time urine is allowed to remain in the bladder) and, therefore, contains relatively higher levels of cellular elements and analytes, such as protein, if present.

The first morning specimen, also called an 8-hour specimen, is collected when the patient first wakes up in the morning, after emptying the bladder, before going to sleep. Alternatively, urine can also be collected over any 8-hour period for patients who have atypical work/sleep schedule.

Proper collection practices and accurate recording of the collection time are important criteria for the first-morning specimen. For this purpose, any urine which is voided from the bladder during the 8-hour collection period should be pooled and refrigerated, so that a true 8-hour specimen is obtained.

Random Specimen

This is the specimen most commonly sent to the laboratory for analysis, primarily because it is easiest to obtain and can be made readily available. This type of specimen is usually submitted for urinalysis and microscopic analysis, although it is not the specimen of choice for either of these tests.

It is due to the reason that random specimen can, sometime, give an inaccurate view of a patient's health, if the specimen is too diluted and analyte values are artificially lowered. Pediatric specimens, which routinely undergo chemistry and microscopic analysis, are generally of this type. As the name implies, a random specimen can be collected at any time. Although there are no specific guidelines for how the collection should be conducted, introduction of contaminants into the specimen should be avoided. This requires explicit instructions to patients so that they do not touch inside of the cup or cup lid.

Timely Collection of Urine

Among the most commonly performed tests requiring **24-hour urine specimen** include proteins, urea, creatinine, uric acid, VMA and 17-ketosteroids, etc., which are affected by diurnal variation. Sometimes, a timed specimen (usually 8-hours) may also be used for this purpose.

For the collection of urine sample over the fixed time, bladder is emptied prior to beginning of the timed collection. Then, for the duration of the designated time period, all urine is collected and pooled into a collection container, with the final collection at the end of the period. Accurate timing is critical for calculations that are conducted to determine analyte concentrations and ratios. Interpretations based on faulty calculations can result in improper diagnosis and medical treatment.

Urine Collection from Catheter

This procedure is conducted when a patient is bed-ridden or cannot urinate, independently. The healthcare provider inserts a Foley's catheter into bladder, through urethra, to collect the urine specimen (specimen may also be collected through an existing Foley's catheter). Specimen may be collected directly from a Foley's catheter into an evacuated tube or transferred from a syringe into a tube or cup.

Urine Collection by Suprapubic Aspiration

This method is used when a bed-ridden patient cannot be catheterized or a sterile specimen is required. The urine specimen is collected by needle aspiration through the abdominal wall into the bladder.

Urine Collection of Infants and Children

For infants and small children, a special urine collection bag is adhered to the skin surrounding the urethral area. Once the collection is complete, urine is poured into a collection cup or transferred directly into an evacuated tube with a transfer straw.

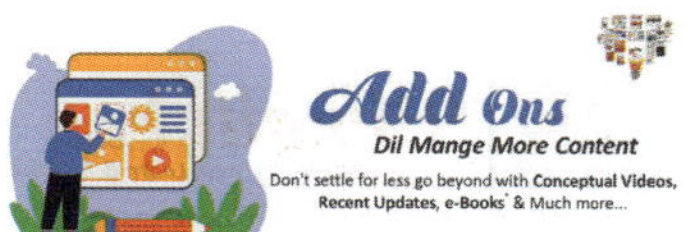

Urine collected from a diaper is not recommended for laboratory testing since contamination from the diaper material may affect test results.

Urine Sample Containers

- Urine collection containers for 24-hour specimen may be of any shape and color but should be of 2–3 L capacity.
- They should be clean and free of particles or interfering substances.
- Urine collection container should have a secure lid and should be leak-proof. This will reduce specimen loss and healthcare worker's exposure to the specimen. It will also protect the specimen from contaminants. For this purpose, it is good to use containers that are made of break-resistant plastic, which is safer than glass.
- Specimen container should not be reused.
- Proper labeling should be applied to the collection container or tube.
- When a preservative is required, it should be added to the collection container before the urine collection begins. If there is more than one acceptable preservative for the analyte to be tested, the least hazardous one should be selected.

Use of Preservatives in Urine Collection

Some common 24-hour preservatives include hydrochloric acid, boric acid, acetic acid and toluene. They allow urine to be kept at room temperature, while still providing results comparable to those of refrigerated urine. Generally, length of preservation ranges from 24 to 72 hours. When the specimen is directly transferred from a collection cup into the preservative tube, it provides a stable environment for the specimen, until testing can be conducted, and reduces the risk of bacterial over growth or specimen decomposition. Non-additive tubes (those not containing any chemical preservative) can be used for urinalysis but must be handled following strict timings and refrigeration guidelines.

NORMAL VALUES OF BIOCHEMICAL PARAMETERS

Normal values (reference range) for various biochemical parameters are a set of values used by the health professionals to interpret a set of clinical chemistry laboratory test results from the biological fluid sample. The test results should always be interpreted using the normal value provided by the laboratory, where the test had been performed.

Regarding the target population, if not otherwise specified, a standard normal value, generally, denotes the healthy individuals, or without any known condition that directly affects the ranges being established. These are likewise established using reference groups from the healthy population and are termed **normal range** or **normal values**.

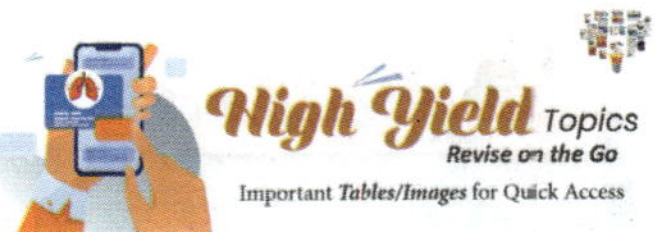

NORMAL VALUES OF COMMON BIOCHEMICAL PARAMETERS IN BLOOD

Normal values of common biochemical parameters in blood are shown in Table 10.2.

TABLE 10.2: Reference range of some constituents in blood

Test	Lower limit	Upper limit	Unit
Sodium (Na)	135	145	mmol/L (mEq/L)
Potassium (K)	3.5	5.0	mmol/L (mEq/L)
Chloride (Cl)	95	105	mmol/L (mEq/L)
Total calcium (Ca)	8.5	10.5	mg/dL
Ionized calcium (iCa)	4.4	5.2	mg/dL
Ceruloplasmin	18	35	µg/dL
Inorganic phosphorus	2.5	4.5	mg/dL
Uric acid (males)	4.5	7.0	mg/dL
Urea	15	45	mg/dL
Creatinine	0.8	1.5	mg/dL
Total proteins	6.3	8.4	g/dL
Albumin	3.5	5.5	g/dL
Globulins	2.3	3.5	g/dL
Bilirubin, total	0.2	0.8	mg/dL
Bilirubin, conjugated	0.0	0.3	mg/dL
Alanine transaminase (ALT)/Glutamate pyruvate transaminase (SGPT)	8	56	IU/L
Aspartate transaminase (AST)/Glutamate oxaloacetate transaminase (SGOT)	8	40	IU/L
Alkaline phosphatase	39	117	U/L
Gamma-glutamyl-transferase (GGT)	5	35	U/L
Creatine kinase (CK)	20	50	IU/L
Triglycerides (Below 40 years of age)	54	110	mg/dL
Triglycerides (Above 40 years of age)	70	150	mg/dL
Total cholesterol	120	200	mg/dL
HDL-cholesterol, male	35	80	mg/dL
HDL-cholesterol, female	40	86	mg/dL
LDL-cholesterol	80	120	mg/dL
Glucose	60	90	mg/dL
Glycated hemoglobin (HbA1c)	4.0	6.0	% of Hb
Lactate dehydrogenase (LDH)	50	150	U/L
Amylase	53	190	U/L
Acid phosphatase	—	3	U/L

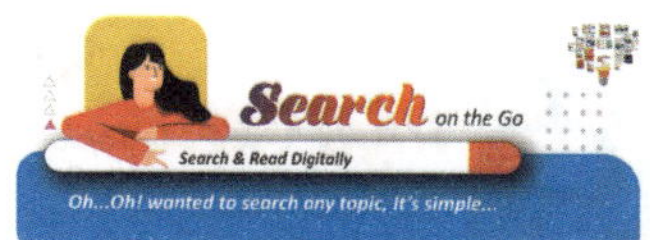

NORMAL VALUES OF ARTERIAL BLOOD GAS PARAMETERS

If arterial/venous is not specified for an acid base or blood gas value, then it generally refers to arterial, and not venous, which otherwise is standard for other blood tests. Acid, base and blood gases are among the few parameters that exhibit substantial difference between the arterial and the venous blood. Normal values of arterial ABG parameters are shown in Table 10.3.

TABLE 10.3: Reference range of ABG parameters

Test	Lower limit	Upper limit	Unit
pH	7.35	7.45	
$[H^+]$	36	44	nmol/L
Base excess	−3	+3	mEq/L
pO_2	75	100	mm Hg
Oxygen saturation	95	100	%
pCO_2	35	45	mm Hg
HCO_3^-	18	23	mmol/L

NORMAL VALUES OF SOME HORMONES IN BLOOD

Normal values of some of the hormones in blood are shown in Table 10.4.

TABLE 10.4: Reference range of some hormones

Test	Lower limit	Upper limit	Unit
Thyroid stimulating hormone (TSH)	0.3	5.0	mIU/L or µIU/mL
Free thyroxine (FT_4)	0.89	1.76	ng/dL
Total thyroxine (T_4)	4.5	12.5	µg/dL
Free triiodothyronine (FT_3)	2.3	4.2	pg/mL
Total triiodothyronine (T_3)	86	187	ng/dL

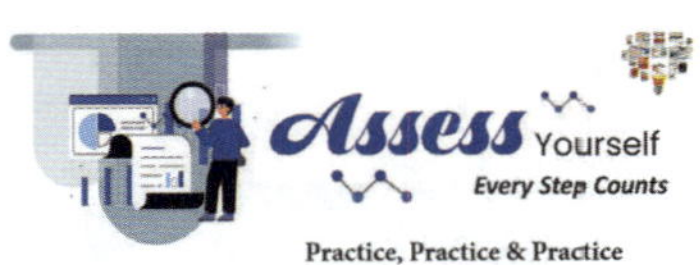

NORMAL VALUES OF SOME BIOCHEMICAL PARAMETERS IN URINE

Normal values of some biochemical parameters in urine are shown in Table 10.5.

TABLE 10.5: **Reference range of some constituents in urine**

Constituent	Normal excretion
D-xylose	1–2 g/5 hrs
Total nitrogen	10–20 g/24 hrs
Creatinine	1.0–2.0 g/24 hrs
Calcium	0.1–0.7 g/24 hrs
Chloride	110–250 mEq/24 hrs
Sodium	40–220 mEq/24 hrs
Potassium	25–125 mEq/24 hrs
Phosphorus	0.4–1.3 g/24 hrs
Urea	25–30 g/24 hrs
Uric acid	0.5–1.0 g/24 hrs

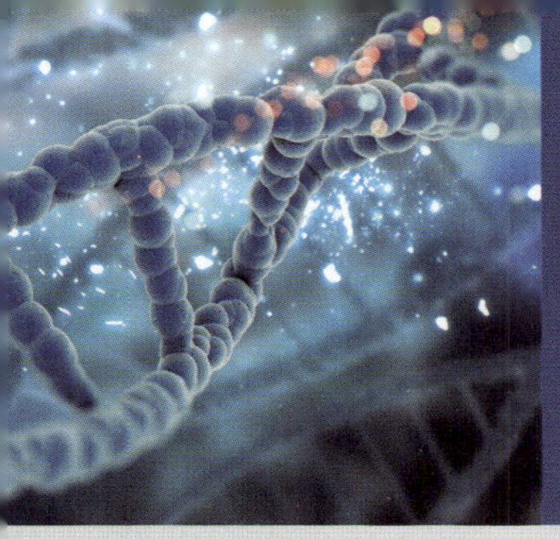

LONG AND SHORT ANSWER QUESTIONS

1. What is an anticoagulant? Describe the role of various anticoagulants in blood collection.
2. What is a vacutainer? Define the principle of working of a vacutainer. Describe the use of various types of vacutainers.
3. **Differentiate between:**
   a. Whole blood, serum and plasma
   b. Vacutainer and venipuncture
   c. Hemolytic, icteric and lipemic serum
4. **Write notes on:**
   a. Vacutainer
   b. Venipuncture
   c. Blood collection on babies
   d. Collection and handling of urine sample

MULTIPLE CHOICE QUESTIONS

1. **Which of the following is a commonly used parameter to assess kidney function?**
   a. Alanine aminotransferase (ALT)
   b. Creatinine
   c. C-reactive protein (CRP)
   d. Thyroid stimulating hormone (TSH)

2. **What does the acronym HDL stand for in context of lipid profiles?**
   a. High density lipoprotein
   b. Human digestive lipase
   c. Hemoglobin detection level
   d. Hypothalamus-derived lipids

3. **Which of the following is a measure of average blood glucose levels over the past 3 months?**
   a. Fasting blood sugar
   b. Glycated hemoglobin (HbA1c)
   c. Random blood sugar
   d. Oral glucose tolerance test (OGTT)

4. **What biochemical parameter is typically used to assess liver function?**
   a. Troponin
   b. Albumin
   c. Amylase
   d. Red blood cell count

ANSWER KEY

1. b   **2.** a   **3.** b   **4.** b

Notes

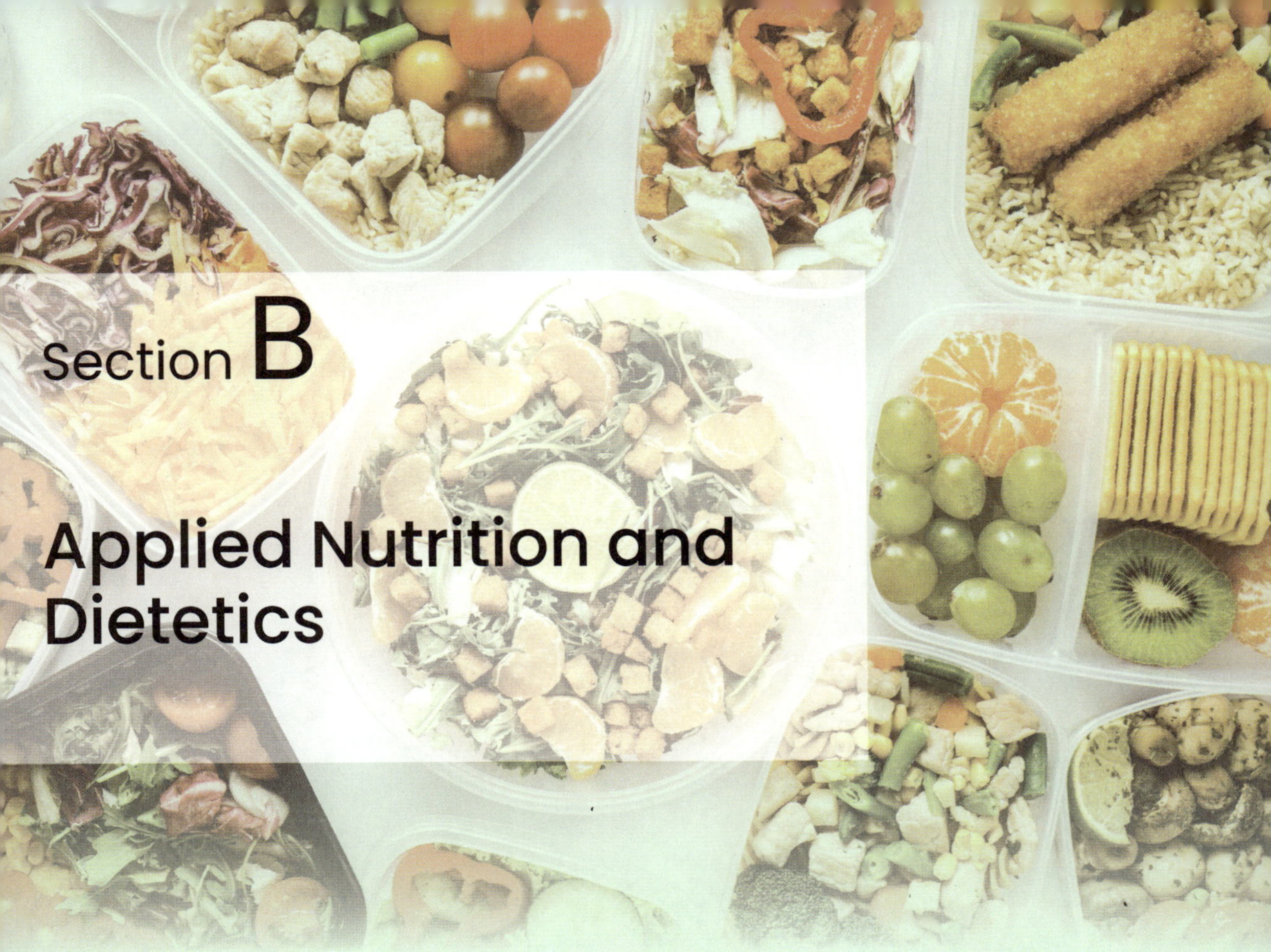

Section B

Applied Nutrition and Dietetics

SECTION OUTLINE

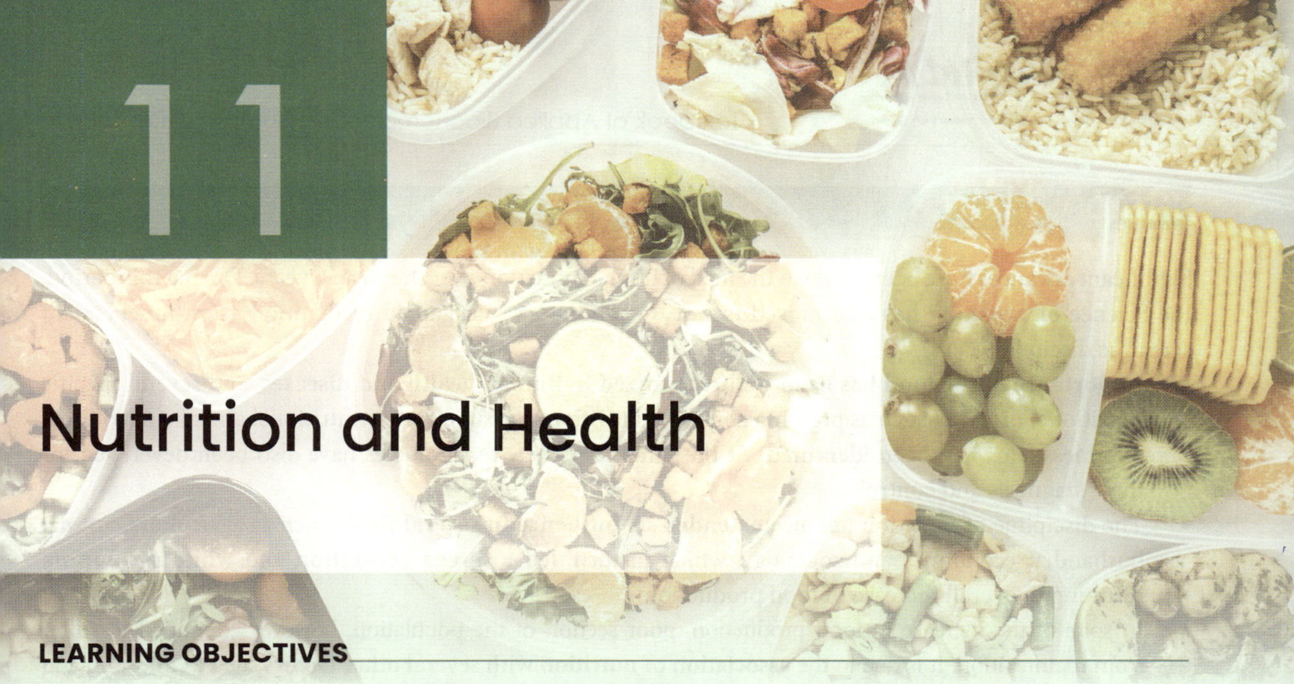

11

Nutrition and Health

LEARNING OBJECTIVES

After the completion of the chapter, the readers will be able to:
- Identify the importance of nutrition in health and wellness.
- Identify macronutrients and micronutrients.
- Describe malnutrition and causes, effects and prevention.

CHAPTER OUTLINE

- Introduction
- Nutrition
- Health
- Malnutrition
- Role of Nutrition in Maintaining Health
- Factors Affecting Food and Nutrition
- Nutrients
- Food

KEY TERMS

Nutritional genomics: Assessing an individual's genetic variations and using this information, coupled to the gene variant-diet and lifestyle-disease associations, to develop therapeutic interventions.

Overnutrition: A condition where an individual consumes more nutrients than he/she requires, leading to an imbalance in diet and potential negative health outcome, such as obesity.

Stretch reflex: Myotatic reflex, which is the contraction of a muscle in response to its passive stretching.

Undernutrition: Lack of proper nutrition, caused by not having enough food or not eating enough food containing substances necessary for growth and health.

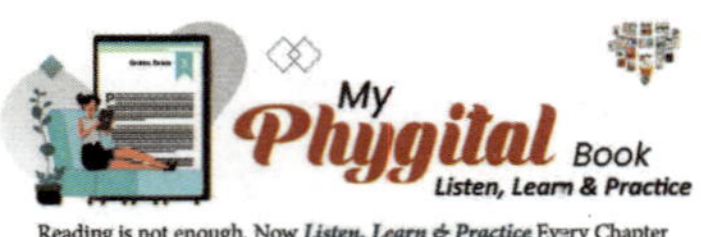

INTRODUCTION

Significant advances have been made in the field of human nutrition over the past 50 years. During this period, the Science of Nutrition has also moved out of the laboratory and gained recognition as an independent scientific discipline.

- **Importance of the food has been well recognized in human health and diseases**, and several specific nutritional diseases, such as protein energy malnutrition, endemic goiter, nutritional anemia, nutritional blindness, etc., had been identified. At the same time, new technologies have also been developed for their diagnosis and control.
- The discipline of nutrition has also **extended its influence in several fields** such as agriculture, animal husbandry, economics and sociology, which in turn, led to **green revolution** and **white revolution**, resulting in overall increase in food production.
- In spite of the increase in food production, poor section of the population, however continued to suffer from malnutrition. It is due to the **association of nutrition with several other factors** such as infection and immunity, fertility, maternal and child health, and family health, which has received further scientific attention.
- It led to the concept that **nutritional problems are multifactorial**. Accordingly, greater emphasis is being paid on **integrating nutrition into primary health care system** and toward the formulation of national dietary goals to promote health.
- More recently, a great deal of interest has been focused on the **role of dietary factors in the pathogenesis of noncommunicable diseases**, such as coronary heart disease, diabetes and cancer.
  With the newer concepts and approaches, the science of nutrition is becoming more dynamic.

NUTRITION

Nutrition is the study of nutrients and their relationship with food and living beings, i.e., it is a science of food and its relationship to health.

Nutrition interprets the interaction of nutrients and other substances in food, in relation to maintenance, growth, reproduction, health and disease of an organism. It includes food intake and absorption, assimilation and catabolism of nutrients, and excretion of waste products.

Diet refers to the food that a person, normally, takes every day. A proper diet is essential from the very early stages of life, for proper growth, development and to remain active. Since people consume food, it is essential to advocate nutrition in terms of foods, rather than nutrients. Apart from supplying nutrients, foods provide a host of other components (non-nutrient phytochemicals), which have a positive impact on health.

Food consumption, which largely depends on production and distribution, determines the health and nutritional status of the population. This is largely determined by the availability and palatability of **food**. For human beings, a healthy diet includes preparation of food and storage methods that preserve nutrients from oxidation, heat or leaching, and reduces the risk of food borne illnesses.

HEALTH

World Health Organization (WHO) defined health as "a state of complete physical, mental and social well-being and not merely the absence of disease or infirmity." In 1986, the WHO made further clarifications

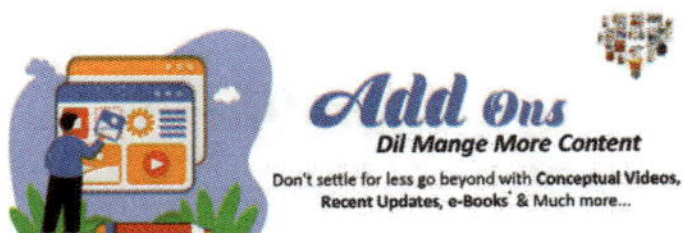

that "Health is a positive concept emphasizing social and personal resources, as well as physical capacities." In 2009, researchers defined health as the ability of a body to adapt to new threats and infirmities. Mental and physical health is the two most frequently discussed types of health.

Physical Health

A person who has good physical health is likely to have bodily functions and processes working at their peak. This is not only due to an absence of disease. Regular exercise, balanced nutrition and adequate rest all contribute to good health.

Mental Health

Mental health refers to a person's emotional, social and psychological well-being.

Wellness includes both physical and mental health. Both of these are important and related to each other. Say, if an individual is not physically healthy, he or she may not also be mentally healthy and may suffer from stress and subsequently, depression. Similarly, if a person is mentally ill, such as under depression, the individual may suffer from weight loss which, in turn, may affect physical ability to perform work. Further, such an individual may not only be performing his/her own work well, but will affect his/her utility for the family as well as society.

Factors Affecting Physical and Mental Health

Wellness (good physical and mental health) is a continuous process and is regulated by several factors, which include:

- **Balanced diet:** One should consume a balanced diet, mostly from the natural sources, every day.
- **Physical activity:** The individual must perform some type of exercise, at least 30 minutes each day for 5 days a week.
- **Life style:** Besides balanced diet and exercise, one must adopt a life style to remain busy to lead a stress free life with a positive outlook.
- **Routine checkup:** One must undergo routine laboratory and medical checkup periodically, particularly, for the life-threatening disease such as weight gain, obesity and cardiovascular disease, or a chronic infection.
- **Social work:** One should contribute to the family and the society, to the best of his/her physical and mental health, and financial status.

MALNUTRITION

Malnutrition means an incorrect or imbalanced intake of nutrients. It may be defined as a pathological state, resulting from a relative or absolute deficiency; or excess of one or more essential nutrient(s). Accordingly, malnutrition may be observed in any of the following forms, i.e., as undernutrition or overnutrition.

Undernutrition

Undernutrition or undernourishment is a result of intake of quantitatively as well as qualitatively inadequate diet. The diet may be either less in quantity (such as in marasmus) or may be lacking in one or more nutrients (such as kwashiorkor, nutritional anemia or vitamin deficiencies). Undernutrition may be a result of poverty and large family size, unhealthy life style and poor health care system, faulty feeding habits, inadequate sanitation (resulting in frequent infections), or migratory population (or people) living in rural areas or urban slums, particularly, those belonging to socially-backward groups, such as scheduled castes and tribes, and landless laborers.

Low birth-weight babies, preschool children, adolescent girls, pregnant and lactating women, and elderly socially-deprived persons are at high risk of developing undernutrition. Undernutrition may result in low birth-weight babies, and clinical and subclinical undernutrition during childhood and adolescence. National surveys indicate that about half of the children below 5 years suffer from subclinical under nutrition, such as underweight (43%), and stunting and wasting (20%), which indicates that under nutrition is of long duration. It has also been shown that there is a steep increase in the prevalence of underweight with increase of age, from 27% at 6 months of age to a high of 45% at 24 months of age. Persistent undernutrition throughout the growing phase of childhood may lead to short stature in adults (Chapter 24).

Overnutrition

Overnutrition means either too many calories or the wrong types of calories such as saturated fats or highly processed sugar, that lead to diet-related chronic diseases, such as obesity and other lifestyle disorders.

India is passing through the phase of economic transition, where, although under nutrition continues to be a major problem, prevalence of over nutrition is also emerging as a significant problem, especially, in urban areas. This is due to the over consumption of energy-rich diets containing increased amounts of fat and sugar, and low in dietary fiber and complex carbohydrates, particularly by the higher income group. Besides, lack of physical activity, sedentary life style, increased consumption of alcohol (empty calories) and use of tobacco are the other contributing factors which lead to increased prevalence of disorders like obesity, hypertension, diabetes and coronary heart disease (Chapter 24).

The prevalence of overweight/obesity is higher among women (10.9%) compared to men (7.8%), in rural areas. The prevalence of Diabetes Mellitus and Coronary Heart Disease (CHD) is higher in urban areas as compared to their rural counterparts. The incidence rate of cancer is comparatively higher among women (123) compared to men (113 for 100,000).

ROLE OF NUTRITION IN MAINTAINING HEALTH

- **Many common symptoms and diseases can often be prevented with better nutrition:** According to US Department of Health and Human Services (2000), several leading causes of death, including cardiovascular diseases (atherosclerotic heart disease and hypertension), cerebrovascular disease (stroke), diabetes and some cancers, have a strong link with the type and amount of food being consumed.
- **Nutritional knowledge** of both, the general public as well as health professionals, is critical, if we are to succeed in reducing morbidity and mortality from the killer diseases. With the advancements in the

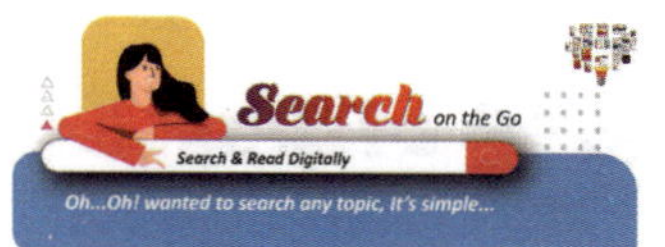

fields of Molecular Biology, Biochemistry and Genetics, it is now well understood that a disease may be genetically biased but is influenced by environmental factors, including nutrition.

- **Nutrition is** not only a basic component of preventive medicine but is **also effective in corrective medicine** for many common health problems.

- **Role of nutrients and other biologically active food components on gene expression is also the focus of exciting field of nutrition**, called **Nutritional Genomics** or **Nutrigenomics**. The expectation is that by analyzing individual's genotypes at birth, disease susceptibilities can be shown from an early age, and categorized into the nutrition and lifestyle choices available to individuals throughout their lives. The Human Genome Project has also been the impetus for this fundamental shift, to integrate genetic principles into health care.

FACTORS AFFECTING FOOD AND NUTRITION

The food we eat, says a lot about our character, personality and where we are from? Food also reflects family history, culture and religious background, economic status, how one feels, where one goes, and what one does, socially. Thus, a number of factors affect food and nutrition:

- **Socioeconomic factors:** Our social existence is, probably, one of the biggest contributors to what we eat. The people, we live with, work with and socialize with, have a great deal of influence over what we eat. For example, some of the foods are considered to be **only for those with low income**, yet these foods are just as nutritious, and can be prepared in as many delicious ways, as the more expensive foods.

- **Cultural factors:** Eating and choosing food, is no longer just about feeding our body what it needs and what tastes good, but food practices are also different from culture to culture and generation to generation. Whether our background is European or African, Asian or Latin American, cultural influences contribute to food, what we eat or bring home. These influences can blend into preparation and serving methods, too. For example, **Mexican dishes** often include abundance of beans, rice and cheese. **Middle Eastern menus** are known for their olives and olive oil, fruits, vegetables and spices. **Chinese foods** include many stir-fry and combination meals. **Indian foods** often are deep-fried and high in fat, etc.

- **Traditions:** Dietary habits and eating patterns form our **family's traditions** make our food habit in young age.

- **Production:** Each region of the country is known for its distinct type of foods, produced in that area. For example, **North East region** is famous for its supply of **seafoods and fresh-fishes**; in the **Western Coast** (with its warm weather and trendy lifestyle) one can often find many **fresh and Asian/Pacific-types of foods**, etc.

- **System of distribution:** A public distribution shop, also known as **fair price shop**, is a part of India's public distribution system, established by the Government of India, which distributes ration at a subsidized price, to the poor. Locally, these are known as **ration shops** and public distribution shops, and **chiefly sell wheat, rice and sugar**, at a price lower than the market price, called **Issue Price**. The basic objective of the public distribution system, in India, is to provide essential consumer goods **at cheap** and **subsidized** price, to the consumers, so as to insulate them from the impact of rising prices of these commodities and **maintain the minimum nutritional status of the population.**

- **Lifestyle: Friends, peers and colleagues have a big influence over food choices. Teens choose fast foods**, like pizza, French fries, hot dogs, shakes and soft drinks, because everyone else is eating these items. On the other hand, some of them even might choose not to eat at all, in order to trim down, like their friends. Some of the foods have more prestigious value than others, and we have to use them as **company foods**, to honor, or impress, our friends, clients or officers, though they may cost more, may be hard to get, take a lot of time to prepare or are unusual.

- **Food habits:** Food habits also have deep psychological roots, and are associated with religious customs and beliefs. For example, even some vegetarians do not consume onion and garlic; Muslims avoid pork, while Hindus avoid beef, etc. Some persons like much of salt while others only a little; some like very sweet food, others do not; some like spicy food while others prefer bland food, etc.

NUTRIENTS

Nutrients are molecules which the body uses to function appropriately and stay in a healthy condition. It includes all the organic and inorganic substances that are obtained from the food which we eat. There are six groups of nutrients called carbohydrate, lipids, protein, vitamins, minerals and water. They are essential to supply energy, build and maintain body cells and regulate metabolic processes. These may be classified in several different ways as macro and micronutrients, organic and inorganic nutrients, or energy-yielding and nonenergy-yielding nutrients.

Macro- and Micronutrients

Macronutrients

Macronutrients are the nutrients which are required by the body in relatively large amounts. These include **carbohydrates** (including **dietary fiber**), **lipids** or **fats** (including **fatty acids** and **cholesterol**), **proteins** (including **amino acids**) and **water** (Table 11.1).

TABLE 11.1: Macro- and micronutrients with their primary functions

Nutrient	Functions
Carbohydrates	Major source of energy
Lipids	Provide large amount of energy, insulation, fat soluble vitamins and essential fatty acids
Proteins	Building and maintenance of tissues, antibodies, enzymes, hormones and other compounds
Vitamins	Facilitate use of other nutrients, used in regulation of growth and several metabolites
Minerals	Help in building bones and teeth, maintenance of acid base balance, muscle functions and nervous system activity
Water	Dissolves and carries nutrients, removes waste products, regulate body temperature

Carbohydrates, lipids and **proteins** are also referred to as the **proximate principles of food**. Together with water, they form bulk of the food in an Indian diet.

- **Carbohydrates:** Carbohydrates are the cheapest sources of energy and are easily available dietary sources. They are the main sources of energy for the body, which provides about 70% of the daily calorie requirements. Carbohydrates, in addition to the supply of energy also serve as the components of cell membrane and receptors. Carbohydrates are very well synthesized in our body from non-carbohydrate sources. Carbohydrates are classified according to their number of sugar units as **monosaccharides** (such as glucose and fructose), **disaccharides** (such as sucrose and lactose) and **polysaccharides** (such as starch, glycogen and cellulose; Chapter 12).

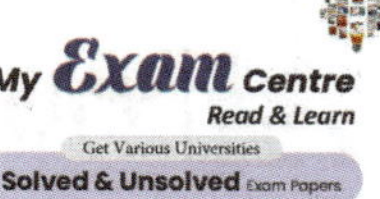

- **Monosaccharides**, i.e., **glucose** and **fructose** (found in fruits, vegetables and honey), and **disaccharides**, i.e., **sucrose** (found in sugar, also called table sugar) and **lactose** (found in milk) are referred to as **simple carbohydrates**.
- **Polysaccharides**, such as **starch** (found in cereals, millets, pulses and root vegetables) and **glycogen** (found in animal foods) are referred to as **complex polysaccharides**.
- **Dietary fibers** include **other complex carbohydrates** which are **resistant to digestion** in the human digestive tract, e.g., **cellulose** (in vegetables and whole grains), and **gums** and **pectins** (in vegetables, fruits and cereals).
  - **Cellulose and stretch reflex:** Cellulose (polysaccharide) materials present in the diet form the bulk (fiber) of the food. It cannot be digested by human beings because of the absence of the enzyme cellulase. The cellulose helps in the movement of the food through the gastrointestinal tract. The cellulose material of the diet absorbs the waste from large intestine and while doing so it stretches the wall of the large intestine and as a result, defecation takes place. This is called stretch reflex.

- **Lipids:** Lipids or fat, include a group of substances which are poorly soluble, or nearly insoluble, in water but are soluble in organic solvents. Over 90% of the **dietary fat** includes **triacylglycerols** (triglycerides), which consist of a molecule of glycerol (glycerine) with three fatty acids attached to it. Fatty acid molecules contain a –COOH group attached to unbranched hydrocarbon chains connected by single bonds alone (**saturated fatty acids**) or by both double and single bonds (**unsaturated fatty acids**). Other types of dietary lipids include **cholesterol, phospholipids, sterols** and **carotenoids**; Chapter 15).
  - Fats and oils are concentrated sources of energy. We consume fat because of its high calorific values (1 g gives 9 kcal) and also that it can be easily stored with less amount of water, therefore, occupy less space.
  - Fat is also essential for **structure and functions of cell** and **cell membranes**.
  - Lipids also act as signaling molecules.
  - Fat is also needed to maintain a stable body temperature and to sustain the health of skin and hair.
  - Fat also contributes to **palatability of food** and is important in cooking and food processing.
  - They are also a good source of **fat soluble vitamins** viz., A, D, E and K.
  - Fats are also taken because of their essential fatty acids (also referred to as polyunsaturated fatty acids or PUFA) content. Essential fatty acids are those which cannot be synthesized in our body, hence they should be supplied through the diet. They are **linoleic acid** and **linolenic acids. Arachidonic acid** is also an essential fatty acid but it **can be synthesized from linolenic acid**. These are essential for the control of blood cholesterol. While a minimum amount of fat should be included in the diet to meet the requirement of EFA, excess of fat is harmful.
  - Plant fats are superior to animal fats because they contain more of polyunsaturated fatty acids, i.e., essential fatty acids and less of cholesterol.
  - The cholesterol in the diet should be restricted because excess intake of cholesterol leads to its deposition in the tissues thereby causing atherosclerosis.

- **Proteins:** Proteins are organic compounds that **consist of amino acids** which are joined by peptide bonds. Proteins are needed for their content of certain amino acids that are essential to human body for the biosynthesis of proteins, body repair in adult, and for body building and body repair in children. Human body proteins are made up of only 20 standard amino acids, out of which nearly 10 amino acids can be synthesized in the body but the remaining 10 cannot be synthesized in the body, hence they have to be supplied through the diet. Therefore, they are known as essential amino acids. **The essential amino acids are** methionine, valine, phenylalanine, isoleucine, tryptophan, leucine, lysine and threonine. Besides, arginine and histidine are referred to as semi essential amino acids. Through digestion, proteins are broken down by proteases into free amino acids; Chapter 14).

- Proteins have more physiological roles than any other nutrient, e.g., they are important for **growth**, **development** and **tissue repair**.
- Proteins provide **structural material**.
- Protein also helps in **maintaining water and pH balance**.
- Protein also **keeps the immune system strong**.
- **Proteins do provide energy**, which means like carbohydrates and fats, proteins can provide energy, when necessary. However, our body does not commonly use them for energy because, if proteins were a primary source of energy, they would be unavailable for these other life-sustaining functions.

    Proteins are in a constant state of flux in the body, with continuously being synthesized and degraded. Foods rich in protein include meat, poultry, fishes, nuts, eggs, milk and milk products. Different foods contain different amounts and combinations of amino acids (the building blocks of proteins). Accordingly, proteins are said to be the:

    - **High quality proteins** are, mainly, obtained from **animals** (e.g., meat, fish, eggs and dairy products). They **contain full range of essential amino acids**, needed by the body. These are also referred to as the **proteins of high biological value**.
    - **Low quality proteins** are obtained from plant sources. They have **low biological value**, since an individual protein may lack one or the other essential amino acid. **Vegans and vegetarians** cannot get all the amino acids they need, from a single source. However, combining the plant foods from different sources provide them good quality protein, e.g., pulses and cereals.

- **Water:** Water is essential for life. Although human can survive for a number of weeks without food, one cannot live without fluid for >2 or 3 days. On an average, water makes up nearly 60% of body weight and is essential for normal functioning of all the cells in the body. **Though, amount of fluid needed varies according to age, time of the year, climate conditions, diet and level of physical activity, on an average an adult person** should drink, at least, eight 8 glasses of water (1500–2000 mL) every day. It is a major nutritional element that helps to:

  - Regulate body temperature
  - Lubricate joints
  - Protect major organs and tissues
  - Transport important substances.

We can obtain our fluid requirements from a number of sources, such as water and other drinks, as well as the food we eat. **Dehydration** (loss of body water) can impair physiological responses and in extreme cases, **can be fatal**. At the same time, it can be dangerous to drink too much water (over hydration), as water intoxication **can lead to hyponatremia**.

Micronutrients

Micronutrients, mainly include vitamins and minerals. They are required comparatively in small quantities, i.e., from milligrams to few grams. These are also referred to as protective foods.

Besides, vitamins and minerals, antioxidants and phytochemicals, too, may be referred to as micronutrients, since they are also required in small quantities and said to protect (or influence) some of the body systems.

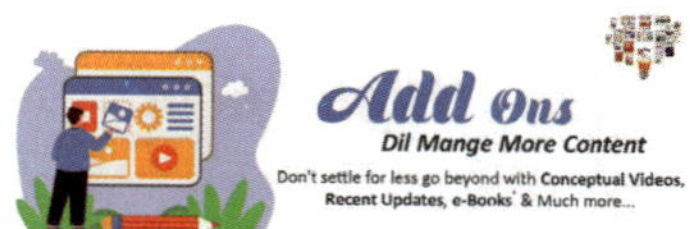

Their essentiality, however, has not been well established like that of vitamins and minerals.

- **Vitamins:** Vitamins are a group of organic compounds and perform a variety of functions in the body. Every vitamin is chemically different from each other. Although they do not yield energy but vitamins enable the body to use other nutrients. Since body is generally unable to synthesize most of the vitamins, hence, they must be provided by food. Vitamins are divided into two groups, as follows:

    i. **Fat soluble vitamins**, which include vitamins A, D, E and K
    ii. **Water soluble vitamins**, which include B vitamins and vitamin C (Chapter 16).

    Although recommended daily allowance for each vitamin differs, but it is important to consume all the vitamins each day, to keep our body healthy. It is due to the reason that:

    - Vitamins are **required** by the body **in small amounts**, for a variety of essential processes.
    - Most vitamins **cannot be made by the body**, so need to be provided in the diet.
    - **Vitamin D can be made** by the body in the skin when **body is exposed to sunlight**.
    - **Requirements** for vitamins **change across life stages**.

- **Minerals:** Minerals are the inorganic substances. These are required by the body in small amounts. **Our body requires different amounts of each mineral; accordingly**, they are divided into two classes (Table 11.2).

    - **Major minerals** include sodium, potassium, calcium, phosphorus, magnesium, sulfur and chloride, which are required in large amounts (milligrams to grams).
    - **Trace minerals** include copper, fluoride, zinc, iron, chromium, selenium, iodine, molybdenum and manganese, which are needed in small amounts (microgram to milligrams; Chapter 17).

All minerals and trace elements are present in healthy tissues, where their concentration remains relatively constant. Besides, there are certain elements like nickel, vanadium, tin, boron, etc., which have not been shown to have any function in human body, thus are not dietary essential.

TABLE 11.2: **Essential minerals and trace elements required by human body**

Minerals	Trace elements
Calcium	Copper
Phosphorus	Chromium
Magnesium	Manganese
Sodium	Molybdenum
Potassium	Selenium
Iron	Iodine
Zinc	
Fluoride	

Organic and Inorganic Nutrients

The presence or absence of carbon is what differentiates organic nutrients from inorganic nutrients. Carbohydrates, lipids, proteins and vitamins have carbon in their structure, making them organic. Water and minerals do not have carbon, so they are inorganic.

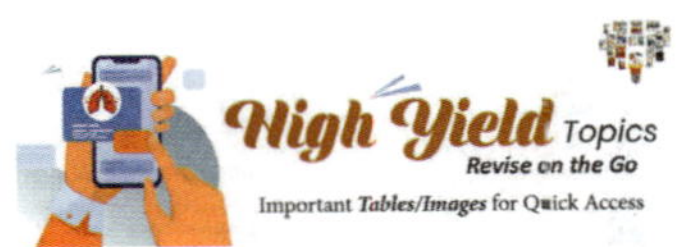

- **Organic nutrients:** The term organic refers to life, and we know that organic nutrients **contain carbon**. Carbon is an important element not only in organic nutrients but for all sort of life on Earth. The organic nutrients are also the **necessary building blocks of various cell** components. These include **macronutrients**, i.e., **carbohydrates**, **protein** and **lipids** as well as **micronutrients**, i.e., **vitamins**. As discussed above, vitamins are required in small amounts and play either the catalytic role or the regulatory role in metabolism.
- **Inorganic nutrients:** Minerals and water (micronutrients) do not contain carbon, so they are referred to as inorganic nutrients. As discussed above, number of minerals (inorganic elements) are essential for the growth of living things. For example, trace amounts of fluorine (as fluoride) is essential for proper tooth formation. Similarly, iodine (as iodide) is required for formation of thyroxine, an important regulatory hormone. Silicon (as silicate) is a prominent component of the outer skeletons and is required for normal growth. Calcium is required as a major component of bone.

Energy Yielding and Non-Energy Yielding Nutrients

- **Energy-yielding nutrients: Carbohydrates**, **fats** and **proteins** (**organic macronutrients**) are referred to as **energy-yielding nutrients** because they contain calories and supply the body with energy. Both, carbohydrate and protein provide 4 kcal/gram, while lipids provide 9 kcal/g.
  - **Carbohydrates** are considered the **most important nutrient for** immediate **energy**. This is because carbohydrates are easily converted to energy. They are the most significant sources of energy in Indian diets, where nearly 65–80% of the total energy intake may be available from carbohydrates. Being cheap source of energy, carbohydrates **form the bulk of an Indian diet**. They may be either simple or complex carbohydrates.
  - **Lipids**, also referred to as fats, are important energy nutrients, as well. In fact, lipids are the **most energy-dense** of the three energy-yielding nutrients, since fat contains more calories per mass, or volume than carbohydrates or proteins. Fat contributes to approximately 10–30% of the total energy intake. The high storage of energy in lipids also makes them a great source of stored energy in the body.
  - **Proteins** contribute to approximately 7–15% of the total energy intake. However, as discussed above, our body does not commonly use protein for energy because they are important for various other life-sustaining functions.
- **Non-energy yielding nutrients:** The non-energy yielding nutrients include **dietary fiber (organic macronutrient)**, and **vitamins** and **minerals (micronutrients)**.
  - **Dietary fiber**, as discussed above, is an important **component of carbohydrate** (a **macronutrient**). It delays and retards absorption of carbohydrates and fats and increases the satiety value. Diet rich in fiber also reduces glucose and lipids in blood and increases bulk of the stool.
  - **Vitamins** do not contain calories and do not, directly, supply our body with energy, but they are indirectly linked to energy. This is because certain vitamins are **necessary for energy metabolism**, which means they help our body convert calorie-containing nutrients into energy. Vitamins serve **other roles** as well, such as **maintaining vision**, **protecting our cells from damage** and **helping our blood clot**.
  - **Minerals**, as discussed above, are the inorganic substances required by the body in small amounts, for a variety of functions such as formation of bones and teeth, and act as essential constituents of body fluids and tissues, components of enzyme systems, and for normal nerve functions.

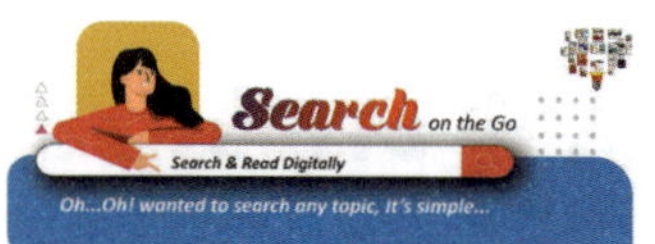

FOOD

Food is **any substance consisting**, essentially, **of carbohydrate, fat, protein and other nutrients** used in the body of an organism **to furnish energy, and sustain growth and vital processes**. The absorption and utilization of food by the body is fundamental to nutrition and is facilitated by digestion, i.e. the substance is **ingested by the organism and assimilated by the cells**.

It may be defined as any solid or liquid substance which, when taken by the body, provides the body with necessary materials to enable it to grow, replace the worn-out and damaged parts, and provide energy to function, normally. Daily intake of food has a direct influence on the health and well-being of an individual. Also, the food is composed of different chemical elements.

Origin of Food

According to their origin, various food stuffs are grouped into two categories, i.e. the food of the **plant origin** or of the **animal origin**.

- **Foods of plant origin:** Most of the food has its origin in plants. Some food is obtained directly from plants. Since even the animals, that are used as food sources, are raised by feeding them foods that are derived from plants. For example, cereal grain is a staple food. It provides more food energy Worldwide, than any other type of crop. Most of the grains that are produced, Worldwide, are also fed to livestock. Foods of the plant origin include:
  - **Seeds:** Majority of the foods consumed by human beings are seed-based. These include **edible seeds** such as cereals, legumes and nuts as well as **oilseeds** that are often pressed to produce rich oils. Oilseeds are, particularly, high in unsaturated fats.
  - **Fruits:** Fruits make up a significant part of the diet in almost every society.
  - **Vegetables:** Vegetables include **root vegetables** (potatoes and carrots), **bulbs** (onion), **leafy vegetables** (spinach), and **other vegetables** like cabbage and cauliflower.
- **Foods of animal origin**: Animal foods are used either directly or indirectly, e.g. **meat, milk and eggs**.
- **Other foods**: Besides there are some food materials which neither come from animals nor from plant sources. For example, various **edible fungi** (especially mushrooms) and **inorganic substances** (such as rock salt).

Food Groups

As mentioned above, various nutrients present in the food are categorized as macronutrients (needed in relatively large amounts) and micronutrients (needed in smaller quantities). These include carbohydrates (including fiber), fats, proteins, vitamins, minerals and water. All these nutrients should be present in our diet, but it is not possible to obtain all the nutrients from one source. They can be obtained from different sources or food groups (Chapter 18).

A food group is a collection of foods that share similar nutritional properties or biological classifications. Most common food groups include:

- **Grains (whole grain cereals and millets):** The group also include any food, which is made from cereal grains, such as bread and pasta, breakfast cereals and popcorn, etc.

- **Vegetables:** Vegetables come in a wide variety of colors, flavors and textures. They are also important sources of vitamins, minerals and fiber. Vegetables are broadly classified into three groups as green-leafy vegetables, roots and tubers, and other vegetables.
- **Fruits:** Fruits include a variety of colors, flavors, nutrients and texture, such as citrus fruits, berries, several fruits which grow on trees (like apricots, cherries, peaches and mangoes), besides figs, raisins and pineapples, etc. Fruits are good sources of carbohydrates, vitamins and minerals. Some fruits contain glucose, while others contain fructose or pentose. Most of the fruits are also good sources of potassium.
- **Dairy (milk and milk products):** Dairy includes milk and milk products as milk is used either as such or in the preparation of several products like curd, cheese, ice cream, butter, ghee and sweets. It is considered to be a complete food. Thus, milk is an ideal food for infants and children. It is also a good supplementary food for adults.
- **Condiments and spices:** Condiments and spices are used as seasoning or flavoring agents in food to increase its acceptability. Since condiments and spices are used in small quantities, they do not add substantially to the nutritive value of the food but improve taste and flavor of the cooked food. After they act on the mucous membrane of the mouth, stomach and intestine, they stimulate secretion of digestive juices.
- **Beverages:** Various beverages such as water, milk, coffee and tea, fruit juices and alcoholic beverages have different effects.

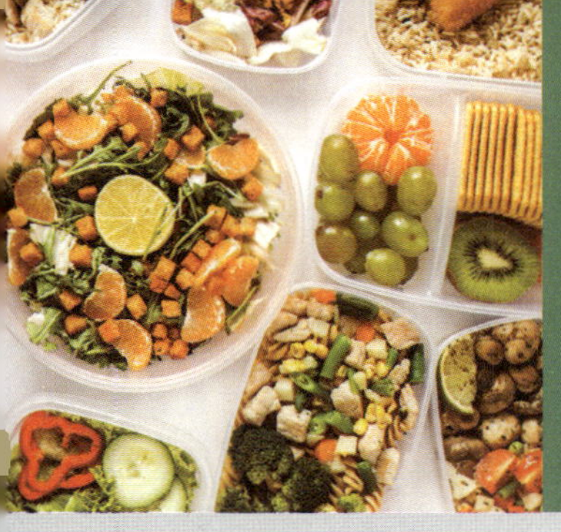

STUDENT ASSIGNMENT

LONG AND SHORT ANSWER QUESTIONS

1. Define nutrition. Describe the role of nutrition in maintaining health.
2. What is malnutrition? Describe undernutrition and overnutrition.
3. What is a nutrient? Describe various dietary nutrients.
4. Define food. Give classification of foods according to origin.
5. **Differentiate between:**
   a. Undernutrition and overnutrition
   b. Macro and micronutrients
   c. Organic and inorganic nutrients
   d. Energy yielding and non-energy yielding nutrients
6. **Write notes on:**
   a. Malnutrition
   b. Undernutrition
   c. Overnutrition
   d. Factors affecting food and nutrition
   e. Macronutrients
   f. Micronutrients
   g. Foods of plant origin
   h. Foods of animal origin

MULTIPLE CHOICE QUESTIONS

1. **Which macronutrient is the main source of energy for the body and includes monosaccharides like glucose and fructose, as well as polysaccharides like starch and cellulose?**
   a. Lipids
   b. Proteins
   c. Carbohydrates
   d. Water

2. **Which macronutrient is essential for the structure and function of cell membranes, provides a high calorific value, and includes fatty acids such as linoleic and linolenic acids?**
   a. Carbohydrates
   b. Proteins
   c. Lipids
   d. Vitamins

3. **Which food group is primarily known for providing a significant source of fiber, vitamins, and minerals, and is broadly classified into green-leafy vegetables, roots and tubers, etc.?**
   a. Fruits
   b. Dairy
   c. Vegetables
   d. Grains

4. **Which of the following food groups is used in the form of food items like bread, pasta, and popcorn, and is known for being a major source of carbohydrates?**
    a. Condiments and spices   b. Beverages
    c. Dairy   d. Grains

12

Carbohydrates

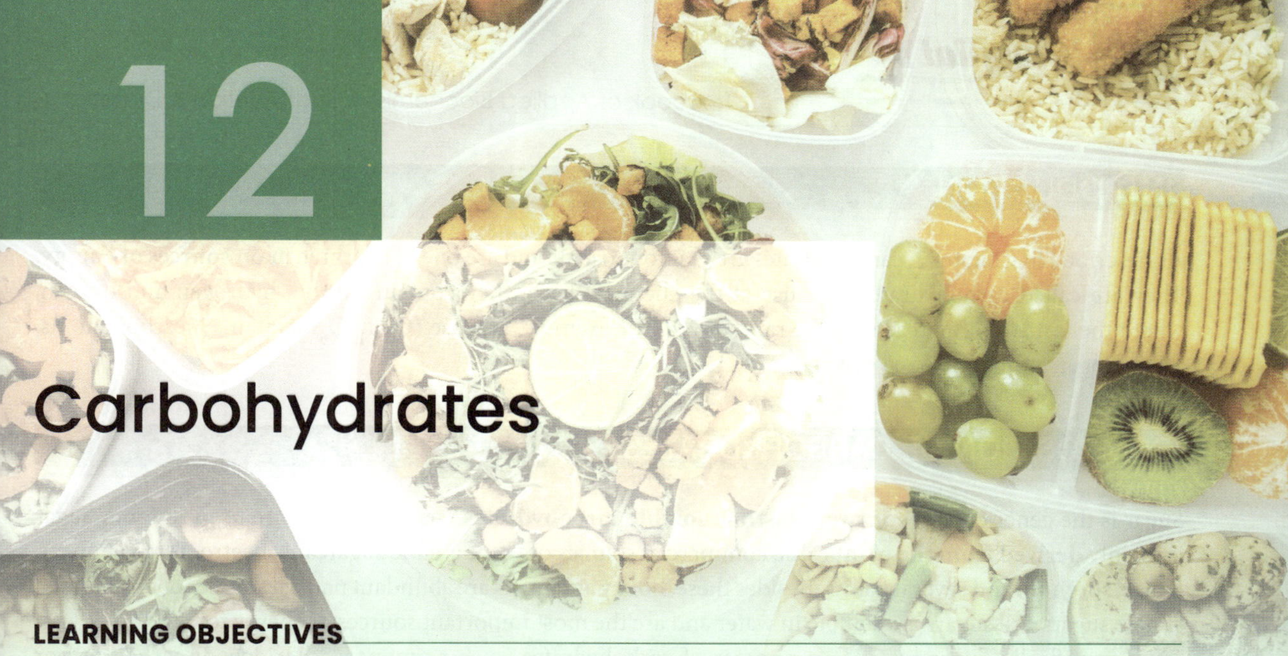

LEARNING OBJECTIVES

After the completion of the chapter, the readers will be able to:
- Learn composition of starches, sugar and cellulose.
- Learn recommended daily allowance (RDA) of carbohydrates.
- Learn dietary sources.
- Explain functions of carbohydrates.

CHAPTER OUTLINE

- Introduction
- Composition of Carbohydrates
- Classification of Carbohydrates According to Nutritional Significance
- Dietary Fiber
- Good Carbohydrates versus Bad Carbohydrates
- Calorific Value of Carbohydrates
- Recommended Daily Allowances of Carbohydrates
- Dietary Sources
- Functions of Carbohydrates

KEY TERMS

Amylose: A polymer that can be found in starch. It is made up of hundreds to thousands of glucose molecules in a linear chain. It is water-soluble.

Calorific value: The amount of heat energy released during complete combustion of a unit mass of a fuel. It is expressed in kcal/100 g.

Type 2 diabetes: A condition that happens because of a problem in the way the body regulates and uses sugar as a fuel.

INTRODUCTION

As described in Chapter 2, carbohydrates are macronutrients and are one of the three **main sources of energy**. They are called carbohydrates, because at the chemical level, they contain carbon, hydrogen and oxygen, where the last two are present in the ratio of 2:1. For example, glucose ($C_6H_{12}O_6$) contains 6 carbon atoms, 12 hydrogen atoms and 6 oxygen atoms $(CH_2O)_6$.

COMPOSITION OF CARBOHYDRATES

Sugar is the generic name for **sweet-tasting, soluble carbohydrates**, many of which are **used in food**. Sugar is mainly **derived from the plants**. The commercial sources of sugar are the sugarcane, beetroot, maple sugar, maize, sorghum and several palms. Besides these, honey and fruits are abundant natural sources of unbounded simple sugars. All sugars are soluble in water and are the most important sources of energy for cells.

Scientifically, sugar refers to a number of carbohydrates, such as monosaccharides, disaccharides, or oligosaccharides.

- **Monosaccharides:** Monosaccharides are also called **simple sugars**. Common monosaccharides include glucose, galactose and fructose. They share the same molecular formula, i.e., as $C_6H_{12}O_6$. Because of their six carbon atoms, each is a **hexose**:
  - The most important being **glucose**, as blood sugar. It is the immediate source of energy for cellular respiration.
  - **Galactose**, a sugar in milk (and yogurt)
  - **Fructose**, a sugar found in honey.

  Monosaccharides, in a closed-chain form, **can form glycosidic bonds with other monosaccharides**, **creating disaccharides** (such as sucrose) and **polysaccharides** (such as starch). Monosaccharides may be further converted into **structural polysaccharides such as cellulose** and pectin for cell wall construction, or into **energy reserves in the form of storage polysaccharides, such as starch** and glycogen.

- **Disaccharides:** Disaccharides are formed by linking two monosaccharides with the removal of a molecule of water. Commonly available disaccharides include **lactose**, **maltose** and **sucrose**.
  - **Lactose** is formed when a molecule of **glucose** is linked to **galactose**. It is also called **milk sugar**, since it is found naturally in milk. Lactose is **synthesized in the mammary glands during lactation** and is secreted into the milk. During digestion, lactose is **hydrolyzed** to its monosaccharide units, i.e., glucose and galactose **by the intestinal enzyme** referred to as **lactase**.
  - **Maltose** is formed when a molecule of **glucose** is linked to another molecule of **glucose**. It is obtained during hydrolysis of starch. During digestion, maltose is hydrolyzed to its monosaccharide units, i.e., glucose and glucose by the intestinal enzyme referred to as maltase.
  - **Sucrose** is formed when a molecule of glucose is linked to fructose. It is also referred to as **table sugar** since it is commonly used on the table for routine use in home-made drinks. Sucrose is also referred to as cane sugar since it is obtained from the stems of sugarcane and roots of sugar beet. During digestion, sucrose is split into its constituent monosaccharides glucose and fructose by the enzyme **sucrase** (also called **invertase**).

    Sucrose is used by people as a sweetener for foods (e.g., toast and cereal) and beverages (e.g., coffee and tea).

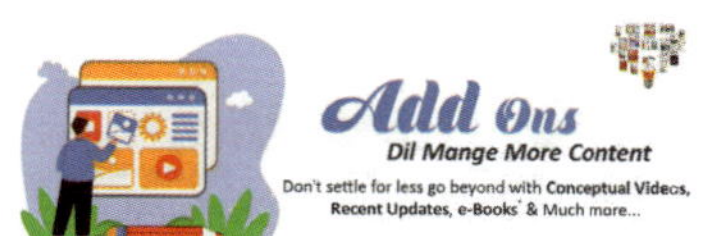

- **Polysaccharides:** Polysaccharides are made up of many monosaccharide molecules. Examples of polysaccharides are **starch**, **glycogen** (the form in which glucose is stored in the body), and **cellulose** and pectin (components classed as dietary fiber), etc.

  - Starches: **Starch** or **amylum** is a polymeric carbohydrate consisting of numerous glucose units joined by glycosidic bonds. This **polysaccharide is produced by most green plants as energy storage**. Starch molecules arrange themselves in the plant in semi-crystalline granules. Each plant species has a unique starch granular size, e.g., rice starch is relatively small while potato starches have larger granules. **Starch content of different foods varies, e.g., potatoes 15%, wheat 55%, corn 65% and rice 75%.**

    Starch is a mixture of two polymers, i.e., amylose and amylopectin. Natural starches consist of about 10–30% amylose and 70–90% amylopectin.

    - **Amylose** is **a linear polysaccharide,** composed entirely of D-glucose units joined by the α-1,4-glycosidic linkages.

    - **Amylopectin** is **a branched-chain polysaccharide,** composed of glucose units linked primarily by α-1,4-glycosidic bonds but with occasionally α-1,6-glycosidic bonds, which are responsible for the branching. A molecule of amylopectin may contain many thousands of glucose units with **branch points occurring after about every 25–30 units.**

    In the human body, several enzymes known collectively as **amylases degrade starch** sequentially into usable glucose units. Alpha-amylases are found in plants and animals. **Human saliva is rich in amylase** and the **pancreas also secretes the enzyme**.

    The complete hydrolysis of starch yields, in successive stages, glucose:

    $$Starch \rightarrow Dextrin \rightarrow Maltose \rightarrow Glucose$$

    Starch is the **most common carbohydrate in the human diet** and is contained in many staple foods. The major sources of starch intake worldwide are the cereals **(rice, wheat and maize)** and the root vegetables **(potatoes and cassava)**. Widely used prepared foods containing starch are bread, pancakes, cereals, noodles and pasta.

  - **Glycogen:** Glycogen is the energy reserve carbohydrate of animals including humans, hence is also referred to as **animal starch**. Like starch in plants, glycogen is found as granules **in liver** (4–8% by weight of tissue) **and in skeletal muscle cells** (0.5–1.0%). When fasting, humans draw on these glycogen reserves during the first day without food to obtain the glucose needed to maintain metabolic balance.

    Glycogen is **structurally quite similar to amylopectin**, although glycogen is more branched (8–12 glucose units between branches) and the branches are shorter. Enzyme **phosphorylase catalyzes the breakdown of glycogen to glucose**, when energy is needed, by a process called glycogenolysis.

  - **Cellulose:** Cellulose is a **polysaccharide (homopolysaccharide)** like amylose, but it differs from amylose in the way that **glucose molecules**, in cellulose **are linked together by β-1,4-glycosidic linkages** instead of α-1,4-glycosidic linkages present in amylose. Cellulose is found in plants, as a structural component of their cell wall. **We are**, however, **unable to digest cellulose** due to the reason that **human beings do not contain enzyme β-amylase**, which is required for the digestion of cellulose.

CLASSIFICATION OF CARBOHYDRATES ACCORDING TO NUTRITIONAL SIGNIFICANCE

According to their significance in nutrition, carbohydrates are classified as simple sugars and complex carbohydrates including fiber.

- **Simple sugars:**
  - **Intrinsic sugars**, which are incorporated into the cellular structure of foods, e.g., **glucose, fructose, pentose**, etc., the sugars **found in whole fruits** and **vegetables**.
  - **Extrinsic sugars,** which are not bound into a cellular structure, e.g., **lactose (milk sugar) found in dairy products, sucrose (table sugar) found in** confectionery, etc.
- **Complex carbohydrates:**
  - **Starch:** It is found in potatoes, bread, rice and pasta.
  - **Dietary fiber:** These are the carbohydrate polymers, which are neither digested nor absorbed in the small intestine, e.g., cellulose, pectin, etc.

DIETARY FIBER

Dietary fiber refers to indigestible carbohydrates, such as cellulose and hemicellulose, pectin, lignin, gums and mucilage. Pectin, gums, mucilages and some of the hemicelluloses are soluble in water and, hence, are also called **soluble fibers**. On the other hand, cellulose, various hemicelluloses and lignin are insoluble in water and are referred to as **insoluble fibers** (Chapter 19).

Fiber cannot be digested by human beings due to the absence of the required digestive enzymes but is essential for digestion. Fiber promotes healthy bowel movement and decreases the risk of chronic diseases, such as coronary heart disease and diabetes. However, unlike sugars and starches, fiber is not absorbed in the small intestine and is not converted to glucose. Instead, fiber passes into the large intestine, relatively intact, where it is converted to hydrogen, carbon dioxide and fatty acids. Sources of fiber include fruits, grains and vegetables, especially, legumes.

Significance of Dietary Fiber

High intake of dietary fiber has many **health benefits**. For example, diets rich in fiber decreases risk of obesity, type 2 diabetes, colon cancer, cardiovascular disease and gastrointestinal disorders:

- Diets rich in fiber are, usually, low in fat and provide lesser calories. Since such a diet forms bulk of the food, which takes longer to eat, and gives a feeling of fullness. Dietary fiber not only regulates body weight but also **lowers the risk of obesity**.
- Higher intake of soluble fiber also delays stomach emptying and, thus regulates blood glucose level. This in turn also **reduces the risk of type 2 diabetes**.
- Diet rich in fiber also lowers the risk of certain types of cancer. It is due to the reason that food with large amounts of fruits and vegetables, provides antioxidants, which protect our body against cell damage and **cancer**.
- Soluble fiber also lowers serum cholesterol, thus, **reduces the risk of a cardiovascular disease**.

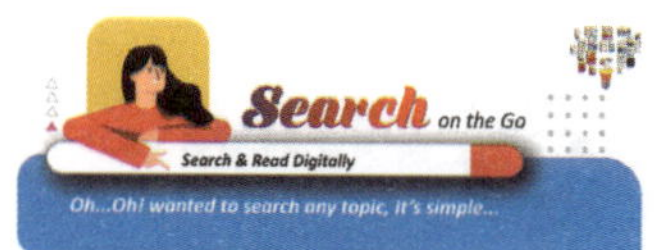

- Diet rich in insoluble fiber also adds bulk to feces and softens stool for its easy passage. Thus, dietary fiber helps in **prevention of constipation and hemorrhoids**, particularly, when fluid intake is high.
- **Excess of fiber** in the diet may, however, cause deficiency of some minerals, such as zinc, calcium, magnesium and iron. It is due to the reason that dietary fiber binds these minerals and thus, reduces their absorption.

GOOD CARBOHYDRATES VERSUS BAD CARBOHYDRATES

Carbohydrates form the basis of most diets, making up half of total energy (calorie) intake. Dietary carbohydrates can be separated into two types, as complex (good) carbohydrates and simple (bad) carbohydrates.

- **Good carbohydrates:** Carbohydrates, usually, considered to be **good** includes complex carbohydrates such as those obtained from whole grains, fruits, vegetables, beans and legumes. They contain larger chains of sugar molecules and take longer to digest than processed grains. They are not only processed slowly, but also contain a bounty of other nutrients (Fig. 12.1).

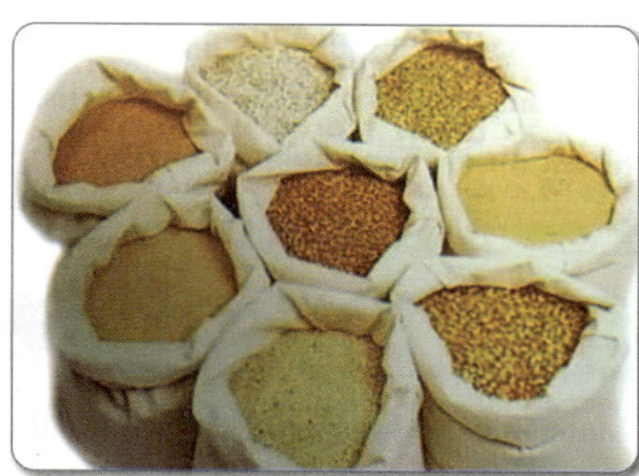

Fig. 12.1: Sources of good carbohydrates

  Good carbohydrates are:
  - Low or moderate in calories
  - High in nutrients
  - Devoid of refined grains and sugar
  - High in naturally occurring fiber
  - Low in sodium
  - Low in saturated fat
  - Very low in or devoid of, cholesterol and trans fat

- **Bad carbohydrates:** Carbohydrates, usually, considered **bad** include refined sugars, such as those obtained from pastries, white sugar, honey, fruit juices and soda, highly processed foods, white rice, white bread and other white-flour foods (Fig. 12.2).

  They are digested more quickly by the body. This makes them a faster source of energy. Also, these types of carbohydrates do not offer as many additional nutrients.

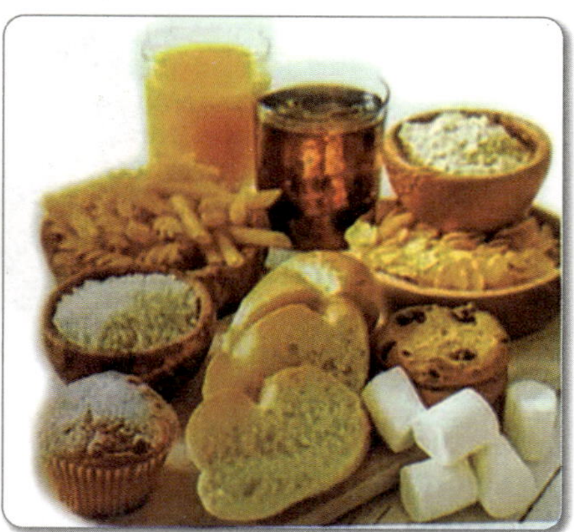

Fig. 12.2: Sources of bad carbohydrates

  Bad carbohydrates are:
  - High in calories
  - Full of refined sugars
  - Low in many nutrients
  - Low in fiber
  - High in sodium
  - High in saturated fat, cholesterol and trans fat

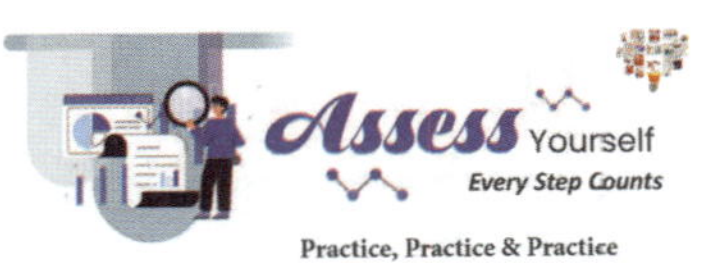

CALORIFIC VALUE OF CARBOHYDRATES

Calorific value or caloric value of the food is the amount of heat produced by combustion of one gram of fuel. It is expressed in terms of calories per gram or joules/kg. Calorific value of carbohydrate is 4 kcal/g.

RECOMMENDED DAILY ALLOWANCES OF CARBOHYDRATES

The ICMR-NIN (2020) Expert Group has recommended that 55–60% of the dietary energy intake should be derived from carbohydrates. The minimum requirement for carbohydrate has been recommended as 100 g/day for normal healthy adults. Minimum requirement during pregnancy has been recommended as 135 g/day while during lactation carbohydrate intake should be 155 g/day.

It is further recommended that dietary free sugar should be restricted to 5–7% of energy intake.

DIETARY SOURCES

Main dietary sources of carbohydrates include grains, vegetables and fruits. Complex carbohydrates are present in whole grains (such as cereals and rice), bran, beans, bread and pasta. Milk and milk products provide lactose, while beverages, jams, jellies and candies provide refined sugar, such as glucose and fructose (Fig. 12.3).

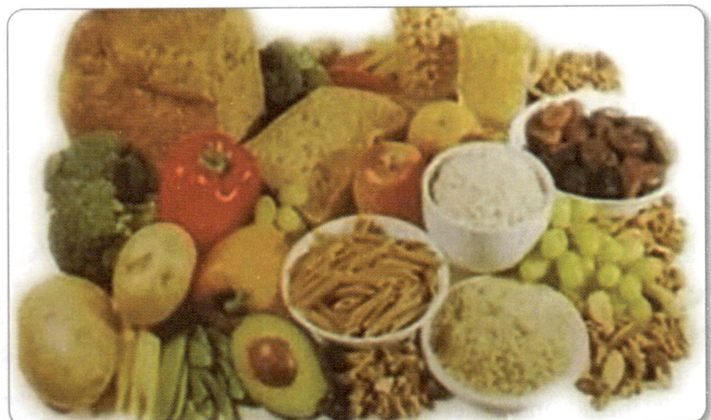

Fig. 12.3: Dietary sources of carbohydrates

Foods which are rich in carbohydrates include:

- **Dairy:** Milk, yogurt and ice cream
- **Fruits:** Whole fruits and fruit juice
- **Grains:** Cereal grains, bread and rice
- **Legumes:** Beans and pulses
- **Starchy vegetables:** Potatoes and corn
- **Sugary sweets:** Soda (when fluid intake is high), candy, cookies and other desserts.

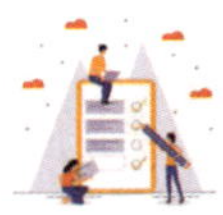
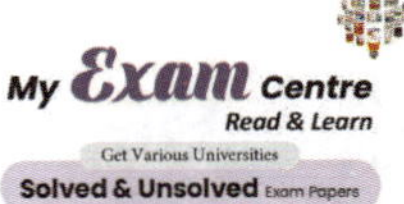

FUNCTIONS OF CARBOHYDRATES

Carbohydrates are necessary for good health and give a variety of benefits:

- **Brain health:** Carbohydrates are important for brain functions. They are a quick source of energy and have influence on mood and memory.
- **Weight loss:** Although, carbohydrates are often blamed for weight gain, the right kind of carbohydrate can actually help to maintain a healthy weight. This can happen due to the consumption of many good carbohydrates, especially, whole grains and vegetables with skin, which contain fiber.
- **Good sources of nutrients:** Whole, unprocessed fruits and vegetables are well known for their nutrients contents. Due to the same reason, some of the food stuffs are even considered as super foods, such as the green leafy vegetables, sweet potatoes, berries, citruses and apples. Whole grains also have significantly higher amounts of fiber, energy and polyunsaturated fats, as well as all micronutrients (except vitamin B_{12} and sodium). Further, whole grains have also been shown to contain antioxidants.
- **Heart health:** Fiber also helps to lower cholesterol. This is due to the reason that the digestive process requires bile acids, which are made, partly, from cholesterol. As the digestion improves, liver pulls cholesterol from blood, to form more bile acid, thereby, reducing the amount of LDL (the bad cholesterol).

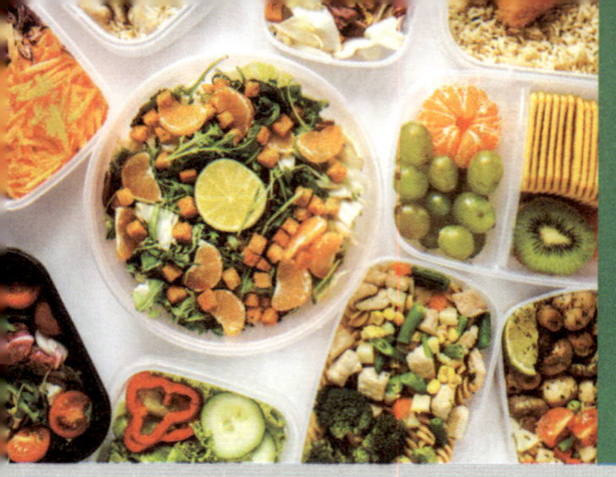

LONG AND SHORT ANSWER QUESTIONS

1. Define carbohydrates. Describe the classification of carbohydrates.
2. Describe calorific value, RDA, dietary sources and functions of carbohydrates.
3. **Differentiate between:**
   a. Simple sugars and complex carbohydrates
   b. Good carbohydrates and bad carbohydrates
4. **Write notes on:**
   a. Dietary fiber
   b. Starches
   c. Cellulose
   d Functions of carbohydrates

MULTIPLE CHOICE QUESTIONS

1. **Which of the following is considered a good carbohydrate?**
   a. White bread
   b. Whole grain bread
   c. Sugary cereal
   d. Cookies
2. **Which of the following is a characteristic of bad carbohydrates?**
   a. High in fiber
   b. Low glycemic index
   c. Quickly raise blood sugar levels
   d. Provide sustained energy
3. **Which of the following is a dietary source of carbohydrates?**
   a. Chicken breast
   b. Olive oil
   c. Sweet potatoes
   d. Salmon
4. **What is the primary function of carbohydrates in the body?**
   a. Building and repairing tissues
   b. Providing energy
   c. Aiding digestion
   d. Regulating hormone levels

ANSWER KEY

1. b	2. c	3. c	4. b

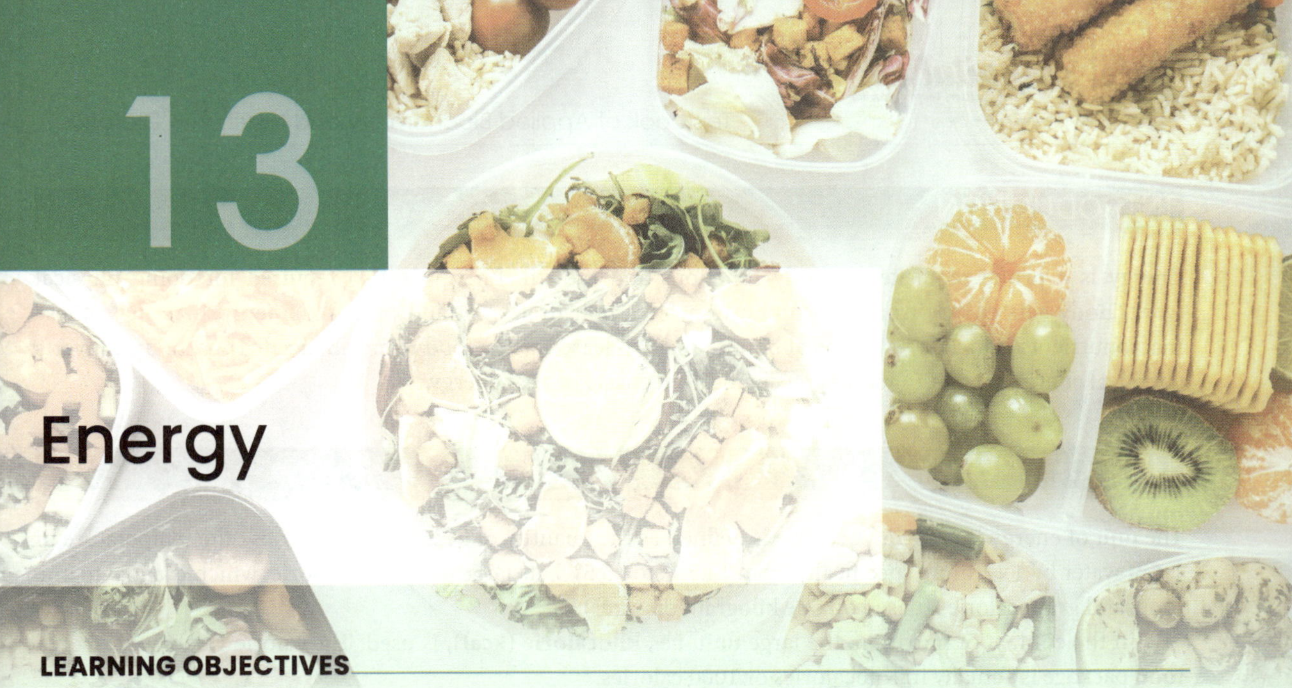

13

Energy

LEARNING OBJECTIVES

After the completion of the chapter, the readers will be able to:
- Explain unit of energy.
- Explain basal metabolic rate (BMR).
- Explain factors affecting BMR.
- Explain energy requirements for different categories of people.

CHAPTER OUTLINE

- Introduction
- Unit of Energy
- Significance of Dietary Energy
- Energy Requirements
- Dietary Sources of Energy
- Energy Requirements for Different Categories of People
- Measurement of Energy
- Body Mass Index
- Basal Metabolic Rate

KEY TERMS

Basal metabolic rate: The number of calories our body burns to perform basic (basal) life-sustaining functions.

Calorimetry: A process that quantifies the heat release from metabolism of cellular fuels. It provides assessment of caloric energy present in foods and allows for measurement of energy expenditure to determine adequate calorie requirement.

Dietary energy: Metabolizable energy which is the amount of energy available to the body from food after accounting for the obligatory energy losses, mostly in stool and urine.

Dietary fiber: Roughage or bulk that includes the parts of plant foods that body cannot digest or absorb.

Energy equilibrium: The state at which the number of calories eaten equals the number of calories used. Energy balance is affected by physical activity, body size, amount of body fat and muscle, and genetics.

INTRODUCTION

Energy is a prime requisite for body functions and growth. Energy is also required for doing physical work. Body gets energy from the combustion of carbohydrates, fat and proteins. Energy, present in these macronutrients is locked in chemical bonds, and is released when food is metabolized. Thus, body converts chemical energy present in food to mechanical, electrical or heat energy.

UNIT OF ENERGY

The unit of energy is **calorie**. A calorie is defined as the quantity of heat, required to raise the temperature of 1 g of water by 1°C, more specifically from 14.5°C to 15.5°C. Its large unit is kilocalorie, which is equal to one thousand gram calories (based on one kilogram of water).

In the context of nutrition, the large unit, i.e., **kilocalorie (kcal),** is used. The calorie value, we see on a **food** package is actually in Kilocalories or 1000 calories.

The SI unit of energy is **joule (J)**. One calorie is approximately 4.2 J.

SIGNIFICANCE OF DIETARY ENERGY

Dietary energy is **required for performing several functions** in the body. These include:
- **Maintenance of body temperature**
- **Growth**
- Performing **metabolic activities** such as digestion of food, absorption of the dietary nutrients, etc.
- Performing daily **physical activities**

ENERGY REQUIREMENTS

Energy requirements (needs) of an individual is defined as the **level of energy intake** in relation to **energy expenditure (output)**.
- **Energy intake:** Energy intake refers to the total **amount of energy** (calorie) **consumed** from the diet.
- **Energy output:** Energy output refers to the **amount of energy** (calorie) **used** (expenditure) by the body to meet its requirements.

Factors Affecting Energy Requirement

As discussed above, energy requirement is determined in terms of energy expenditure. Several factors affect energy requirements. These include:
- Age
- Sex
- Physiological state such as pregnancy or lactation
- Level and duration of physical activities.

Energy intake and energy output of normal healthy individuals are finely balanced.

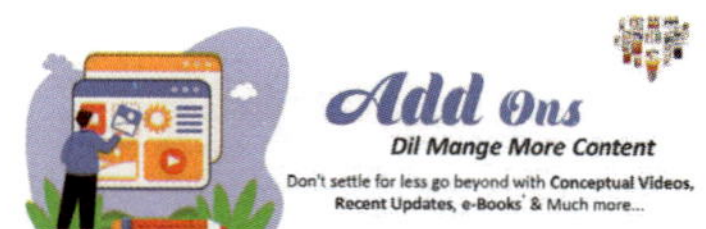

Energy Balance

The relationship between energy intake and energy expenditure is referred to as energy balance.

Energy balance refers to balance of energy intake and expenditure, i.e., when energy intake is equal to energy output. It results in no change in body weight over a period of time, and is referred to as **energy equilibrium (energy balance)**. Most adults maintain energy equilibrium.

- **Positive energy balance:** When energy intake is more than the body needs, it is referred to as positive energy balance. Positive energy balance leads to weight gain. Any surplus of energy intake than the requirement, is stored as fat, and continuous excess intake of energy leads to obesity.
- **Negative energy balance:** When energy intake is less than the expenditure, it is referred to as negative energy balance. If an adult fails to meet the requirement, he loses weight. When a child's intake of food falls below a standard reference, growth slows down.

Components of Energy Requirement

Total energy requirement for different categories of people, is made up of three components, which include:

1. **Basal energy expenditure:** The total amount of energy used, over the period of 24 hours, in the state of complete physical and mental rest, at comfortable environment (temperature and humidity), is referred to as **energy requirement during resting condition**. It is also referred to as **basal energy expenditure.** It is the amount of energy spent by the body for performing various activities, which are necessary to sustain normal body functions and homeostasis, such as respiration, blood circulation, synthesis of several substances for use in the body, pumping of ions across the membranes as well as maintenance of body temperature. It is expressed in terms of **basal metabolic rate (BMR)**.

2. **Requirement for physical activities:** It is the most variable component of energy expenditure. Energy expenditure for physical activities varies from 30% to 100% of the basal requirement. It depends upon the duration, type and intensity of physical activity, including the energy expenditure for occupational work. According to the type of occupational work, various individuals are classified into 3 categories as:
   i. Light workers (such as those doing office work)
   ii. Moderate workers (like a student)
   iii. Heavy workers (such as those performing manual physical labor, rickshaw pullers, etc.)
   Amounts of energy expenditure for different types of physical activities, as per National Institute of Nutrition, Indian Council of Medical Research (NIN–ICMR, 2011) are shown in Table 13.1.
   ICMR-NIN (2020), while defining the **energy expenditure using physical activity estimations**, have **suggested three terms** which include:
   i. **Physical Activity Ratio (PAR):** It is expressed as the **ratio of the energy cost of an individual activity per minute to the cost of BMR per minute**.
   ii. **Physical Activity Level (PAL):** PAR values **calculated** as above, **for the various activities performed in a day** can be aggregated to a 24-hour period to get the physical activity level. It is actually the **ratio of the energy expenditure in 24 hours and the value of BMR for 24 hours**.
   PAL value is proposed as 1.4, 1.8 and 2.3 for the sedentary, moderate and heavy work, respectively.
   iii. **Total Energy Expenditure (TEE):** TEE is **calculated based on the multiplication of basal metabolic rate (BMR) to the physical activity level** (PAL), i.e.:
   $$\text{TEE} = \text{BMR} \times \text{PAL}$$
   TEE values are particularly **given for infants**.

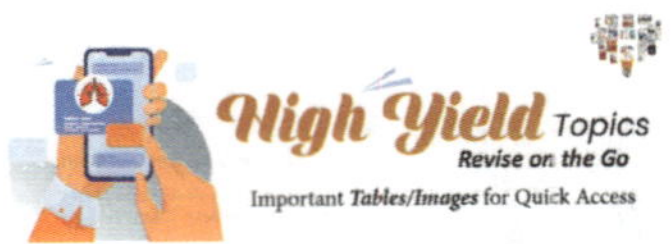

TABLE 13.1: Energy expenditure for different types of physical activities

Activity zones	Type of activities	Energy expenditure* (kcal/min)
1	Sleeping, resting or relaxing	1.0
2	Sitting (light activities); eating, reading, writing, listening or talking	1.5
3	Standing, standing (light activity); washing face, shaving, combing, or watering plants	2.3
4	Walking (slow), driving, dusting, bathing. dressing, marketing or childcare	2.8
5	Light manual work, sweeping, cleaning utensils, washing clothes or other house chores	3.3
6	Warm-up and recreational activities, walking up/down stairs, cycling or fetching water	4.8
7	Manual work (moderate pace), loading/unloading, walking with load, harvesting, carpentry or plumbing	5.6
8	Practice of noncompetitive sport/games, cycling (15 km/hr), gymnastics, swimming or digging	6.0
9	High intense manual work and sports activities—tournaments, wood cutting, carrying heavy loads, running or jogging	7.8

*NIN-ICMR (2011)

3. **Requirement on account of specific dynamic action of food:** It refers to energy expenditure associated with the consumption of food. Body spends some energy to digest, absorb and metabolize dietary nutrients. It depends upon the type and amount of various nutrients consumed. **Specific dynamic action (SDA)** is also referred to as **diet-induced thermogenesis or thermogenic effect of food.** SDA is more after the consumption of carbohydrates and proteins than fat. This is due to the reason that fat is metabolized more efficiently compared to proteins. On an average, for a mixed diet, SDA value constitutes about 10% of total energy expenditure.

DIETARY SOURCES OF ENERGY

As we know, main dietary sources of energy in our diet include **carbohydrates, fats and proteins**.

Recently ICMR-NIN (2020), in its report, has also emphasized the importance of **dietary fiber** and has suggested that dietary fibers, both soluble and insoluble, undergo fermentation in the large intestine and in turn produce short chain fatty acids. These fatty acids are used by the cells of the colon and the liver, as a source of energy. And thus, dietary fiber also provides **2 kcal/g**. Hence, the metabolizable energy available from the dietary components (macronutrients) should be accounted for as shown in Table 13.2.

TABLE 13.2: Amount of metabolizable energy available from different dietary components

Dietary component	Metabolizable energy available (kcal/g)*
Carbohydrates	4
Fats	9
Proteins	4
Dietary fiber	2

*ICMR-NIN (2020)

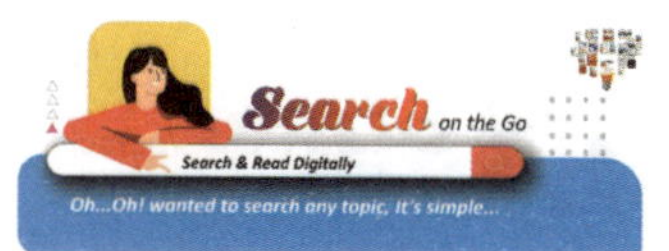

ENERGY REQUIREMENT FOR DIFFERENT CATEGORIES OF PEOPLE

As discussed above, several factors determine energy requirement such as basal metabolic rate, level and duration of physical activity, age and physiological state (pregnancy and lactation), and SDA (processes involved in the extraction of energy from food). Besides, it also depends upon the source of energy.

- Energy requirements have been laid down by various expert groups of the FAO/WHO and these standards are revised from time to time in light of the newer knowledge.
- For Indian people, ICMR-NIN (2020) Expert Group has assessed the energy requirement in terms of energy expenditure instead of energy intake.
- The Committee has recommended dietary intake of energy for a healthy, well-nourished and active population.
- The Committee has further suggested that while computing the requirement of energy, the source of energy should also be considered. In Indian diets, major sources of energy are, the plant-based foods which consist of carbohydrates, fats and proteins.
- Energy requirement for adults with sedentary activity has been lowered, due to the lowered BMR.
- Further, it is also suggested that **55–60% of dietary energy should be derived from carbohydrates, 20–30% from fats and 10–15% from proteins**.

Average daily energy requirement for people of different age groups and the type of work performed by them is shown in Table 13.3.

Children

Because of their rapid growth, young children require proportionately, more energy for each kilogram of body weight than adults.

Children **above the age of 13 years** need as much energy as adults. This is because they show a good deal of physical activity, almost equal to the work done by adults. This is also the age when puberty sets in, and there is a spurt in growth and increase in metabolic rate.

Adults

Energy requirement decreases with age because of fall in BMR and decrease in physical activity. ICMR-NIN (2020) has recommended that, on an average, **a moderate male worker requires 2710 kcal/day** while a **female** performing the same type of work **needs 2130 kcal/day**.

Pregnant and Lactating Women

Energy requirement for women is increased during pregnancy (+350 kcal/day) and lactation (+600 kcal/day during first 6 months, i.e., between 0 and 6 months, and +520 kcal/day during the next 6 months, i.e., between 7 and 12 months), over and above their normal requirement. This is to meet extra energy needs that are associated with the deposition of tissues and for secretion of milk, consistent with good health.

TABLE 13.3: Energy requirements for Indians*

Population/group	Category of worker/period	Body weight (kg)	Energy requirement** (kcal)
Adult men (18+)	Sedentary		2110
	Moderate	65	2710
	Heavy		3470
Adult women (18+)	Sedentary		1660
	Moderate	55	2130
	Heavy		2720
Pregnant women	2nd trimester	(+) 10	(+) 350
	3rd trimester		(+) 350
Lactating women	0–6 months		(+) 600
	7–12 months		(+) 520
Infants	0–6 months***	5.8	530
	7–12 months	8.5	680
Children	1–3 years	12.9	1110
	4–6 years	18.3	1360
	7–9 years	25.3	1700
Adolescents	Boys 10–12 years	34.9	2220
	Boys 13–15 years	50.5	2860
	Boys 16–18 years	64.4	3320
	Girls 10–12 years	36.4	2050
	Girls 13–15 years	49.6	2400
	Girls 16–18 years	55.7	2500

* ICMR-NIN (2020)
** Estimated average requirement
*** Adequate intake

MEASUREMENT OF ENERGY

Measurement of Energy Content of Food

As we know that all foods and drinks contain calories. Some foods such as lettuce contain few calories. Other foods like peanuts, contain a lot of calories. We can find out how many calories are present in a food by looking at the components of the food, i.e., how many grams of carbohydrates, proteins and fat the diet contains, as these are the major dietary sources of energy. On an average they supply energy at the following rates, i.e., carbohydrates and proteins, 4 kcal/g, and fat, 9 kcal/g.

To calculate the amount of energy available from food, quantity of carbohydrates, proteins and fat is multiplied 4, 4 and 9, respectively, and thereafter, the results are added up. For example, if one consumes a meal, such as a parantha with cheese or butter, that contains 40 g of carbohydrates, 10 g of proteins and 15 g of fat.

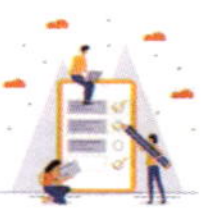
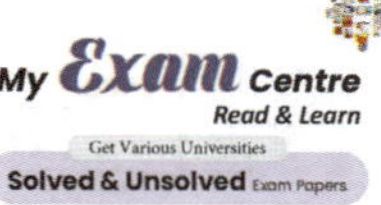

Total energy available from this meal will be:

$$= (\text{g of carbohydrates} \times 4) + (\text{g of proteins} \times 4) + (\text{g of fat} \times 9)$$
$$= 160 + 40 + 135 \text{ kcal}$$
$$= 335 \text{ kcal}$$

Measurement of Heat Given-Off

Measurement of the amount of heat given-off by an individual, i.e., the total energy expenditure is called **calorimetry**. The amount of energy expenditure, in relation to oxygen consumed, can be measured directly or indirectly.

Direct Calorimetry

Direct calorimetry measures the amount of heat production, by the body, which is proportional to the total energy use. For this purpose, the subject is put in a small insulated chamber that is surrounded by the circulating water. Thereafter, rise in temperature of the water is measured, which is directly related to energy consumed by the subject. Although, direct calorimetry provides a measure of energy expenditure in the form of heat, it does not provide any information on the kind of food consumed (fuel oxidized). Further, it is very cumbersome procedure, thus, it is not commonly used.

Indirect Calorimetry

Indirect calorimetry refers to the determination of energy expenditure, by the body without measuring heat production, indirectly. It is comparatively easier and less expensive than the direct calorimetry.

Indirect calorimetry estimates energy expenditure by determining the amount of oxygen consumed, in relation to the amount of carbon dioxide produced by an individual, over a given period of time. Data obtained from indirect calorimetry are used for the calculation by using **respiratory quotient**.

Respiratory Quotient

Respiratory quotient (RQ) refers to the moles of CO_2 expired in relation to the moles of O_2 consumed, i.e.,

$$\textbf{RQ} = \text{Moles of } CO_2 \text{ expired/moles of } O_2 \text{ consumed.}$$

The value, thereafter is converted into kcal (heat produced) per square meter of body surface area/hour, and is extrapolated to energy expenditure per 24 hours.

Value of RQ depends upon the type of food consumed:

- **RQ for carbohydrates** is 1. It is due to the reason that the number of moles of carbon dioxide produced from 1 gram of carbohydrate is equal to the number of moles of oxygen consumed.
- **RQ for protein** is 0.82.
- **RQ for fat** is 0.7.
- **RQ for the mixed diet** is 0.85.

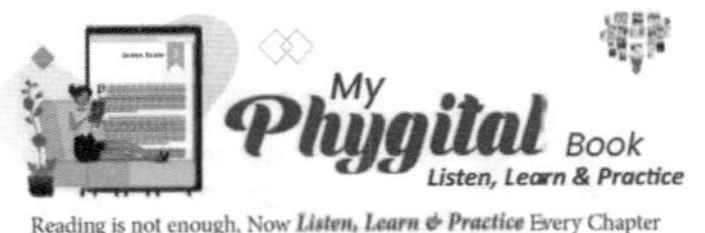

BODY MASS INDEX

Body mass index (BMI) is computed by dividing the weight in kilograms by the square of the height in meters (Chapter 20).

The ideal ranges of weights for a given height are provided by WHO, which is useful for categorizing persons as normal (ideal), undernourished and overweight (or obese).

- BMI ranging from **18.5 to 25** is considered to be **normal**
- A person with a BMI ≥**25** is considered **overweight**
- A person with a BMI of **30 or more** is, generally considered **obese**.

BASAL METABOLIC RATE

Basal metabolic rate **(BMR)** is the amount of energy expenditure at rest, in a neutrally temperate environment, in the post-absorptive state, by indirect calorimetry in the laboratory setting.

The amount of energy at complete physical and mental rest meets the requirement for the functioning of vital organs, i.e., the heart, lungs, kidneys, nervous system, intestine, liver, sex organs, muscles and skin, etc.

Determination of BMR

The BMR is measured, when a person is lying at complete rest but awaken, from a normal overnight sleep, 10–12 hours after the last meal, and performing no physical activity.

The BMR remains constant throughout the day under normal conditions and constitutes about 50–75% of the total energy expenditure by an individual. It is expressed in terms of kcal/hr.

Factors Affecting BMR

- **Body mass:** Lean body mass refers to the portion of the body, exclusive of the stored fat, i.e., the fat-free mass (metabolically active tissue). Muscles, various other organs, bones and body fluids, make up most of the lean body mass. An individual, with a large lean body mass has higher resting energy expenditure than the one with same weight but having higher proportion of body fat.
- **Age:** BMR is highest during the period of rapid growth, mainly within first two years of life. It is reduced thereafter, but again reaches a peak during puberty and adolescence. BMR is further reduced, by about 2–3% per decade, in adults. This is due to the reason that whereas lean body mass tends to decrease, fat content increases with age.
- **Sex:** Metabolic rate is higher in men (by about 50 kcal/day) than women. This is due to the reason that women have less active muscle mass, for each kg of body weight. Women generally have less lean body mass. Resting metabolic rate also varies during menstrual cycle. It fluctuates from the low point from about one week before ovulation to the high point, just before the onset of menstruation.
- **Other factors:** These factors, however, may be less consistent of shorter duration and limited to individual situations (Table 13.4).

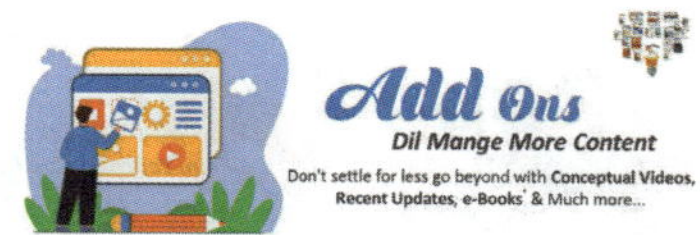

TABLE 13.4: Factors affecting BMR

Factors that increase BMR	Factors that decrease BMR
• Total body weight • Increased lean body mass • Large body surface area • Rapid growth • Hot and cold temperature • Stress • Hyperthyroidism • Caffeine • Pregnancy and lactation • Smoking • Fever	• Growing age • Female gender • Starvation • Hypothyroidism • Sleep

- BMR falls by about 10% during **sleep**.
- It rises during the period of rapid **growth,** such as in infancy and adolescence.
- **Hormones,** especially, thyroxin and norepinephrine, regulate BMR. Hypothyroidism slows BMR, while hyperthyroidism increases BMR.
- **Excitement and stress**, which cause release of epinephrine, increase cellular activity and, thus, BMR.
- **Pregnancy:** BMR is decreased in early stages of pregnancy, whereas later in pregnancy BMR is increased because of uterine, placental and fetal growth.
- Fever increases BMR by about 7%, for each degree increase in **body temperature** (above 98.4°F).
- **Environment temperature** also affects BMR. During exposure to cold, BMR increases. People living in tropical climate, usually, have higher BMR than those living in the temperate areas.
- During **starvation BMR** declines, as body slows basic functions to conserve energy.
- Some unknown **genetic factors** have also been attributed to the variations in BMR.

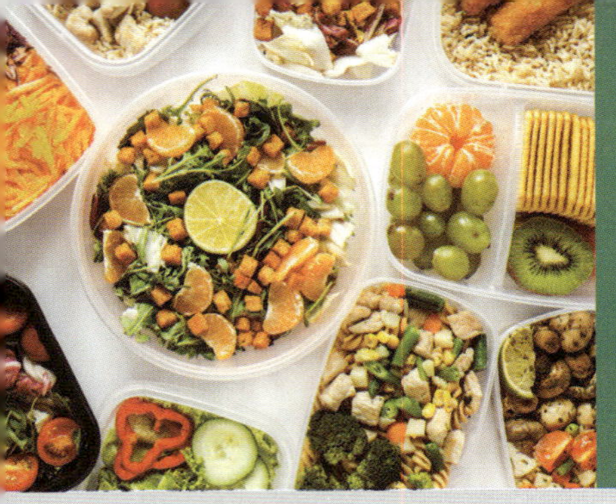

STUDENT ASSIGNMENT

LONG AND SHORT ANSWER QUESTIONS

1. Define energy. Describe the unit of energy.
2. Define basal metabolic rate (BMR). Describe various factors which affect BMR.
3. **Write notes on:**
   a. Energy
   b. Unit of energy
   c. Energy balance
   d. Energy requirement and its components
   e. Measurement of energy content of food
   f. Body mass index
   g. Basal metabolic rate

MULTIPLE CHOICE QUESTIONS

1. **What is BMR?**
   a. Basal metabolic rate
   b. Blood-based metabolic response
   c. Body mass ratio
   d. Bone mineral density

2. **Which of the following factors can increase BMR?**
   a. Aging
   b. Fasting or calorie restriction
   c. Low levels of thyroid hormone
   d. High levels of lean muscle mass

3. **Which of the following factors can decrease BMR?**
   a. Cold weather
   b. Overhydration
   c. Chronic stress
   d. Pregnancy

4. **Which of the following is not a factor that affects BMR?**
   a. Age
   b. Gender
   c. Height
   d. Blood type

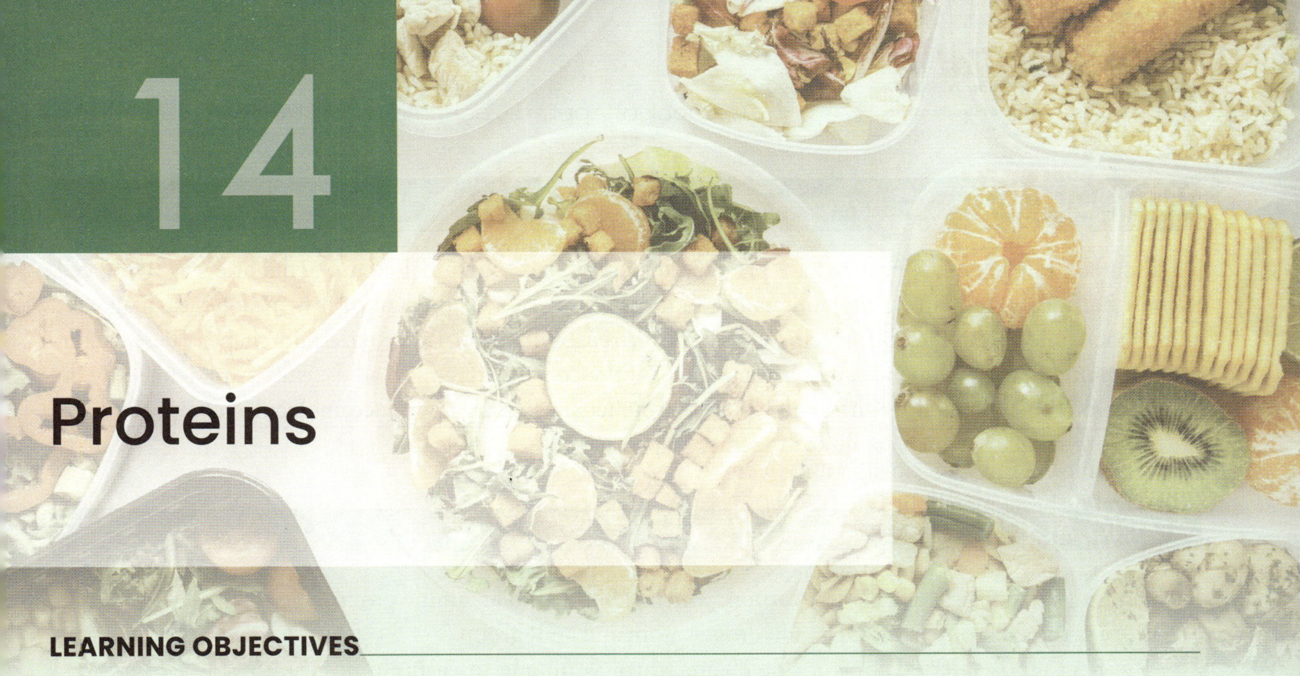

14

Proteins

LEARNING OBJECTIVES

After the completion of the chapter, the readers will be able to:
- Learn composition of proteins and essential amino acids.
- Describe functions, dietary sources and protein requirements-RDA.

CHAPTER OUTLINE

- Introduction
- Amino Acids
- Classification of Proteins
- Complementary Action of Proteins
- Functions of Proteins
- Dietary Sources of Proteins
- Protein Requirements

KEY TERMS

Essential amino acids: Amino acids which cannot be synthesized in the body and must be taken in diet are called essential amino acids, e.g., valine, leucine, phenylalanine, etc.

Nonessential amino acids: Amino acids which can be synthesized in the body are known as nonessential amino acids.

Semi-essential amino acids: Growth-promoting amino acids such as arginine and histidine. These are not essential for a normal adult but are essential for growing children, pregnant women, and lactating women.

INTRODUCTION

As discussed in Chapter 4, proteins are primary structural and functional components of every living cell. Almost half of the protein in our body is in the form of muscle and the rest of it is in bone, cartilage and skin. Biochemical activities of proteins are characterized by their structure, size and shape. These factors are determined by the sequence and characteristics of the constituent amino acids, which are defined by the sequence of gene encoded by the genetic code. Proteins are the organic macromolecules composed of 20 different amino acids, which are linked together by peptide bonds.

AMINO ACIDS

Each amino acid consists of a central carbon, which is bonded to an amine group ($-NH_2$), a carboxyl group ($-COOH$), a hydrogen atom and an R group.

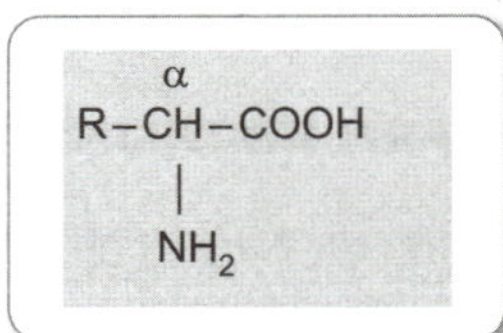

The R group is referred to as a side chain, which is unique to each amino acid. The side chain may vary from a hydrogen atom (H) to some complex group (Fig. 14.1).

Fig. 14.1 An amino acid

Classification of Amino Acids

There are 20 different amino acids, commonly, found in all proteins. From the nutritional point of view, amino acids are classified into three groups, referred to as essential or indispensable amino acids, semi-essential or conditionally indispensable amino acids and nonessential or dispensable amino acids (Table 14.1).

TABLE 14.1: Classification of amino acids according to dietary requirements

Essential	Semi-essential	Nonessential
• Methionine	• Arginine	• Glycine
• Threonine	• Histidine	• Alanine
• Tryptophan		• Serine
• Valine		• Cysteine
• Isoleucine		• Tyrosine
• Leucine		• Aspartate
• Phenylalanine		• Glutamate
• Lysine		• Asparagine
		• Glutamine
		• Proline

- **Essential amino acids:** Certain amino acids, which are termed **essential**, have to be obtained from proteins in the diet, since they are not synthesized in the human body. Adult human body can maintain nitrogen equilibrium on a mixture of eight (pure) amino acids, as its sole source of nitrogen. Thus, these are defined as essential or indispensable amino acids. These include **leucine, isoleucine, lysine, methionine, phenylalanine, threonine, tryptophan** and **valine.**
- **Semi-essential amino acids:** Semi-essential (conditionally indispensable) amino acids are the amino acids that can be synthesized by an adult under normal healthy condition. However, under other

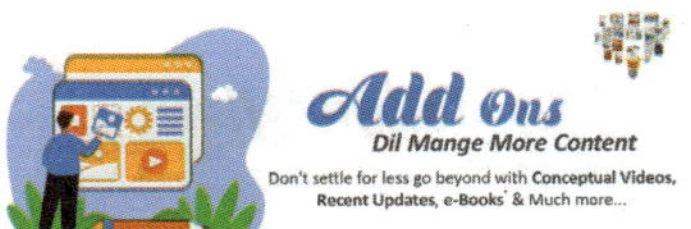

circumstances, when either they cannot be synthesized or are synthesized in insufficient amounts, due to their increased demand, they become dietary essential, e.g.:

- **In infants and children—Arginine and histidine** are considered to be essential (indispensable) amino acids, since infants and children cannot synthesize them.
- **In premature infants, tyrosine**, and in preterm and term infants, **cysteine** are considered to be dietary essentials.
- **In certain disease states:** There are certain disease states during adult life, when the demand of a particular amino acid is increased by the body, and thus, it becomes dietary essential, e.g.:
    - **In a liver disease** cysteine requirement cannot be met by the body, due to diminished trans-sulfuration capacity of the liver. Thus, cysteine becomes dietary (conditionally) essential.
    - **In chronic renal failure** concentration of tyrosine, and its ratio to phenylalanine, becomes consistently low, owing to reduced synthesis of tyrosine from phenylalanine. Thus, under these circumstances, tyrosine becomes dietary essential.
    - **During episodes of infections**, inflammation, other types of catabolic states or malnutrition, glutamine is considered to be conditionally essential.
    - **During catabolic stress and uremia** taurine is postulated as an indispensable substrate and potent antioxidant.
- **Nonessential amino acids:** All the other remaining amino acids are referred to as **nonessential amino acids,** since they can be synthesized in the body to build proteins.

CLASSIFICATION OF PROTEINS

Proteins may be classified either based on the source or the nutritional value.

Classification of Proteins Based on their Source

Proteins are, generally, obtained from either animal sources or plant sources. They are also of different types with respect to structure and functions.

- **Animal proteins:** Animal proteins may be grouped as fibrous proteins or globular proteins:
    - **Fibrous proteins:** These are found in the protective and supportive tissues, e.g., **keratin** (chief protein of hair), **collagen** (of connective tissue), **fibrin** (of blood clot), and **myosin** (of muscle).
    - **Globular proteins:** These are found in tissue fluids, e.g., **casein** (in milk), and **albumin** and **globulins** (in milk, blood and egg white).
- **Plant proteins:** Plant proteins may be grouped as glutelins and prolamins:
    - **Glutelins:** These include glutenin from wheat, hordenine from barley, oryzenin from rice, etc.
    - **Prolamins:** These include gliadin from wheat and zein from maize.

Classification of Proteins Based on their Nutritional Quality

Nutritional quality of a protein is defined with respect to its amino acids content. Accordingly, proteins may be divided into two groups, as high quality proteins and poor quality proteins:

1. **High quality proteins:** A high quality protein is the one that provides all the essential amino acids. These are referred to as **complete proteins** or the **proteins with high biological value**. Generally, animal proteins are of high quality, as they provide all the essential amino acids in right proportions, e.g., from meat, fish, eggs, milk and cheese.
2. **Poor quality proteins:** An incomplete protein is the one that is low in one or more essential amino acids. Plant or vegetable proteins are not of the same quality, because of their lower contents of some of the essential amino acids. Thus, proteins form plant based foods, e.g., whole grains, rice, corn, beans, legumes, oatmeal and peas, etc., are called **incomplete proteins** or **proteins with poor biological value**.

In the past, this difference has led to the concept of **first-class** and **second-class proteins**, for proteins from animal foods and plant foods, respectively.

COMPLEMENTARY ACTION OF PROTEINS

Complementary action of proteins refers to the pattern of amino acids, from the combination of proteins from two different plant sources. As a result of it, the limiting amino acid from one source is compensated from the other, when the foods from two different sources are taken together, such as cereals (e.g., chapati or rice) and pulses (e.g., lentils or beans). The two protein sources together make a high biological value protein. Thus, if vegetarians (and vegans) eat a variety of vegetable proteins in combination, there is no reason why the quality of protein cannot be as good as in a diet comprising of meat, milk, fish, eggs, soybeans or other foods that contain high quality protein.

In Indian subcontinent, where protein intake is low, complementary action of proteins plays an important role in helping individuals to meet their amino acids requirements.

FUNCTIONS OF PROTEINS

Proteins perform a variety of functions, within organisms, including metabolic reactions, DNA replication, respond to stimuli and transport of molecules from one location to another.

- Proteins are fundamental **structural and functional elements** within every cell of the body and are involved in a wide range of metabolic interactions.
- All cells and tissues contain proteins, which are **essential for growth** and **repair of tissues,** and **maintenance of good health**.
- Proteins also provide the body, approximately, 10–15% of its dietary energy and it is the second most abundant compound in the body, following water.

Caloric Value of Proteins

Caloric value of proteins is similar to carbohydrates but nearly half of the fat. Accordingly, each gram of protein provides 4 kcal.

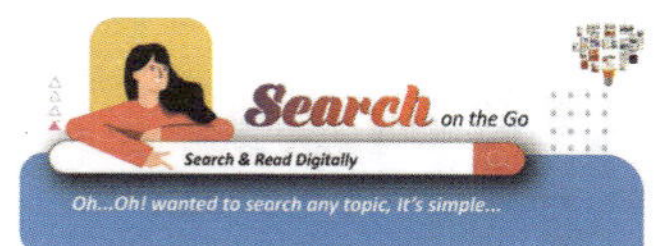

DIETARY SOURCES OF PROTEINS

Animal foods, like milk, meat, fish and eggs, and **plant foods**, such as pulses and legumes, are rich sources of proteins (Fig. 14.2).

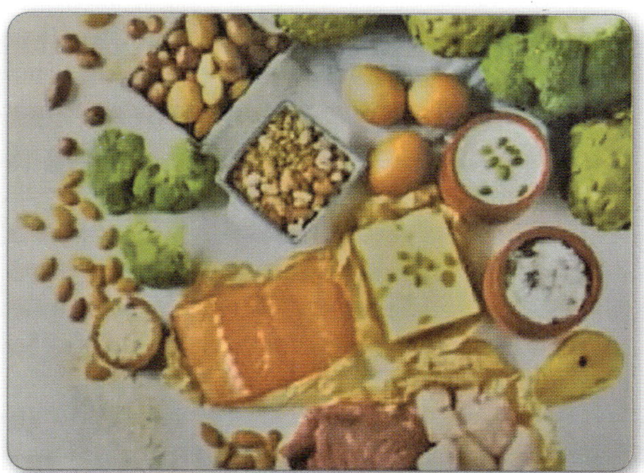

Fig. 14.2: Dietary sources of proteins

PROTEIN REQUIREMENTS

Recommended daily allowances (RDA) of proteins vary with age, physiological status and stress. More proteins are required by growing infants and children, pregnant women and by the individuals during infections, illness or stress. RDAs for protein for different category of persons, as per NIN–ICMR (2020), are shown in Table 14.2.

- **For healthy adults:** RDA for proteins, for adults has been suggested to be 54 g/day for men and 46 g/day for women. This pre-supposes the use of first class protein (high in essential amino acids) with adequate energy supply.
- **For infants and children:** The estimates of daily protein requirements for infants have been defined as 8 g/day **during the first 6 months of life,** and 10.5 g/day **for next 6 months. After the first year of life**, the requirements are believed to fall, progressively, to the adult level.
- **During pregnancy:** On an average, the pregnant woman should receive an additional 9.5 g of protein during the second trimester and 22 g during the third trimester of pregnancy.
- **During lactation:** During lactation, additional 16.9 g of protein has been recommended during the first 6 months and 13.2 g during 7–12 months.
- **In disease conditions:** In some diseases, protein intake must be controlled, e.g., **acute liver failure** (when the intake has to be restricted in order to avoid hepatic coma) and in **uremia** (where the capacity to excrete nitrogenous end products is limited).

TABLE 14.2: Recommended daily allowances of protein for Indians*

Population/group	Category of worker/age	RDA (g)
Adult men (18+)	Sedentary	
	Moderate	54
	Heavy	
Adult women (18+)	Sedentary	
	Moderate	46
	Heavy	
Pregnant women	2nd trimester	(+) 9.5
	3rd trimester	(+) 22
Lactating women	0–6 months	(+) 16.9
	7–12 months	(+) 13.2
Infants	0–6 months**	8
	7–12 months	10.5
Children	1–3 years	12.5
	4–6 years	16
	7–9 years	23
Adolescents	Boys 10–12 years	32
	Boys 13–15 years	45
	Boys 16–18 years	55
	Girls 10–12 years	33
	Girls 13–15 years	43
	Girls 16–18 years	46

* ICMR-NIN (2020)
** Adequate intake

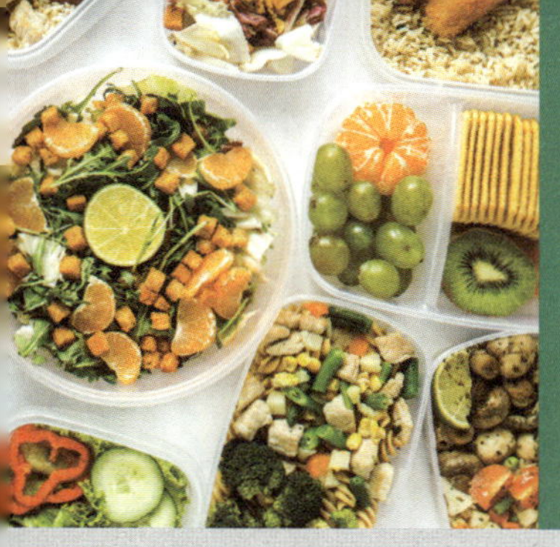

STUDENT ASSIGNMENT

LONG AND SHORT ANSWER QUESTIONS

1. Define proteins. Describe composition of proteins.
2. What are amino acids? Classify amino acids.
3. Describe functions, caloric value, RDAs and dietary sources of proteins.
4. Describe RDAs of proteins for different age groups.
5. **Differentiate between:**
   a. Essential and nonessential amino acids
   b. High and low biological value proteins
   c. Plant proteins and animal proteins
6. **Write notes on:**
   a. Essential amino acids
   b. Classification of proteins based on their nutrition quality
   c. Complimentary action of proteins

MULTIPLE CHOICE QUESTIONS

1. **What is the primary function of proteins in the body?**
   a. Providing energy
   b. Regulating hormones
   c. Building and repairing tissues
   d. Aiding in digestion

2. **What is the caloric value of proteins?**
   a. 4 Calories per gram
   b. 7 Calories per gram
   c. 9 Calories per gram
   d. 12 Calories per gram

3. **What does RDA stand for in the context of protein intake?**
   a. Recommended daily allowance
   b. Recommended dietary assessment
   c. Required dietary amount
   d. Recommended digestive allocation

4. **Which of the following is a dietary source of protein?**
   a. Broccoli
   b. Olive oil
   c. Chicken breast
   d. White rice

ANSWER KEY

1. c   **2.** a   **3.** c   **4.** c

Notes

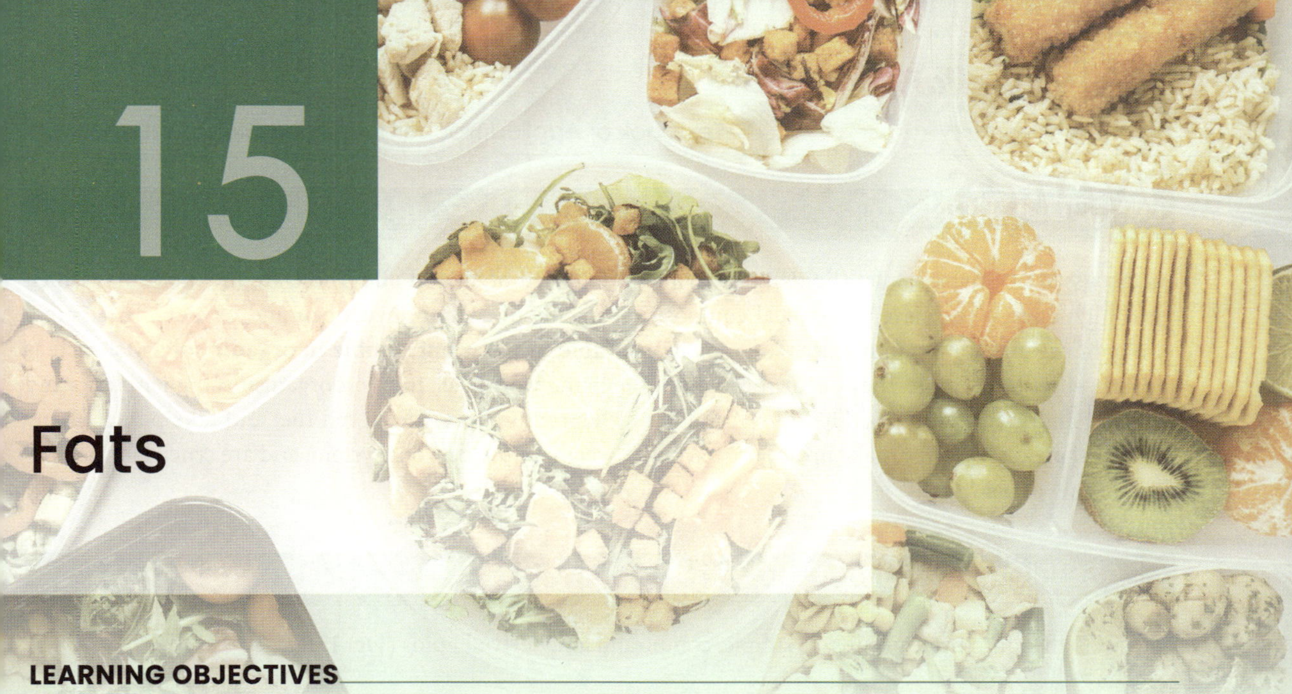

15

Fats

LEARNING OBJECTIVES

After the completion of the chapter, the readers will be able to:
- Explain saturated and unsaturated fats.
- Describe calorie value, functions and dietary sources of fat and fatty acids.
- Describe fat requirements-RDA.

CHAPTER OUTLINE

- Introduction
- Classification of Fat
- Dietary Fat

KEY TERMS

Compound lipids: Esters of fatty acids with alcohol (mostly glycerol) along with a few additional groups such as phosphorus, sugars, proteins, etc.

Derived lipids: When both simple and compound lipids combine and undergo the process of hydrolysis, the produced chemical is known as the derived lipids.

Neutral fat: The esters of three molecules of fatty acids and one molecule of trihydric alcohol glycerol. Hence, they are also called triglycerides.

Thrombogenicity: Tendency of a material to generate blood clotting and/or thrombus, when in contact with the blood.

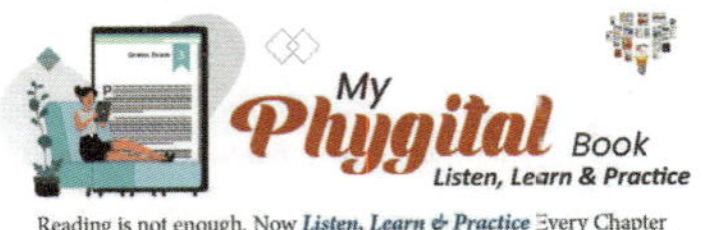

INTRODUCTION

As discussed in Chapter 3, fat (lipids), primarily is composed of fat and oils. These are the molecules which yield high energy and have a chemical composition mainly of **carbon**, **hydrogen** and **oxygen**. These are a family of organic compounds which are mostly **insoluble in water** but **soluble in organic solvents**, such as alcohol, ether or acetone. They occur throughout the living world, i.e., in microorganisms, higher plants and animals, and in all cell types. Lipids contribute to cell structure, provide stored fuel and take part in many biological processes. They make up about 70% of dry weight of the nervous system, and are crucial for healthy functioning of nerve cells.

CLASSIFICATION OF FAT

Fat is classified into three groups, as simple, compound and derived lipids (Fig. 15.1).

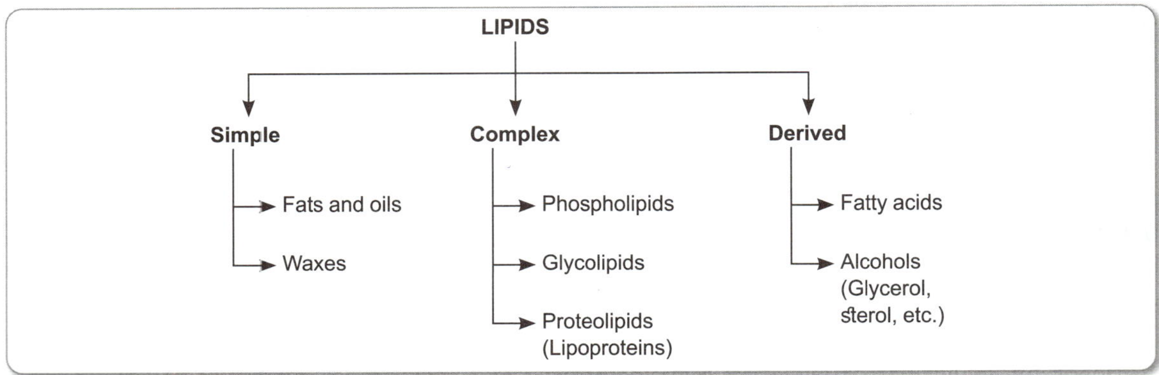

Fig. 15.1: Classification of lipids

- **Simple lipids:** Simple lipids are the esters of fatty acids with alcohol. These include **neutral fat** (**triacylglycerols** or **triglycerides**), and oils and waxes.
    - **Neutral fat:** Neutral fat is also referred to as **triacylglycerols** or **triglycerides**. These are the **esters of fatty acids with glycerol**, a trihydroxyalcohol.
        - The presence of a specific fatty acid influences its characteristics, such as melting point and digestibility.
        - A triacylglycerol has three fatty acids attached to glycerol. Three fatty acids attached to glycerol may be similar or different.
        - They make more than 95% of the total lipids in our diet.
        - Triacylglycerols are commonly found in vegetable oils, butter, whole milk, cheese, cream, fried foods and some meats.
        - Naturally occurring triacylglycerols are also found in foods such as avocados, olives, corn and nuts. A **fat** differs from oil in the way that fat is solid whereas oil is liquid at room temperature.
    - **Waxes:** Waxes are the esters of fatty acids with high molecular weight monohydroxyalcohols, e.g., beewax, carnauba wax, etc.
- **Compound lipids:** Compound lipids are the esters of fatty acids with alcohol and some additional groups, e.g., **phospholipids**, proteolipids (**lipoproteins**), etc.

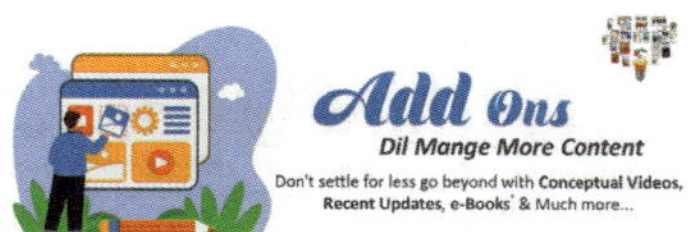

- **Phospholipids:** Phospholipids, also called **phosphatides**, are **lipids conjugated with phosphoric acid**.
    - Phospholipids contain two fatty acids, glycerol, phosphoric acid and a nitrogenous base, or some other substituent, e.g., phosphoglycerides, phosphoinositides and phosphosphingosides.
    - They possess a hydrophilic head and non-polar tails. Hence, these are called **polar lipids** and are **amphipathic** in nature. They are water soluble and are found both, in plants and animals.
    - Phospholipids make up about 2% of the dietary lipids.
    - They are crucial in the body to form cell and organelle membranes, the structures in which fat is enclosed and transported throughout the bloodstream.
- **Lipoproteins:** As **fat** (fatty acids, triglycerides, cholesterol, etc.) is not soluble in water, it is transported in blood (the aqueous environment), **in combination with proteins**, in the form of coated-capsules, called **lipoproteins**. These include chylomicrons, **very low density lipoproteins (VLDL)**, **low density lipoproteins (LDL)** and **high density lipoproteins (HDL)**.
    - **Chylomicrons transport exogenous fat** (dietary lipids) from the intestine.
    - **VLDL transports endogenous fat** which is synthesized in the liver.
    - **LDL transports cholesterol from liver to various tissues**. **High blood level of LDL-cholesterol** (referred to as **bad cholesterol**) results in the **accumulation of lipids in the aorta** and may **cause atherosclerosis**.
    - **HDL transports excess of the cholesterol from the tissues to the liver for its utilization**. So, **HDL-cholesterol** (also called **good cholesterol**) **prevents atherosclerosis**.
- **Derived lipids:** Derived lipids are the substances derived from simple and compound lipids, by hydrolysis. These include, mainly, **cholesterol** and **fatty acids** (fat).
- **Cholesterol:** Cholesterol is a derivative of **cyclopentanoperhydrophenanthrene ring**, also called **steroid nucleus.** Cholesterol is a most abundant steroid found in animals. It has **27 carbons**, a **hydroxyl group**, a **double bond**, **two methyl groups** and a **side chain**. Because of the presence of the OH group, cholesterol is called a steroid alcohol (sterol). Due to the presence of this group cholesterol can form an ester with a long-chain fatty acid and form cholesterol esters.
    - Cholesterol is **synthesized in various tissues** in the body. Nearly 0.3 g of **cholesterol is also absorbed** from the diet, daily. Ingested cholesterol is absorbed with other lipids and is incorporated into chylomicrons and VLDL. More than 80% of it is esterified in the intestinal mucosa and is transported with lipoproteins. About 50% of the normal intake of dietary cholesterol is absorbed by the small intestine while the rest of it is excreted in the feces.
    - Egg, meat, and milk are the important dietary sources of cholesterol. It is also synthesized in the body by nearly all cells. The amount of cholesterol synthesized each day, in man is at least three times to that what is ingested in the diet.
    - An adult man contains about 1 g of cholesterol/kg body weight. Nearly 25% of it is present in membrane of the nervous system, as a major **component of myelin sheath**. It is also a major **component of plasma membrane**. **Cholesterol** is also a metabolic **precursor** of various substances, such as **steroid hormones** (glucocorticoids and mineralocorticoids), **vitamin D**, and **bile acids and salts**.
- **Fatty acids:** Fatty acids are the **building blocks of fat**. They constitute more than 90% of dietary fat.
    - A fatty acid is made up of a chain of carbon atoms, with a methyl group ($-CH_3$) at one end and an acid group ($-COOH$) at the other end.

- All types of fats are built of carbons and hydrogen, and have a similar chemical structure, i.e., a fatty acid has a chain of carbon atoms bonded to hydrogen atoms. However, what makes one fat different from another is the length and shape of the carbon chain, and the number of hydrogen atoms connected to the carbon atoms.
- Seemingly slight differences in structure translate into crucial differences in its form and functions.

DIETARY FAT

Dietary fat is important for making healthy cells. It produces hormones and other signaling molecules and is a source of energy and energy storage. Fat is not just a nutrient essential to our body, it is also a key player in healthy cooking. It carries heat and helps cook foods quickly and evenly. It also coats our taste buds, making flavor linger longer.

- Dietary fat is a major source of energy for our body.
- It also helps absorb some vitamins and essential fatty acids.
- Dietary fat is also needed to build cell membranes and sheaths surrounding nerves.
- It is also essential for blood clotting, muscle movement and inflammation.
- For long-term health, some fats are better than others.

Types of Dietary Fat

There are, mainly, two types of dietary fat, referred to as **saturated fat** and **unsaturated fat**.

Besides these two, however, there is also another type of fat, which is referred to as trans-fat. Though all these have the same amount of calories but different effects on our health. Trans-fat is most harmful for our health.

We need to aim for a good balance between the different dietary fats to optimize our health and reduce health risks (Table 15.1).

TABLE 15.1: Types of fat and their impact on our health

Type of fat	Food types	Impact on our health
Saturated fat	Generally solid at room temperature. Animal sources such as meat and dairy (butter, cheese, cream, etc.), and some vegetable oils including coconut oil and palm oil.	Less healthy. Diets high in saturated fats have been linked to raised levels of LDL, which is a risk factor for heart disease. Saturated fat should be consumed in smaller amounts only (about 7–10% of total fat intake).
Unsaturated fat	Vegetable oils like olive oil, sunflower oil and rapeseed/canola oil, and nuts and avocados.	Improves insulin sensitivity, and lowers LDL and triacylglycerol levels, thus, reduces the risk of heart disease.
Trans fat	Trans fat is found in the processed foods. It is widely used by fast food outlets.	Trans fats increase bad cholesterol, reduce good cholesterol and, thus, are bad for our health.

Saturated Fat

Fats that are **tightly packed with no double bonds** between the fatty acids are called saturated fats. Because those carbon chains are so full with hydrogen atoms, the chains are stiffer, i.e., less flexible. This is the reason

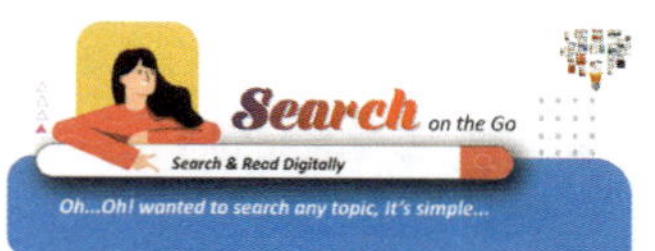

that saturated fats are **solid at room temperature**. They have a negative impact on our health. They are the naturally occurring **bad fats** and are found in butter, hard cheeses, fatty meat and meat products, cream, lard, suet and some plant oils including coconut oil and palm oil.

- Saturated fats fall somewhere in the middle, i.e., **in between the trans fats (bad fat) and the unsaturated fat (good fat)**.
- Most nutrition experts recommend **limiting saturated fat to fewer than 10% of calories** a day.
- **High intake** of saturated fatty acids is known to **increase serum total cholesterol** and **LDL-cholesterol** levels, **reduce insulin sensitivity**, **enhances thrombogenicity**, which will **raise the risk for heart disease** and **type 2 diabetes**.
- Common sources of saturated fat include red meat, whole milk and whole-milk dairy foods such as cheese, coconut oil and many commercially prepared baked goods and other foods.

Unsaturated Fat

Structurally, unsaturated fats differ from saturated fats by having fewer hydrogen atoms bonded to their carbon chains, i.e., their fats are loosely packed. They tend to be liquid at room temperature. These will have a positive impact on our health and are said to be good fats. Foods that are rich in unsaturated fats include oils that are liquid at room temperature, i.e., vegetable, nut and seed oils, oily fish such as salmon, tuna, trout, etc.

Within the category of unsaturated fats, there are two main subcategories, which include **monounsaturated fats (MUFA)** and **polyunsaturated fats (PUFA)**. Both MUFA and PUFA have heart-health benefits, though PUFA has a slight edge over MUFA.

1. **Monounsaturated fats:** Monounsaturated fats (MUFA) have a single carbon-to-carbon double bond. The result is that it has two fewer hydrogen atoms than a saturated fat and a bend at the double bond. They are, usually, liquid at room temperature.

   Good sources of monounsaturated fats are olive oil, peanut oil, canola oil, avocados and most nuts, as well as high-oleic acid containing safflower oil and sunflower oil.

2. **Polyunsaturated fats:** Polyunsaturated fats (PUFA) have more than one double bond in the molecule and are liquid at room temperature. PUFA are **essential fats** and are required for normal body functions. Since our body cannot make them, so we must get them from food.

   PUFA are present only in plant foods. Soybean oil, corn oil and safflower oil, and walnuts and sunflower seeds are good sources of PUFA. Fatty acids obtained from plant seeds usually contain **two or more double bonds**, which, generally, occur after every three carbon atoms. Three PUFA, i.e., linoleic acid, linolenic acid, and arachidonic acid, form **essential** component of the diet since they are necessary for **growth** as well as **normal health**. Hence, they are also called essential fatty acids.

Nomenclature of an Unsaturated Fatty Acid

Nomenclature of an unsaturated fatty acid may be given in two ways, i.e., either according to the **delta (δ) system** or the **omega (ω) system**.

- **Delta system of nomenclature:** According to the delta (δ) system of nomenclature, carbon atoms in a fatty acid are numbered beginning with the carboxyl carbon (–COOH) as carbon number 1. The next carbon, to which the carboxyl group is attached, is designated as carbon number 2. This is also called α-carbon atom. Accordingly, carbon 3 is referred to as the β carbon, and so on.
- **Omega system of nomenclature:** According to the omega (ω) system of nomenclature, carbon atoms are numbered beginning with the methyl terminal (CH_3–) end, where a double bond first appears. This carbon atom, i.e., the carbon atom of the terminal CH_3 group is called omega (ω) carbon.

Recently, replacement of the symbol ω by the letter "n" has also been recommended.

Most important of the polyunsaturated fatty acids are ω-3 and ω-6 fatty acids.

- **ω-3 fatty acids:** α-Linolenic acid (ALA) is referred to as omega-3 fatty acid (ω-3 fatty acid). It is beneficial to our body. The body cannot synthesize ω-3 fatty acids and we have to get them from food. Soybean oil, rapeseed oil and mustard oil contribute significant amount of α-linolenic acid. Legumes/pulses, mustard and fenugreek seeds, and green-leafy vegetables are also good sources of α-linolenic acid. **ω-3 fatty acids** help prevent heart disease and stroke.

  Fish and fish oils provide long chain η-3 fatty acids, which are biologically more active than the α-linolenic acid, which is present in plant foods. It helps to reduce inflammation (redness, swelling and irritation), which, in turn, helps in the prevention of a wide range of diseases, including arthritis and heart disease. If this type of fat is missing from our diet, we might experience fatigue, poor memory, dry skin, depression, heart problems and poor blood circulation.

- **ω-6 fatty acid:** Linoleic acid is referred to as ω-6 fatty acid, since the first double bond from the ω-end is present after the sixth carbon atom. Elongation and desaturation of linoleic acid can form arachidonic acid, which acts as a precursor for a series of 20-carbon compounds called eicosanoids (Fig. 15.2).

  Omega-6 fatty acids have also been linked to protection against heart disease. Foods rich in linoleic acid and other omega-6 fatty acids include vegetable oils such as safflower, soybean, sunflower, walnut and corn oils.

$$\overset{1}{C}H_3 - (CH_2)_7 - \overset{9}{C}H = CH - (CH_2)_7 - COOH$$

Oleic acid
(ω-9 fatty acid, a nonessential fatty acid)

$$\overset{1}{C}H_3 - (CH_2)_4 - \overset{6}{C}H = CH - CH_2 - CH = CH - (CH_2)_7 - COOH$$

Linoleic acid
(ω-6 fatty acid, an essential fatty acid)

$$\overset{1}{C}H_3 - \overset{2}{C}H_2 - \overset{3}{C}H = CH - CH_2 - CH = CH - CH_2 - CH = CH - (CH_2)_7 - COOH$$

α-Linolenic acid
(ω-3 fatty acid, an essential fatty acid)

Fig. 15.2: Nonessential and essential fatty acids

Essential Fatty Acids

Linoleic acid (ω-6 fatty acid) and **linolenic acid** (ω-3 fatty acid) are referred to as **essential fatty acids.** They help to control inflammation, blood clotting and brain development.

Significance of Essential Fatty Acids

- Essential fatty acids (EFA) are the **components of cell membranes**. While n-6 PUFA are predominant in all cells, the nerve tissue has high levels of long chain n-3 PUFA.
- An appropriate balance of the two PUFA, namely, linoleic acid and α-linolenic acid in the diet are **essential for the functioning of vascular, immune, nervous and renal systems, and for early brain development.**

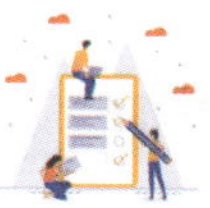
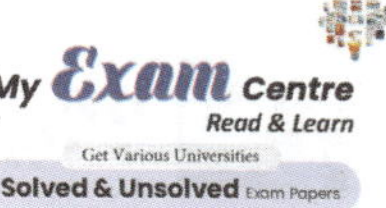

- They are also used for **esterification of cholesterol** and thus, help in its transport and metabolism. Particularly, consumption of the fat containing ω-**6 fatty acids** helps in **lowering plasma cholesterol**.
- Diets rich in ω-**3 fatty acids** promote **reduction in plasma triacylglycerols.**
- **Arachidonic acid** also acts as a **precursor of eicosanoids**, such as **prostaglandins**, **thromboxanes**, and **leukotrienes**.

Trans Fat

Besides the saturated and unsaturated fats, there is also a third type of dietary fat, which is referred to trans fat. Trans fats are a form of unsaturated fat that rarely exists in natural food but are associated with partially hydrogenated vegetable oils. Trans fat is said to be bad fat, since it is **more hazardous than even the dietary cholesterol.** Trans fats, as cooking oils, have been banned in some regions because of their impact on cardiovascular health. They are **found in commercially fried** and **processed foods** (Fig. 15.3).

Trans fat is **formed from the chemical process called hydrogenation.** Hydrogenation is used to turn healthy oils into solids and to prevent them from becoming rancid.

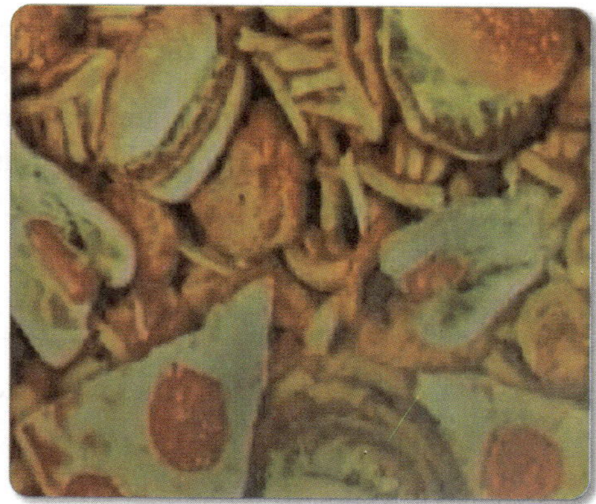

Fig. 15.3: Source of trans fats

- Trans fat is said to be bad fat, since it has no nutritional value and is harmful to our health. Our **body is unable to metabolize trans fat**, causing it to accumulate.
- Eating **foods rich in trans fat increases the amount of bad cholesterol** (LDL-cholesterol) in the blood and **reduces the amount of good cholesterol** (HDL-cholesterol).
- Trans fats create inflammation, which is linked to heart disease, stroke, diabetes and other chronic conditions.
- It also contributes to insulin resistance, which increases the risk of developing type-2 diabetes.
- Even small amounts of trans fats can harm health to the extent that for every 2% of the calories from trans fat consumed daily, the risk of heart disease increases by 23%.
- WHO recommends that trans fat **should not be consumed**. Alternatively, the intake of trans fat should not exceed 1% of total energy intake from fat.
- Trans fat is often found in fried foods, processed snacks and baked goods.

Cholesterol

As discussed above, cholesterol is a type of fat that is needed by the body to form cell membrane. Besides, **cholesterol** also serves as a **precursor** of **steroid hormones, vitamin D,** and **bile acids and salts.** Cholesterol can be synthesized by the body as well as consumed through diet. Cholesterol is **synthesized in various tissues** in the body. Whereas, nearly 0.3 g of **cholesterol is absorbed** from the diet, almost three times of it (about 1.0 g) is synthesized in the body, daily.

Cholesterol is a most abundant in animal products. Important dietary sources include eggs, meat and milk. It is transported from blood to various tissues in the form of lipoproteins. It is mainly present in low density lipoproteins (LDL) and high density lipoproteins (HDL). LDL-cholesterol is referred to as bad cholesterol since it is deposited in the arteries. On the other hand, HDL-cholesterol is referred to as good cholesterol due to the reason that HDL removes cholesterol from tissues to the liver for its utilization and removal.

Triacylglycerols

Triacylglycerols or triglycerides, also referred to as neutral fat, are the **esters of fatty acids with glycerol** (a trihydroxyalcohol). A triacylglycerol may have three similar or different fatty acids. Triglycerides make up more than 95% of the total dietary lipids. Important sources of triacylglycerols include oils, butter, whole milk, cheese, cream, fried foods and some meats. Triacylglycerols are also found in avocados, olives, corn and nuts. Excessive deposition of triacylglycerols in the liver, may be due to protein deficiency or lack of lipotropic factors such as choline, results in fatty liver.

Caloric Value of Fat

Fat is a concentrated source of energy providing 9 kcal/g.

Functions of Fat

Dietary fat, generally, has a bad reputation, but fat is vital for your health. The body actually needs fat for energy and for many critical processes such as the absorption of certain vitamins and minerals.

- Fat contributes to texture, flavor and taste, and increases the palatability of the diet.
- Fat is also essential for meeting some of the nutritional needs, like that of essential fatty acids (linoleic, n-6 and α-linolenic, n-3). EFA are metabolized at various sites in the body, to generate a group of biologically active compounds which perform several important physiological functions.
- Fat also serves as a rich source of energy.
- Fat also promotes the absorption of fat soluble vitamins (A, D, E and K).
- Fat also imparts a feeling of fullness and satisfaction, and, thus, delays the onset of hunger.
- Fat, along with proteins, constitutes major components of body fluids and cell membranes.
- Fat also serves as structural component of cell membrane, functions as energy storehouse, and provides insulation, cellular communication and protection.

Dietary Sources of Fat

As mentioned above, dietary fats are derived from two sources, viz. the visible fat and invisible fat. The total fat (both, visible and invisible) in the diet comes from three groups of foods, i.e., fats and oils; meat, poultry and fish; and dairy foods (Fig. 15.4).

Visible Fat

Fats and oils, which include cooking oils, butter, margarine and cream, etc., are referred to as visible fat, because they are easily seen and identified.

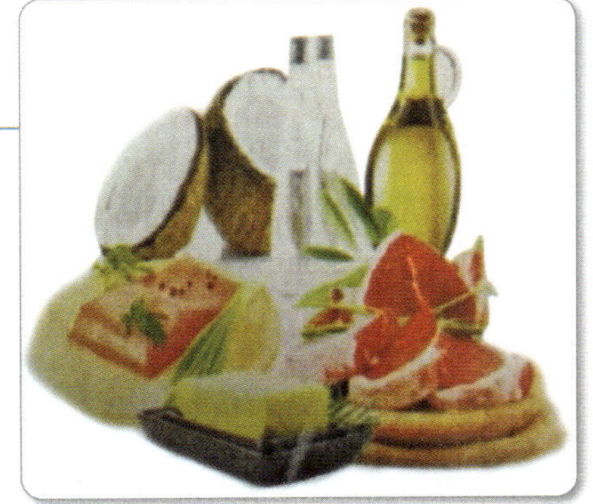

Fig. 15.4: Dietary sources of fat

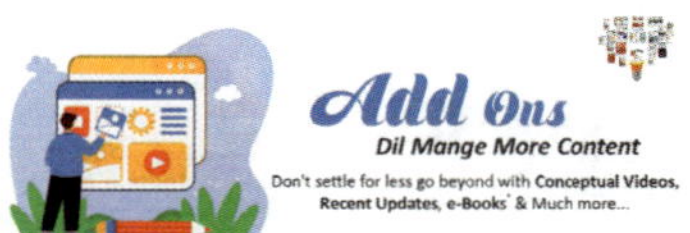

Invisible Fat

The other group contains invisible fat, because they cannot be easily separated from the food.

Difference between visible and invisible fat can be described by looking at meat, as an example. After trimming the outer layer of fat (the visible fat) from the meat, 20–40% of its calories still come from the fat (the invisible fat), which is present in the lean portion of the meat. Other examples of invisible fat include, the fats found in baked goods, nuts, peanut butter, processed meats and deep-fried foods, such as potato chips.

Visible fat should include various types, viz. saturated, monounsaturated and polyunsaturated.

- **Saturated fats** are found in animal products, such as butter, cheese, whole milk, ice cream, cream and meat. They are also found in some vegetable oils, such as coconut oil and palm oil.
- **Unsaturated fats** are found in most vegetable oils (with the exceptions of coconut oil and palm oil). Out of these, **monounsaturated** fatty acids are found in olive oil and canola oil, whereas **polyunsaturated fatty acids** are found in safflower oil, sunflower oil, corn oil and soybean oil, and fish.

  Seeds and nuts are rich in ω-3 **fatty acids**, whereas vegetable oils, such as soybean oil and canola oil, are good sources of, both, ω-3 and ω-6 **fatty acids**.

Requirement of Fats

According to ICMR-NIN (2020), **total fat** (visible and invisible) should provide between 20 and 30% of total calories.

- The upper limit for visible fat intake for healthy adult moderate workers has been suggested as 30 g/day for males and 25 g/day for females.
- Total visible fat intake has been suggested as 30 g/day during pregnancy as well as lactation.
- Older children and adolescents should consume, nearly, 25–50 g of cooking oils/ghee.
- Minimum level of total fat has been suggested as 40–60% of the total energy intake for infants between 0-6 months of age, which can be met from breast milk.
- Minimum level of total fat has been suggested as 35% of energy for infants between 7 and 12 months of age. It is further suggested that visible fat intake should be 25 g/day.
- Visible fat intake during pregnancy and lactation should be 30 g/day. The higher fat and EFA requirements during pregnancy and lactation are to meet the increased needs of the fetus and young infants, in view of their crucial role in physical and neuronal growth and development.
- Diet of young children and adolescents should contain about 30–50 g/day.
- Healthy adults, over the age of 19 years, should get not >**25–30% of daily calories from fat**. Young children (age 1–2 years) may be given up to 40% of their daily calories in the form of fat.
- Dietary fat, with an appropriate proportion of saturated, monounsaturated and polyunsaturated fatty acids, is most desirable.
- **Saturated fat should be limited to less than 10% of our daily calorie intake** since they are the biggest dietary cause of high LDL-cholesterol level (bad cholesterol).
- The remaining should be divided, evenly, between monounsaturated and polyunsaturated fat. To get a good proportion of all the classes of fatty acids, it is advisable to consume more than one type of vegetable oils.
- ω-6 Fatty acid (linoleic acid) should provide only about 2% of calories.
- ω-3 Fatty acid (α-linolenic acid) should provide between 1.0 and 1.5% of total calories intake.
- Recommended intake value for cholesterol is 200–300 mg/day.

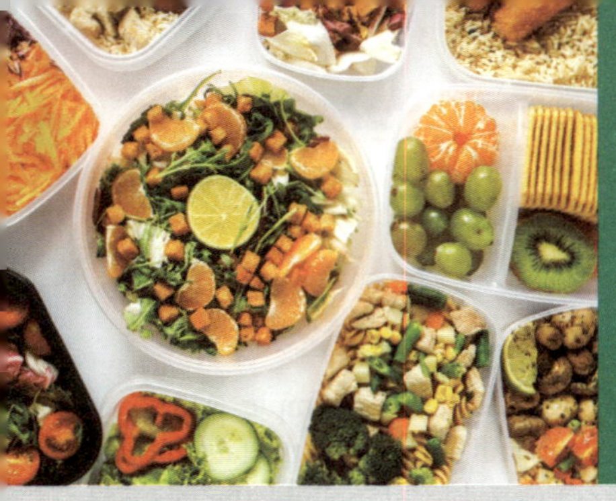

STUDENT ASSIGNMENT

LONG AND SHORT ANSWER QUESTIONS

1. Define fats. Give classification of fats.
2. Describe caloric value, functions, dietary sources and RDA of fats.
3. **Differentiate between:**
   a. Saturated and unsaturated fats
   b. ω-3 and ω-6 fatty acids
4. **Write notes on:**
   a. Essential fatty acids
   b. Trans fat

MULTIPLE CHOICE QUESTIONS

1. **Which type of fat is known to increase the levels of "good" HDL cholesterol in the body?**
   a. Trans fats
   b. Saturated fats
   c. Monounsaturated fats
   d. Polyunsaturated fats

2. **What is the caloric value of fats?**
   a. 2 Calories per gram
   b. 4 Calories per gram
   c. 7 Calories per gram
   d. 9 Calories per gram

3. **Which is a primary function of fats in the body?**
   a. Providing quick energy
   b. Building muscle mass
   c. Insulating organs
   d. Regulating blood sugar levels

4. **Which of the following is a dietary source of healthy fats?**
   a. Butter
   b. Coconut oil
   c. Processed meats
   d. Potato chips

ANSWER KEY

1. d   2. d   3. c   4. b

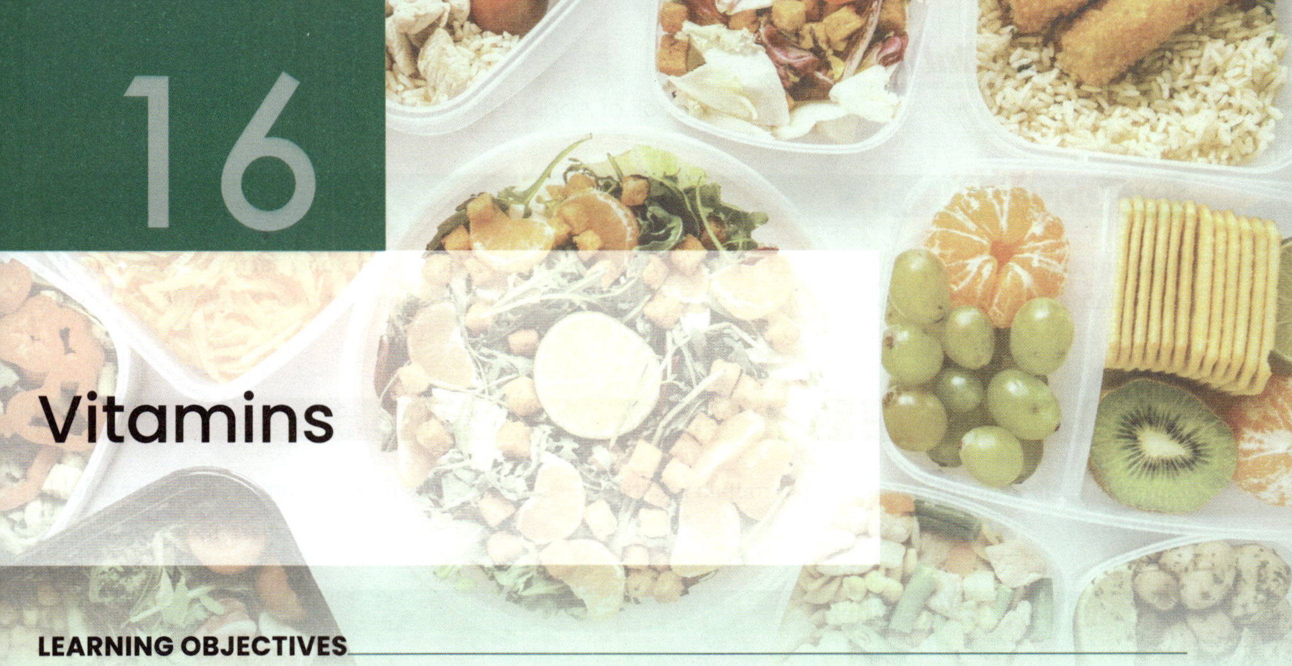

16

Vitamins

LEARNING OBJECTIVES

After the completion of the chapter, the readers will be able to:
- Describe the classification of vitamins.
- Explain the fat soluble vitamins, their functions and sources.
- Explain the water soluble vitamins, their functions and sources.

CHAPTER OUTLINE

- Introduction
- **Classification of Vitamins**
- Fat Soluble Vitamins
- Water Soluble Vitamins

KEY TERMS

Pellagra: A systemic disease caused by a severe deficiency of niacin (vitamin B_3). It affects the whole body and can eventually lead to death.

Recommended daily allowance: The average daily dietary intake level that is sufficient to meet the nutrient requirement of nearly all (97–98%) healthy individuals in a particular life stage and gender group.

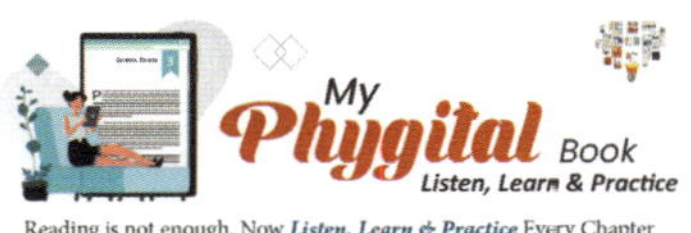

INTRODUCTION

Vitamins are the organic constituents of food, called **protective accessory food factors**. These are the micronutrients which are essential for life and well-being. Vitamins, in general, cannot be synthesized by the body and have to be supplied in the diet.

CLASSIFICATION OF VITAMINS

Based on their solubility, vitamins are grouped into two categories, as **fat soluble vitamins** and **water soluble vitamins**.

FAT SOLUBLE VITAMINS

Fat soluble vitamins include vitamin A, vitamin D, vitamin E and vitamin K. These are absorbed from the gastrointestinal lumen, in the presence of **dietary fat** (triacylglycerols) and **bile salts**. **Precursors** of vitamin A and vitamin D are called **provitamins** and are found, mostly, in plant sources.

Due to their solubility in fat, fat soluble vitamins can be **stored** in various organs such as liver and adipose tissue. Their large dietary intakes for a fairly long duration may result in toxic symptoms (**hypervitaminosis**).

Fat soluble vitamins are elaborated in Table 16.1.

TABLE 16.1: Fat soluble vitamins, their biological functions, deficiency diseases, sources and RDA for adults

Vitamin	Provitamin	Biological functions	Sources	RDA*	Deficiency diseases
Vitamin A (Retinol)	β-Carotene (Carotenoids)	In vision cycle, growth and maintenance of epithelium	Liver oil, fish oil and vegetable oils	840–1000 µg	Night blindness; disorders of mucous membrane, bone, nerves; and reproduction
Vitamin D (Calciferol)	7-Dehydro-cholesterol	Regulation of serum, calcium and phosphorus	Fish oil	600 IU	Rickets and osteomalacia
Vitamin E (Tocopherols)	—	As antioxidant	Seed oils	8–10 mg	Hemolytic anemia in infants and muscular dystrophy
Vitamin K (Phylloquinone)	—	In blood coagulation	Seed oils	55 µg	Blood clotting failure

*ICMR-NIN (2020)

Vitamin A

Vitamin A refers to a **group of three compounds, collectively called retinoids. Vitamin A includes retinol** (vitamin A alcohol), **retinal** (vitamin A aldehyde or retinaldehyde) and **retinoic acid** (vitamin A acid).

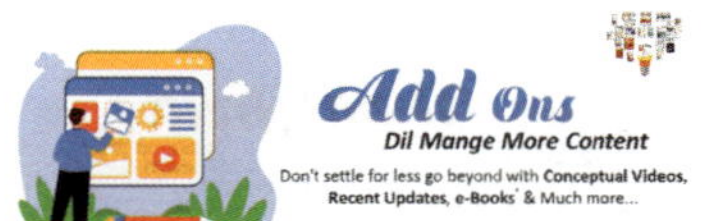

Besides, **plants contain a group of compounds called carotenoids**. They yield retinoids, when metabolized in the body and, thus, are referred to as **provitamin A (precursors of vitamin A)**, e.g., β-carotene**.**

Functions of Vitamin A

- **Vitamin A** is essential to the normal structure and functions of the skin and mucous membranes such as eyes, lungs and digestive system. It is, therefore, **vital for vision, embryonic development**, **growth** and **cellular differentiation**, and **immune system**. Besides,
  - **Retinal** is essential for **night** and **color vision.**
  - **Retinol** is required in **reproduction** and **bone health.**
  - **Retinoic acid** is important for **cell growth** and **differentiation**.
- **Provitamin A** (carotenoids) functions as a potent **antioxidant** and **prevents** damaging effects of **free radicals**. Thus, carotenoids help to **prevent damage from chemical carcinogens** and **lower the risk of certain types of cancer**.

Dietary Sources of Vitamin A

- **Vitamin A:** Animal foods, such as liver, cod liver oil, egg yolk and milk are rich sources of vitamin A (**retinoids**).
- **Provitamin A:** Dark green and yellow-orange vegetables such as carrots, spinach and broccoli, and orange colored fruits like peaches, apricots and mango are good sources of provitamin A (**carotenoids**).

Recommended Daily Allowances of Vitamin A

- Vitamin A requirement is expressed in terms of **retinol equivalents** (RE).
- One RE represents one mg of retinal or 12 mg of β-carotene.
- Vitamin A intake can also be expressed in terms of **international units** (IU).
- One IU of vitamin A is equivalent to 0.3 mg of retinal or 3.6 mg of β-carotene.
- Average daily requirement (RDA) of vitamin A for adults is 840–1000 µg.
- Its requirement is increased up to 900 µg during pregnancy and 950 µg during lactation.

Vitamin D

Vitamin D is a sterol (**steroid alcohol**), also called **sunshine vitamin**. Although several forms of vitamin D have been shown to exhibit **antirachitic** properties, most important of these are:

- **Vitamin D$_2$ (ergocalciferol)** found in plant foods
- **Vitamin D$_3$ (cholecalciferol)** found in animal foods and synthesized in the skin.

Vitamin D is classically a **prohormone**. It acts as a precursor to the hormone, calcitriol (1,25-dihydroxy-cholecalciferol), involved in calcium homeostasis, that is essential for bone mineralization and neuromuscular functions.

Functions of Vitamin D

- Primary role of vitamin D is to **regulate blood calcium** level. Calcitriol, the hormone synthesized from vitamin D, directly as well as with parathyroid hormone (PTH) and calcitonin, regulates blood calcium levels through its action on bone, kidneys and small intestine.

- Receptors for calcitriol are also found in a variety of other tissues, hence, vitamin D has also been shown to **inhibit cell proliferation** and **enhance cell differentiation**.

Dietary Sources of Vitamin D

Most of the vitamin D required by the body is **obtained through the action of sunlight on skin**.

Major dietary sources of vitamin D include cod liver oil, fish oil, egg yolk and liver. Other sources include fortified milk and foods.

Recommended Daily Allowances of Vitamin D

- Exclusively breast-fed infants, who receive little exposure to sunlight, need about 5 mg (200 IU) of vitamin D per day (1 mg = 40 IU).
- For elder people recommended daily intake (RDA) is 600 IU.

Vitamin E

Vitamin E refers to a group of several lipid soluble compounds synthesized by plants, such as tocopherols and tocotrienols. Commercially available form of the vitamin is called dl-α-tocopherol.

Functions of Vitamin E

Vitamin E performs several functions:

- Vitamin E acts as an **antioxidant**.
- It **stabilizes cell membrane** and **defends cells against oxidative damage from free radicals**. Since cells damaged by free radicals, are prone to mutations, thus, vitamin E **helps to prevent cancer**.
- Vitamin E also **maintains antioxidant status of β-carotene**.

Dietary Sources of Vitamin E

Wheat germ oil is the richest source of vitamin E. Foods containing large amounts of polyunsaturated fatty acids are also rich in vitamin E. Accordingly, vegetable oils such as safflower oil, cottonseed oil and sunflower oil, and nuts and seeds, are good sources of vitamin E.

Recommended Daily Allowances of Vitamin E

- Vitamin E requirement is expressed in terms of IU.
- One IU of vitamin E, from natural sources, is equivalent to 0.67 mg of α-tocopherol.
- One IU of synthetic (commercially available) vitamin E is equivalent to 0.45 mg of α-tocopherol.
- Its requirement is related to body size, physical activity, psychological stress, exposure to environmental pollutants and intake of polyunsaturated fatty acids.
- Normally, 0.8 mg of vitamin E is required per g of PUFA intake.
- Average daily requirement (RDA) of α-tocopherol, for adults, is 8–10 mg.

Vitamin K

Vitamin K refers to a family of compounds known as naphthoquinones.

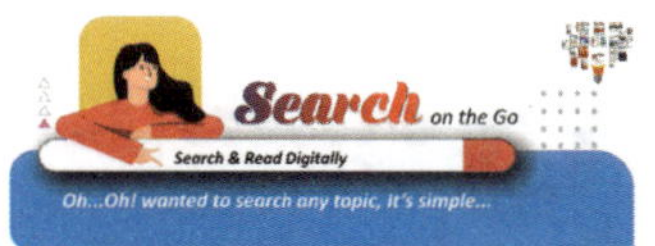

These include:

- **Vitamin K$_1$** (**phylloquinone**, obtained from plant sources).
- **Vitamin K$_2$** (**menaquinone**, obtained from animal sources and synthesized by intestinal bacteria).
- **Vitamin K$_3$** (**menadione**, the water soluble form, available commercially).

Amongst the three, phylloquinone is the most biologically active form.

Functions of Vitamin K

- Vitamin K plays a key role in the **formation of blood clot**. It is required for many reactions in the blood-clotting cascade, which involves the production of a series of proteins, such as prothrombin, factor VIII, factor IX and factor X, and fibrin.
- Vitamin K also **helps in bone formation**, where it is required in the carboxylation of osteocalcin, which is required for mineralization and maturation of bone.

Dietary Sources of Vitamin K

Intestinal bacteria can synthesize and meet about 10–15% of the daily requirement of vitamin K.

- Green leafy vegetables (spinach, broccoli, etc.) and vegetable oils (soybean oil, cottonseed oil, etc.) are good **sources of phylloquinone**.
- Animal products, such as dairy products and meat, contain limited amounts of **menaquinone**.

Recommended Daily Allowances of Vitamin K

Average daily intake (RDA) of vitamin K (phylloquinone), for adults, is 55 µg.

WATER SOLUBLE VITAMINS

Water soluble vitamins include B vitamins (vitamin B complex) and vitamin C. As these are soluble in water, they are rapidly absorbed from the gastrointestinal lumen. Water soluble vitamins are used as **coenzymes** in various metabolic reactions. Due to their water solubility, most of the water soluble vitamins are **not stored** in the body. Since, they cannot be stored, a dietary **deficiency quickly becomes manifest**. Typical deficiency symptoms for most of the water soluble vitamins, particularly, those of vitamin B complex, include dermatitis, glossitis, cheilosis and diarrhea, besides some of the neurological symptoms, such as peripheral neuropathy and malaise.

Water Soluble Vitamins

Water soluble vitamins consist of several **B-vitamins** (vitamin B complex) and **vitamin C**. They are susceptible to destruction by heat and alkalinity. Some cooking practices also destroy these vitamins (Table 16.2).

TABLE 16.2: Water soluble vitamins, their coenzyme forms, major biochemical functions, RDA for adults and deficiency diseases

Vitamins	Coenzyme forms	Major biochemical functions	RDA[*]	Deficiency diseases
Vitamin B complex				
Thiamine (B_1)	TPP	Oxidative decarboxylation	1.4–2.3 mg	Beriberi
Riboflavin (B_2)	FMN, FAD	Oxidation-reduction with flavoproteins	1.9–3.2 mg	Lesions on lips, cheilosis
Niacin (B_3)	NAD^+, $NADP^+$	Hydrogen acceptor for dehydrogenases	11–23 mg	Pellagra
Pantothenic acid (B_5)	Coenzyme A	Formation of CoA, component of the acyl carrier protein	5 mg	Muscle cramps, burning feet
Pyridoxine (B_6)	Pyridoxal-5-PO_4	Transamination decarboxylation	1.9–3.1 mg	Peripheral neuritis
Biotin (B_7)	Carboxybiocytin	Cocarboxylase	25 µg	Anemia, dermatitis
Folate (B_9)	FH_4	Carrier of one-C moiety	220–300 µg	Megaloblastic macrocytic anemia
Cobalamin (B_{12})	Cobamide coenzymes	Transmethylation with FH_4	2.2 µg	Pernicious anemia
Vitamin C (Ascorbic acid)	L-Ascorbate	Hydroxylation	65–80 mg	Scurvy

*ICMR-NIN (2020)

B-Vitamins

The B-vitamins or vitamin B complex consists of various vitamins, which are generally referred by their names. These include:

- Thiamine (vitamin B_1)
- Riboflavin (vitamin B_2)
- Niacin (vitamin B_3)
- Pantothenic acid (vitamin B_5)
- Pyridoxine (vitamin B_6)
- Biotin (vitamin B_7)
- Folate (vitamin B_9)
- Vitamin B_{12}

Most of the B-vitamins are synthesized in the GIT by the intestinal flora. They primarily act as coenzymes and help in catalyzing various metabolic reactions, particularly, energy producing reactions.

Thiamine

Thiamine is **also referred to as vitamin B_1 or antiberiberi factor**.

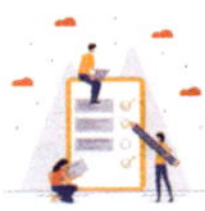
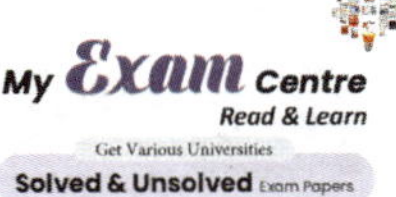

Functions of Vitamin Thiamine

- Thiamine is a coenzyme for several energy yielding metabolic pathways, as a component of the **coenzyme thiamine pyrophosphate (TPP)**. Accordingly, thiamine requirement is related to the amount of energy consumed.
- **Vitamin B$_1$** is also involved in the normal **functioning of the nervous system** and other excitable tissues, such as **skeletal muscle** and the **heart**.

Dietary Sources of Thiamine

Pork and wheat germ are the richest sources of thiamine. Whole grains, nuts, meat (especially pork), fruits and vegetables and fortified breakfast cereals, are also good sources of thiamine in the diet.

Recommended Daily Allowances of Thiamine

- Daily requirement (RDA) for vitamin B$_1$ varies from 1.4 mg/day to 2.3 mg/day.
- Its RDA depends upon calorie intake, and has been defined as 0.6 mg/1000 kcal.
- Requirement of thiamine is increased in hypermetabolic states, such as in fever, hyperthyroidism, alcohol intake and during pregnancy.

Riboflavin

Riboflavin is also referred to as **vitamin B$_2$**. It is also called **lactoflavin**, due to its presence in milk. It is needed for the normal structure and function of mucous membranes and the skin.

Functions of Riboflavin

- Riboflavin, as a component of **coenzymes flavin mononucleotide (FMN)** and **flavin adenine dinucleotide (FAD)**, acts as electron and hydrogen acceptor, and participates in several oxidation reduction reactions in the citric acid cycle, β-oxidation of fatty acids, and oxidative deamination.
- Thus, vitamin B$_2$ is required to release energy from proteins, carbohydrates and fat.

Dietary Sources of Vitamin B$_2$

Milk, organ meat (such as liver and kidney), mushrooms and cotton-cheese are good sources of riboflavin.

Recommended Daily Allowances of Vitamin B$_2$

- Average daily requirement (RDA) for vitamin B$_2$ is 1.9–3.2 mg/day. Like thiamine, requirement of riboflavin also depends upon calories intake and has been defined as 0.6 mg/1000 kcal.
- Its requirement is increased during pregnancy and lactation.

Niacin

Nicotinic acid and **nicotinamide** (or niacinamide) refers to two, similarly functioning, compounds that have niacin (also referred to as **vitamin B$_3$**) activity. It is also known as **pellagra preventive factor**.

Functions of Niacin

As a component of **nicotinamide adenine dinucleotide (NAD)** and **nicotinamide adenine dinucleotide phosphate (NADP)**, nicotinic acid participates in oxidation reduction reactions.

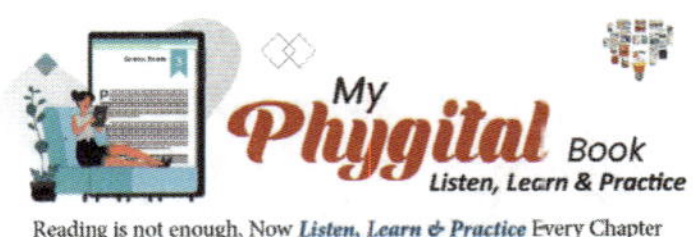

- **NAD** accepts electrons and hydrogen, and is reduced to NADH, that carries electrons to the electron transport chain.
- **NADP** is reduced to NADPH, which is used in the synthesis of fatty acids, cholesterol and steroid hormones.

Dietary Sources of Niacin

Good sources of niacin include rice polishing, wheat, mushrooms, peanuts, eggs, milk and dairy products, liver meat and seafood.

NAD is also synthesized from tryptophan in the body.

Recommended Daily Allowances of Niacin

- Requirement of niacin is expressed in terms of niacin equivalents, to include both the preformed vitamin as well as that is synthesized from tryptophan in the body.
- Its requirement (RDA) has been defined as 11–23 mg/day.

Pantothenic Acid

Pantothenic acid, also referred to as **vitamin B$_5$**, is the combination of pantoic acid and β-alanine. It is essentially required for the synthesis of coenzyme A (CoA), which is essential for fatty acid metabolism as well as to synthesize and metabolize proteins, carbohydrates and fats.

Functions of Pantothenic Acid

As an integral part of the **coenzyme A** (CoA) and acyl carrier protein (ACP), pantothenic acid is used in energy producing reactions and fatty acid synthesis.

Dietary Sources of Pantothenic Acid

Chicken, liver, egg yolk, broccoli, potatoes, oats and whole grains are good sources of pantothenic acid.

Recommended Daily Allowances of Pantothenic Acid

Average daily requirement (RDA) of pantothenic acid for adults is 5 mg.

Pyridoxine

Pyridoxine, also called **vitamin B$_6$**, refers to three different compounds (vitamers), which include:

- **Pyridoxine**
- **Pyridoxal**
- **Pyridoxamine**.

Vitamin B$_6$ has a central role in the metabolism of amino acids. Together with folate and vitamin B$_{12}$, pyridoxine is also required for the maintenance of blood homocysteine level, whose raised level is a risk factor for cardiovascular disease.

Functions of Vitamin B$_6$

- Vitamin B$_6$ is converted to its coenzyme, called **pyridoxal-5-phosphate** (**PLP**), which is used as a coenzyme with different enzymes that are involved in the transfer of amino group (NH$_2$), carboxyl group (COOH) or water.

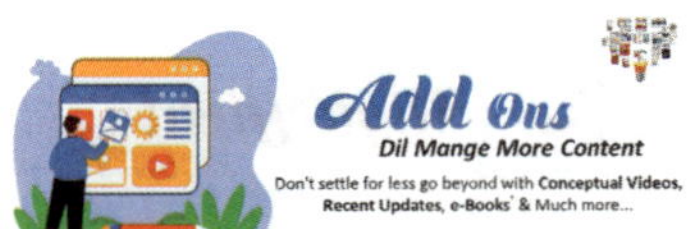

- PLP also plays a role in the **synthesis of nonessential amino acids**.
- It also **promotes gluconeogenesis** and facilitates glycogenolysis.
- Vitamin B_6 also helps in the **production of several neurotransmitters**, such as serotonin, γ-aminobutyric acid, dopamine and norepinephrine.
- It also **helps in the conversion of tryptophan to niacin**.
- Vitamin B_6 is also important in the **synthesis of hemoglobin.** It also helps in the binding of oxygen to hemoglobin.
- Dietary vitamin B_6, **along with folate and vitamin B_{12}, lowers blood homocysteine levels**, which, in turn, is associated with the risk of cardiovascular disease.

Dietary Sources of Vitamin B_6

Eggs, fish, green-leafy vegetables and cereals are rich sources of pyridoxine. Banana, watermelon, potato and sunflower seeds are also good sources of the vitamin.

Recommended Daily Allowances of Vitamin B_6

Vitamin B_6 requirement (RDA) for an adult is 1.9–3.1 mg/day.

Biotin

Biotin, also referred to as **vitamin B_7**, is involved in a wide range of metabolic processes, primarily, related to the utilization of fats, carbohydrates and amino acids.

Functions of Biotin

Biotin, as a component of biotin-containing enzymes, is important in carboxylation reactions, in which carbon dioxide is added to a substrate, e.g., in the conversion of pyruvate to oxaloacetate, propionyl CoA to succinyl CoA and acetyl CoA to malonyl CoA.

Dietary Sources of Biotin

Good sources of biotin include rice polishing, whole cereals, cauliflower, peanut, cheese and liver. Egg yolk, though, is good source of biotin, but avidin, present in raw egg-white, binds biotin and the avidin-biotin complex prevents its absorption.

Recommended Daily Allowances of Biotin

Average daily intake (RDA) of biotin, for adults, is 25 µg.

Folate

Folate (folic acid), also called **vitamin B_9**, refers to a group of derivatives of **pteroylglutamic acid**. It is the synthetic form of folate and is used in supplements and food fortification.

Functions of Folate

- Folate as a component of its **coenzyme**, tetrahydrofolate (**FH_4**), is important in **one-carbon metabolism**.
- It plays an important role in **amino acid metabolism,** particularly, in the metabolism of serine and methionine, and in purine synthesis.
- Folate **with vitamin B_{12} also helps in the formation of red blood cells**.

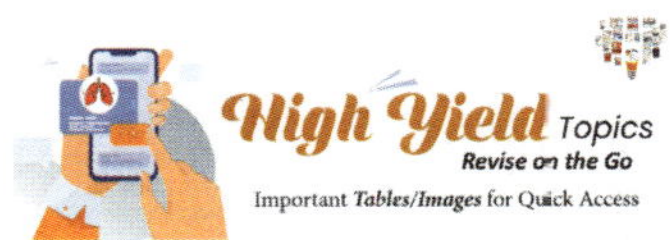

- It is also required **for** normal **cell division**, structure of the **nervous system**, specifically, in the **development of the neural tube**, which develops into the spinal cord and skull, in the embryo.
- Folate **with vitamins B$_6$** and **B$_{12}$** is also required for **the maintenance of blood homocysteine level**.

Dietary Sources of Folate

Spinach and other dark green-leafy vegetables, broccoli, orange, banana, wheat germ, sunflower seeds, brown rice, peas and legumes, and liver are good sources of folic acid.

Recommended Daily Allowances of Folate

- Average daily requirement (RDA) for folate for a normal adult is 220–300 μg.
- Its requirement is 330 μg and 570 μg during lactation.

Vitamin B$_{12}$

Vitamin B$_{12}$, also called **cyanocobalamin**, refers to a family of cobalamin-containing compounds, which include **cyanocobalamin** and **hydroxycobalamine**.

Functions of Vitamin B$_{12}$

- Vitamin B$_{12}$ is a constituent of the **cobamide coenzymes**, which include **deoxyadenosylcobalamin** and **methylcobalamin**.
- It is also **important for the nervous system**, formation of red blood cells and metabolism of folic acid.
- Deoxyadenosylcobalamin **with folic acid plays a key role in one-carbon metabolism**.
- Methylcobalamin is also **essential in amino acid metabolism, DNA synthesis** and **cell multiplication**.
- Vitamin B$_{12}$ also **helps to maintain myelin sheath**.
- It is also **required in propionate metabolism**, i.e., in the conversion of methylmalonyl CoA to succinyl CoA.

Dietary Sources of Vitamin B$_{12}$

Vitamin B$_{12}$ is found in almost all foods of animal origin such as meat, fish, poultry, and milk and milk products.

Recommended Daily Allowances of Vitamin B$_{12}$

Average requirement (RDA) of vitamin B$_{12}$ for a normal adult is 2.2 μg/day.

Vitamin C

Vitamin C is also referred to as **ascorbic acid**. It cannot be synthesized in human beings.

Functions of Vitamin C

Vitamin C performs several functions in the body. These include:

- **Collagen synthesis:** Vitamin C plays an important role in hydroxylation reactions. Hydroxylation of proline and lysine is important in the synthesis of collagen, a fibrous protein found in the connective tissues, which binds cells and tissues together. Collagen is a most abundant protein present in skin, bone, tendons, cartilage and teeth.

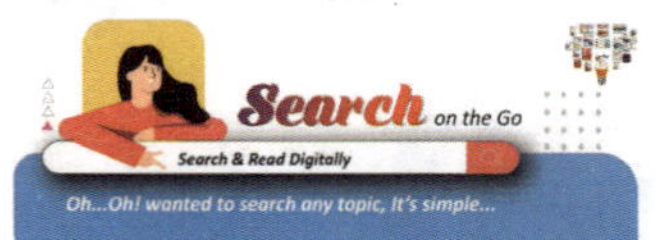

- **Antioxidant activity:** Vitamin C also acts as an antioxidant and prevents damage caused by free radicals. Thus, vitamin C, in turn, reduces the risk of certain chronic diseases such as heart disease, cancers and cataract.
- Vitamin C also helps in recycling of the oxidized form of **vitamin E** for its reuse within the cells.
- Vitamin C also stabilizes the reduced form of folic acid.
- **Absorption of iron:** As a reducing agent, vitamin C also enhances the absorption of non-heme iron from plant foods.
- **Synthesis of vital compounds:** Vitamin C also helps in the synthesis of carnitine, norepinephrine, epinephrine, serotonin, thyroxin, bile acids, steroid hormones and purines.
- **Immune functions:** Vitamin C also enables lymphocytes and other cells of the immune system to function properly. High doses of vitamin C may reduce severity and duration of cold-related symptoms.

Dietary Sources of Vitamin C

Amla (goose berry), citrus fruits, tomatoes, guava, strawberries, spinach and other leafy vegetables, and potatoes are good sources of vitamin C.

Recommended Daily Allowances of Vitamin C

- Average daily requirement (RDA) for vitamin C for adult men is 65–80 mg.
- Women need more vitamin C during pregnancy and lactation.
- Smokers also need more vitamin C, as smoke increases metabolic turnover of the vitamin.

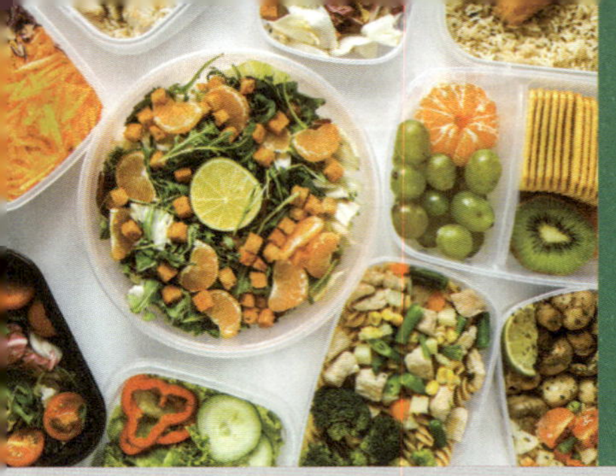

STUDENT ASSIGNMENT

LONG AND SHORT ANSWER QUESTIONS

1. What are vitamins? Give classification of vitamins.
2. Describe functions, dietary sources and RDA of vitamin A.
3. Describe functions, dietary sources and RDA of vitamin D.
4. Describe functions, dietary sources and RDA of thiamine.
5. Describe functions, dietary sources and RDA of folic acid.
6. Describe functions, dietary sources and RDA of vitamin C.
7. **Write notes on:**
   a. Fat soluble vitamins
   b. Water soluble vitamins
   c. Vitamin E
   d. Vitamin K
   e. Vitamin B_2
   f. Nicotinic acid
   g. Vitamin pyridoxine
   h. Vitamin B_{12}

MULTIPLE CHOICE QUESTIONS

1. **Which of the following vitamins is fat soluble?**
   a. Vitamin B_{12}
   b. Vitamin C
   c. Vitamin K
   d. Vitamin B_6

2. **Which of the following is the primary function of vitamin D in the body?**
   a. Aiding in the absorption of calcium
   b. Supporting the immune system
   c. Boosting energy levels
   d. Regulating blood sugar levels

3. **Which of the following vitamins is water soluble?**
   a. Vitamin A
   b. Vitamin E
   c. Vitamin C
   d. Vitamin D

4. **What is the recommended dietary allowance (RDA) for vitamin B_{12} for adults?**
   a. 1–2 µg/day
   b. 50 µg/day
   c. 100 µg/day
   d. 500 µg/day

ANSWER KEY

1. c   2. a   3. c   4. a

17

Minerals

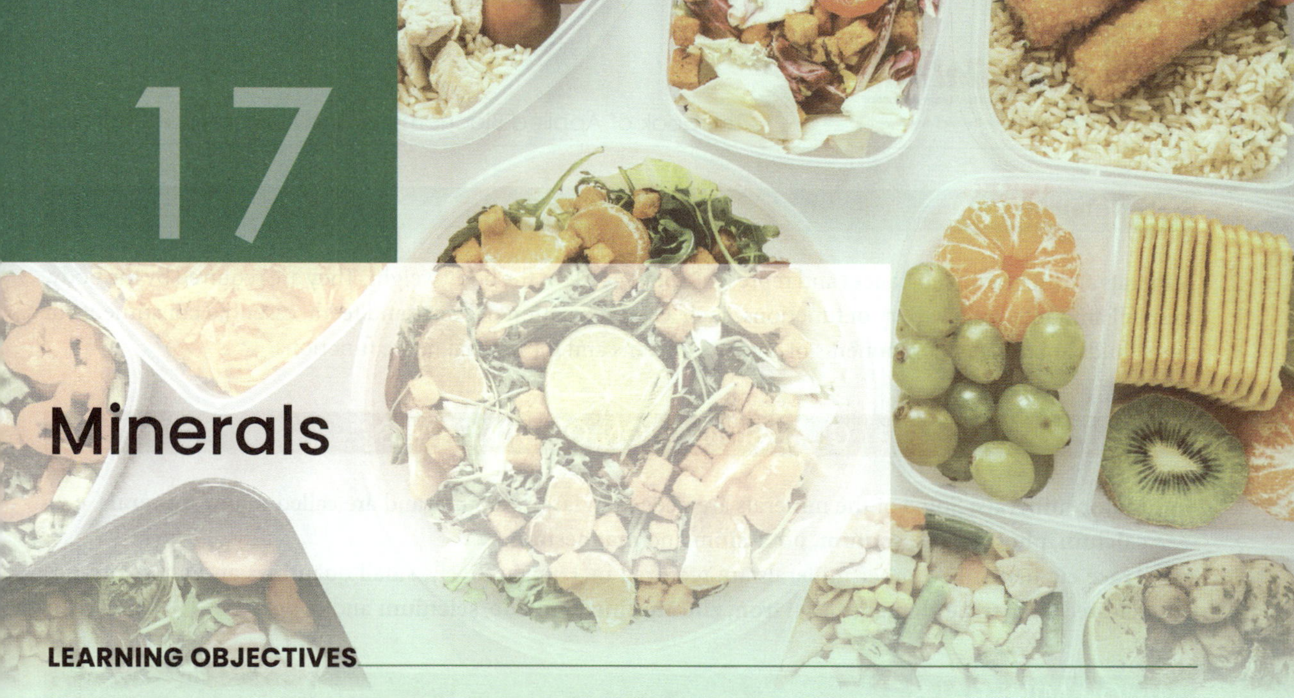

LEARNING OBJECTIVES

After the completion of the chapter, the readers will be able to:
- Explain major minerals (calcium, phosphorus, sodium, potassium, and magnesium) and trace elements.
- Explain functions; dietary sources; requirements—RDA.

CHAPTER OUTLINE

- Introduction
- **Classification of Minerals**
- Major Minerals
- Trace Elements

KEY TERMS

Cretinism: A condition of severe physical and mental retardation due to iodine deficiency, and specifically due to deficiency of thyroid hormones during early pregnancy.

Endemic goiter: Iodine deficiency characterized by abnormal cold sensitivity, excessive fatigue, insomnia, low blood pressure.

Extracellular fluid: All body fluids outside the cells of any multicellular organism.

Nonheme proteins: Contain strongly bound functional iron atoms attached to sulfur, but they do not contain porphyrins such as ferredoxins, hemerythrin. All of them have a role in electron transfer.

Oxidation-reduction reaction: A type of chemical reaction in which reduction and oxidation occur at the same time.

INTRODUCTION

Minerals are inorganic substances and represent about 4–5% of the body weight. They are required by the body, in small amounts, for a variety of functions, such as for formation of bones and teeth, essential constituents of body fluids and tissues, components of enzyme systems and for normal nerve functions.

CLASSIFICATION OF MINERALS

- **Major minerals:** Some of the minerals are needed in large amounts and are called **major minerals**, e.g., **calcium**, **phosphorus**, **sodium**, **potassium** and **magnesium**.
- **Trace elements:** Few other minerals are required in, comparatively, small quantities and, therefore, are referred to as **trace elements**, e.g., **iron**, **zinc**, **iodine**, **fluoride**, **selenium** and **copper**.

MAJOR MINERALS

Major minerals are the ones that the body requires in amounts of at least 100 mg/day. These include **calcium**, **phosphorus**, **sodium**, **potassium** and **magnesium**.
- Major minerals travel through the body in various ways.
- The key task of sodium and potassium is to maintain proper balance of water in the body.
- Calcium, phosphorus and magnesium are important for healthy bones.
- Having too much of one major mineral can result in a deficiency of another. These sorts of imbalances are usually caused by overloads from supplements, not food sources.

Calcium

Calcium (Ca) is the most abundant mineral, found in the body. It is found in highest concentration in the body and is needed by all the cells. Adult human body contains, nearly, 1.0–1.5 kg of calcium, out of which about 99% is found in bones and teeth, and 1% in the extracellular fluid. Calcium level in the blood is regulated by balancing calcium absorption from the gut, excretion via kidneys, and mobilization and deposition in the bone. These sites are regulated by feedback mechanisms, which are controlled by several hormones, including parathyroid hormone (PTH) and active vitamin D.

Functions of Calcium

Calcium performs several functions in the body:
- **Bones and teeth:** Formation of bone and teeth. Bones are reservoir of Ca in the body.
- **Muscle contraction:** Ca mediates excitation and contraction of muscle fibers. Ca also interacts with troponin-C to trigger muscle contraction. Ca also activates ATPase and increases interaction between actin and myosin.
- **Nerve conduction:** Transmission of nerve impulses from presynaptic to postsynaptic region.
- **Secretion of hormones:** It mediates the secretion of insulin, PTH, calcitonin and vasopressin.
- **Second messenger:** Ca and cyclicAMP are second messengers of different hormones, such as glucagon.

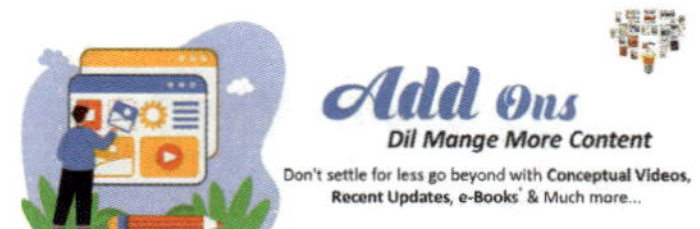

- **Membrane integrity and permeability:** Calcium influences transport of number of substances across the membranous barrier.
- **Blood coagulation:** Calcium is essential for factor IV in blood coagulation cascade and in the conversion of prothrombin to thrombin
- **Action on heart:** Ca prolongs systole. High Ca concentration also increases myocardial contractility.
- **Activation of enzymes:** Calmodulin (Ca-binding regulatory protein) binds with 4 Ca ions and leads to activation of several enzymes.

Dietary Sources of Calcium

Milk, cheese and other dairy products are rich sources of calcium. Eggs, dry fruits, legumes, green-leafy vegetables (such as broccoli and cabbage), fortified soya products and fish eaten with the bones (such as tinned salmon and whitebait) are also good sources of calcium.

Recommended Daily Allowances of Calcium

An adult requires nearly 1000 mg of calcium/day. Its requirement (RDA) is increased to about 1200 mg/day during lactation.

Phosphorus

A normal adult body contains nearly 600–800 g of phosphorus. About 85% of it is present in skeleton and teeth, as calcium phosphate crystals. It is essential for the structure of cell membranes, as phospholipids. Phosphorus, in the cells, contributes to a number of processes associated with energy metabolism.

Functions of Phosphorus

- Phosphate with calcium forms hydroxyapatite, the major inorganic molecule in teeth and bones.
- As part of phospholipids, phosphorus is present in every cell membrane in the body. Numerous phospholipid molecules also act as secondary messengers, within the cytosol.
- As a part of phosphate buffer, it is important in intracellular fluid and kidney tubules, where phosphate functions in the excretion of hydrogen ions.
- As phosphates, phosphorus participates in numerous essential functions of the body, e.g., as a component of DNA and RNA, ATP and other high energy phosphate compounds, such as creatine phosphate, glucose-6-phosphate, phosphoenolpyruvate, etc.

Dietary Sources of Phosphorus

Phosphorus is found in foods containing phosphoproteins, nucleoproteins, phospholipids and glycerophosphates, as well as in the form of inorganic phosphates (chiefly of Ca and Na). Phosphorus is abundant in red meat, dairy products, fish, poultry, bread, rice and oats, and is usually found in foods that also contain calcium.

Recommended Daily Allowances of Phosphorus

Daily requirement (RDA) of phosphorus for adults is 1000 mg/day.

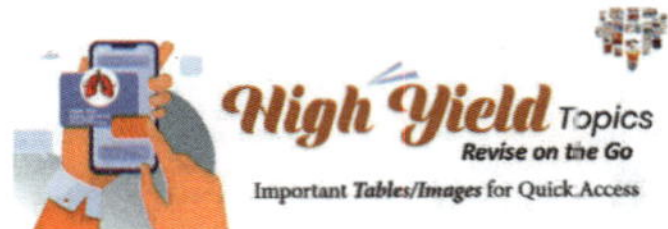

Sodium

The adult human body contains $\approx$100 g of sodium, as sodium ions (Na$^+$). About half of this is found in the extracellular fluid while the remaining half in the cells and bone. Sodium is the **major cation in the ECF**. Normal serum sodium concentration is 136–145 mEq/L. Intestinal secretions such as bile and pancreatic juice contain substantial amounts of sodium.

It exists in the body in association with several anions such as chloride, bicarbonate, phosphate, lactate and proteinate. High concentration of Na$^+$ along with low K$^+$ in the extracellular fluid is maintained by Na$^+$/K$^+$-ATPase (Na$^+$/K$^+$-pump). Dietary sodium is a component of common salt, known as sodium chloride (NaCl).

Functions of Sodium

Sodium performs several functions, as:
- **Regulation of osmotic pressure:** Sodium plays a dominant role in the maintenance of osmotic pressure of different body fluids and protects body against excessive fluid loss.
- **Regulation of acid-base balance:** Sodium salts with the corresponding weak acids form chief buffer system of the extracellular fluid and, play an important role in the regulation of pH of the body fluids.
- **Absorption of monosaccharides and amino acids:** Na$^+$ also plays an important role in the absorption of monosaccharides as well as amino acids from the small intestine.
- **Nerve transmission:** Sodium is also important in the maintenance of neuromuscular irritability and excitability.
- **Maintenance of blood viscosity:** Sodium is also important in the maintenance of blood viscosity.
- **Electrolytes and water balance:** Sodium is also important in the maintenance of water and electrolytes balance.
- Na$^+$ also acts as **a cofactor** for some enzymes, such as Na$^+$, K$^+$-ATPase.
- Sodium, as salt is an essential ingredient of food and enhances its taste. It is also used as a preservative.

Dietary Sources of Sodium

All food substances contain sodium, but added salt (sodium 40%, chloride 60%) is the major source of sodium in our diet. Cereals, pulses, vegetables, and animal and sea foods are the major sources of sodium.

Preserved foods (such as pickles), sun dried foods (like papads, sauces/ketchup) and canned foods contribute to higher intake of salt.

Recommended Daily Allowances of Sodium

Sodium requirements depend on its losses through urine, faeces and sweat. The sweat loss varies according to climatic conditions. High ambient temperature and vigorous physical exercise increase sodium loss through sweat.

Requirement (RDA) for sodium has been suggested as 2000 mg/day.

Potassium

Potassium is a major cation of the intracellular fluid. It is present in small amount in the extracellular fluid. Normal serum potassium concentration is 3.5–5.0 mEq/L.

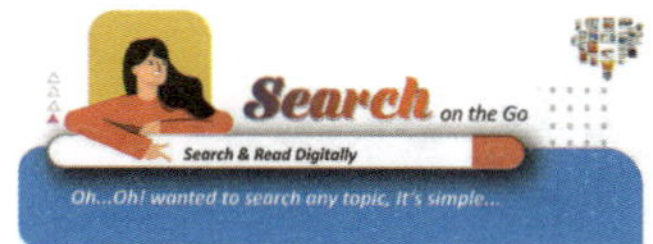

Functions of Potassium

- Potassium is essential for water and electrolyte balance, and normal functioning of the cells, including nerves.
- Potassium, with sodium, is involved in maintaining normal water balance, osmotic equilibrium and acid-base balance.
- In addition to calcium, potassium is important in the regulation of neuromuscular activity.
- Concentrations of sodium and potassium determine membrane potential in nerves and muscle.
- Potassium also promotes cellular growth.
- Potassium also has an integral role in Na/K-ATPase pump.

Dietary Sources of Potassium

Potassium is present in almost all foods, but fruits, vegetables, fresh meat and dairy products are good sources of potassium.

Recommended Daily Allowances of Potassium

Adequate intake (RDA) of potassium for adults is 3500 mg/day.

Magnesium

Magnesium is an essential mineral present in all human tissues, especially, in bones. It has both physiological and biochemical functions, and has important relationship with calcium, potassium and sodium. It is needed for the activation of many enzymes, e.g., those concerned with the replication of DNA, synthesis of RNA, and for the secretion of parathyroid hormone which is involved in bone metabolism.

Functions of Magnesium

- Magnesium is a cofactor for >300 enzymes involved in the metabolism of food components, and the synthesis of many metabolic products. Among the important reactions, requiring magnesium, are those catalyzing synthesis of fatty acids and proteins, phosphorylation of glucose and its derivatives in the glycolytic pathway, and transketolase reactions.
- Magnesium also plays a role in neuromuscular transmission and activity.
- Magnesium also acts as a physiologic calcium channel blocker.

Dietary Sources of Magnesium

Magnesium is widely available from, both, plant and animal cells, and is the mineral present in chlorophyll, the green pigment in plants. Whole grain, cereals, potatoes and sea-foods are good sources of magnesium. Beverages, such as coffee, tea and cocoa, also contain large amounts of magnesium.

Recommended Daily Allowances of Magnesium

Average daily requirement (RDA) of magnesium, for adults, is 370–440 mg.

TRACE ELEMENTS

The minerals that the body requires in amounts <100 mg/day are referred to as trace elements. These include **iron**, **iodine**, **fluoride**, **copper**, **zinc**, **manganese**, **chromium**, **selenium**, **cobalt** and **molybdenum**.

Trace elements perform a variety of functions. For example:

- Iron is best known for ferrying oxygen throughout the body.
- Fluoride strengthens bones and wards off tooth decay.
- Zinc helps blood clot, is essential for taste and smell, and bolsters the immune response.
- Copper helps form several enzymes, one of which assists with iron metabolism and the creation of hemoglobin, which carries oxygen in the blood.
- The other trace minerals perform equally vital jobs such as helping to block damage to body cells and forming parts of key enzymes or enhancing their activity.

Iron

Total quantity of iron (Fe), in normal adult human body is about 4 g. Iron may be incorporated in the protoporphyrin ring, both in the Fe^{2+} and Fe^{3+} forms. Fe^{2+}-protoporphyrin complex is called **heme**, while Fe^{3+}-protoporphyrin complex is designated as **hematin**. Heme-containing proteins include hemoglobin, myoglobin and several enzymes, such as catalase and peroxidases. **Nonheme** proteins include ferritin, transferrin, cytochromes and iron-sulfur proteins.

Functions of Iron

- As a component of hemoglobin, iron has a role in the transport of oxygen and carbon dioxide.
- Myoglobin, also a heme-containing protein, serves as an oxygen reservoir within muscle.
- Iron also an active component of cytochromes (enzymes), is involved in the processes of cellular respiration and energy (ATP) generation.
- It also forms a component of ribonucleotide reductase, the rate-limiting enzyme in DNA synthesis.
- Iron is also involved in immune functions and cognitive performance.
- It is also involved in functions and synthesis of neurotransmitters.

Dietary Sources of Iron

Dietary iron is found in two forms, i.e., as **heme iron** (from animal sources) and **nonheme iron** (from plant sources).

- Food, cooked in iron cookware is the best source of iron.
- **Animal foods** such as meat, fish and egg, are good sources of heme iron. It is the most bioavailable form of iron.
- Green-leafy vegetables, cereals, legumes, pulses and beans (whole grains), nuts and fruits, are good sources of nonheme iron, the predominant form of iron found in plant foods.

Recommended Daily Allowances of Iron

Recommended daily allowance (RDA) for iron is about 19 mg for normal adult males. For females, the requirement is increased to 29 mg (due to loss) during menstruation, and during pregnancy and lactation, due to increased demand of the body.

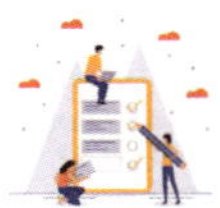
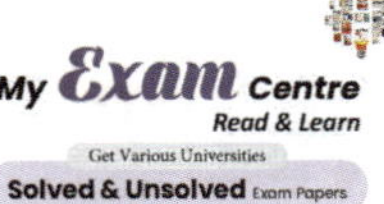

Zinc

Total body content of zinc in an adult man, is about 2.0 g. Choroid of the eye, liver, prostate gland and prostate fluid contain high concentration of zinc.

Functions of Zinc

- Zinc, primarily, an intracellular ion, functions with >300 enzymes. It also participates in the metabolism of carbohydrates, lipids, proteins and nucleic acids.
- In the nucleus, zinc stabilizes RNA and DNA structure, and is required for the activity of RNA polymerases.
- Zinc also functions in chromatin proteins, involved in transcription and replication.
- It is also involved in the integrity of subcellular organelles, in transport processes, immune functions and expression of genetic information.

Dietary Sources of Zinc

Zinc is present in many foods, but is most readily absorbed from meat. Colostrum is a rich source of zinc. It is also present in milk, cheese, eggs, shellfish, wholegrain cereals, nuts and pulses.

Recommended Daily Allowances of Zinc

Daily intake (RDA) of zinc is about 13–17 mg.

Copper

Adult human body contains 100–150 mg of copper, out of which, nearly 50% is found in muscles and 25% in bones.

Functions of Copper

- Copper is a component of many enzymes, particularly, those which require vitamin C, such as cytochrome oxidase, ferroxidase (ceruloplasmin), tyrosinase, ascorbic acid oxidase, superoxide dismutase, etc.
- It is also a constituent of α-amino-levulinate synthase and ferroxidase I, and thus, helps in the metabolism of iron and biosynthesis of hemoglobin.
- Copper is also an important constituent of several other proteins, such as erythrocuprein, cerebrocuprein and hepatocuprein, which are present in the bone marrow, brain and liver, respectively.
- It also helps in the formation of bone and elastin fibers, and maintenance of myelin sheath.
- Copper is also important for infant growth, brain development, immune system and strong bones.

Dietary Sources of Copper

Nuts, leafy vegetables, dried legumes, egg yolk, and fish and liver meat, are good sources of copper.

Recommended Daily Allowances of Copper

A normal adult's RDA for copper is 1.5–1.7 mg.

Iodine

Nearly 20–30 mg of iodine is present in adult human body. It is an essential component of the thyroid hormones, which are vital regulators of basal metabolic rate, and physical and mental development.

Functions of Iodine

Important function of iodine is the synthesis of the thyroid hormones T_3 and T_4, which are formed in the thyroid gland. These hormones function in the regulation of basal metabolic rate in adults, and are required for growth and development in children.

Dietary Sources of Iodine

Iodine requirement is mostly fulfilled from drinking water. Adequate supply of iodine can also be met from iodized salt. Seafoods, fruits, vegetables, cereals and meat are good sources of iodine.

Recommended Daily Allowances of Iodine

Daily requirement (RDA) for iodine is about 140 µg.

Fluoride

Fluoride is present in traces, in several tissues, mainly bones, teeth, thyroid gland and skin.

Functions of Fluoride

- Main function of fluoride is in the mineralization of bones and teeth.
- Fluoride also acts as an antibacterial agent, in the oral cavity and protects teeth from dental caries.

Dietary Sources of Fluoride

Drinking water is an important source of fluoride, in a human diet. Besides, fluoride can also be obtained from tea and fish.

Recommended Daily Allowances of Fluoride

Daily requirement (RDA) of fluoride is 2–3 mg.

Selenium

Selenium is present in high amounts in renal cortex, pancreas, pituitary and liver.

Functions of Selenium

The main function of selenium is as a component of some of the important antioxidant enzymes (e.g., glutathione peroxidase) therefore, to protect the body against oxidative damage.

- It is also necessary for the use of iodine in thyroid hormone production, immune system and reproductive functions.

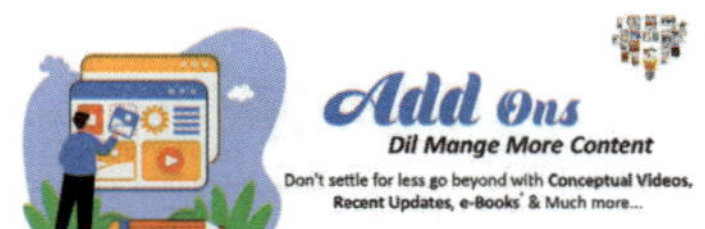

- Selenium, as selenomethionine, or selenocysteine, exists in several proteins that are widely distributed in the body.
- Antioxidant effects of selenium and vitamin E may reinforce each other, by the overlap of their protective actions against oxidative damage. Whereas, glutathione peroxidase (GSH-Px) acts in the cytosol and mitochondrial matrix, vitamin E exerts its action within the cell membrane.

Dietary Sources of Selenium

Selenium is found in a variety of foods, especially, Brazil nuts, bread, fish, meat and eggs. The selenium content of cereals is directly proportional to the selenium content of the soil. Thus, plant foods, cereals, fish and meat are rich in selenium.

Recommended Daily Allowances of Selenium

Daily requirement (RDA) for selenium is about 40 µg.

Manganese

Total body manganese (Mn) content of an adult man is about 10–12 mg. It is mainly concentrated in the bone, liver and kidney.

Functions of Manganese

Manganese is required for bone formation and energy metabolism. It is also a constituent of an antioxidant enzyme, which helps to prevent free radical mediated damage to cells.

- Manganese is a component of many enzymes, including glutamine synthetase, pyruvate carboxylase and mitochondrial superoxide dismutase.
- Manganese is also associated with the formation of connective and skeletal tissues, growth and reproduction, and carbohydrate and lipid metabolism.

Dietary Sources of Manganese

Nuts, whole grain cereals, legumes and leafy vegetables are good sources of manganese. Tea is also a rich source of manganese.

Recommended Daily Allowance of Manganese

Daily requirement (RDA) of manganese is about 4 mg.

Chromium

Total body chromium (Cr) content of adult men varies between 5 and 10 mg. Trivalent form of chromium (Cr^{3+}) is biologically active. An organic compound of chromium, termed **glucose tolerance factor**, potentiates the effects of insulin, may be by facilitating its binding to the cell-receptor sites. Thus, it is important in the removal of ingested glucose.

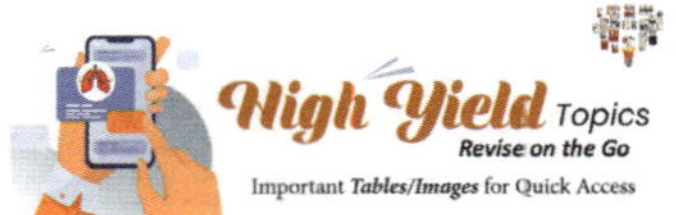

Functions of Chromium

- Chromium potentiates insulin action and as such influences carbohydrates, lipid and protein metabolism.
- As a glucose tolerance factor (GTF), chromium regulates the synthesis of a molecule that potentiates insulin action.
- It is also required in the regulation of gene expression.

Dietary Sources of Chromium

Sources of chromium include meat, nuts, cereal grains, Brewer's yeast and molasses. Besides mushroom, black pepper, meat (liver) and cheese are also good sources of chromium.

Recommended Daily Allowances of Chromium

Daily requirement (RDA) of chromium is about 50 µg.

Molybdenum

Adult human body contains nearly 5 mg of molybdenum (Mo). Liver and kidney contain large amount of it.

Functions of Molybdenum

Molybdenum is a prosthetic group for several enzymes, such as xanthine oxidase, aldehyde oxidase and sulfite oxidase, which catalyze oxidation-reduction reactions. Sulfite oxidase is also important in the degradation of cysteine and methionine, and catalyzes the formation of sulfate from sulfite.

Dietary Sources of Molybdenum

Pulses, cereals, green leafy vegetables and meat are good sources of molybdenum.

Recommended Daily Allowances of Molybdenum

Daily requirement (RDA) for molybdenum is about 100–200 µg.

Cobalt

Adult human body contains 2–3 mg of cobalt. It is mainly present in the liver and kidneys.

Functions of Cobalt

Cobalt is a component of vitamin B_{12} (cobalamin), which is essential for the maturation of red blood cells and for the normal functioning of all cells.

Dietary Sources of Cobalt

Liver meat is a rich source of cobalt.

Recommended Daily Allowances of Cobalt

Requirement (RDA) of cobalt is 1–2 µg/day.

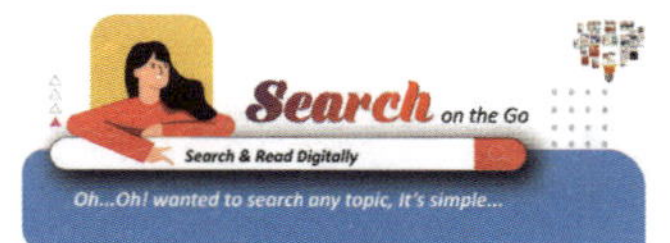

Recommended daily allowances, dietary sources, functions and deficiency diseases of different minerals are shown in Table 17.1.

TABLE 17.1: Recommended daily allowances for adults, dietary sources, functions and deficiency diseases of minerals

Minerals	Recommended daily allowances*	Dietary sources	Functions	Deficiency diseases
Calcium	1000 mg	Milk and milk products, eggs, dry fruits, legumes, cabbage and cauliflower	Calcification of bones and teeth, blood coagulation, cofactor for adenylate cyclase. Ca^{2+}-ATPase, and protein kinases	Rickets in children and osteomalacia in adults
Phosphorus	1000 mg	Milk and milk products, eggs, meat, legumes and cereals	Calcification of bones and teeth, component of nucleic acids, regulation of blood pH and activator for enzymes involved in phosphorylation/ dephosphorylation	Neural, muscular, skeletal, hematological and renal abnormalities
Sodium	2 g	Common salt	Water and electrolyte balance	
Potassium	3.5 g	Fruits, vegetables and dairy products	Acid-base balance	Cardiac arrhythmia
Magnesium	370–440 mg	Whole grain cereals, potatoes and seafoods	Cofactor for various ATP-dependent enzymes required in the synthesis of fatty acids and proteins, phosphorylation of glucose and its derivatives in the glycolytic pathways and transketolase reactions	Tremors, muscle spasms, personality changes, anorexia, nausea and vomiting, tetany, convulsions and coma
Iron	19–29 mg	Meat, fish, eggs, green-leafy vegetables, cereals and legumes	Component of heme and nonheme proteins, such as hemoglobin, catalase and cytochromes	Iron deficiency anemia, reduced work capacity and immunocompetence
Zinc	13–17 mg	Meat, seafoods, eggs legumes and milk	Cofactor for various enzymes that participate in reactions involving either synthesis or degradation of carbohydrates, lipids, proteins and nucleic acids	Short stature, hypogonadism, mild anemia and reduced immune functions
Copper	1.5–1.7 mg	Nuts, leafy vegetables, dried legumes, egg-yolk, fish and liver meat	Component of several enzymes, such as cytochrome oxidase, ferroxidase (ceruloplasmin), tyrosinase, ascorbic acid oxidase and superoxide dismutase	Anemia, neutropenia, skeletal abnormalities and Menke's syndrome

Contd...

Minerals	Recommended daily allowances*	Dietary sources	Functions	Deficiency diseases
Iodine	140 µg	Drinking water, iodized salt, sea-foods, fruits, vegetables, cereals and meat	Synthesis of iodine-containing hormones (T3 and T4), regulation of BMR in adults, growth and development in children	Endemic goiter and cretinism
Fluoride	2–3 mg	Drinking water and tea	Development of tooth enamel and as antibacterial agent	Dental caries and osteoporosis
Selenium	40 µg	Plant-foods, cereals, fish and meat	Component of selenoproteins, such as glutathione peroxidase and selenoprotein-P	Liver necrosis
Manganese	4 mg	Nuts, whole grain cereals, legumes and leafy-vegetables	Component of many enzymes, such as glutamine synthetase, pyruvate carboxylase and superoxide dismutase	Sterility, skeletal abnormalities and ataxia in offspring
Chromium	50 µg	Brewer's yeast, mushroom, black pepper, liver, whole grains, nuts and cheese	Potentiates insulin action and influences carbohydrate, lipid and protein metabolism	Insulin resistance and lipid abnormalities
Molybdenum	100–200 µg	Pulses, cereals, green-leafy vegetables and meat	Component of enzymes, such as xanthine oxidase, aldehyde oxidase and sulfite oxidase	Mental changes, abnormalities of sulfur and purine metabolism
Cobalt	1–2 µg	Food from the animal origin	Component of vitamin B_{12}	Macrocytic anemia and pernicious anemia

*ICMR-NIN (2020)

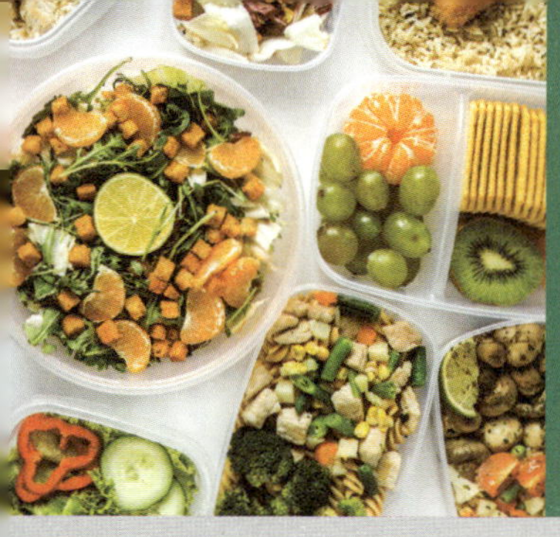

STUDENT ASSIGNMENT

LONG AND SHORT ANSWER QUESTIONS

1. **Describe dietary sources and functions of:**
   a. Sodium
   b. Potassium
   c. Calcium
   d. Magnesium
   e. Iron
   f. Phosphorus
   g. Zinc
2. **Write short notes on:**
   a. Major minerals
   b. Trace elements

MULTIPLE CHOICE QUESTIONS

1. **Which mineral is essential for the formation of healthy bones and teeth?**
   a. Iron
   b. Zinc
   c. Calcium
   d. Magnesium

2. **What is a good dietary source of potassium?**
   a. Red meat
   b. Bananas
   c. Cheese
   d. White bread

3. **Which mineral is important for the proper functioning of enzymes in the body?**
   a. Iodine
   b. Copper
   c. Phosphorus
   d. Selenium

4. **What is the function of iron in the body?**
   a. Helps in blood clotting
   b. Supports immune function
   c. Aids in energy production
   d. Regulates fluid balance

Notes

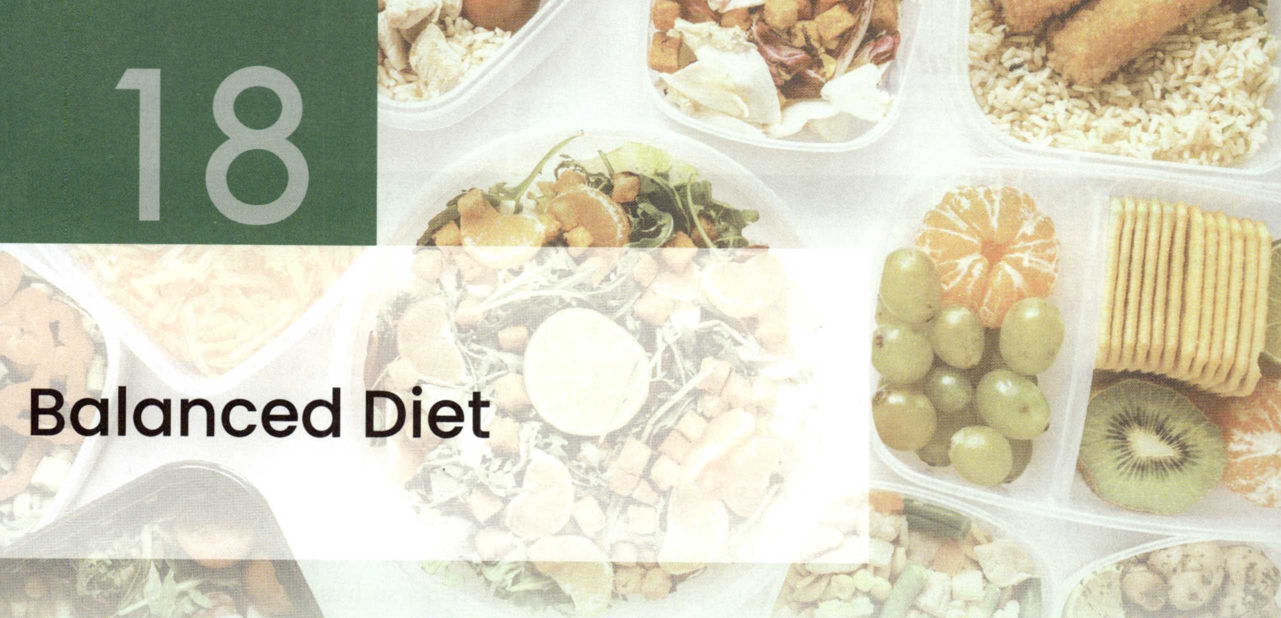

18

Balanced Diet

KEY TERMS

Antioxidants: Compounds that inhibit oxidation, a chemical reaction that can produce free radicals. Free radicals may play a part in cancer, heart disease, stroke, and other diseases of aging.

Essential nutrients: Ones that cannot be synthesized by the body and, therefore, must be supplied from foods. These nutrients are essential for normal body functions and for growth.

Food exchange system: Refers to the food items on a particular list which may be substituted with any other food item on the same list.

Highly processed food: These foods go through multiple processes (extrusion, molding, milling, etc.), contain many added ingredients and are highly manipulated. Examples are soft drinks, chips, chocolate.

Protective food: Vitamin and mineral-rich foods.

INTRODUCTION

A balanced diet is defined as the diet that contains all the food constitutes in proper proportion to meet the energy and nutritional requirements of the individual. The components of a balanced diet will vary depending on age, sex, physiological needs such as pregnancy and lactation, and nature of physical activity. In addition, a balanced diet ought to offer bioactive phytochemicals like dietary fiber, antioxidants and nutraceuticals that have positive health advantages. While designing the quality and quantity of a balanced diet, the total calories are distributed among three classes of food in the following proportion:

1. Carbohydrates (the energy yielding substances): 50–70%
2. Fats (to yield energy and act as insulating materials): 20–30%
3. Proteins (to act as building materials, and bear the wear and tear of the body): 10–15%

    In addition, a balanced diet should also provide other non-nutrients, such as **dietary fiber**, **antioxidants** and **phytochemicals**, which have positive health benefits.

    - **Dietary fiber**, includes complex carbohydrates, such as those obtained from whole grains, fruits, vegetables, beans and legumes. They are low or moderate in calories, and are devoid of refined grains and sugar. Dietary fiber promotes healthy bowel movement and decreases the risk of chronic diseases, such as coronary heart disease and diabetes.
    - **Antioxidants**, such as vitamins C and E, beta-carotene, riboflavin and selenium, protect the body from free radical damage. Spices, like turmeric, ginger, garlic, cumin and cloves, are rich in antioxidants.
    - **Phytochemicals**, such as polyphenols, flavones, etc., also afford protection against oxidative damage.

A balanced diet is good for our physical and mental health. Sometimes we eat because we enjoy the taste and experience of different foods. Sharing food and meals are also important social events. But other than for pleasure, we need food to get nutrients, vitamins, minerals and energy. Very few foods are either all good or all bad. By having an idea of the balance in our diet, it should be easier to enjoy food and be healthy.

PRINCIPLES IN PLANNING A BALANCED DIET

Balanced diet is planned according to the kinds of food produced in the region, economic capacity, religion, customs, taste and habit of the people.

- **According to kinds of food produced:** Planning a balanced diet, according to kinds of food produced, should be aimed that the diet must contain various groups of foodstuffs such as **energy yielding foods**, **body building foods** and **protective foods** in the correct proportions.
    - **Energy yielding foods:** Energy yielding foods should include foods from different groups:
        - This group contains high carbohydrates and also pure fats and carbohydrates. **They are divided into two groups:**
            i. Cereals, roots and tubers
            ii. Pure carbohydrates and fats.
        - Cereals provide proteins, certain minerals and vitamins in addition to energy in the diets of the low-income groups.
        - Roots and tubers provide some amounts of proteins, minerals and vitamins.
        - Pure carbohydrates and fats provide only energy.

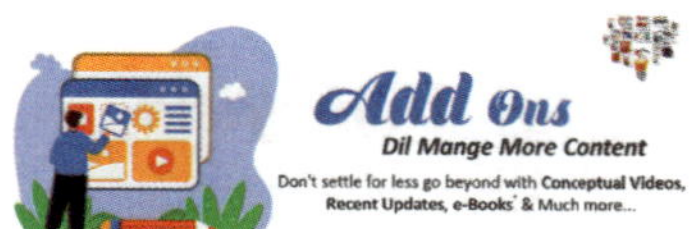

- **Body building foods:** These contain high protein and are divided into two groups:
    i. Milk, egg, meat and fish
    ii. Pulses, oilseeds and nuts.
- **Protective foods:** The protective foods are rich in proteins, vitamins and minerals. These are classified into two groups:
    i. Foods rich in vitamins, minerals and proteins of high biologic value, e.g., milk, egg, fish and liver.
    ii. Foods rich in certain vitamins and minerals only, e.g., green-leafy vegetables and some fruits.
- **According to economic capacity:** According to economic capacity, balanced diet may be planned for **high cost**, **moderate cost** or **low cost**, as follows:
  - **Balanced diets at high cost:** Balanced diets at high cost may include large amounts of costly foods such as milk, eggs, meat, fish and fruits, and moderate quantities of cereals, pulses, nuts and fats.
  - **Balanced diets at moderate cost:** Balanced diets at moderate cost may include moderate amounts of milk, egg, meat, fish, fruits, fat, and large amounts of cereals, pulses, nuts and green-leafy vegetables.
  - **Balanced diets at low cost:** Balanced diets at low cost may include small amounts of milk, egg, meat, fish, fat, and large amounts of cereals, pulses, nuts and green-leafy vegetables.

Points to be Considered in Planning a Balanced Diet for Indians

For planning the balanced diets, following points should be considered:
- For all nutrients, minimum RDA must be met. For energy, the total calories can be RDA ± 50. Energy derived from cereals should not be >75%. It is better to include two cereals in one meal, like rice and wheat, or millets and rice. Whole grain cereals, par-boiled grains or malted grains give higher nutritive value. Flour should not be sieved, as it reduces bran content. Minimize the use of refined cereals, like white flour (maida).
- Variety of foods should be used in the menu. No single food has all the nutrients. Ideally, each meal should consist of all the food groups.
- To improve the protein quality from plant sources, ratio of proteins from cereals to pulses should be nearly, 4:1. In terms of the grains, it may be eight parts of cereals and one part of pulses. Two to three servings of pulses should be taken every day. Germinated pulses are more nutritious. One egg can be served along with cereals and pulses, to improve the quality of proteins. Alternatively, one serving of poultry/fish can be included.
- Choose a diet low in fat, particularly, saturated fat, trans fat and cholesterol. Nearly, 15–20% of the total calories (energy) should be derived from fat and oils, and 5% from sugar and jaggery. It is better to use more than one type of oil. Combination of oils should be there to have proper balance of ω-3 and ω-6 fatty acids. Fried food should not be planned, even if oil allowance is less, or in low calories diets.
- Food rich in fiber should be included in the diet. Green-leafy vegetables should be taken more than one serving. For this purpose, colored vegetables and fruits should be preferred. Five servings of colorful fruits and vegetables should be included in a day's diet to meet the requirement of antioxidants.
- Every meal should contain at least one medium size raw fruit. Taking juice out of it may cause loss of some nutrients, like vitamin C.
- About two glasses of low-fat milk should be included. Curd should be consumed to provide probiotics.
- Use salt and sugar in moderation.

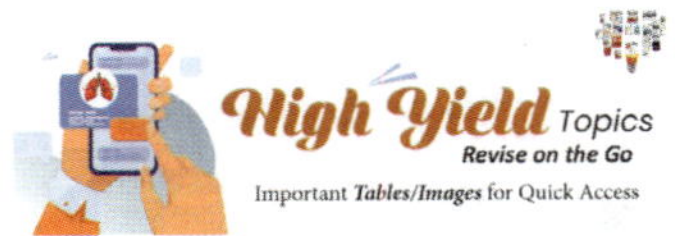

- Water should be taken in adequate quantity.
- Usually, the number of meals should be four. For very young children and patients, number of meals can be more.
- One-third of the nutritional requirement, at least for calories and proteins, should be met by lunch and dinner.
- For quick calculations, food exchange list can be used. If possible, meals should be planned, at a time, for several days.
- Use processed and ready to eat foods only judiciously, since processed food contains a variety of food additives.
- To children and patients, whose nutritional requirements are high, supplementary foods can be given.

Steps to Choose a Balanced Diet

A balanced diet does not mean giving up or cutting out our favorite foods, but choosing a balance of foods that are important to eat from a wide variety of different foods each day. **The important factors are:**

- **Energy value:** The average caloric requirement of an adult male and female should be met by the food provided daily.
- **Quality and quantity of the constituents of food:**
  - **Primary foods (proteins, fats and carbohydrates):** Proteins, fats and carbohydrates are, generally, consumed in the ratio of 1:1:4. Further, it is advised that 10–15% of the total calories should be obtained from protein, 20–30% from fat and 50–70% from carbohydrate.
  - **Secondary foods (vitamins and minerals):** These are essential in the diet but in very minute quantities to enable utilization of primary foods.
  - **Water:** Although water is not a food, it is ordinarily consumed in the diet and serves a prime role in the health of the body. Hence, it is one of the components of food.
- **Variation in the diet:** There is a risk of missing some essential elements or vitamins in a varied diet.
- **Digestibility of the food:** The food is of no use if it is not digested in the alimentary canal. Digestibility is more concerned with absorbability. When fats and starch are largely used, vegetables and animal proteins are not absorbed. Absorption is enhanced with a mixed diet when the substance is taken alone.
- **Cooking:** Food consistency is considerably changed on cooking. Harmful organisms are destroyed. Cooking breaks down the connective tissue fibers of meat and makes meat easier to masticate, and helps in the digestion. Overcooking shrinks the coagulated protein and decreases the digestibility.

  Cooking also increases water content and digestibility of vegetables. Cellulose frame work is loosened and starch from starch grains is liberated. Fats are not changed much upon cooking. Cooking enhances the flavor of the food. However, B-vitamins and vitamin C are destroyed when vegetables are cooked.
- **Psychological factors:** Appetite is reduced by worry and anxiety. Digestion is also upset due to imperfect mastication and secretion of digestive juices. Consumption of food is increased while taken in pleasant surroundings and good company with different items.
- **Cost:** Dietary food is much influenced by family income. When the income is good, consumption is high with all the protective foods. A poor income has poor protective foods. Lowest income group having low protective foods suffer from rickets and nutritional anemia. They are less resistant to infectious diseases.

  Based upon the above factors, it has been suggested that a balanced diet should contain proteins (70 g), fats (50 g), carbohydrates (440 g), calcium (0.8 g), phosphorus (1.4 g), iron (40 mg), vitamin A

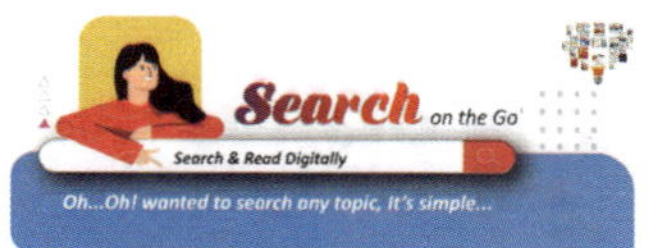

(1300 IU), vitamin B$_1$ (1.8 mg) and vitamin C (200 mg). In addition to this, 2–3 L of water and other elements must be included in the daily diet.

Essential nutrients, approximate percentage of daily calories intake, their functions and sources for a healthy balanced diet are shown in Table 18.1.

TABLE 18.1: Essential nutrients and approximate percentage of daily calories intake, their functions and sources for a healthy balanced diet

Nutrients	% of daily calories intake*	Functions	Sources
Carbohydrates	55–60%	Provide energy	Grains (both, refined and unrefined) such as wheat, maize, corn, millet, oats, rice, flour, pasta, noodles; potatoes; sweet potatoes, and fruits
Protein	10–15%	Tissue growth and maintenance	Meat, fish, nuts, eggs, beans and pulses
Fat	20–30%	Energy, essential fatty acids, fat soluble vitamins	Nuts, oilseeds, vegetable oils, dairy products (milk, cheese, etc.)
Fiber	15 g/1000 kcal	Regulates blood sugar levels and bowel health	Peas, beans, vegetables, fruits, whole grain cereals
Vitamins and minerals		Regulation of metabolism and other biochemical functions	Specific to each vitamin/mineral. Fruits and vegetables, lean meat, nuts and whole grain cereals
Water		For maintaining hydration and regulation of body temperature	Drinking water and beverages. About 20% of water intake comes from food

*ICMR-NIN (2020)

FOOD GUIDE

A balanced diet, as discussed above, should contain all the nutrients, i.e., carbohydrates, proteins, fat, vitamins, minerals and water, which are essential for daily life. To meet the requirement of all the nutrients which are essential for good health, one need to eat a variety of foods that may be selected from different food groups.

A **food group** is a collection of foods that share similar nutritional properties or biological specifications. Foods are grouped together because they provide similar amounts of the key nutrients of that food group. For example, the key nutrients of the milk, yogurt, cheese and alternatives food group include calcium and protein, while the fruit group is a good source of vitamins, especially, vitamin C. Recent developments on dietary advice suggest basic four food groups.

"Dietary guidelines suggest that the nutrients must be obtained through a judicious choice and combination of a variety of foodstuffs from different food groups, as per food pyramid, also referred to as food guide pyramid (Fig. 18.1).

Food Guide Pyramid

Food guide pyramid (food pyramid) is a graphic representation of the number of servings, from the four major food groups, needed daily to form a healthful diet. The pyramid is divided into four levels of foods according to recommended consumption, i.e.:

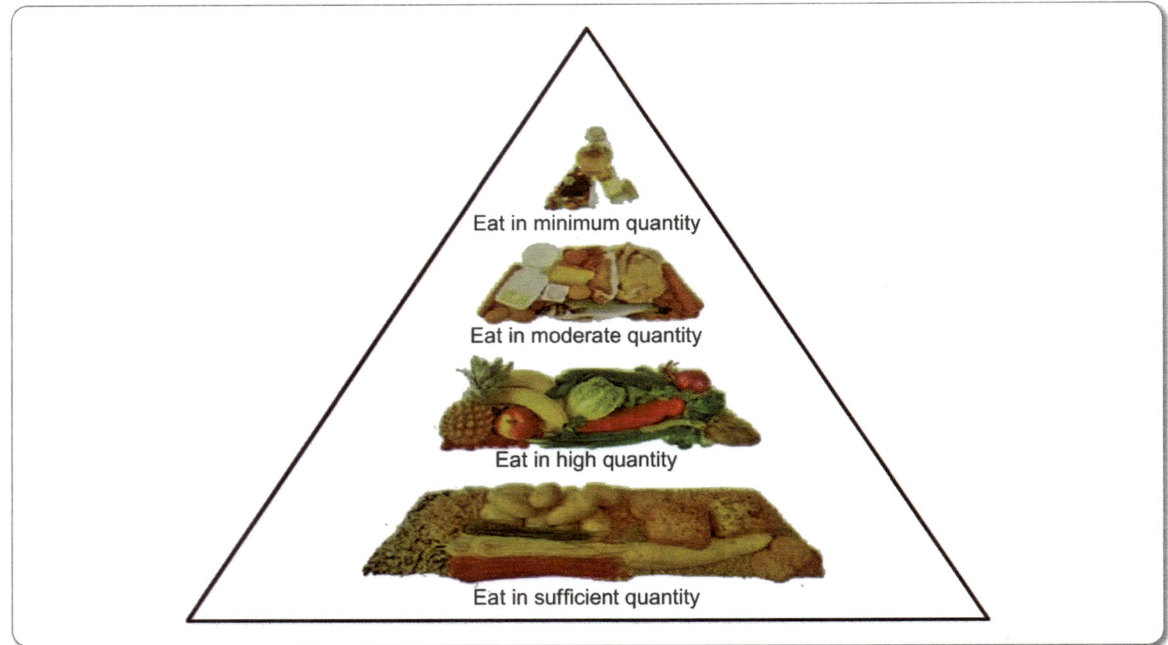

Fig. 18.1: Food pyramid

1. **At the base,** the foundation of a healthful diet is the group of **cereals and legumes/beans,** which should be eaten in sufficient quantity.

   Foods in this group are the **sources of complex carbohydrates** and provide **important vitamins, minerals and fiber.** Dietary fiber delays and retards absorption of carbohydrates and fats, and increases the satiety value. Diets rich in fiber also reduce glucose and lipids in blood, and increase the bulk of the stools. Thus, diets rich in complex carbohydrates are healthier than low-fiber diets, based on refined and processed foods.

2. **On the second level** (going up the pyramid) are **vegetables and fruits,** which should be eaten liberally. Vegetables **provide vitamins** (such as vitamin A, vitamin C and folate) and the **minerals** (like iron and magnesium) and carbohydrates, including fiber. Fruits also are good sources of vitamins A and C. Vitamins are essential for numerous body processes and for the maintenance of the structure of skin, bone, nerves, eyes, brain, blood and mucous membrane. Minerals are required for the maintenance and integrity of skin, hair, nails, blood and soft tissues. They also govern nerve cell transmission, acid/base and fluid balance, enzymes and hormones activity as well as the blood-clotting processes.

3. Next up, **on the third level,** are dairy foods along with meat and meat alternatives (e.g., nuts, eggs and legumes), i.e., **foods and oils from the animal sources,** which should be eaten moderately. Dairy products **provide proteins, vitamins** (especially, riboflavin, vitamin A and vitamin D) **and minerals** (particularly, calcium and phosphorus). Meat and meat substitutes are good sources of proteins, some of the B-vitamins, iron and zinc. Animal proteins are of high quality as they provide all the essential amino acids, in right proportions, while proteins from plants or vegetable sources are not of the same quality because of their low content of some of the essential amino acids. However, a combination of cereals, millets and pulses provides most of the amino acids, which complement the deficiencies from each other, to provide better quality protein.

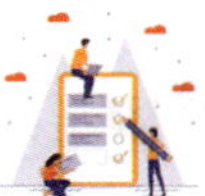
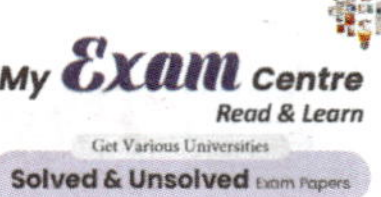

4. **The upper part** of the pyramid (at the apex) contains fats and sweets, i.e., the **highly processed foods**, which should be eaten sparingly.

   Excess of these substances could lead to obesity, diabetes, cardiovascular disease and cancer.

   Accompanying the pyramid there is also a recommendation to **do regular physical activity**, and **warnings against smoking and drinking alcohol**.

   The pyramid, thus, is an easy way to use guidelines that helps us to select a variety of foods.

BASIC FOUR FOOD GROUPS

There is no single perfect food that provides all nutritional needs for everyone. All the required nutrients (as mentioned above), which form a balanced diet, occur in very different proportions in different foods. Therefore, a variety, within each group is essential. Basic four food groups include:

1. **Cereals, millets and pulses: Cereals**, such as rice and wheat, and **millets**, like jowar, bajra, ragi, etc., are the **most widely eaten staple foods in India**.

   - These are the cheapest **sources of calories** and constitute as much as 70–80% of the calories in the diet of majority of population, in our country.
   - Most cereal grains also contain 6–12% **proteins**. In general, cereal proteins are deficient in the essential amino acid lysine. Rice protein, however, is rich in lysine, compared to other cereals.
   - Whole grain cereals are also important sources of **B-vitamins**, especially, **thiamine** and **niacin**, which are present in the outer bran layer of the grain. Excessive milling and polishing of rice removes the outer covering and, hence, decreases its thiamine content.
   - Cereal grains do not contain vitamin A, except yellow maize, which contains some amount of β-**carotene**.
   - Total fat content, in cereals, varies from 2% to 5%.
   - On an average, 400 g of cereals are consumed per person, per day, in India.
   - Commonly used legumes include grams, peas and beans.
   - Dried **pulses and legumes** are rich in **proteins** (about 19–24%). They are good sources of **lysine** and **threonine**, which are deficient in most of the cereals. Pulses are, however, poor sources of sulfur-containing amino acids.
   - **Pulses** are also good sources of several B-vitamins and minerals, such as **thiamine**, **riboflavin** and **phosphorus**.
   - Legumes, however, contain some **natural toxins**, which can be removed by soaking and normal cooking procedures. This, however, may result in loss of some B-vitamins.
   - Legumes are **good for young children**, provided these are cooked, finely mashed and mixed with other food items.
   - Germination or **sprouting increases vitamin C**, riboflavin and niacin contents of legumes.

2. **Vegetables and fruits:** Vegetables and fruits provide vitamins, minerals and fiber, they should be included in meals and snacks each day. One must choose a variety of fruits and vegetables (including of different colors, textures and flavors) to provide a wide range of vitamins and minerals.

   - **Vegetables** are broadly classified into three groups, as green-leafy vegetables, roots and tubers, and other vegetables.

     i. **Green-leafy vegetables:** Many types of green leaves, such as spinach (palak), amaranth, fenugreek leaves (methi), drumstick leaves, mint, coriander, mustard leaves, colocasia leaves, radish and

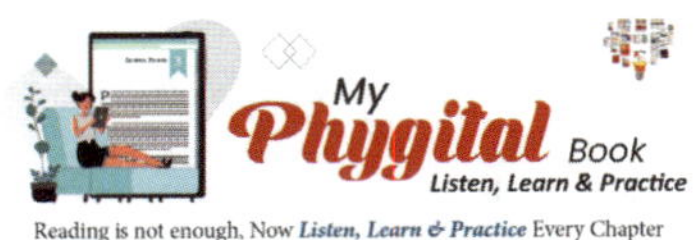

turnip leaves, and bathua, are rich sources of iron, β-carotene, vitamin C, riboflavin, folic acid and calcium. They also provide dietary fiber and antioxidants, and proteins (about 2–7%). Green-leafy vegetables, however, contain oxalic acid, which, in turn, interferes with the absorption of calcium.

ii. **Roots and tubers:** Roots and tubers, such as potatoes, sweet potatoes, carrots, etc., are good sources of starch. They also contain small amount of proteins, some B-vitamins and vitamin C. Yellow sweet potatoes and carrots are also rich sources of carotene.

iii. **Other vegetables:** These include green peas and beans, pumpkin, gourds, ladies finger, brinjal, etc. Green peas and beans are good sources of protein and some B-vitamins. They are also fair sources of vitamin C and certain minerals.

- **Fruits** are good sources of different carbohydrates, vitamins and minerals.
  - Fresh fruits are, generally, good sources of vitamins. **Amla** (gooseberry) is, especially, rich in **vitamin C.**
  - **Yellow fruits**, like mango and papaya, contain β-carotene.
  - **Dried fruits**, like dates and raisins, are rich sources of **iron.**
  - Banana is rich in carbohydrates. Some fruits contain glucose, while others contain fructose or pentose.
  - Most of the fruits are also good sources of potassium.
  - Fruits also contain pectins, which provide bulk to the diet and help in bowel movement.
  - Drying of fruits results in loss of carotene. Other procedures cause loss of thiamine. Canning of fruit juices results in loss of vitamin C.

3. **Milk and milk products**, **eggs**, **meat and fish:**
- **Milk and milk products:** Milk is either used as such or in the preparation of several products, such as curd, cheese, ice-cream, butter, ghee and a variety of sweets.
  - **Milk is an ideal food for infants and children**. It is also a good supplementary food for adults. Milk contains **good quality proteins** (3.2–4.3%). It is also rich in **calcium** and several other nutrients in proper proportions, and, thus, milk is considered to be a complete food. Milk is, however, deficient in vitamin C and iron. Composition of milk varies widely, from its source. For example, human milk contains more lactose, while buffalo milk contains more fat.
  - Milk, yoghurt and cheese are the most common dairy foods, and main dietary sources of calcium. Having enough calcium is important for healthy bones and teeth. Full-cream, milk is recommended for children aged one to two years, while reduced-fat plain milk is suitable for adults.
  - Pasteurization of milk results in loss of vitamin C, while prolonged boiling results in loss of thiamine, vitamin B_6 and vitamin B_{12}.
- **Eggs and poultry:** Eggs contain about 13% **proteins** and 13% fat. Egg proteins are good sources of **all essential amino acids** and have high nutritive value. Egg is also a rich source of **vitamin A** and **some B-vitamins**. Egg, however, does not contain vitamin C and is a poor source of calcium. Egg consists of egg white and egg yolk.
  - **Egg white** contains about 11% proteins, mainly **albumin**. Besides, egg white is also a good source of **riboflavin** but devoid of fat and vitamin A. Raw egg white also contains a heat labile factor, called **avidin**, which binds biotin and makes it unavailable.
  - **Egg yolk** contains about 15% of **proteins** and 30% of **fat**. It is a rich source of **riboflavin, vitamin A, iron** and **phosphorus**. Egg yolk is also rich in **cholesterol**. It is used as a supplement to the diet of infants.
  - **Poultry meat** is a good source of proteins, containing all essential amino acids.

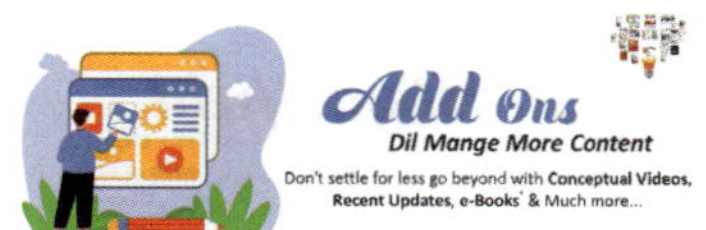

- **Meat and fish:** This group includes red meat (such as beef and lamb), white meat (such as pork and chicken) and fish. They are rich in proteins, iron and zinc.
    - **Meat: Proteins** content of flesh foods is around 20%. Meat is also a good source of several B-vitamins and minerals, particularly, **vitamin B_{12}, iron** and **phosphorus**. Flesh foods, generally, are not good sources of vitamin A with the exception of liver, which is very rich in **vitamin A**.
    - **Fish:** Fish contains **polyunsaturated fatty acids** (PUFA), which protect us against cardiovascular diseases. Fish is also rich in **proteins**, but a fair source of B-vitamins. Fatty fish also contains **vitamin A** and **vitamin D**. Small fishes are good source of **calcium**, since these are eaten with bones. Large fishes are rich in **phosphorus**.
    Canning of meat and poultry results in loss of various B-vitamins, particularly, thiamine.

4. **Oils and fats, and nuts and oilseeds:**
    - **Oils and fats:** Oils and fats are the main sources of **energy** as well as **essential fatty acids** and **fat soluble vitamins**.
        - **Fats of animal origin** contain **cholesterol**, but are a poor source of vitamin E and essential fatty acids.
        - On the other hand, **fats of vegetable origin** such as sunflower oil, soybeans oil, cottonseed oil, etc., are a good source of essential fatty acids and vitamin E.
        - **Frying destroys vitamin A**, vitamin E and essential fatty acids.
        - **Rancidity** results in the formation of peroxides, which, in turn, affect intestinal flora and have irritating effects on the intestine.
    - **Nuts and oilseeds:** Nuts and oilseeds such as peanut, groundnut, soybean and oilseeds, are rich sources of **proteins**. They contain about 18–40% protein. They are also rich sources of **fat**, several **B-vitamins** and **vitamin E**.
        - **Groundnut** contains about 20–30% **proteins** and 40–50% **fat**. Though limiting in lysine, threonine and methionine, groundnut is a good source of **thiamine, niacin, pantothenic acid** and **phosphorus**. When harvested under moist conditions, groundnut may get contaminated with *Aspergillus flavus*, which may produce aflatoxin. Roasting destroys trypsin inhibitors and improves its nutritive value.
        - **Soybeans** contain nearly 35–45% **proteins** and 15–20% **fat**. Soybean proteins are good sources of all **essential amino acids** except methionine. It is also a good source of **thiamine** and **niacin**. Soybean, however, contains hemagglutinins and trypsin, and certain growth inhibitors, which can be inactivated by pressure-cooking. Soybean is mainly used in soy-flour, milk substitutes and infant foods.

RECOMMENDED DIETARY ALLOWANCES

The recommended dietary allowance (**RDA**) is the average daily dietary intake level that is sufficient to meet the nutrient requirement of nearly all (97–98%) healthy individuals in a particular gender and life stage group (life stage considers age and, when applicable, pregnancy or lactation).

The RDAs are the levels of intake of essential nutrients that, on the basis of scientific knowledge, are judged by the Food and Nutrition Board to be adequate to meet the known nutrient needs of practically all healthy persons. RDA is neither minimal requirement nor necessarily optimal level of intake, rather, RDA is the safe and adequate level, which incorporates margin of safety, intended to be sufficiently generous to encompass the presumed variability in requirements among individuals and meet the needs of almost all healthy people, in a given population.

RDA for Indians

Dietary Recommendations for Indians

In India, first attempt to define nutrient requirements and desirable dietary intakes of nutrients for Indians to maintain good health **was made by** the Nutrition Advisory Committee of the Indian Research Fund Association, now **Indian Council of Medical Research** (ICMR) **in 1944**.

- Thereafter, **in the wake of reports by** the Food and Agriculture Organization (**FAO**) **on energy and protein**, **requirements for these were revised** by the Committee **in 1958**.
- Subsequently, the Committee **revised requirements for all the nutrients except energy in 1968 and 1978**.
- Further, based on the international data provided by FAO/WHO/UNU 2004 expert committee, the ICMR **Committee further revised and upgraded** the required dietary allowances **(RDA)** recommendations for Indians **in 2010**.

  At this stage, the Committee, however, derived only the RDA and not the estimated average requirement (EAR).

  - **Recently**, the Indian Council of Medical Research-National Institute of Nutrition (ICMR-NIN) Expert Group has further **revised and defined nutrient distribution and requirements** for normal individuals of all age and physiological groups along with the different physical activity groups of Indian population **in 2020**.

    The Group has given recommendations for all the nutrients including **energy, carbohydrates, dietary fiber, fats and oils, proteins, fat soluble vitamins** (vitamins A, D, E and K), **water soluble vitamins** (Vitamin B complex, i.e., thiamine, riboflavin, niacin, pantothenic acid, pyridoxine, biotin, folate and cyanocobalamin, and vitamin C), **minerals** (calcium and phosphorus, iron, magnesium, sodium and potassium, zinc, copper, chromium, manganese, selenium and iodine), **water** and **antioxidants.**

General Considerations to Estimate Nutrient Requirements for Indians

ICMR-NIN (2020) Expert Group considered following points for giving its recommendations of various nutrients for Indians:

- **Recent data on energy expenditure and protein metabolism**
- **Available data on minerals and vitamins losses**, and **absorption**.
- In order to derive a single value for the requirement of various nutrients, the group **used two features of the distribution of requirements**, i.e., either the median of the distribution of requirements (referred to as **estimated average requirement,** EAR) or the 97.5th percentile of the distribution (called **recommended daily allowance,** RDA).
- **Requirements** of various nutrients **have been suggested for different age** and **physiological categories, based on sex, body weight** and **physical activity level.**

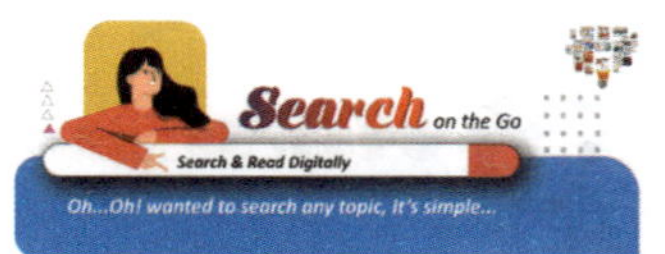

- Taking several factors into consideration, **energy requirements** have been **calculated with respect to the BMR values for normal healthy individuals** and have been **expressed in terms of kcal/day**.
- **Carbohydrate intake** has been suggested **based on the minimum level of glucose required for utilization by the brain** and has been expressed **in grams per day**.
- For the first time, the group has recommended the **requirement of dietary fiber. Based on energy intake**, the **safe intake of dietary fiber** has been suggested **in grams per day**.
- We know that **fat provides essential fatty acids** and **is necessary for** the **absorption of fat-soluble vitamins.**

  The group has suggested the **upper limit for visible fat intake in grams per day.** Further, it is also recommended that **a minimum of 20% of the dietary energy should be derived from fat**, out of which **10%** of the dietary energy should be **from visible fat**. The group further suggested that as a source of visible fat, a **correct combination of oils should be used.**
- The group has calculated the **protein requirement** according to the value of net-protein utilization (NPU) of dietary proteins **by taking the NPU values of the mixed vegetable proteins** contained in Indian diets and the safe intake has been expressed in grams per day. **This is due to the reason** that although, both, animal foods (milk, meat, fish and eggs) and plant foods (pulses and legumes) are rich sources of proteins, the **animal proteins are of high quality** (as they provide all the essential amino acids and in right proportions) **compared to the proteins from the** plant or **vegetable sources** (which are not of the same quality because of low contents of some of the essential amino acids). But **a combination of proteins from cereals, millets and pulses provides all the essential amino acids**, i.e., they **complement each other so as to provide better quality protein.**

  So, **to define protein requirement the Group has introduced** a newer protein quality index referred to as **Digestible Indispensable Amino Acid Score** (DIAAS).

  Further, RDA for protein has been suggested based on body weight and varies for different age categories.
- **RDA for vitamins B_1, B_2, niacin, pantothenic acid, vitamin B_6 and vitamin C** have been **expressed in mg** (milligrams) per day; for **biotin, folate, vitamin B_{12} and vitamin A in µg/day**; while for **vitamin D in IU** (international units) per day.

  Further, **RDA for niacin has been calculated in terms of niacin equivalent (NE)** by taking into account the **contribution of tryptophan** and assuming that 60 mg of tryptophan forms 1 mg of niacin in the body.

  RDA **for folate** has been given **in terms of** the **dietary folate equivalent** (DFE).

  The Group has also suggested that **vitamin B_{12} is derived, entirely, from the foods of the animal origin.**

  The requirement for **vitamin A has been expressed in terms of retinol equivalents (RE)**, considering a **conversion factor of 12:1 for α-carotene** and **6:1 for β-carotene**.

  Based on the consumption of extra calories, additional requirements for vitamins B_1, B_2 and B_6 have been suggested during pregnancy and lactation.
- **RDA for calcium, phosphorus, magnesium, sodium, potassium, iron, zinc, copper** and **manganese** are expressed **in mg (milligrams)/day** while for **chromium, selenium and iodine in µg** (micrograms) per day.

  Due to the increasing incidence of hypertension, intake of sodium has been recommended as safe intake.

RDA for iron has been suggested **based on the consideration that nearly 8% of iron is absorbed from food** in healthy adults, and **menstrual losses in women** during the reproductive age.

- **RDA during pregnancy and lactation has been suggested as additional intakes**. This requirement is **over and above** the **normal requirement of the nonpregnant adult women**.
- **For infants and children**, RDA values for energy, protein, iron, thiamine, riboflavin and niacin have been **expressed in terms of per kg body weight per day**.
- **Total water requirement** has been suggested **based on energy requirement** (estimated average ratio, 2020) **and the WHO guidelines of 1.5 mL/kcal ingested**.

ICMR–NIN 2020 Dietary Recommendations for Indians

As per recommendations of the ICMR-NIN (2020), RDA for Indians for various nutrients, for different age and sex groups are shown in Tables 18.2 to 18.4.

TABLE 18.2: RDA of macronutrients for Indians (ICMR-NIN, 2020)

Population/group	Category of worker/period	Carbohydrates (g)	Dietary fiber* (g)	Visible fat (g)	Protein (g)
Adult men (18+)	Sedentary	100	30	25	
	Moderate	100	40	30	54
	Heavy	100	50	40	
Adult women (18+)	Sedentary	100	25	20	
	Moderate	100	30	25	46
	Heavy	100	40	30	
Pregnant women	2nd trimester	135		30	(+) 9.5
	3rd trimester	135		30	(+) 22
Lactating women	0–6 months	155		30	(+) 16.9
	7–12 months	155		30	(+) 13.2
Infants	0–6 months**	55*			8
	7–12 months	95*		25	10.5
Children	1–3 years	100	15	25	12.5
	4–6 years	100	20	25	16
	7–9 years	100	26	30	23
Adolescents	Boys 10–12 years	100	33	35	32
	Boys 13–15 years	100	43	45	45
	Boys 16–18 years	100	50	50	55
	Girls 10–12 years	100	30	35	33
	Girls 13–15 years	100	36	40	43
	Girls 16–18 years	100	38	35	46

* EAR

** = AI

TABLE 18.3: RDA of vitamins for Indians (ICMR-NIN, 2020)

Population/ group	Category of worker/period	Thiamine (mg)	Riboflavin (mg)	Niacin (mg)	Pantothenic acid* (mg)	Pyridoxine (mg)	Biotin* (µg)	Folate* (µg)	B12 (µg)	Vitamin C (mg)	Vitamin A (µg)	Vitamin D (IU)
Adult men (18+)	Sedentary	1.4	2	14	5	1.9	25	300	2.2	80	1000	600
	Moderate	1.8	2.5	18	5	2.4	25	300	2.2	80	1000	600
	Heavy	2.3	3.2	23	5	3.1	25	300	2.2	80	1000	600
Adult women (18+)	Sedentary	1.4	1.9	11	5	1.9	25	220	2.2	65	840	600
	Moderate	1.7	2.4	14	5	1.9	25	220	2.2	65	840	600
	Heavy	2.2	3.1	18	5	2.4	25	220	2.2	65	840	600
Pregnant women	2nd trimester	2	2.7	(+) 2	5	2.3	25	570	(+) 0.25	(+) 15	900	600
	3rd trimester	2	2.7	(+) 2	5	2.3	25	570	(+) 0.25	(+) 15	900	600
Lactating women	0–6 months	2.1	3	(+) 5	(+) 2	(+) 0.26	(+) 5	330	(+) 1	(+) 50	950	600
	7–12 months	2.1	2.9	(+) 5	(+) 2	(+) 0.17	(+) 5	330	(+) 1	(+) 50	950	600
Infants	0–6 months*	0.2*	0.4*	2*	2	0.1*	4	25*	1.2	20*	350*	400*
	7–12 months	0.4*	0.6*	5*	2	0.6*	5	85	1.2	30*	350	400*
Children	1–3 years	0.7	1.1	7	2	0.9	7	120	1.2	30	390	600
	4–6 years	0.9	1.3	9	3	1.2	9	135	2.2	35	510	600
	7–9 years	1.1	1.6	11	4	1.5	12	170	2.2	45	630	600
Adolescents	Boys 10–12 years	1.5	2.1	15	5	2	15	220	2.2	55	770	600
	Girls 10–12 years	1.4	1.9	14	5	1.9	16	225	2.2	50	790	600
	Boys 13–15 years	1.9	2.7	19	5	2.6	20	285	2.2	70	930	600
	Girls 13–15 years	1.6	2.2	16	5	2.2	20	245	2.2	65	890	600
	Boys 16–18 years	2.2	3.1	22	5	3	25	340	2.2	85	1000	600
	Girls 16–18 years	1.7	2.3	17	5	2.3	25	270	2.2	70	860	600

*Adequate intake

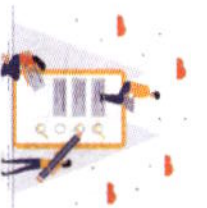

TABLE 18.4: RDA of minerals for Indians (ICMR-NIN, 2020)

Population/ group	Category of worker/period	Calcium (mg)	Phospho-rus (mg)	Magnesi-um (mg)	Sodium* (mg)	Potassi-um* (mg)	Iron (mg)	Zinc (mg)	Copper (mg)	Chromi-um (µg)	Manga-nese (mg)	Seleni-um (µg)	Iodine (µg)
Adult men (18+)	Sedentary	1000	1000	440	2000	3500	19	17	1.7	50	4	40	140
	Moderate	1000	1000	440	2000	3500	19	17	1.7	50	4	40	140
	Heavy	1000	1000	440	2000	3500	19	17	1.7	50	4	40	140
Adult women (18+)	Sedentary	1000	1000	370	2000	3500	29	13	1.5	50	4	40	140
	Moderate	1000	1000	370	2000	3500	29	13	1.5	50	4	40	140
	Heavy	1000	1000	370	2000	3500	29	13	1.5	50	4	40	140
Pregnant women	2nd trimester	1000	1000	440	2000	3500	27	14.5					220
	3rd trimester	1000	1000	440	2000	3500	27	14.5					
Lactating women	0–6 months	1200	1200	400	2000	3500	23	14.1					280
	7–12 months	1200	1200	400	2000	3500	23	14.1					
Infants	0–6 months*	300**	450**	30**	500	900							100**
	7–12 months	300**	450**	75**	650	1100	3	2.5					130**
Children	1–3 years	500	500	90	1000	1750	8	3.3	0.6	22	1.8	16–18	90
	4–6 years	550	550	125	1300	2250	11	4.5	0.9	28	2.9	29–32	90
	7–9 years	650	650	175	1600	2825	15	5.9	1	31	3.6	36–42	90
Adolescents	Boys 10–12 yrs	850	850	240	2000	3500	16	8.5	1.28	36	4.7	51	100
	Girls 10–12 yrs	850	850	250	2000	3500	28	8.5	1.15	34	4.1	45	100
	Boys 13–15 yrs	1000	1000	345	2000	3500	22	14.3	1.43	41	5.1	58	140
	Girls 13–15 yrs	1000	1000	340	2000	3500	30	12.8	1.3	37	4.6	52	140
	Boys 16–18 yrs	1050	1050	440	2000	3500	26	17.6	1.8	44	6.1	71	140
	Girls 16–18 yrs	1050	1050	380	2000	3500	32	14.2	1.54	38	4.7	55	140

*Safe intake
**Adequate intake

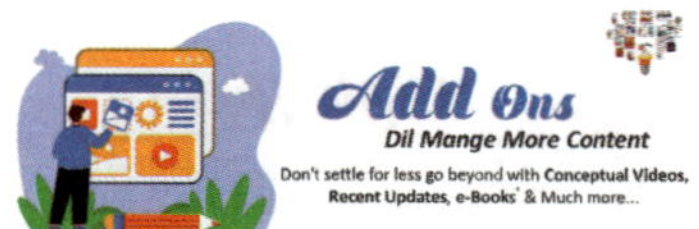

RDA for Normal Healthy Adults

Based on the recommendations of the ICMR-NIN (2020), RDA for various nutrients, for adult moderate workers are described as follows:

- **Energy: RDA for calories for adult moderate workers** has been suggested as **2710 kcal/day for males** and **2130 kcal/day for females**.

  It is further suggested that since 70–80% of the total dietary calories in India are derived from carbohydrates that are present in plant foods such as cereals, millets and pulses, the **recommendation** for **cereals and millets is 400 g** and for **pulses 80 g/day**.

- **Carbohydrates:** It is recommended that a **minimum of 100–130 g of carbohydrates should be consumed per day**.

- **Dietary fiber: Safe intake of dietary fiber** has been suggested as **15 g per 1000 kcal/day**.

- **Fats:** The **upper limit for visible fat intake for healthy adult moderate workers has been suggested as 30 g/day for males** and **25 g/day** for **females**.

- **Protein: Safe intake of protein** has been suggested as **0.83 g/kg/day**.

- **Vitamins:**

  - **Thiamin: RDA for thiamine for** adult moderate workers has been suggested as **1.8 mg/day for males** and **1.7 mg/day for females**.

  - **Riboflavin: RDA for riboflavin** for adult moderate workers has been suggested as **2.5 mg/day for males** and 2.4 mg/day for females.

  - **Niacin: RDA for niacin (NE)** for adult moderate workers has been suggested as **18 mg/day for males** and **14 mg/day for females**.

  - **Pyridoxine: RDA for pyridoxine** for adult moderate workers has been suggested as **2.5 mg/day for males** and **1.9 mg/day for females**.

  - **Folate: RDA for folate** for adult moderate worker has been suggested as **300 µg/day for males** and 220 µg/day for females.

  - **Vitamin B_{12}: RDA for vitamin B_{12}** for adult moderate male and female workers has been suggested as 2.2 µg/day.

  - **Vitamin C: RDA for vitamin C** for adult moderate workers has been suggested as **80 mg/day for males** and **65 mg/day for females**.

  - **Vitamin A: RDA for vitamin A** (RE) for adult moderate workers has been suggested as **1000 µg/day for males and 840 µg/day for females**.

- **Minerals:**

  - **Calcium** and **phosphorus:** RDA for calcium for adult moderate workers has been suggested as **1000 mg/day** for males and females.

    Additional 200 mg/day has been suggested **for women during postmenopause**.

    Similar values have been recommended for phosphorus.

  - **Magnesium: Estimated average requirement** for magnesium for adult moderate workers has been recommended as **440 mg/day for males** and **370 mg/day for females**.

  - **Sodium** and **potassium: Safe intake of sodium** has been suggested as **2000 mg/day**. Accordingly, the **salt intake** has been recommended as **5 g/day**.

    Potassium intake has been suggested as **3500 mg/day**.

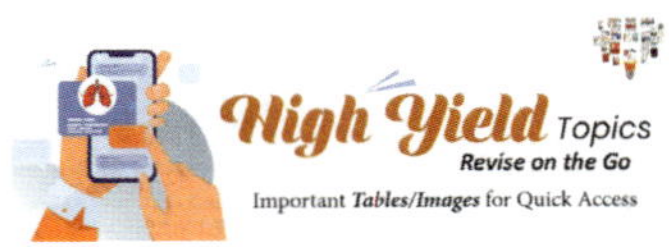

- **Iron: RDA for iron** for adult moderate workers has been suggested as **19 mg/day for males and 29 mg/day for females.**
- **Water:** Total water requirement for adult moderate workers has been suggested as 4050 mL/day for males and 3200 mL/day for females.

Limitations of RDA

Recommended daily allowances, as discussed above, are the levels of intake of essential nutrients that, on the basis of scientific knowledge are judged, by the Food and Nutrition Board, to be adequate to meet the known nutrient needs of practically all healthy persons. RDA is neither minimal requirement nor necessarily optimal level of intake, rather, RDA is the safe and adequate level, which incorporates margin of safety, intended to be sufficiently generous to encompass the presumed variability in requirements among individuals and meet the needs of almost all healthy people, in a given population. Accordingly, RDA has various limitations:

- There are variations among individuals. Nutrient requirement of an individual and the dietary allowance for a group or a population are distinctly different. RDA takes into account the variability that exists in the requirement of a given nutrient between individuals in a given population group only.
- Projections from RDA *via* corresponding balanced diets to national food supplies do enable policy decisions, but do not solve the problem of equitable distribution according to nutritional need.
- The RDA for a nutrient is a value to be used as a goal for dietary intake by healthy individuals. It is not intended to be used to assess the diets of either individuals or groups, or to plan diets for groups.
- There is no evidence to suggest that nutrients consumed at the recommended intake present a risk of adverse effects to the general population.
- The effects of nutrients from fortified foods or supplements may differ from those of naturally occurring constituents of foods because of several factors, i.e., the chemical form of the nutrient, the timing of the intake and amount consumed in a single bolus dose, the matrix supplied by the food and the relation of the nutrient to the other constituents of the diet.
- RDAs are based on limited data. They over-state the needs of most individuals and are limited to the needs of healthy people.
- The nutrient requirements of specific individuals are ordinarily unknown. Therefore, as there is no practical way of identifying whose needs are high and whose are low, RDAs should not be interpreted as requirements of specific individuals. The basis for estimating RDAs is such that even if a person habitually consumes less than the RDA, his or her diet is not necessarily inadequate. However, the farther the habitual intake falls below the RDA and the longer the low intake continues the greater is the risk of deficiency.
- The RDAs do not take into account special needs arising from infections, metabolic disorders, or chronic diseases. In addition, large doses of some nutrients may have some drug-like action.
- RDAs have not been established for all essential nutrients. RDAs are established when there is sufficient scientific evidence to recommend a specific level of consumption. Of the approximately 50 known essential nutrients, RDAs have been established for only 25. The Board states that additional nutrients may someday be proven essential. To ensure that these unrecognized nutritional needs are met, the Board recommends the RDA be provided from as varied a selection of foods as is practicable on the assumption that a varied diet will do this. However, the RDAs can serve as a guide such that a varied diet meeting RDAs will probably be adequate in all other **nutrients**.

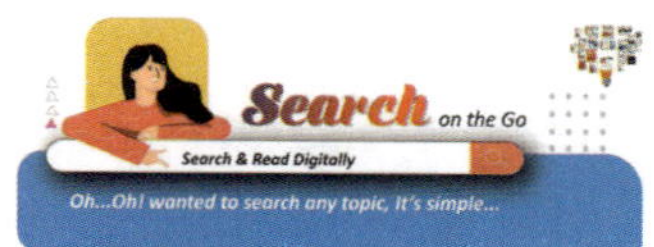

- Since the RDAs are the basis of most nutrition efforts, they must be expanded and supported by more nutrition research. There is a need to identify and to set priorities of research needs, to improve the basis and expand the coverage of the RDAs.
- There are also losses during cooking.

Uses of RDAs

The RDA represents the level of the nutrient to be consumed daily to meet all the requirements of most of the individuals in a given population. The various uses of RDAs include:
- Modifying nutrient requirements in clinical management of diseases
- To help public health nutritionists to compose diets for schools, hospitals, prisons, etc.
- For health care policy makers and public health nutritionists to design, develop nutrition intervention programs and policies
- For planning and procuring food supplies for population groups
- For evaluating the adequacy of food supplies in meeting national nutritional needs
- For interpreting food consumption records of individuals and population
- For establishing Standards for the national feeding programs implemented by the Governments for its vulnerable population
- For designing nutrition education programs for the masses
- For developing new food products and dietary supplements by the industry
- Establishing guidelines for the national labelling of packaged foods [by Food Standards Safety Authority of India (FSSAI)].

FOOD EXCHANGE SYSTEM

The food exchange system was created by the American Diabetic Association in 1950, in coordination with the American Dietetic Association and the US Public Health Services to establish guidelines to help target issues within the American eating habits. Its goal was to develop an educational tool for persons with diabetes that would provide uniformity in meal planning and allow for the inclusion of a wider variety of foods. It was again revised and republished in 2013.

The food exchange system is based on principles of good nutrition that apply to everyone and helps people learn how to eat more balanced and nutritious, while providing a wide variety of foods. The food exchange system includes six groups of food, each group of foods are placed in a food exchange list. The food exchange lists are **fruits**, **vegetables**, **milk**, **starches**, **fats**, **meats** and **meat substitutes**. The foods in each individual group have a similar amount of calories and nutrients such as carbohydrates, fat and protein. The **number of servings**, or **exchanges**, from a group that one can consume each day depends on how many calories one needs. A dietitian can help determine our nutrition needs, including total calories and proportion of carbohydrates, protein, fats that one should consume.

The food exchange system is an easy way to begin counting carbohydrates for diabetics to help them regulate their blood sugar level. For example, one chapati (approximately 20 g) provides nearly 2 g protein, 15 g carbohydrate and 70 kcal of energy. It may be exchanged with similar low glycemic index foods such as one large slice of bread or 3 table spoon of cooked rice or one idly, etc. each one of which provide nearly the same amount of protein, carbohydrates and energy. Similarly, any of the pulses or legumes, to have a variety of foods, can be exchanged with the other since 100 g of Bengal gram, black gram, green gram, red gram or horse gram, etc., each provides nearly 24 g protein, 60 g carbohydrate and 340 calories.

CALCULATION OF NUTRITIVE VALUE OF FOODS

Nutritive value of foods can be calculated by making the list of the kind and amount of every foodstuff, including sugar, butter, coffee, etc., as well as the foods that are eaten in between the meals.

Nutritive values are the averages of many samples of foods that are analyzed in laboratories. Several factors determine the nutritive value of foods, which include:

- Conditions of growing the crop
- Handling of the produce from farm to market to consumer
- Care given to the food in home
- Manner in which the food is cooked.

Average nutritive values of some of the foods are given in Table 18.5.

TABLE 18.5: Average nutritive values of some of the foods (per 100 g)*

Foodstuffs	Protein (g)	Fat (g)	Carbohydrates (g)	Calories (kcal)
Cereals	9.9	2.3	71.0	344
Bread	7.8	0.7	51.9	245
Salt biscuits	6.6	32.4	54.6	534
Sweet biscuits	6.4	15.2	71.9	450
Pulses	22.6	2.0	58.4	342
Green leafy vegetables	3.8	0.6	6.0	45
Roots and tubers	1.2	0.2	16.0	70
Other vegetables	2.2	0.3	6.3	36
Nuts and oilseeds	15.2	46.6	20.4	578
Condiments and spices	9.8	6.6	40.6	261
Fruits	1.1	0.4	7.6	79
Meat	21.0	4.9	0.8	131
Eggs	13.3	13.3	0.0	173
Milk	3.6	5.8	4.7	85
Curd	3.1	4.0	3.0	60
Butter	0.0	81.0	0.0	29
Ghee	0.0	100.0	0.0	900
Oil	0.0	100.0	0.0	900
Sugar	0.1	0.0	99.4	398
Honey	0.3	0.0	79.5	319
Jaggery	0.4	0.1	95.0	383
Sago	0.2	0.2	87.1	351

*NIN-ICMR (1998)

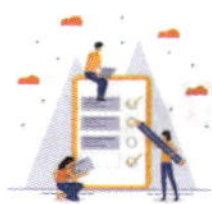
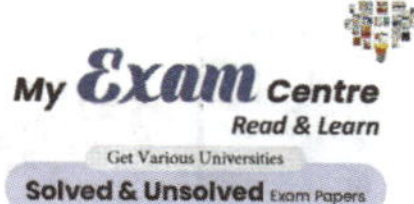

Nutritive Value of an Average Indian Diet

An average Indian diet is highly cereal-based, particularly, of the weaker economic sections, where cereals form bulk of the diet and provide 80% of the calories. They are, however, deficient in pulses, green leafy vegetables, oils and fats, and fruits. Most staple foods used are rice in Southern parts and wheat in North India. The trend of mixed cereals consumption is, however, emerging.

- These predominant cereal diets have little or no visible fats. They, however, consist of significant quantity of invisible fat, which contributes to nearly 6% energy, in an adult diet with 2400 kcal.
- These diets can be improved by eating mixed cereals or by adding coarse cereals (millets), locally grown leafy vegetables, butter milk and increased use of pulses and local fruits.
- Another improvement which can be affected, is improvement of cooking practices, e.g., not to discard cooking water. It is advisable to use minimum of water or to utilize cooking liquid in either soups or gravies.
- It is not advisable to peel and cut the vegetables long before they are ready for boiling.
- Excessive washing of rice should be avoided to save vitamin B_1 (thiamine). The rice kanji, which is strained away during cooking, also carries with it, thiamine and nicotinic acid.
- Tamarind can be added to cooking water to preserve vitamins.

Table 18.6 enlists nutritive values of some foods from different food groups, with their nutrient contents.

TABLE 18.6: **Nutritive values of some of the common foods**

Nutrients	Food groups	Foodstuffs	Nutrient content* (per 100 g of the edible portion)
Energy (kcal)	Cereals and tubers	Rice, wheat and tapioca	340
	Nuts and oilseeds	Almonds, cashew nuts, coconut (dry) and groundnut	600
	Oil and ghee	Vegetable oil, ghee and vanaspati	900
Protein (µg)	Pulses and legumes	Bengal gram, black gram, green gram, lentil and red gram	22
	Nuts and oilseeds	Groundnuts, cashew nuts and almonds	23
	Fish		20
	Meat and poultry	Meat	22
		Egg white	11
	Milk product	Cheese, khoa, skimmed milk powder and whole milk powder	30
Vitamin A (µg)	Fats and edible oils	Butter, ghee and hydrogenated oil (fortified)	700
β-carotene (mg)	Leafy vegetables	Coriander leaves, spinach, mint and radish leaves	2–6
		Other leafy vegetables such as amaranth, curry leaves and fenugreek leaves	7–15
	Other vegetables	Pumpkin and green chilies	1.0
		Carrots	6.5
	Fruits	Ripe mango	2.0
		Papaya	0.9

Contd...

Nutrients	Food groups	Foodstuffs	Nutrient content* (per 100 g of the edible portion)
Vitamin C (mg)	Green leafy vegetables	Cabbage, coriander leaves, drumstick leaves and knol khol (green)	112–220
	Other vegetables	Giant chilies (capsicum)	137
		Green chilies	117
	Fruits	Amla	600
		Guava	212
Thiamine (mg)	Cereal grains and grain products	Bajra, barley, ragi, wheat germ and wheat bread (brown)	0.2
	Pulses and legumes	Bengal gram, black gram, green gram, lentil, red gram and soybean	0.2
Riboflavin (mg)	Leafy vegetables	Amaranthus, carrot leaves, colocasia leaves, curry leaves, fenugreek leaves, mint, radish leaves and spinach	0.25
	Nuts and oilseeds	Mustard seeds, sunflower seeds, almonds and walnuts	0.3
	Condiments and spices	Chilies (dry), chilies green, coriander and cumin seeds	0.35
	Fruits	Apricot (dried) and papaya	0.23
	Meat and poultry	Sheep liver	1.7
		Egg	0.26
Folic acid	Milk and milk products	Skimmed milk powder and whole milk powder	1.5
	Green leafy vegetables	Amaranth, mint and spinach	120
	Pulses	Bengal gram, black gram, green gram and red gram	130
	Oilseeds	Soybean	180
Iron (mg)	Green leafy vegetables	Amaranth, Bengal gram leaves, cauliflower (green) and radish leaves	18–40
	Cereals and legumes	Ragi, Bengal gram (whole), horse gram (whole), rajmah and soybean	200–340
	Green leafy vegetables	Amaranth, cauliflower (green), curry leaves and knol khol leaves	500–800
Calcium (mg)		Colocasia leaves	1540
	Nuts and oilseeds	Coconut (dry), almond, mustard seeds and sunflower seeds	130–490
		Cumin seeds	1080
	Fish	Bacha, katla, mrigal, prawn and rohu	320–650
	Milk and milk products	Buffalo milk, cow milk, goat milk and curd	120–210
		Cheese, khoa, skimmed milk powder and whole milk powder	790–1370

*NIN-ICMR (1998)

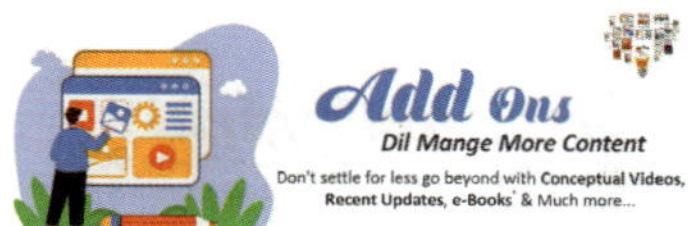

DIETARY FIBER

Dietary fiber, also known as **roughage**, is the **indigestible part of plant foods**. Fiber includes nonstarch polysaccharides such as cellulose, dextrins, inulin, lignin, chitins, pectins, beta-glucans, waxes and oligosaccharides. Fiber is mostly in vegetables, fruits, whole grains and legumes.

Health Benefits of Dietary Fiber

Dietary fiber has a host of health benefits including reducing the risk of heart disease and type 2 diabetes. It is also crucial for keeping the gut healthy:

- **Protection against heart disease:** Several studies, over the past several decades, have examined the effect of dietary fiber on heart health, including preventing cardiovascular disease and reducing blood pressure. It has been suggested that people eating high fiber diets had significantly reduced risk of cardiovascular disease and lower mortality from these conditions. These heart protective effects could be because fiber reduces total cholesterol and low density lipoprotein-cholesterol (LDL), also called bad cholesterol, which is a major risk for heart conditions.

- **Better gut health:** Fiber is important for keeping the gut healthy. Eating enough fiber can prevent or relieve constipation, helping waste to move smoothly through the body. It also encourages healthy gut microbes. It increases the bulk of stool, helps promote regular bowel movements and reduces the time that waste spends inside the intestines. Further, dietary fiber has a positive impact on gastrointestinal disorders, including colorectal ulcer, gastroesophageal reflux disease, diverticular disease and hemorrhoids. Dietary fiber intake may also reduce the risk of colorectal cancer.

- **Reduced diabetes risk:** Adding more fiber to the diet may also have benefits for diabetes. Fiber can help slow down the absorption of sugar, helping to prevent blood sugar spikes after meals. It is reported that people who ate high fiber diets, especially cereal fiber, had a lower risk of developing type 2 diabetes and a reduction in blood glucose levels.

- **Weight management:** For people aiming to lose weight, a diet high in dietary fiber can help regulate weight loss. High fiber foods help a person feel fuller for longer and may help people adhere to a diet. It is reported that people who increased their dietary fiber intake increased their weight loss and adherence to their dietary caloric restriction.

Types of Dietary Fiber

There are two types of dietary fiber, referred to as soluble and insoluble. Both form an essential part of a healthful diet. Most high fiber containing foods have both insoluble and soluble fiber, so people do not need to think much about the difference. Instead, they can focus on overall fiber intake.

1. **Soluble fiber:** Soluble fiber dissolves in water and forms a gel-like substance in the stomach. Bacteria later break the gel down in the large intestine. Soluble fiber provides some calories to the individual. Soluble fiber provides the following benefits:

   - **Lowering LDL cholesterol** in the blood by affecting how the body absorbs dietary fat and cholesterol.
   - Slowing absorption of other carbohydrates through digestion, this can **help regulate blood sugar level**.

   Good sources of soluble fiber include beans, fruits, oats, nuts and vegetables.

2. **Insoluble fiber:** Insoluble fiber does not dissolve in water and passes through the gastrointestinal tract, mostly intact. It does not provide calories.
    - Insoluble fiber helps build bulk in the stool, helping a person pass stool more quickly.
    - It can also help prevent constipation.

    Good sources of insoluble fiber include fruits, nuts, vegetables and whole grain foods.

RDA for Dietary Fiber

Safe intake of dietary fiber has been suggested by ICMR-NIN (2020) as **15 g/1000 kcal/day**.

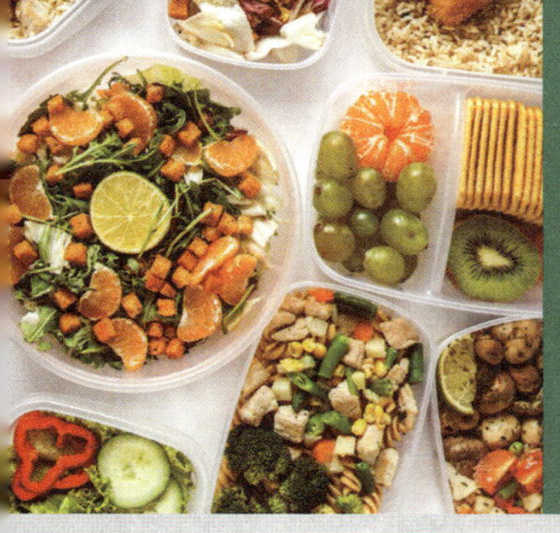

STUDENT ASSIGNMENT

LONG AND SHORT ANSWER QUESTIONS

1. Define a balanced diet. Describe principles and steps in formulation of a balanced diet.
2. Define RDA. Describe limitations and uses of RDAs.
3. Define nutritive value of foods. How will you calculate the nutritive value of food?
4. **Write notes on:**
   a. Food guides
   b. Basic four food groups
   c. Recommended daily allowances
   d. Food exchange system
   e. Nutritive value of foods
   f. Dietary fiber

MULTIPLE CHOICE QUESTIONS

1. **Which of the following is a key principle in formulating a balanced diet?**
   a. Eliminating all carbohydrates
   b. Including a variety of foods from different food groups
   c. Focusing only on high-protein foods
   d. Consuming only one type of fruit

2. **How many food groups are mainly involved in formulating a balanced diet?**
   a. 2
   b. 4
   c. 6
   d. 8

3. **Which step in formulating a balanced diet involves calculating the individual's daily calorie needs?**
   a. Assessing nutrient requirements
   b. Identifying food sources
   c. Planning meals and snacks
   d. Evaluating and adjusting the plan

4. **What is the final step in the formulation of a balanced diet plan?**
   a. Evaluating and adjusting the plan
   b. Assessing nutrient requirements
   c. Identifying food sources
   d. Planning meals and snacks

Notes

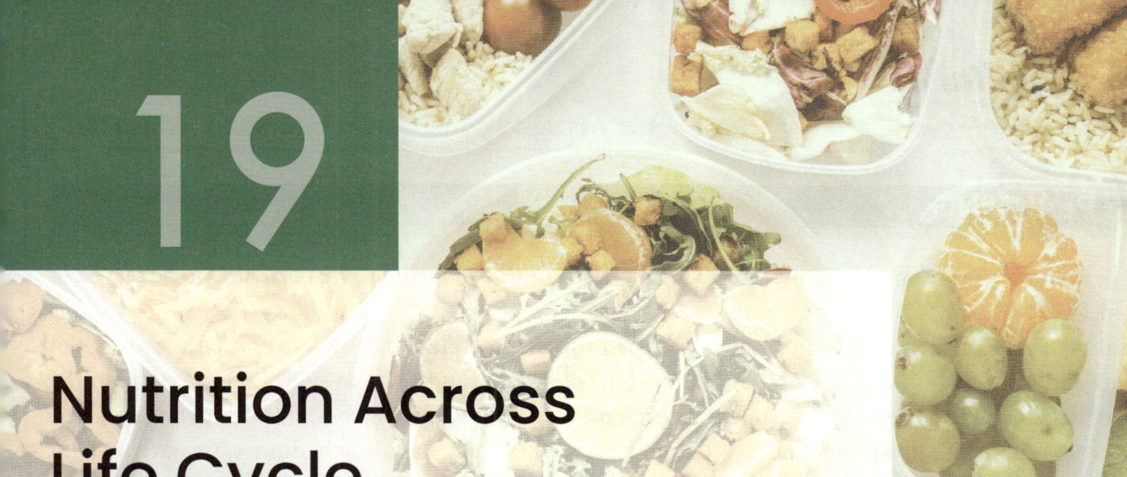

19

Nutrition Across Life Cycle

LEARNING OBJECTIVES

After the completion of the chapter, the readers will be able to:
- Identify nutritional needs of different age groups.
- Describe meal planning, their principles and steps.
- Describe infant and young child feeding.

CHAPTER OUTLINE

- Meal Planning

Infant and Young Child Feeding
- Breastfeeding
- Recommended Dietary Allowance
- Infant Foods

Diet Plan for Different Age Groups
- Diet Plan for Children and Adolescents

- Diet Plan for Elderly
- Diet in Pregnancy
- Anemia in Pregnancy
- Nutrition in Lactation
- Complementary Feeding
- Weaning

KEY TERMS

Complementary feeding: When children receive foods to complement breast milk or infant formula such as cereals with added iron.

Diet plan: Tailored according to an individual's health status, weight and lifestyle, along with their weight loss and health goals.

Folate deficiency anemia: Occurs when a lack of vitamin B_{12} or folate causes the body to produce abnormally large red blood cells that cannot function properly.

Meal planning: Any strategy that is used to map out what an individual is going to eat during a particular day, week, or month.

Supplementary nutrient: A substance or product that is added to a person's diet to make sure they get all the nutrients they need. It may include vitamins, minerals, proteins, or fats, and may be given by mouth, by tube feeding, or into a vein.

MEAL PLANNING

A **meal** or **menu** is a list of specific foods offered for a specific period. It includes a list of dishes to be served in a given meal.

Meal planning or **menu planning** is defined as a process which involves application of knowledge of food, nutrients, food-habits, and like and dislike to plan wholesome and attractive meals. So, it refers to the practice of deciding what one would like to eat for each meal, including main dishes, side dishes and desserts. It is the process of listing down the foods which can be served for breakfast, lunch, dinner or snacks. Menu plans may be for a day, week or month. It is also a way to make sure that one is eating a balanced diet, meeting one's nutritional needs.

Principles of Meal/Menu Planning

The planned food needs to be tasty and palatable with its nutritive value. For this, the following principles are to be followed during meal planning:

- **It should give maximum nutrients:** To follow the principle of nutrition is an important principle of meal planning. For example, a family may have members of all age groups like infant, adolescent, adult, pregnant lady, old person, etc., and that the nutritional requirement of each member may be different. Hence, it is necessary to consider the daily nutritional requirement of each member.

  It is also important to include some foods from each food group. Foods selected from only one food group are neither nutritionally balanced nor likeable, e.g., a meal having egg, curd and kheer will be rich in protein, but deficient in minerals and vitamins due to the absence of fruits, vegetables and salad. Therefore, the complete menu should supply not only adequate calories, fat and protein but also minerals, vitamins, water and roughage, all of which are essential for the physical well-being of each member of a family. Further, nutritive value of the food can also be enhanced by adopting certain practices like sprouting, fermentation and use of other practices that can also minimize the loss of nutrients during processing and cooking.

- **It must suit the family:** Meal should be planned in such a way that it fulfills the needs of all the family members. As we know that the requirements of several nutrients vary with age, occupation and life style, so, a family meal should cater to the needs of all the family members, such as for infants and children of various ages, the pregnant and lactating women, the elderly, and for the specific health needs. For example, enough fat and flexibility in calorie density is essential to meet the energy needs of children. A young child requires soft and bland diet, whereas adolescents need rich food to satisfy appetite. Pregnant women require more greens in the diet. A heavy worker requires more calories and B-vitamins. It should also provide suitable nutrients for different situations, like during sickness, deficiencies or diabetes, etc.

  Thus, the food should be in accordance with the requirements of different members of the family. This, however, does not mean that separate food has to be cooked for each member. Requirements of each family member can be met by making a few changes in the meal, e.g., dal water can be served as soup, and dal can be served to a patient of hypertension by reducing the amount of salt in it. Non-fried dal can be served to a patient and rest of the members can enjoy fried dal. Apart from this, number of meals taken in a day by the family also differs. For example, if a family takes two main meals in a day, then the maximum nutritional requirements should be met by these two meals, in case if meals are taken thrice a day, the quantity of food in each meal can be accordingly adjusted.

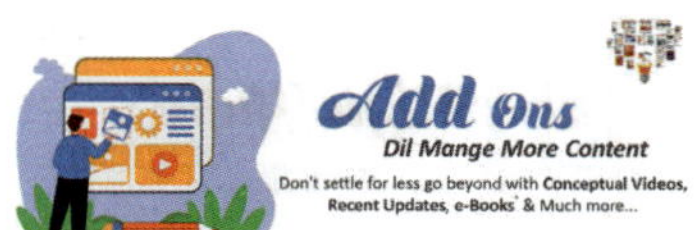

- **It should provide variety:** During menu planning one must consider psychological and cultural habits of the family members. For example, nobody likes a rigid meal pattern every day. Variety in meal can be brought by selecting different foods from various food groups, by blending color, flavor, taste and texture into it, and by using different methods of cooking:

    - **Selection of foods from different food groups:** As we know, a group of foodstuffs having same nutrients are called a Food Group. Foods selected from a single food group are neither acceptable nor balanced, e.g., a person has milk, cheese, sandwich and milk pudding in breakfast may not relish his breakfast, but on the other hand if foods from different groups are selected, e.g., vegetable sandwich fruits and milk are served, it will definitely bring variety and also enhance the taste and nutritive value of the meal.

    - **Variety in color combination:** Blending of different colors will make food attractive and likeable, on the other hand, food will appear dull if all foods are of the same color, e.g., a meal consisting of urad dal, plain curd, plain rice, onions and radish salad does not appeal despite of being nutritious. But if a meal has whole urad dal, dam aloo, onion, tomato, radish and carrot salad decorated with green coriander, mint chutney and rice pulao, it will appeal anyone because of beautiful colors. So, use foods that complement each other in color, and avoid all meals of one color. Such a meal also enhances appetite.

    - **Variety in texture:** Texture in food refers to its state of being soft, solid, crisp or liquid. A meal would not be enjoyable if all the foods are of the same texture. Combine soft food with crisp and chewy food. For example, a meal should have some solid foods which can be consumed raw like salads, fruits, etc., some crispy foods like chips, papad, etc., and some soft foods like custard, pudding, dal, etc.

    - **Variety in taste and flavor:** A meal will be very stimulating if its flavor can water our mouth. So, blending of different flavors is also essential for a good meal planning. All the tastes like salty, sour, sweet and bitter add novelty to food. For example, one would not relish the meal if all the foods in it are very spicy. A bland meal will also not be very likeable. Good combination of foods, generally, enhances the flavor of each other, e.g., bread with butter, pakoras with mint chutney, etc.

    - **Variety in methods of cooking:** Texture, taste and flavor of foods can also be changed by using different methods of cooking. In addition to the traditional cooking methods like frying, boiling, roasting, baking, steaming, etc., novelty to the food can be added by fermentation and sprouting. For example, potato can be served in different forms like cutlets, chips, etc., in place of simple potato vegetable.

    Specific dishes offered, should also consider the environmental temperatures, e.g., special hot foods can be offered on cold rainy days and vice versa.

- **Meals should provide satiable value:** Food which provides satiety and does not cause hunger between two meals is known as satiable food. Protein and fat rich foods have higher satiety value as compared to carbohydrates. In meal planning, interval between two meals should be considered while selecting protein and fat foods so that one does not feel hungry very soon, e.g., the interval between dinner and breakfast is long, and therefore, protein-rich breakfast will be more satiable.

- **It should save the time, energy and money:** Once meals are planned for a day or week, then first prepare a list of items and these should be procured in time. This saves unnecessary trips to the market and thus, saves time, energy and money. For this:

    - Foods can be purchased at reasonable prices. For this, rates can be compared at different shops or can be procured from wholesale dealers. Items purchased at the last moment in a hurry cost more.

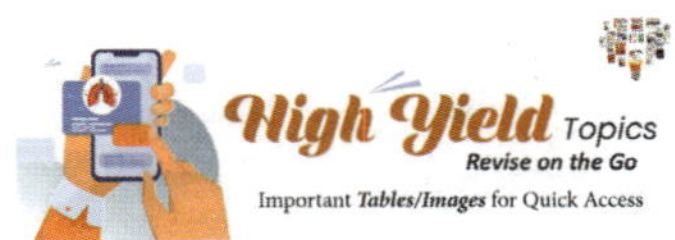

- The cost of the meal can also be reduced by bulk purchasing, and using seasonal fruits and vegetables. Foods in a bigger pack cost, however, should be purchased only when there is proper provision for its storage.
- Shopping should be done at times the markets are not very crowded.
- Kitchen items should be arranged thematically near the work place so as to avoid fatigue while working in the kitchen.
- Time and labor saving kitchen devices like mixer, fridge, cooker, solar cooker, etc., should be used.
- Meal planning can also save time in pre-preparation of food, e.g., if rajma is to be cooked in lunch, these can be soaked overnight. Soaked grains are easy to cook and save time and fuel.

Steps of Meal/Menu Planning

- It is recommended that the daily requirement of all the nutrients should be arranged in three meals, which should provide selection of foods that most nearly suit the needs, preferences, habits and activities of all family members.
- Basic breakfast should provide more than 25% of the daily requirement. It may consist of fruits, cereals, milk, bread and eggs.
- Dinner should be a lighter meal than lunch, although foods included may be same. The dinner menu should be made after planning the menu for breakfast and lunch.
- The meal should be satisfying and provide the desired nutrition to the whole family.

INFANT AND YOUNG CHILD FEEDING

Infant and Young Child Feeding **(IYCF)** is a key area to improve child survival and promote healthy growth and development.

- According to WHO and UNICEF, under nutrition is estimated to be associated with 2.7 million child deaths annually or 45% of all child deaths. The first 2 years of a child's life are particularly important, as optimal nutrition during this period lowers morbidity and mortality reduces the risk of chronic disease and fosters better development overall.
- **A global strategy for IYCF** was issued jointly by the World Health Organization **(WHO)** and the United Nations Children's Fund **(UNICEF)** in 2002, to reverse the disturbing trends in infant and young child feeding practices. In 2004, infant and young child feeding practices were assessed using the WHO assessment protocol and rated poor to fair. To address these problems on infant and young child feeding practices, the first National IYCF Plan of Action was formulated. It aimed to improve the nutritional status and health of children, especially, the under-three and consequently reduce infant and under-five mortality. Specifically, its objectives were to improve, protect and promote infant and young child feeding practices, increase political commitment at all levels, provide a supportive environment and ensure its sustainability.
- **IYCF chapter of Indian Academy of Pediatrics** invited a group of experts for National Consultative Meet for discussing and contributing on latest scientific advances and developments. Various partners from WHO, UNICEF, Ministry of Child Welfare Department, Ministry of Health and Family Welfare, Ministry of Chemical and Fertilizers of Government of India, Human Milk Banking Association of India, Indian Medico-Legal and Ethics Association, Nongovernmental organizations and academicians from various states of India contributed to these guidelines. The guidelines were finalized at New Delhi in August, 2015.

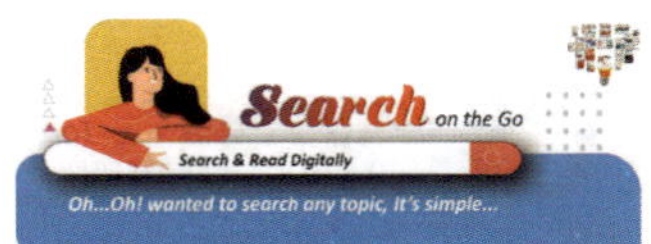

Guidelines for IYCF:

- Initiation of breastfeeding as early as possible after birth, preferably within 1 hour.
- Exclusive breastfeeding in the first six months of life and no other foods or fluids.
- Appropriate and adequate complementary feeding after completion of 6 months. Complementary foods should not be confused with the supplementary foods.
- Handwashing with soap and water at critical times, including before eating or preparing food and after using the toilet.
- Avoid junk food. Home food should be preferred over artificial, commercial, tinned or packaged food.
- Promote and establish Human Milk Banks.
- Full immunization and vitamin A supplementation with deworming.
- Effective home-based care and treatment of children suffering from severe acute malnutrition.
- Adequate nutrition and anemia control for adolescent girls, pregnant and lactating mothers.
- Effective implementation and monitoring of Infant Milk Substitute (IMS) Act and other laws related to child nutrition.

BREASTFEEDING

Babies usually double their length and triple their weight between birth and 1 year of age.

- It is recommended that infants be exclusively breastfed up to around 6 months of age.
- Breast milk, generally, supplies a baby with the required amounts of nutrients, fluids and energy up to about six months of age. Besides, it also contains many protective and immunological factors that benefit the baby's development.

Composition of Breast Milk

Composition of breast milk is given in Table 19.1.

Advantages of Breastfeeding

- Early initiation of breastfeeding, within 1 hour of birth, protects the newborn from acquiring infections and reduces newborn mortality. The risk of mortality due to diarrhea and other infections can increase in infants who are either partially breastfed or not breastfed at all.
- Exclusive breastfeeding for 6 months has many benefits for the infant and mother. Chief among these is protection against gastrointestinal infections, which is observed not only in developing but also industrialized countries.
- Breast-milk is also an important source of energy and nutrients in children aged 6–23 months. It can provide half or more of a child's energy needs between the ages of 6 and 12 months, and one third of energy needs between 12 and 24 months.
- Breast-milk is also a critical source of energy and nutrients during illness, and reduces mortality among children who are malnourished.
- Children and adolescents, who were breastfed as babies, are less likely to be overweight or obese. Additionally, they perform better in intelligence tests and have higher school attendance.

TABLE 19.1: Nutrient contents of breast milk

Nutrient	Content/100 mL
Calories	67 kcal
Proteins	1.1 g
Fat	3.5 g
Lactose	7.0 g
Sodium	0.9 mEq
Potassium	1.4 mEq
Calcium	35 mg
Phosphorus	15 mg
Iron	30–50 µg
Zinc	120 µg
Vitamin A	60 µg
Vitamin C	5.2 mg

- Longer durations of breastfeeding also contribute to the health and well-being of mothers. It reduces the risk of ovarian and breast cancer and helps space pregnancies. Exclusive breastfeeding of babies under 6 months has a hormonal effect which often induces a lack of menstruation.
- Mothers and families need to be supported for their children to be optimally breastfed.
  - Breast-milk contains all the nutrients, which are essentially required for infants.
  - **Colostrum**, the milk secreted during the first 3–4 days after child birth, is **rich in proteins, minerals, vitamins** (especially, vitamin A) and **antibodies**.
  - Breast-milk also has several special components, such as **growth factors, enzymes, hormones and anti-infective factors**.
  - Breast-milk also provides **good quality proteins, fat, vitamins, calcium, iron** and **other minerals** necessary to meet the requirements up to 4–6 months.
  - Breast-milk also has high content of docosahexaenoic acid (**DHA**), which plays an important role in **brain development**.
  - Breast-milk also has immunoglobulin A (**IgA**), **lactoferrin, lactoperoxidase** and the **complements**, which protect the infant from several infections.
  - Breast-milk, however, is not adequate for the infant beyond 6 months of age.

RECOMMENDED DIETARY ALLOWANCE

RDA During First Six Months of Age

- **Energy:** For infants with the average body weight of 5.8 kg, **adequate intake** of energy has been suggested as **530 kcal/day**.

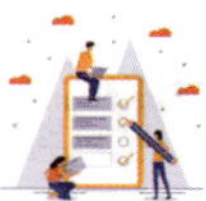
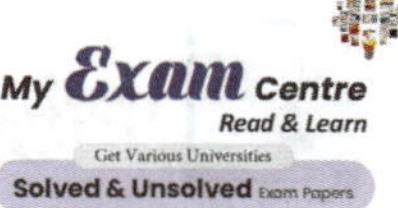

- **Fat:** Minimum level of total fat has been suggested as **40–60% of the total energy intake**.
- **Protein:** RDA for protein has been suggested as **8.0 g/day**.
- **Vitamins:**
  - **Thiamine:** RDA for thiamine has been suggested as **0.2 mg/day**.
  - **Riboflavin:** RDA for riboflavin has been suggested as **0.4 mg/day**.
  - **Niacin:** RDA for niacin has been suggested as **2.0 mg/day**.
  - **Vitamin B_6:** RDA for vitamin B_6 has been suggested as **0.1 mg/day**.
  - **Folate:** RDA for folate has been suggested as **25 µg/day**.
  - **Vitamin B_{12}:** RDA for vitamin B_{12} has been suggested as **1.2 µg/day**.
  - **Vitamin C:** RDA for vitamin C has been suggested as **20 mg/day**.
  - **Vitamin A:** RDA for vitamin A has been suggested as **350 µg/day**.
  - **Vitamin D:** RDA for vitamin D has been suggested as **400 IU/day**.
- **Minerals:**
  - **Calcium:** RDA for calcium has been suggested as **300 mg/day**.
  - **Magnesium:** RDA for magnesium has been suggested as **30 mg/day**.
  - **Iodine:** RDA for iodine has been suggested as **100 µg/day**.
- **Water:** Total water requirement has been suggested as 600 mL/day, which is available from breast milk.

  Further, it has also been suggested that, since **breast milk contains all these nutrients** which are essentially required for infants, and that the **requirements of these nutrients, for infants between 0 and 6 months of age, can be met from breast milk**, thus, breastfeeding should, essentially, be promoted at least for six months.
  - Breast milk also **provides several special components** such as **growth factors, enzymes, hormones** and **anti-infective factors**.
  - It also has a **high content of** docosahexaenoic acid (**DHA**) which plays an important role in brain development.
  - Breast milk also provides immunoglobulin A (**IgA**), **lactoferrin, lacto-peroxidase and complements** which provide immunity and protects the infant from several types of infections.
  - Besides breast milk, **colostrum** (the milk secreted during the first 3–4 days after childbirth) **is also rich in proteins, minerals, vitamins** (especially vitamin A) and **antibodies**.

RDA During 6–12 Months of Age

- **Energy:** For infants above 6 months of age, with the average body weight of 8.5 kg, **adequate intake** of energy has been suggested as **680 kcal/day**.
- **Fat:** Minimum level of total fat has been suggested as **35% of energy**.
- It is further suggested that **visible fat intake should be 25 g/day**.
- **Protein:** RDA for protein has been suggested as **10.5 g/day**.
- **Vitamins:**
  - **Thiamine:** RDA for thiamine has been suggested as **0.4 mg/day**.
  - **Riboflavin:** RDA for riboflavin has been suggested as **0.6 mg/day**.
  - **Niacin:** RDA for niacin has been suggested as **5.0 mg/day**.
  - **Vitamin B_6:** RDA for vitamin B_6 has been suggested as **0.6 mg/day**.
  - **Folate:** RDA for folate has been suggested as **85 µg/day**.

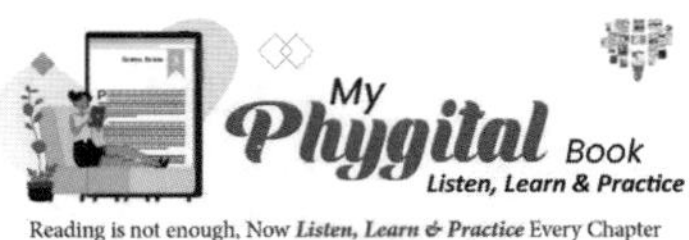

- ■ **Vitamin B$_{12}$:** **RDA** for vitamin B$_{12}$ has been suggested as **1.2 µg/day**.
- ■ **Vitamin C: RDA** for vitamin C has been suggested as **30 mg/day**.
- ■ **Vitamin A: RDA** for vitamin A has been suggested as **350 µg/day**.
- ■ **Vitamin D: RDA** for vitamin D has been suggested as **400 IU/day**.
- **Minerals:**
  - ■ **Calcium: RDA** for calcium has been suggested as **300 mg/day**.
  - ■ **Magnesium: RDA** for magnesium has been suggested as **75 mg/day**.
  - ■ **Iron: RDA** for iron has been suggested as **3 mg/day**.
  - ■ **Zinc: RDA** for zinc has been suggested as **2.5 mg/day**.
  - ■ **Iodine: RDA** for iodine has been suggested as **130 µg/day**.
- **Water:** Total water requirement has been suggested as 1000 mL/day. It can be met from breast milk, water and other fluids.

Further, it has been suggested that these requirements should, partially, be met from breast milk. Accordingly, along with the breast milk, these infants, after six months of age, should be given home-based semi-solid foods. For this purpose:

- In addition to breast milk, **they should be provided the supplementary or complementary foods such as** liquids (like **milk**), semisolids (like **khichdi and kheer**) and solid preparations like **rice**, etc.
- **These can be low-cost food supplements which can be prepared at home from commonly used ingredients,** such as cereals (wheat, rice, ragi, jowar, bajra, etc.), pulses (grams and dals), nuts and oilseeds (groundnut, sesame, etc.), vegetable oils (groundnut oil, sesame oil, etc.), and sugar and jaggery. These foods, in turn, will provide **good quality protein, adequate calories and several protective nutrients**.
- In addition, these infants should also be **given fruits and green leafy vegetables** which are rich sources of vitamins and minerals. However, these should be well cleaned before cooking.

INFANT FOODS

Infancy is a period of rapid growth. Infant, usually doubles the weight at 6 months; triples at the age of 1 year and 4 times at the age of 2 years. Further, the baby measures about 50 cm at birth, 60 cm at 3 months, 70 cm at 9 months and 75 cm at 1 year.

Recommendations for Infant Foods

- In addition to breast-milk, infants should be provided with the supplementary, or complementary foods such as liquids (like milk) or semi-solids (like khichdi and kheer), or solid preparations like rice, etc.
- Low-cost food supplements, which can be prepared at home from commonly used ingredients such as cereals (wheat, rice, ragi, jowar, bajra, etc.); pulses (grams/daals), nuts and oilseeds (groundnut, sesame, etc.), oils (groundnut oil, sesame oil, etc.), and sugar and jaggery, should be prepared and used. These foods will provide good quality proteins, adequate calories and other protective nutrients.
- Infants can also be given fruits and green-leafy vegetables, which are rich source of vitamins and minerals. However, green vegetables should be well cleaned before cooking.
- In addition to the above mentioned foods, infants (0–12-month-old) also require 500 mg of calcium, 25 mg of vitamin C, 25 µg of dietary folate and 0.2 µg of vitamin B$_{12}$ per day, which can be met from breast milk and home-based semi-solid foods.

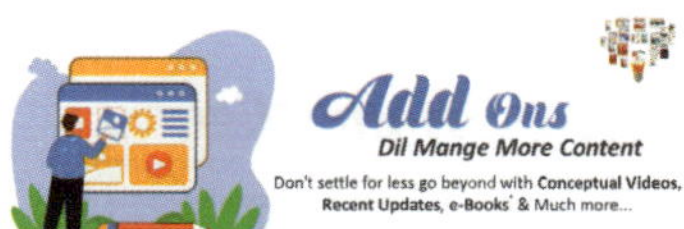

In some families, there may be a traditional pattern to start solid foods to the children; however, the recommended practice is to introduce solid foods at about 6 months of age. For this purpose, babies may be started directly on normal family food. They may be offered a variety of foods but in small portions. The food may comprise of the cereals, meshed vegetables and fruits. Be patient, as the child may take longer or may not even eat at all. Do not force the child and let the taste develop gradually. They may be served with cereal-based foods like rice or bread to meet their calories needs. To meet the requirement of vitamins and minerals, they may be served with meshed fruits like banana or apple and fresh juices. Some of the vegetables, particularly potato may be liked by the children. They may be served with egg, cheese and pulses to meet the requirement of protein. Do not serve the spicy food to the child. As children like sweet taste, so if there is a dessert, hold it on till they had finished the main food.

DIET PLAN FOR DIFFERENT AGE GROUPS

Our dietary requirement changes with the advancing age. Dietary requirements also change with the physiological state of the body and a disease. Accordingly, our diet plan should change with the changing age and stage of life. Thus, it becomes essential to revise our dietary requirements and plan the diet with the changing needs, to remain physically and mentally healthy. With the advancing age, there is not only increased demand of calories and proteins, but also of the micronutrients, i.e., vitamins and minerals. In some of the physiological conditions, such as during adolescence in girls, there is increased demand of iron. On the other hand, dietary protein and calcium requirements increase in elderly people.

DIET PLAN FOR CHILDREN AND ADOLESCENTS

Childhood is the period of continuous growth and development. During childhood, children tend to vary their food intake (spontaneously) to match their growth patterns.
- **During the second year** the child increases in height by 7–8 cm and gains 4 times of its birth weight.
- **During the pre-adolescent period** the child grows, on an average, by 6–7 cm in height and 1.5–3 kg in weight every year, and simultaneously development and maturation of various tissues and organs take place.

Children's food needs vary widely, depending on their growth and level of physical activity. Like energy needs, a child's needs for proteins, vitamins and minerals also increase with age.

Adolescent period, may also be referred to as teenage, commonly, covers the age group between 12 and 18 years. During adolescence there occurs a spurt of growth. Besides physical growth, there also occurs sexual growth due to several endocrine hormones. As a result of development of bones, and physical and sexual growth, body's requirement for almost all the nutrients (both macronutrients as well as micronutrients) is significantly increased. For example, due to increased basal metabolic rate (BMR), body requires extra calories which can be met by increasing the dietary intake of carbohydrates and fat. Growth also increases the demand of protein. Bone growth also needs extra vitamin D, calcium, phosphorus and magnesium. Increased BMR and the extra consumption of carbohydrates and proteins require additional amount of vitamins, particularly, B vitamins (such as thiamin or vitamin B_1, riboflavin or vitamin B_2, niacin and pyridoxine or vitamin B_6). Girls do need extra amount of iron, folate, vitamin B_{12}, vitamin C and protein. Thus, it is essential to plan their diet accordingly.

Dietary Recommendations for Children and Adolescents

Childhood and adolescence are the **periods of continuous growth and development**.

- **During the second year**, a **child increases in height by 7–8 cm** and **gains body weight**, approximately, **to 4 times of its birth weight**.
- **During the pre-adolescent period**, a **child grows, on an average. by 6–7 cm in height** and **1.5–3.0 kg in body weight, every year** and simultaneously, development and maturation of the various tissues and organs takes place.
- **Adolescent period** (teenage) **is spread almost over a decade** and is **characterized by rapid increase in height and weight** along with the hormonal changes, sexual maturation and wide swing in emotions.
  - Adolescent **growth spurt starts at about 10–12 years in girls** and **two years later in boys**.
  - **Annual peak rates for increase in height and weight are 9–10 cm and 8–10 kg**, respectively.
  - During this period, development of the critical bone mass is essential as this forms the ground for maintaining mineral integrity of bone in later life.
  - Pattern and proportion of various body components, like body water, muscle mass, bone and fat, increase during the entire childhood and adolescence to reach adult values by about 18 years.
  - **Adolescent girls** are at greater physiological stress than boys because of menstruation. Their **nutritional needs are of particular importance** as they have to prepare for motherhood. All these rapid anabolic changes require more nutrients per unit body weight.

Accordingly, it is advised that:

- **Growing children and adolescents require more calcium**. It is recommended that they **should consume calcium rich foods** like **milk and milk products, ragi** (fox-tail millet) and **til** (sesame seed), etc.
- **Young children**, below 5 years of age, **should be given** less bulky **foods** that are **rich in energy and protein**, such as **legumes, pulses, nuts, edible oil/ghee, sugar, milk and eggs**.
- **Vegetables**, including **green leafy vegetables**, and locally available **seasonal fruits** should be a part of their daily menu.
- Older children and adolescents **should also consume plenty of milk** to fulfill high calcium requirements.
- They should consume, nearly, **25–50 g of cooking oils/ghee**.
- **Excessive salt intake should be avoided,** particularly, by children having a family history of hypertension.

DIET PLAN FOR ELDERLY

Body composition changes, as we grow old. In general, we lose lean body mass and gain fat mass. Loss of lean tissue compromises strength, reduces resting energy expenditure, and increases the risk of osteoporosis. Perception of taste also declines with age, which may contribute to loss of appetite and poor food intake. In the GIT, reduction in acid and enzyme secretions, further affect nutrient absorption. Immune functions also decline with age. Absorption, transport, storage and use of fat soluble vitamins are also affected by aging. Environmental, pharmacological and psychological stresses often compound age-related changes in body composition, sensory abilities, organ systems and immune functions. Normal aging, thus, causes multiple physiological changes that, accordingly, affect our nutrient needs and nutritional status. Accordingly, adequate nutrition and balanced diet is important to prevent and control the common hazards of aging.

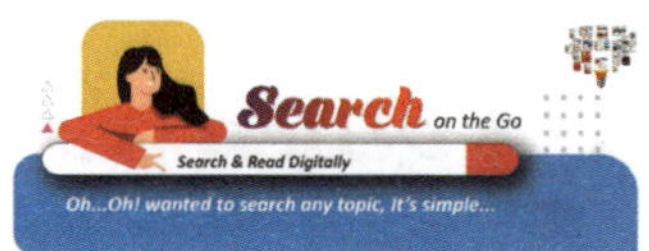

RDA for Elderly Persons

As one grows old, his/her **body composition changes**. In general:

- Elderly person **loses lean body mass** and **gains fat mass.**
- **Loss of lean tissue compromises strength, reduces resting energy expenditure** and increases the **risk of osteoporosis.**
- **Perception of taste** also **declines with age**, which also contributes to **loss of appetite** and **poor food intake**.
- **Reduction in acid and enzyme secretions** further affect nutrient absorption.
- **Immune functions also decline** with age.
- **Absorption, transport, storage and metabolism of fat soluble vitamins are also affected** by aging.

Thus, aging causes **multiple physiological changes**, which, accordingly, **affect our nutrient need as well as nutritional status.**

Accordingly, **ICMR-NIN (2020)** has recommended that, **to maintain regular physical activity, elders should consume nutrient-dense foods,** such as **nuts, oilseeds, fruits, vegetables, legumes and flesh-foods,** to meet their daily requirements of vitamins and minerals.

Recommendations of the group for various nutrients for the elderly persons (more than 60 years of age) are shown in Table 19.2.

TABLE 19.2: RDA of macro and micronutrients for the Elderly

Dietary nutrient	Male (60+)	Female (60+)
Energy (kcal)	1700	1500
Dietary fiber (g)	32	25
Proteins (g)	54	46
Thiamine (mg)	1.4	1.4
Riboflavin (mg)	2	1.9
Niacin (mg)	12	9
Vitamin B_6 (mg)	1.9	1.9
Folate (µg)	300	200
Vitamin B_{12} (µg)	2.2	2.2
Vitamin C (mg)	80	65
Vitamin A (µg)	1000	840
Vitamin D (IU)*	800	800
Calcium (mg)	1200	1200
Magnesium (mg)	440	370
Iron (mg)	19	19
Zinc (mg)	17	13
Iodine (µg)	150	150

* Adequate intake

- **Energy:** Due to a reduction in BMR and the sedentary lifestyle, the group has **suggested** RDA for energy in terms of **estimated average requirement** (EAR).

  EAR for energy has been suggested as **1700 kcal/day for elderly males** (with average body weight of 65 kg) and **1500 kcal for elderly females** (with average body weight of 55 kg).
- **Dietary fiber:** RDA for dietary fiber has been suggested as **30 g/day for elderly males** and **25 g/day for elderly females**.
- **Protein:** RDA for protein has been suggested as **54 g/day for elderly males** and **46 g/day for elderly females**.
- **Vitamins:**
  - **Thiamine:** RDA for thiamine has been suggested as **1.4 mg/day for elderly males as well as females.**
  - **Riboflavin:** RDA for riboflavin has been suggested as **2.0 mg/day for elderly males** and **1.9 mg/day for elderly females.**
  - **Niacin:** RDA for niacin (NE) has been suggested as **14 mg/day for** elderly **males** and **11 mg/day for elderly females.**
  - **Vitamin B_6:** RDA for vitamin B_6 has been suggested as **1.9 mg/day for elderly males as well as females.**
  - **Folate:** RDA for dietary folate has been suggested as **300 µg/day for elderly males** and **200 µg/day for elderly females.**
  - **Vitamin B_{12}:** RDA for vitamin B_{12} has been suggested as **2.2 µg/day for elderly males as well as females.**
  - **Vitamin C:** RDA for vitamin C has been suggested as **80 mg/day for elderly males** and **65 mg/day for elderly females.**
  - **Vitamin A:** RDA for vitamin A (RE) has been suggested as **1000 µg/day for elderly males** and **840 µg/day for elderly females.**
  - **Vitamin D:** RDA for vitamin D has been suggested as **800 IU/day for** elderly **males as well as females.**
- **Minerals:**
  - **Calcium:** RDA for calcium has been suggested as **1200 mg/day for elderly males as well as females.**
  - **Magnesium:** RDA for magnesium has been suggested as **440 mg/day for elderly males** and **370 mg/day for elderly females.**
  - **Iron:** RDA for iron has been suggested as **19 µg/day for elderly males as well as females.**
  - **Zinc:** RDA for zinc has been suggested as **17 mg/day for elderly males** and **13 mg/day for elderly females.**
  - **Iodine:** RDA for iodine has been suggested as **140 µg/day for elderly males as well as females.**
- **Water:** Water is essential for various body functions. In elderly persons, decreased thirst response and reduced concentrating capacity of the kidney may lead to dehydration. Moreover, use of diuretics, alcohol and caffeine increase fluid excretion and further contribute to dehydration. With the increasing dietary fiber intake, it is also essential to consume adequate fluid, ideally water, to avoid dehydration and constipation.

  Accordingly, total water requirement has been suggested as 2800 mL/day for elderly males and 2550 mL/day for elderly females.

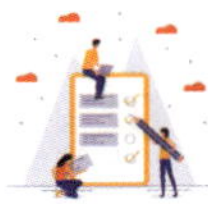
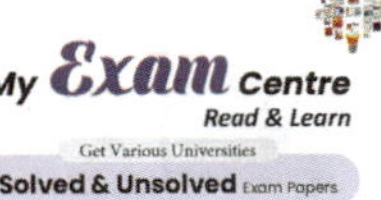

DIET IN PREGNANCY

Pregnancy is the time of tremendous physiological changes that demands healthful dietary and lifestyle choices. This is also a process of growth and development that affects, both, the mother as well as the fetus. Guided by changing levels of hormones, body of the mother undergoes various changes during pregnancy. Various maternal tissues, including the breasts, uterus and adipose stores, increase in size and blood volume is expended. At the same time, gastrointestinal motility is slowed, as a result of which food moves more slowly through the intestinal tract. Due to vomiting and loss of appetite, during the early months of pregnancy, food intake is also generally reduced. Thus, pregnancy is the demanding physiological state.

Nutritional Requirement in Pregnancy

According to ICMR-NIN (2020), nutritional requirements (RDAs) in pregnancy are as follows:

- **Energy:** Due to change in body weight during pregnancy, the group has suggested a proportionate increase in energy requirement.

   Accordingly, **additional 350 kcal/day** have been suggested **during pregnancy**.
- **Carbohydrates:** Carbohydrate intake has been suggested as **135 g/day during pregnancy**.
- **Fat: Total visible fat intake** has been suggested as **30 g/day during pregnancy**.
- **Protein: Additional requirement** of protein has been recommended as **9.5 g/day during the second trimester** and **22 g/day during the third trimester of pregnancy**.
- **Vitamins:**
  - **Thiamine:** RDA for thiamine has been suggested as **2.0 mg/day during pregnancy**.
  - **Riboflavin:** RDA for riboflavin has been suggested as **2.7 mg/day during pregnancy**.
  - **Niacin: Additional 2 mg/day** of niacin has been suggested **during pregnancy**.
  - **Pantothenic acid:** RDA for pantothenic acid is suggested as **5.0 mg/day during pregnancy**.
  - **Vitamin B_6:** RDA for vitamin B_6 has been suggested as **2.3 mg/day during pregnancy**.
  - **Biotin: RDA** for biotin has been suggested as **25 µg/day during pregnancy**.
  - **Folate: Additional** intake of dietary folate has been suggested as **270 µg/day during pregnancy**. Further, it is recommended that to reduce the risk of congenital malformations and increase in birth weight of the fetus, folate should be taken throughout the pregnancy.
  - **Vitamin B_{12}: Additional** intake of vitamin B_{12} has been suggested as **0.25 µg/day during pregnancy**.
  - **Vitamin C: Additional** intake of vitamin C has been suggested as **15 mg/day during pregnancy**.
  - **Vitamin A: RDA** of vitamin A has been suggested as **900 µg/day during pregnancy**. It is further suggested that a **minimum 50% of the vitamin A** (retinol equivalent, RE) requirement **should be met from animal sources**.
  - **Vitamin D: RDA** of vitamin D has been suggested as **600 IU/day during pregnancy**.
- **Minerals:**
  - **Calcium:** It is well known that calcium is essential during pregnancy for proper formation of bones and teeth of the offspring, to prevent osteoporosis in mothers. RDA for calcium has been suggested as **1000 mg/day during pregnancy**.
  - **Phosphorus:** RDA for phosphorus is **similar to that for calcium**.
  - **Magnesium: RDA for magnesium has been suggested as 440 mg/day during pregnancy**.

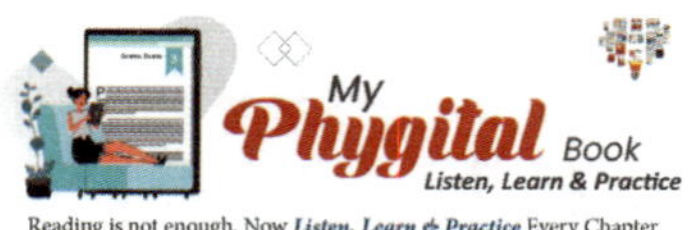

- **Iron:** Extra iron is required by the mother as well as the growing fetus to meet the increased demand for erythropoiesis (formation of RBC).
  Accordingly, RDA for iron has been suggested as **27 mg/day during pregnancy.**
  - **Zinc:** RDA for zinc has been suggested as **14–15 mg/day during pregnancy.**
  - **Iodine:** RDA for iodine has been suggested as **220 μg/day during pregnancy.**
- **Water:** Total water requirement has been suggested as 3700 mL/day during pregnancy.

Balanced Diet Plan in Pregnancy

To meet the above requirements, the group has suggested that the **pregnant woman should eat a wide variety of foods** to make sure that her own nutritional needs as well as those of the growing fetus are met. Though, there is no particular need to modify the usual dietary pattern, the quantity and frequency of usage of different foods should be increased. Furthermore, it is suggested that:
- Maximum amount of **energy can be derived from rice, wheat and millets.**
- A **proper combination of cereals, pulses and nuts can be used to provide adequate protein.**
- **Mineral and vitamin requirements can be met by consuming** a variety of seasonal vegetables, particularly, **green leafy vegetables, milk and fresh fruits.**
- In addition, they are also advised to take daily **supplement of iron, folic acid, vitamin B** and **calcium.**
- These women should also choose **foods rich in dietary fiber,** like whole grain cereals, pulses and vegetables, to avoid constipation.
- Besides, they should take **plenty of fluids,** including 8–12 glasses of water per day.
- **Salt intake should also be restricted** to prevent pregnancy-induced hypertension and pre-eclampsia.
- She should take regular supplement of iron, folate and vitamin B_{12}.

ANEMIA IN PREGNANCY

It is normal to have mild anemia during pregnancy, but one may have more severe anemia from low iron or vitamin levels, or from other reasons. As a result of it, the body does not have enough healthy red blood cells to carry oxygen to the tissues and the baby. Anemia can leave one feeling tired and weak. If it is severe and goes untreated, it can increase the risk of serious complications like preterm delivery.

Types of Anemia

Several types of anemia can develop during pregnancy. These include:
- **Iron-deficiency anemia:** This type of anemia occurs when the body does not have enough iron to produce adequate amount of hemoglobin, the protein in the red blood cells that is required for oxygen transport from the lungs to the rest of the body. It is the most common cause of anemia in pregnancy. Severe or untreated iron-deficiency anemia during pregnancy can increase the risk of having a preterm or low-birth-weight baby, postpartum depression, baby with anemia, or the child with developmental delays.
- **Folate-deficiency anemia:** Folate is a type of B-vitamin body needs to produce new red blood cells, including healthy red blood cells. It is important three months before and in the first trimester of pregnancy to avoid neural tube defects (like spina bifida) in the baby. Folate deficiency can also increase the risk of having a preterm or low birth weight baby.

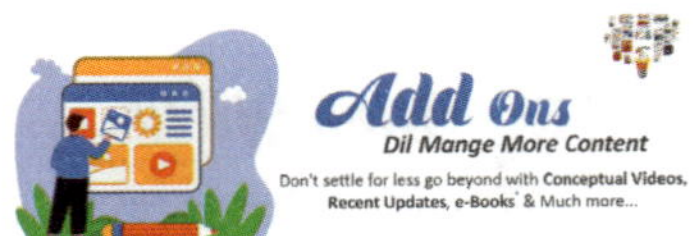

- **Vitamin B_{12} deficiency:** The body also needs vitamin B_{12} to form healthy red blood cells. When a pregnant woman does not get enough vitamin B_{12} from the diet, her body cannot produce enough healthy red blood cells. Women, particularly those, who are vegetarians and vegans, and do not eat meat, poultry, dairy products or eggs, have a greater risk of developing vitamin B_{12} deficiency. Untreated vitamin B_{12} deficiency may contribute to birth defects such as neural tube abnormalities and could lead to preterm labor.

Besides the deficiency of iron, folate and vitamin B_{12}, **blood loss during and after delivery** can also cause anemia.

Diagnosis of Anemia

During the first prenatal appointment and subsequently, during every visit, pregnant females should get a blood test done, to check if one has anemia. These include:

- **Hemoglobin test:** It measures the amount of hemoglobin in the body.
- **Hematocrit test:** It measures the percentage of red blood cells in a sample of blood.

Diet for Anemic Pregnant Women

Anemic pregnant women are suggested to add more foods that are high in iron and folic acid, to the diet.

- To prevent anemia during pregnancy, make sure that the pregnant lady gets enough iron. She should eat well-balanced meals and add more foods that are high in iron, to the diet. Aim for at least three servings a day of iron-rich foods such as dark-green leafy vegetables like spinach, broccoli, fenugreek (methi) and mustard leaves; iron-enriched cereals and grains; beans and lentils; tofu; nuts and seeds; eggs, lean red meat, poultry and fish.
- Foods that are high in vitamin C help the body to absorb more iron. These include citrus fruits and juices, strawberries, kiwis, tomatoes and bell peppers. One can also drink a glass of orange juice and eat an iron-fortified cereal for breakfast.
- Also, choose foods that are high in folate to help prevent folate deficiency. These include green-leafy vegetables, citrus fruits and juices, dried beans and breads and cereals fortified with folic acid.

Supplementation and Counseling

Nutrients for which there are increased requirements during pregnancy include folate, iron, vitamin B_{12} and iodine. Accordingly, **iron supplements** are advised during pregnancy. Increasing **vitamin C intake helps increase iron absorption** from foods. During pregnancy, women also need extra folate, for which **folic acid supplementation** is recommended. Vegetarians and vegan females may also be recommended **vitamin B_{12}** supplementation during pregnancy. **Iodine** supplements are also often advised during pregnancy to meet the increasing needs, as the food sources (such as seafood, iodized salt and bread) are unlikely to provide enough iodine. Iodine is important for normal growth and development of the baby.

Since, both, direct as well as passive smoking is associated with growth retardation, increased risk of spontaneous abortion, stillbirths, placental complications and low birth weight, it is advised to avoid smoking in pregnancy.

NUTRITION IN LACTATION

Nutrition requirement is increased during lactation as the lactating mother not only has to nourish herself but also the infant who is being breastfed. Breastfeeding mothers need a significant amount of extra energy. This extra energy should come in the form of nutrient-dense foods to help meet the extra nutrient requirements that also occur when breastfeeding. Vegan mothers who are breastfeeding should also take a vitamin B_{12} supplement.

Nutritional Requirement in Lactation

According to ICMR-NIN (2020), nutritional requirements (RDAs) for lactating women are as follows:

- **Energy:** An increase in energy requirement has been suggested during lactation, because of utilization of energy in milk production. Accordingly, **additional** energy requirement of a woman who exclusively breastfeeds, has been recommended as **600 kcal/day during the first 6 months of lactation** and **520 kcal/day during 7–12 months of lactation.**
- **Carbohydrates:** Carbohydrate intake has been suggested as **155 g/day during lactation.**
- **Fat: Total visible fat intake** has been suggested as **30 g/day during lactation.**
- **Protein: Additional** protein **requirement for lactating women** has been recommended as **16.9 g/day during the first 6 months** and **13.2 g/day during 7–12 months of lactation.**
- **Vitamins:**
  - **Thiamine:** RDA for thiamine has been suggested as **2.1 mg/day during lactation.**
  - **Riboflavin:** RDA for riboflavin has been suggested as **3 mg/day during the first 6 months** and **2.9 mg/day during 7–12 months of lactation.**
  - **Niacin: Additional 5 mg/day of niacin has been suggested during lactation.**
  - **Pantothenic acid: Additional 2 mg/day** has been recommended **during lactation.**
  - **Vitamin B_6: Additional** recommendations of **0.26 mg/day during 0–6 months of lactation** and **0.17 mg/day during 7–12 months of lactation** have been made for **vitamin B_6.**
  - **Biotin: Additional 5.0 µg/day of biotin** has been suggested **during lactation.**
  - **Folate: Additional** intake of dietary folate has been suggested as **110 µg/day during lactation.**
  - **Vitamin B_{12}: Additional** intake of vitamin B_{12} has been suggested as **1.0 µg/day during lactation.**
  - **Vitamin C: Additional** intake of vitamin C has been suggested as **50 mg during lactation.**
  - **Vitamin A: RDA** of vitamin A has been suggested as **950 µg/day during lactation.**
    It is further suggested that a **minimum 50% of the vitamin A** (retinol equivalent, RE) requirement **should be met from animal sources.**
  - **Vitamin D: RDA** of vitamin D has been suggested as **600 IU/day during lactation.**
- **Minerals:**
  - **Calcium:** It is well known that calcium is essential during lactation for its secretion in breast milk. Accordingly, an **additional 200 mg/day** has been suggested **during lactation.**
  - **Phosphorus:** Recommendations for phosphorus is **similar to that for calcium.**
  - **Magnesium: RDA for magnesium has been suggested as 400 mg/day during lactation.**
  - **Iron:** RDA for iron has been suggested as **23 mg/day during lactation.**
  - **Zinc: RDA** for zinc has been suggested as **14–15 mg/day during lactation.**

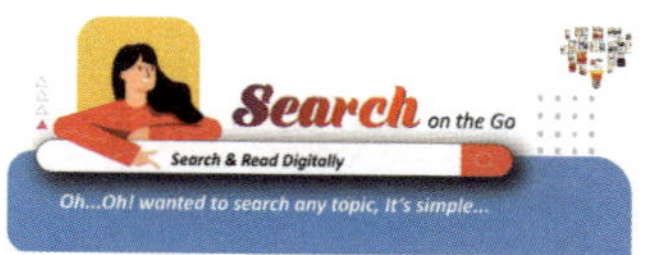

- **Iodine: RDA** for iodine has been suggested as **280 µg/day during lactation**.
- **Water:** Total water requirement has been suggested as 4100 mL/day during lactation.

Diet for Lactating Mothers

To meet the above requirements, the lactating woman should eat a wide variety of foods. Though, there is no particular need to modify the usual dietary pattern, the quantity and frequency of usage of different foods should be increased.

- To meet the calories requirement, lactating mothers should consume extra amount of cereal grains such as rice, wheat and millets.
- They should also consume extra milk, eggs, and legumes and pulses to meet the extra demand of protein. These are also good sources of calcium and other minerals.
- The lactating mothers should also consume fresh fruits and vegetables to fulfill the requirement of vitamins and minerals.
- They should also consume green leafy vegetables to meet the needs of iron and folate.
- The requirement of vitamin A can be obtained by consuming carrots, pumpkin, mangoes and other yellow colored fruits and vegetables, besides eggs and meat.
- They should also take supplements of folate, vitamin B_{12} and iron.
- At the same time, they should take large quantity of water and other beverages (nearly 2–3 L), whereas salt intake should be in limited amount only (below 5 g/day).

COMPLEMENTARY FEEDING

Around the age of 6 months, an infant's need for energy and nutrients starts to exceed, which is provided by breast milk, and complementary foods are necessary to meet those needs. An infant of this age is also developmentally ready for other foods. If complementary foods are not introduced around the age of 6 months, or if they are given inappropriately, an infant's growth may falter.

During the second year, the increase in height is about 10 cm and weight gain about 2.5 kg. During 3–6 years, height gain is 6–7 cm and weight gain is 1.5–2 kg. As growth proceeds during childhood, there are changes in proportion of water, muscle tissues, fat deposition and the skeletal structure. During the second year of life, the child starts developing a sense of individuality which is distinct from his mother. Preschool age is age of imitation and sex identification.

Guiding Principles

- Continue frequent, on-demand breastfeeding until 2 years of age or beyond.
- Start complementary feeding at 6 months with small amounts of food and increase gradually as the child gets older.
- Gradually increase food consistency and variety.
- Increase the number of times that the child is fed, viz., 2–3 meals/day for infants 6–8 months of age and 3–4 meals per day for infants 9–23 months of age with 1–2 additional snacks as required.

- Use fortified complementary foods or vitamin-mineral supplements, as needed.
- Practice responsive feeding, e.g., feed infants directly and assist older children.
- Feed slowly and patiently, encourage them to eat but do not force them, talk to the child and maintain eye contact.
- Practice good hygiene and proper food handling.
- During illness, increase fluid intake including more breastfeeding and offer soft, favorite foods.

WEANING

Weaning is the process of gradually introducing a young child to food other than the breast milk. As described above, the first 2 years of a child's life are particularly important, as optimal nutrition during this period lowers morbidity and mortality, reduces the risk of chronic diseases and fosters better development. For most of the children, growing physical capacities and the desire for independence lead to self-weaning, but some may need added encouragement from parents. The expert groups recommend that:

- Requirements for physical growth can be met by human milk throughout first year of life, but addition of a variety of solid foods help developing a loving and trusting relationship between the parents and the child.
- Continue, on-demand, frequent breastfeeding until 2 years of age.
- During the weaning period, infants may be given modified cow's milk, supplemented by vitamin D.
- Also, gradually introduce solid foods at about six months of age.
- Add iron-fortified infant cereals, progressing to wheat and mixed cereal grains.
- Add strained fruits and vegetables, progressing to finger foods such as small pieces of biscuit, etc.
- Thereafter, gradually delete strained foods and introduce routine table foods like chopped and well-cooked vegetables, eggs and chopped fruits, which should be without salt or sugar.
- Foods with high risk of chocking and aspiration may be delayed.
- Offer a variety of foods, one by one. After a taste, put new food aside, if not taken then try again later to help develop broad tastes.
- Also help the child to drink water or fruit juice by cup.
- Use fortified complementary foods or vitamin-mineral supplements, as needed.

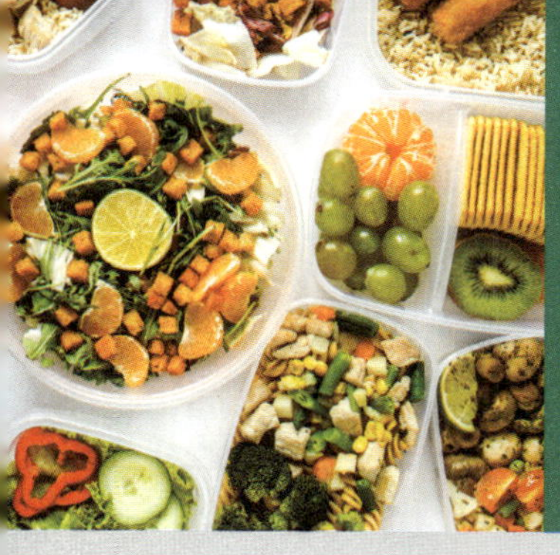

STUDENT ASSIGNMENT

LONG AND SHORT ANSWER QUESTIONS

1. Define meal planning. Explain principles and steps in meal planning.
2. **Describe diet plan for:**
   a. Children
   b. Adolescents
   c. Elderly persons
3. Describe nutritional requirements and balanced diet plan in pregnancy.
4. Describe nutritional requirements and diet for lactating mothers.
5. **Write notes on:**
   a. Infant and young child feeding
   b. Breast feeding
   c. Infant foods
   d. Diet plan for children
   e. Anemia in pregnancy
   f. Complementary feeding
   g. Weaning

MULTIPLE CHOICE QUESTIONS

1. **Which of the following is a key principle in meal planning?**
   a. Including foods only from one food group
   b. Balancing macronutrients in each meal
   c. Consuming the same meal every day
   d. Skipping meals to reduce calorie intake

2. **Growing children and adolescents should consume more:**
   a. Fat
   b. Carbohydrates
   c. Calcium
   d. Nonproteinacious food

3. **A pregnant woman should consume additional _______ kcal of energy/day.**
   a. 10
   b. 100
   c. 600
   d. 350

4. **During first six months of lactation, women should consume additional _______ kcal of energy.**
   a. 100
   b. 600
   c. 350
   d. 1000

ANSWER KEY

1. b   **2.** c   **3.** d   **4.** b

Notes

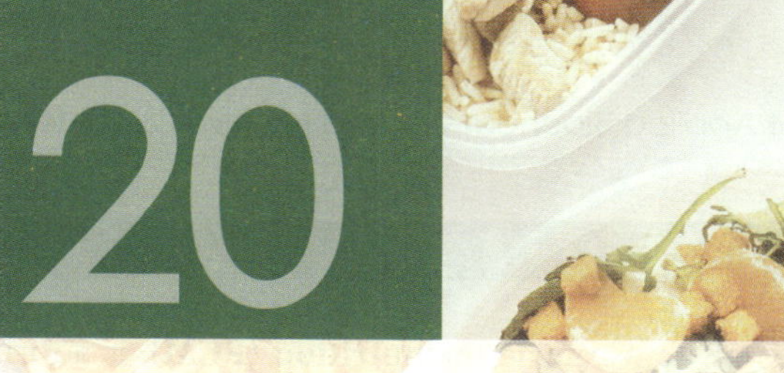

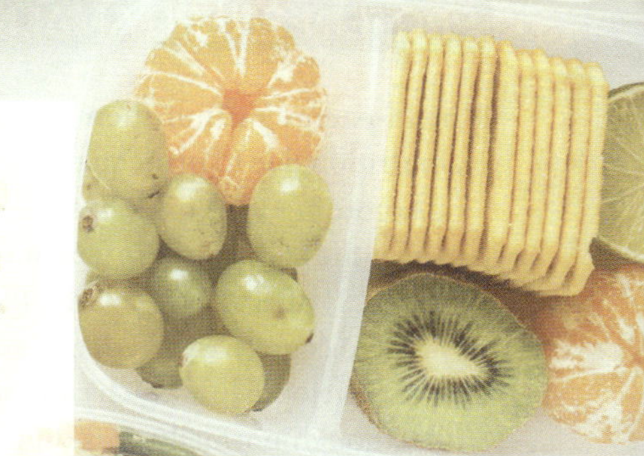

20

Common Nutritional Deficiency Disorders

LEARNING OBJECTIVES

After the completion of the chapter, the readers will be able to:
- Understand magnitude of the problem of PEM.
- Explain severe acute malnutrition (SAM).
- Explain childhood obesity.
- Understand vitamin deficiency disorders.
- Understand deficiency diseases of iron.
- Understand iodine and calcium deficiencies.

CHAPTER OUTLINE

- Protein-Energy Malnutrition
- Severe Acute Malnutrition
- Childhood Obesity

Vitamin Deficiency Disorders
- Vitamin A Deficiency Disorders
- Vitamin D Deficiency Disorders
- Vitamin B Deficiency Disorders
- Vitamin C Deficiency Disorders

Deficiency Diseases of Minerals
- Deficiency Diseases of Iron
- Deficiency Diseases of Iodine
- Deficiency Diseases of Calcium

KEY TERMS

Deficiency diseases: Diseases that are caused by the lack of certain essential nutrients, especially vitamins and minerals, in one's diet over a prolonged period of time.

Endemic neuritis: A disease caused by deficiency of thiamine, characterized by neurological symptoms, cardiovascular abnormalities, and edema.

Protein-energy malnutrition: A form of malnutrition that is defined as a range of conditions arising from coincident lack of dietary protein and/or energy (calories) in varying proportions.

Severe acute malnutrition: Very low weight-for-height/length (Z-score below −3 SD of the median WHO child growth standards), or a mid-upper arm circumference <115 mm, or by the presence of nutritional edema.

PROTEIN-ENERGY MALNUTRITION

Protein-energy malnutrition (**PEM**) also referred to as **protein-calorie malnutrition (PCM)**, is a form of malnutrition due to inadequate intake of calories and/or proteins.

According to World Health Organization, protein energy malnutrition (PEM) refers to **an imbalance between the supply of protein and energy and the body's demand for them to ensure optimal growth and function**. It affects particularly, the preschool children (<6 years) with its dire consequences ranging from physical to cognitive growth and susceptibility to infection. This affects the child at the most crucial period of time of development, which can lead to permanent impairment in later life.

Although normally, it is difficult to separate protein intake and energy intake, since a diet adequate in energy, usually has adequate protein. Similarly, a diet which lacks energy, also limits the use of dietary protein for the synthesis of various proteins, required by the body.

Although PEM can occur at any stage of life, it is most common during childhood, when extra protein is needed for rapid growth. PEM occurs in all parts of the world, but is most common in South East Asia, Africa, South and Central America, and Middle East countries. It is seen most often in population living in poverty, elderly people and hospitalized patients having some associated condition, such as anorexia nervosa, AIDS, cancer or malabsorption syndrome.

Magnitude of the Problem of PEM

In the findings about worldwide distribution of protein energy malnutrition, based on nationally representative cross-sectional data gathered between 1980 and 1992, in 79 developing countries in Africa, Asia, Latin America, and Oceania, confirm that more than a third of the world's children are affected. PEM is measured in terms of underweight (low weight for age), stunting (low height for age) and wasting (low weight for height). For all the indicators (wasting, stunting and underweight) the most favorable situation, i.e., low or moderate prevalence occur in Latin America while Asia, and other countries have high or very high prevalence. The prevalence of stunting among under five is 48% (moderate and severe), wasting is 20% (moderate and severe), with an underweight prevalence of 43% (moderate and severe), which is the highest in the world. The majority of children suffering from undernutrition (80%) are the mild and the moderate forms, which go unnoticed and the early ages are affected more, which makes the process irreversible.

The PEM is a major public health problem in India. Estimates indicate that the prevalence of stunting among under five is about 62% (moderate and severe), wasting is nearly 20% (moderate and severe) and with an underweight prevalence of around 64% (moderate and severe). This affects the child at the most crucial period of time of development, which can lead to permanent impairment in later life.

Classification of PEM

Classification of PEM is based on deficit in body weight for age and presence or absence of edema. The two main clinical syndromes of the extreme forms of PEM are referred to as **marasmus** and **kwashiorkor**, although a **mixed picture** is also seen frequently. These two are differentiated on the basis of clinical findings, with the primary distinction between kwashiorkor and marasmus, being the presence of edema in **kwashiorkor**.

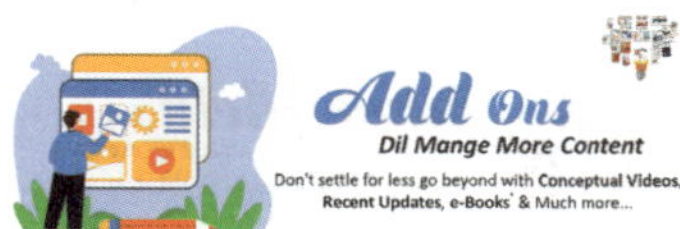

Kwashiorkor

Kwashiorkor, usually develops when diet is low in proteins. Symptoms include edema (swelling of body tissues due to accumulation of fluid), usually in the feet and legs. Belly becomes bloated due to accumulation of fat in the liver (fatty liver). Other features include growth retardation (stunted weight and height), increased susceptibility to infections, dry and fleshy skin, dry and brittle hair, and changes in skin color (pigmentation). Kwashiorkor usually develops in children between 18 to 24 months of age, at the time when weaning occurs. Protein deficiency also impairs digestion and absorption of other nutrients (Fig. 20.1).

The term **kwashiorkor** (means the sickness of the weaning) comes from a word used in Ghana, which means "a **disease of a baby deposed from the breast, when the next one is born**". It is most serious and prevalent **form of malnutrition** in the world, especially, in industrially underdeveloped countries.

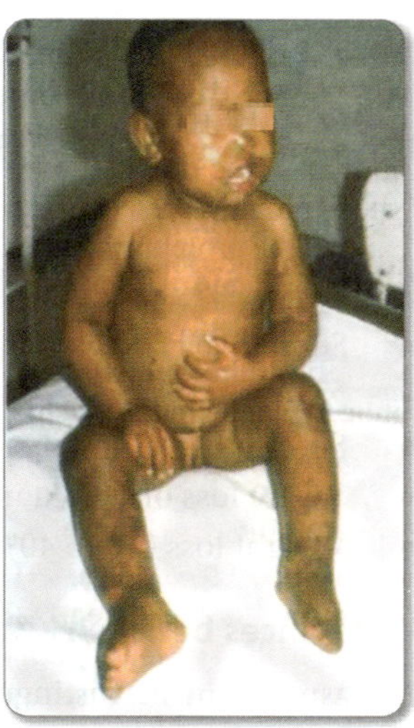

Fig. 20.1: Kwashiorkor

Causes of Kwashiorkor

It is said that kwashiorkor, usually develops when a baby is weaned from the protein-rich breast milk and switched to a protein-poor food. It tends to occur mainly in older infants and young children, and results from a **diet with inadequate protein** but reasonably **normal calorie intake**, often **exacerbated by superimposed infection**. A common scenario is when the older infant or toddler is displaced from breastfeeding, by the birth of a younger sibling and has to wean rapidly, but is unable to increase protein intake adequately. The term sugar baby also has been used to describe these children, as their typical diet is low in protein but high in carbohydrate.

Signs and Symptoms of Kwashiorkor

- Edema with swollen legs
- Pot belly (enlarged liver)
- Mild to moderate growth retardation
- Some weight loss and low subcutaneous fat
- Muscle atrophy
- Round face (moon-like face)
- Dry, flaky peeling skin
- Thin, dry and easily plucked hair

Marasmus

Marasmus results from the body's physiologic adaptation to starvation in response to **severe deprivation of calories and all nutrients**, i.e., proteins, energy and all other nutrients, intakes are grossly inadequate, depleting body fat reserves and severely wasting muscle tissue. Growth slows and children are both short and thin for their age. Their hairs are sparse and fall out easily. It can also reduce brain development and leads to learning disabilities. Marasmus occurs, most often in infants and children between 6 to 18 months of age, particularly in those who are given diluted milk (Fig. 20.2).

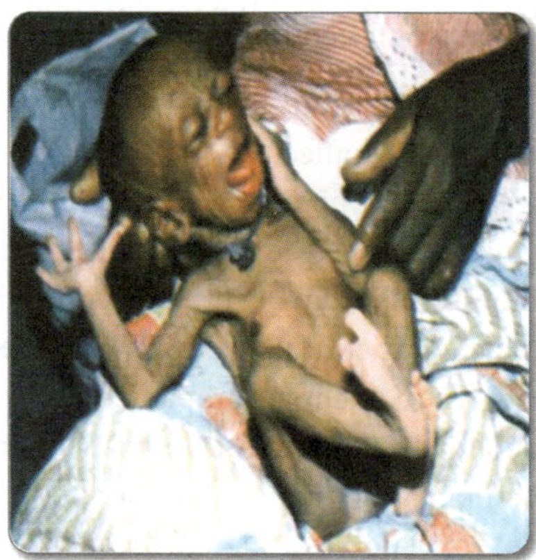

Fig. 20.2: Marasmus

Causes of Marasmus

Marasmus is a form of undernutrition caused by inadequate intake of calories. It affects infants, mainly, between the age of 6 and 18 months, as a result of failure of breastfeeding or a debilitating condition, such as chronic diarrhea.

Signs and Symptoms of Marasmus

- Severe weight loss
- No edema
- Severe growth failure
- Severe loss of subcutaneous fat
- Weight loss (up to 40%)
- Severe muscle atrophy
- Wrinkled face, like old man's face
- Rare skin changes
- Common hair changes

Differences between Kwashiorkor and Marasmus

Marasmus can be distinguished from **kwashiorkor** in the way that, kwashiorkor is a protein deficiency with adequate energy intake, whereas **marasmus** is inadequate energy and protein. Besides, there are other differences between the two conditions, as shown in (Table 20.1).

TABLE 20.1: Differences between kwashiorkor and marasmus

Kwashiorkor	Marasmus
<ul><li>Scaly skin</li><li>Distended abdomen (pot belly)</li><li>Swollen ankles (edema)</li></ul>	<ul><li>Wrinkled (dry and lose) skin</li><li>Severe muscle wasting (particularly, loss of fat from the buttocks and thighs)</li><li>Old person's face</li><li>Hair loss</li></ul>

SEVERE ACUTE MALNUTRITION

Severe acute malnutrition **(SAM)** is defined by a very low weight for height (below −3z scores of the median WHO Growth Standards), by visible severe wasting, or by the presence of nutritional edema characterized by swollen feet, face and limbs. It is the most extreme and visible form of undernutrition. About two-thirds of these children live in Asia and almost one third live in Africa. It is a life-threatening condition requiring urgent treatment.

Severe acute malnutrition kills, at least, an estimated one million children each year, and has been reported to affect an estimated 20 million children under the age of 5, worldwide, who urgently need treatment. Children with severe acute malnutrition are nine times more likely to die than well-nourished children. These deaths are the direct result of malnutrition itself, as well as the indirect result of childhood illnesses like diarrhea and pneumonia that malnourished children are too weak to survive. These settings are plagued by chronic poverty, lack of education, poor hygiene, limited access to food and poor diets.

The SAM is accompanied by significant physiopathological disorders including metabolic disturbances, anemia, compromised immunity leading to susceptibility to infections often difficult to diagnose, etc. The complications are frequent and potentially life-threatening. Mortality rates may be elevated in the absence of appropriate medical management.

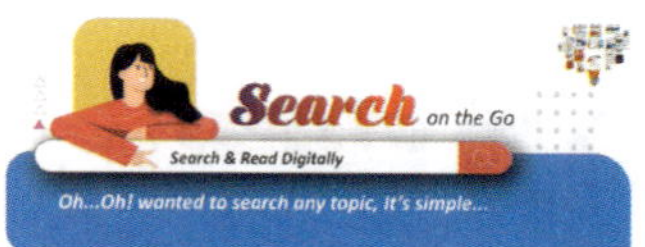

Management and Prevention of Severe Acute Malnutrition

The approach combines **community-based care** for severely malnourished children with traditional **hospital-based treatment**. In both the cases, nurse's role is important.

- Ending acute malnutrition is a complex social and political challenge. Prevention and long-term solutions involve:
  - Dismantling unequal power structures.
  - **Improving equitable access to health services and nutritious foods.**
  - **Promoting breastfeeding**, and **optimal infant and young child feeding (IYCF) practices.**
  - **Improving water and sanitation.**
  - **Ensuring access to quality foods, improved water and sanitation systems and hygienic practices.**
  - **Strengthening and improving access to health services**.
- World Health Organization (**WHO**), the World Food Programme (**WFP**), the United Nations Standing Committee on Nutrition (**UNSCN**) and United Nations Children's Fund (**UNICEF**) have **suggested** that **about three-quarters of children** with severe acute malnutrition, those who have a good appetite and no medical complications, **can be managed at home with highly fortified, ready-to-use therapeutic foods (RUTFs)**.
- **Ready-to-use therapeutic food:** Ready-to-use therapeutic food (RUTF) is a **high-energy, micronutrient enhanced paste** used to treat children under age 5, who are affected by severe acute malnutrition. As its name implies, RUTF **does not need to be cooked** or prepared before consumption. This makes it a practical solution where cooking facilities and fuels are limited. RUTF **has a long shelf life** and is **safe for use even in the absence of clean drinking water**, thereby, reducing the risk of bacterial infection. Therefore, RUTF provides the nutrients required to treat a severely malnourished child at home without refrigeration and even where hygiene conditions are not perfect.
  - The use of RUTF has transformed the treatment of severe acute malnutrition, in part, because it allows those **children without medical complications to be cured right in their own homes and communities**. This approach is referred to as the **community-based management** of severe acute malnutrition.
  - In this approach, **community health workers are trained in the technique of early detection** to recognize cases of severe acute malnutrition and provide RUTF and **routine medical care**.
  - At the same time, **health workers learn to recognize medical complications** and refer those children to hospitals and health centers for further in-patient treatment.
  - Many children with severe acute malnutrition also have infections, including HIV, and make interactions with health workers. So, it is important to have voluntary HIV testing and treatment counseling.

CHILDHOOD OBESITY

Childhood obesity is a serious medical condition where **excess body fat** negatively affects **children and adolescent's health** or well-being. The **problem is global** and is steadily affecting many low and middle-income countries, particularly in urban settings. Childhood obesity is one of the most serious public health challenges of the 21st century and its prevalence has increased at an alarming rate. Globally, in 2016, the number of overweight children, under the age of five, was estimated to be over 41 million. Almost half of these lived in Asia and one quarter in Africa. Due to the rising prevalence of obesity in children and its many adverse health effects, it is being recognized as a serious public health concern.

Obese children are **above the normal weight for their age and height**. Excess intake of energy is stored in the body as fat, which over the time may result in an individual becoming overweight and obese (Fig. 20.3).

Therefore, **the term overweight** rather than obese **is often used**, when discussing childhood obesity. **Overweight and obese children are likely to stay obese in their adulthood too**. Females are more likely to be obese as compared to males, owing to inherent hormonal differences.

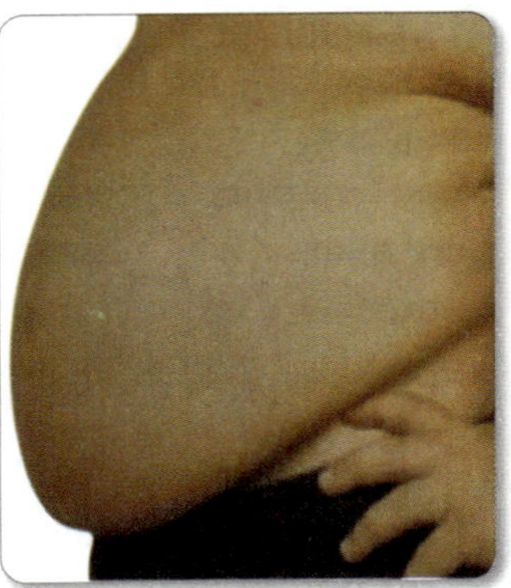

Fig. 20.3: Obesity

Reasons of Obesity

Children become overweight and obese for a variety of reasons:

- The **most common causes are genetic factors, lack of physical activity** and **sedentary behavior, unhealthy eating patterns such as increased intake of energy-dense foods**, which are **high in fat and sugars** but **low in vitamins, minerals and other healthy micronutrients**, or a combination of these factors.
- **Genetic factors:** When both the parents are obese, it is likely that their children may also be obese.
- **Social influences:** Social factors have important influence on the development of childhood obesity. Abundance of calories, highly palatable food and social enjoyment of eating create pressure to overeat and lead to obesity.
- In rare cases, it may be caused by a medical condition, such as a **hormonal problem**.

Consequences of Obesity

Childhood obesity is a multi factorial problem and there are several health consequences of it.

- Childhood obesity is particularly troubling because the **extra weight gain often takes the children on the path to health problems**, which were once considered adult problems, such as **insulin resistance and type-2 diabetes, hypertension** and hyperlipidemia (Fig. 20.4).

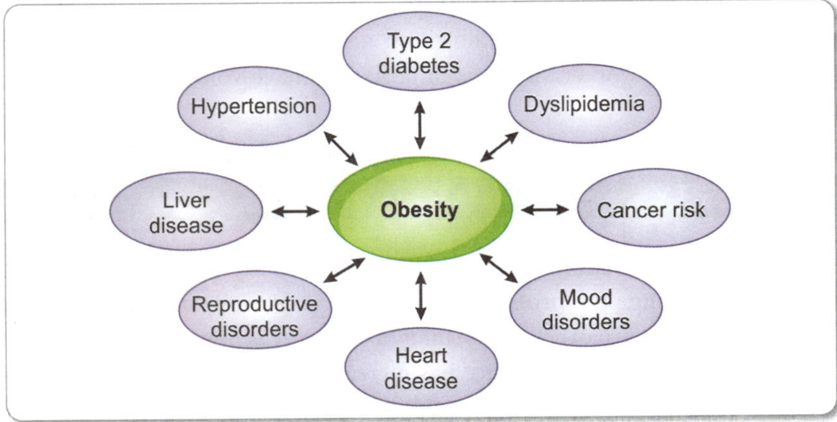

Fig. 20.4: Health problems associated with obesity

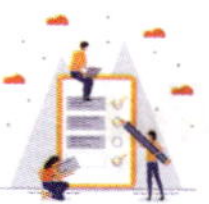
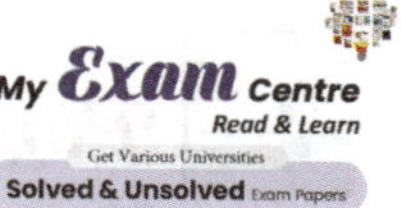

- Childhood obesity can also lead to **poor self-esteem** and **depression**.
- It may also predispose to liver and renal diseases, and reproductive dysfunction.
- Excessive body weight also increases the risk of gallstones, certain types of cancers and osteoarthritis.

Assessment

- **Biochemical features of obesity:** Biochemical features of obesity include:
  - Marked elevation of serum free fatty acids, cholesterol and triacylglycerols, irrespective of the dietary intake of fat.
  - Other findings may include higher fasting blood glucose, decreased glucose tolerance, and in some cases, other hormonal alterations.
- **Clinical assessment of obesity:** Clinical assessment of obesity is made by skin-fold thickness, or ideally by body mass index (BMI).

  BMI is computed by dividing the weight in kilograms by the square of the height in meters and the value is compared to standard values with respect to child's age and growth patterns, i.e.,

$$\textbf{BMI} = \text{Weight (kg)} \div [\text{Height (m}^2)]$$

  The normal range of BMI in children varies with age and sex. The ideal ranges of weight for a given height are provided by WHO, which are useful for categorizing persons as normal (ideal), undernourished and overweight or obese. A person with a **BMI ≥25 is considered overweight** while a person with a **BMI of 30 or more is**, generally, **considered obese**.

  While a BMI above the 85th percentile is defined as overweight, a BMI greater than or equal to the 95th percentile of their peers is considered to be obese.

  The **prevalence of overweight and obesity in adolescents** is defined according to the WHO growth reference for school-aged children and adolescents as:

Overweight = One standard deviation body mass index for age and sex

Obese = Two standard deviations body mass index for age and sex

However, it is suggested that **BMI** should be supplemented with additional screening tools such as **adipose tissue** or **skin fold measurements**.

- A **physical examination** and **some blood tests** can also rule out the possibility of a medical condition as the cause for obesity.
- Obesity invariably predisposes to **reduced levels of high-density lipoproteins (good cholesterol)** and **increased levels of low-density lipoproteins (bad cholesterol)**, and **triglycerides**, besides an **abnormal increase in glucose** and **insulin** levels in blood.

Management and Prevention

There are **no medications currently approved for the treatment of obesity** in children.

- Obesity in children is generally **treated with dietary changes** and **physical activities**. Dieting and missing meals should, however, be discouraged.

- Bariatric surgical procedures are also increasingly being used amongst adolescents with severe adolescent obesity to promote weight loss.

   Overweight and obesity, as well as their related diseases, are largely preventable.

Prevention of childhood obesity, therefore needs high priority.

- One of the best strategies to reduce childhood obesity is to improve the eating and exercise habits of the entire family.
- Limit child's consumption of sugar-sweetened beverages, or avoid them.
- Provide plenty of fruits and vegetables.
- Eat meals as a family, as often as possible.
- Limit eating out, especially, at fast-food restaurants. If one eats out, teach the child how to make healthier choices.
- Adjust portion sizes appropriately for age.
- Limit TV and other screen time to <2 hours a day for children older than 2, and do not allow television for children younger than 2, while taking a meal.
- Treating and preventing childhood obesity help to protect child's health now and in the future.
- Be sure that the child gets enough sleep.

VITAMIN DEFICIENCY DISORDERS

VITAMIN A DEFICIENCY DISORDERS

Vitamin A deficiency is the leading cause of preventable childhood blindness, afflicting 2,50,000–5,00,000 malnourished children in the developing world each year, about half of whom die within a year of becoming blind, as vitamin A deficiency also weakens the immune system.

Causes

- Vitamin A deficiency is more prevalent in vegetarians and often occurs along with the zinc deficiency.
- Faulty feeding practices and weaning
- Infectious diarrhea
- Use of skimmed milk (totally devoid of vitamin A)
- PEM

Signs and Symptoms

Although Vitamin A deficiency affects many tissues, it is most detrimental for the eyes. Young children (below the age of 3 years), and pregnant and lactating women are most vulnerable to vitamin A deficiency. In India, nearly 0.8–1.0% of the preschool children show signs of Bitot's spots and night blindness.

- **Xerophthalmia:** Deficiency of vitamin A results in xerophthalmia, i.e., drying of the conjunctiva and the cornea, followed by destruction of the cornea and blindness. Xerophthalmia occurs when body store of vitamin A is exhausted and supply fails to meet the requirement (Fig. 20.5).

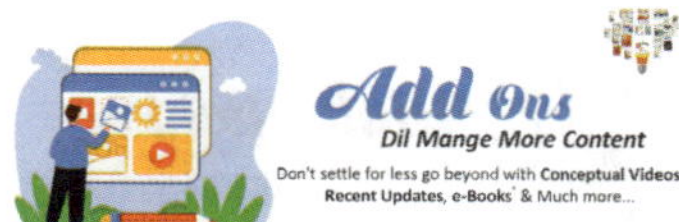

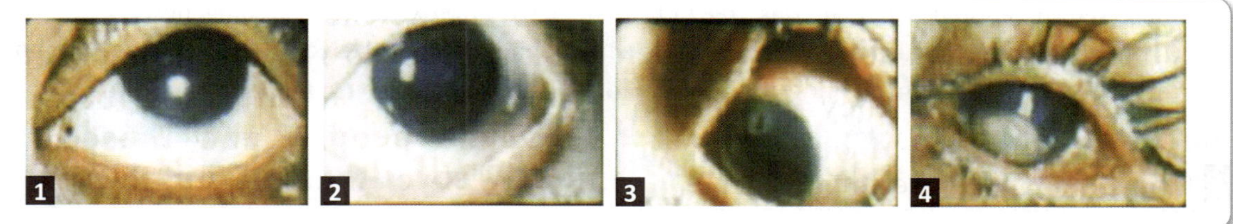

Fig. 20.5: Manifestations of xerophthalmia
(1—Bitot's spot; 2—Corneal xerosis; 3—Keratomalacia and 4—Corneal scar)

- The first symptom of xerophthalmia is **night blindness**, i.e., an individual cannot see to get around after dark or in a dark room. It responds rapidly to vitamin A therapy.
- If untreated, **Bitot's spots** (accumulation of foamy/cheesy material) develop on the conjunctiva. Although these spots may differ in size, location and shape, they have a similar appearance.
- When the cornea becomes dry, the condition is called **xerosis**.
- If the disease is not treated, it can progress within hours to an ulcer of the cornea.
- A **corneal ulcer** can lead to melting or wasting of the cornea, called **keratomalacia**. It indicates destruction of a part or of the complete corneal stroma, resulting in permanent structural alteration. Keratomalacia can lead to perforation of the cornea. At this stage, a **corneal scar** remains in the eye. The sooner the disease is treated, the smaller is the ulcer and smaller is the scar which however, remains forever.

The various stages of development of eye conditions are shown in Figure 20.6.

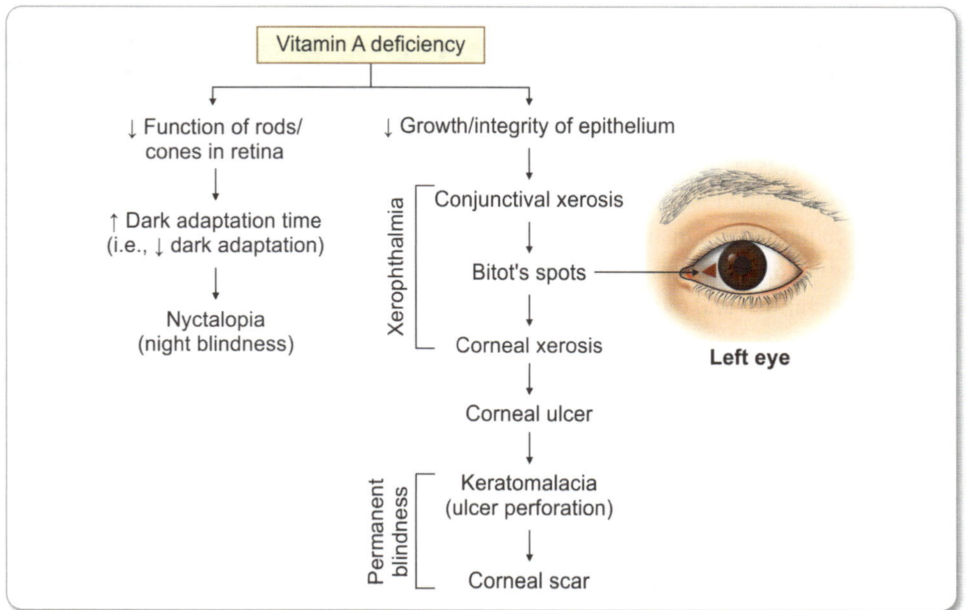

Fig. 20.6: Effect of vitamin A deficiency on the eyes

- Deficiency of vitamin A may also result in **xerosis and keratinization of various extraocular epithelial surfaces** including the mucous membrane, i.e., skin (becomes dry and rough), urogenital tract (chances of urolithiasis, infertility, degeneration of the testes, abortion and production of malformed off-springs), etc.

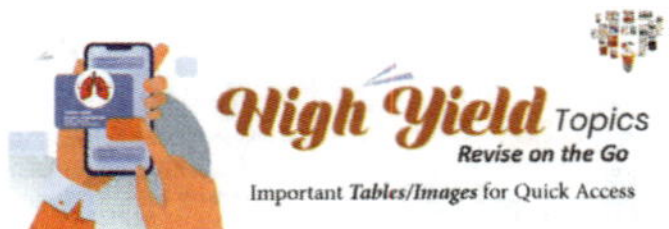

- Increased susceptibility to infections, free radical mediated cytotoxicity and carcinogenesis.
- Vitamin A deficiency also affects osteoblastic activity and results in defective resorption of the bone, thereby affecting growth of children.

Management and Prevention

- **Short-term action: Oral administration of large dose of vitamin A** (Retinol palmitate)
  - Immediately after diagnosis, administer 2 lac IU of vitamin A
  - Followed by, another dose of 2 lac IU 1–4 weeks later.
- **Medium term action:**
  - **Food fortification** with vitamin A, e.g., milk, ghee, etc.
  - **Administration of supplemental dose of vitamin A**
    - **6–11 months:** 1 dose of 1 lac IU
    - **1–5 years:** 2 lac IU, biannually
- **Long-term strategy:** Consumption of dark green leafy vegetables, promotion of breast feeding, improvement in environment health, and immunization against measles.
- Promotion of regular intake of vitamin A-rich foods
  - Feeding locally available foods
  - Kitchen gardening of vitamin A-rich foods

A nurse plays an important role in the management of vitamin A deficiency, both in long-term and medium-term actions, in the administration of large as well as supplemental doses of the vitamin.

VITAMIN D DEFICIENCY DISORDERS

Vitamin D deficiency occurs due to lack of sunshine. Vitamin D deficiency means that one does not has enough vitamin D in the body. It is typically diagnosed by measuring the concentration of the 25-hydroxyvitamin D [25(OH)D] in plasma, which is the most accurate measure of vitamin D store in the body. Deficiency is defined as less than 10 ng/mL and insufficiency in the range of 10–30 ng/mL.

Fair-skinned individuals and those who are younger, convert sunshine into vitamin D far better than those who are darker-skinned and over age 50.

Causes

Deficiencies can arise if a person does not take in enough vitamin D or his/her skin has an impaired ability to synthesize it from the sun. A person can also become deficient if the body is not able to absorb the vitamin or convert it to its active form in the liver and kidneys. Various causes include:

- **Dark skin**: People with darker skin need more sunlight exposure to produce vitamin D than those with lighter skin. Light-skinned people have less melanin than those with darker skin. Melanin is able to absorb UV-B radiation from the sun and reduce the skin's capacity to produce vitamin D_3 by 95–99%.
- **Obesity and overweight**: Being overweight or obese may put an individual at risk for a vitamin D deficiency. Some people with obesity also spend less time outdoors due to mobility issues. Fat cells keep vitamin D isolated so that it is not released. Obesity often makes it necessary to take larger doses of vitamin D supplements in order to reach and maintain normal D levels.

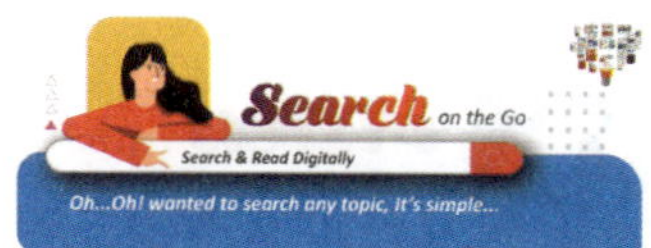

- **Lifestyle factors**: Some people spend little time outdoors due to work, ill health, a lack of outdoor space in their neighborhood, or other factors. These people have less opportunity to expose their skin to sunlight. Those who wear clothes that cover all of their body, whether to protect it from the sun or for cultural or religious reasons, may also have a higher risk of a deficiency. Being that the sun is the primary source of vitamin D, limited exposure to the sun will impact risk for a deficiency.
- **Malabsorption**: People with one of the fat malabsorption syndromes (e.g., Crohn's disease or celiac disease) and people who have had bariatric surgery are often unable to absorb enough of the fat soluble vitamin D.
- **Age**: The ability to convert vitamin D to calcitriol declines with age due to decreased kidney function. As a result, calcium absorption will fall.
- **Kidney and liver diseases**: These diseases reduce the amount of an enzyme needed to change vitamin D to a form that is used in the body. Lack of this enzyme leads to an inadequate level of active vitamin D in the body.
- **Medications and medical conditions**: A wide variety of medications, including antifungal medications, anticonvulsants, glucocorticoids and medications to treat AIDS/HIV can enhance the breakdown of vitamin D and lead to low levels.

Signs and Symptoms

Vitamin D deficiency is a known cause of rickets (skeletal effects) and has been linked to numerous other health problems (nonskeletal effects).

- **Skeletal effects of vitamin D deficiency are:**
  - **Rickets:** Prolonged deficiency of vitamin D during periods of bone growth (in children) leads to rickets. Rickets can cause bone pain, poor growth and deformities of the skeleton, such as bowed-legs, curvature of the spine, and thickening of the ankles, wrists and knees. Ends of the long bones become soft and bulky, characteristic of bowed-legs and knock-knees. There may also be extreme stunting of growth (Figs 20.7A and B).

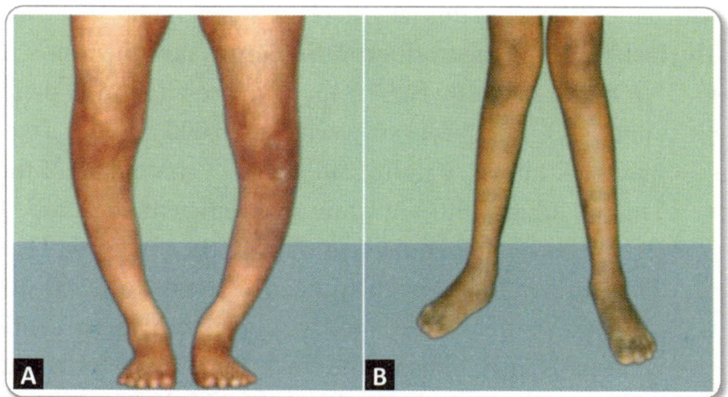

Figs 20.7A and B: Rickets: **A.** Bowed-legs and **B.** Knock-knees

  - **Osteomalacia:** Vitamin D is required to maintain healthy bones. Its deficiency in adults can lead to osteomalacia, also referred to as **adult rickets**. Commonly observed symptoms include increased bone turnover, leading to aching bones and muscles, and proximal muscle weakness.
  - **Osteoporosis:** The bones become thin or brittle. The first sign may be breaking of bone easily as a result of minor trauma. It often affects older people (Fig. 20.8).
- **Nonskeletal effects of vitamin D deficiency**: Vitamin D deficiency may also lead to defects in insulin secretion and impaired glucose tolerance, impaired immunity, carcinogenesis, etc.

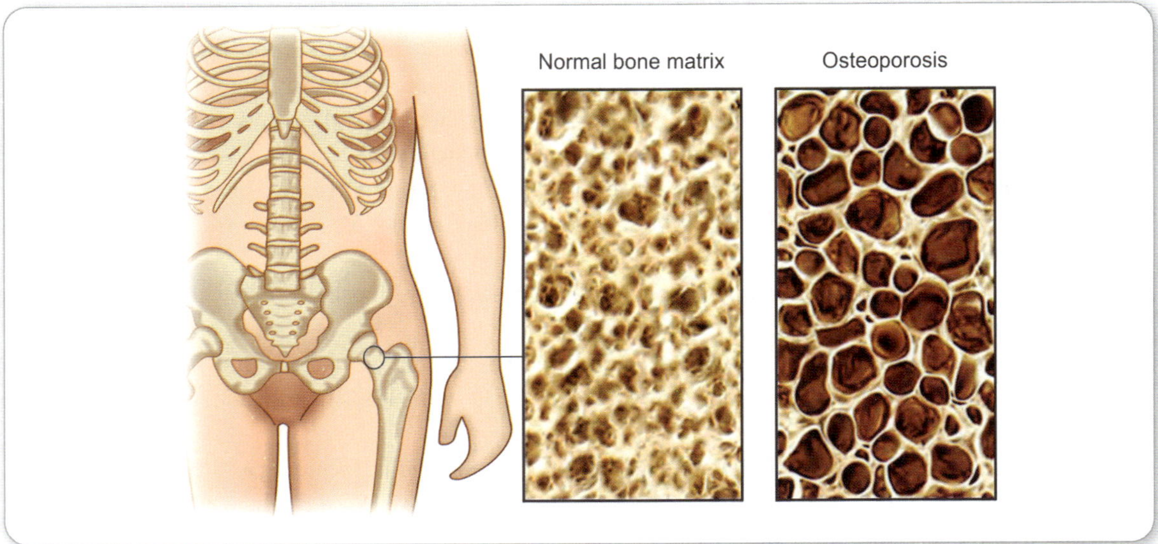

Fig. 20.8: Osteoporosis is characterized by a decrease in bone density (mass per unit volume) and occurs in a fully developed bone, where it appears like 'pores' in the bone, hence the name.

Management and Prevention

Vitamin D_3 has been shown to be the best choice for supplements. Vitamin D supplements should be taken with a meal that contains fat. There are supplements that can be taken on a daily, weekly or monthly basis.

The task force for the Endocrine Society makes the following recommendations:

- For children 1–18 years of age who are vitamin D deficient, recommendation includes 2000 IU/day of vitamin D_3 for at least six weeks; or 50,000 IU once a week for at least 6 weeks to achieve a blood level of 25(OH)D above 30 ng/mL, followed by maintenance therapy of 600–1000 IU/day.
- That all adults who are vitamin D deficient should be given 50,000 IU of vitamin D_3 once a week for eight weeks; or its equivalent of 6000 IU of vitamin D_3 daily to achieve a blood level of 25(OH)D above 30 ng/mL, followed by maintenance therapy of 1500–2000 IU/day.
- In obese patients, patients with malabsorption syndromes and patients on medications affecting vitamin D metabolism, the Task force suggests a higher dose (two to three times higher; at least 6000–10,000 IU/day) of vitamin D to treat vitamin D deficiency, or to maintain a 25(OH)D level above 30 ng/mL, followed by maintenance therapy of 3000–6000 IU/day.

Prevention of Vitamin D Deficiency

Vitamin D (also called **sunshine vitamin**) can be synthesized in human beings from its precursor, called 7-dehydrocholesterol (also referred to as provitamin D), by the action of UV light in the skin. This process is defined as photobiogenesis. Thereafter, vitamin D is converted to its active form in the liver and the kidney. Accordingly, vitamin D deficiency can be prevented by:

- Daily exposure to sunlight for nearly 15–20 minutes.
- Regular check-up and treatment for skin, liver and kidney disorders, besides vitamin D resistant rickets.

- **The Office of Dietary Supplements (ODS) recommends** the following intake each day:
  - **0–12 months**—400 IU (10 µg)
  - **1–70 years**—600 IU (15 µg)
  - **71 years and above**—800 IU (20 µg)
- A nurse plays an important role in the management and prevention of:
  - Vitamin D deficiency as well as
  - Helping in the treatment of other medical condition(s) that may lead to vitamin D deficiency, in a hospital set-up

VITAMIN B DEFICIENCY DISORDERS

The B vitamins are a group of different vitamins, each with unique roles in keeping the body healthy. They are especially important for maintaining cell health and keeping energized. The symptoms of a vitamin B deficiency vary depending on which particular group of B vitamin is deficient. Some foods are high in several B vitamins while certain foods are particularly high in specific B vitamins. Eating a balanced diet is a key for getting all B vitamins our body needs.

Vitamin B$_1$ Deficiency Disorders

Vitamin B$_1$ (thiamine) deficiency is especially common in countries that do not require fortification of wheat and maize flour, and rice to replace the naturally occurring thiamine content lost to milling, bleaching and other processing. Severe deficiency of thiamine causes **beriberi**, which became prevalent in Asia as more people adopted a diet primarily of white rice. Its deficiency is assessed by red blood cell status and urinary output.

The word beriberi comes from a Sinhalese word meaning **"extreme weakness"**, as it can cause severe and even life-threatening symptoms. **Beriberi** became a public health issue in the Far East in the nineteenth century, with the introduction of highly milled (polished) rice. While beriberi is now rare, it still remains a problem in some parts of the world, where rice is the staple food.

There are two main forms of beriberi:

- **Wet beriberi**, which mainly affects the cardiovascular system, causing poor circulation and fluid build-up in the tissues. Its symptoms include enlarged heart, heart failure and severe edema.
- **Dry beriberi**, which primarily affects the central nervous system and causes nerve degeneration, loss of nerve transmission, leading to nervous tingling throughout the body, muscle wasting, poor arm and leg coordination, and deep pain in calf muscles. Primary signs of thiamine deficiency include weakness, irritability and headache, fatigue and depression, and reduced functions associated with brain and nervous system (Fig. 20.9).

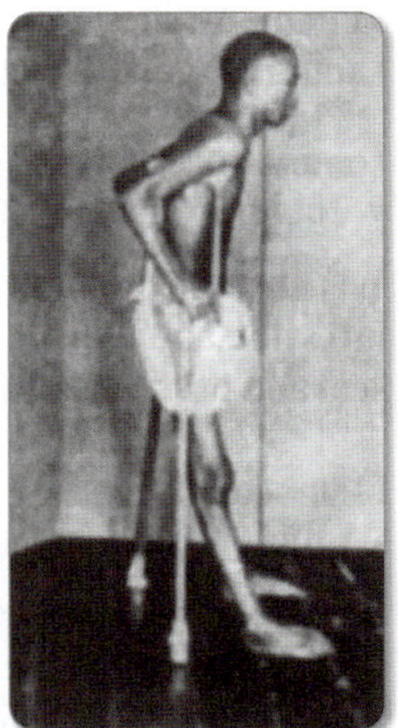

Fig. 20.9: Endemic neuritis (dry beriberi)

Causes

The leading cause of beriberi is either a **diet low in thiamine** or a problem that limits the **body's ability to process thiamine**.

Deficiency of thiamin commonly occurs in:

- Areas where people consume polished-rice, which results in loss of available thiamin. The loss can be decreased by using unpolished or parboiled rice or whole wheat flour.
- Consumption of raw fish in large quantities.
- Chronic alcoholics.
- **Wernicke's encephalopathy:** Alcoholic patients with chronic thiamin deficiency may also have CNS manifestations, ophthalmoplegia, cerebeller ataxia and mental impairment.

Management and Prevention

- **Management of beriberi** includes increased thiamine levels in the body, which may include oral supplements or injections of thiamine, depending on a person's overall health. It may also include taking thiamine supplements to support management.
- **Prevention of beriberi** requires consumption of enough thiamine in their diet. Foods that naturally contain thiamine include meat, nuts and seeds, beans and legumes, seafood and dairy products. Eating fortified bread and cereals, is the most common way for people to reach the recommended daily intake of thiamine. A person who drinks a lot of alcohol should take vitamin B_1, or vitamin B complex, supplement.

Prevention therapy should be given to people with limited intake, malabsorption, or increased requirements lasting more than two weeks. Consumption of about 1 mg of thiamine daily is sufficient to prevent thiamine deficiency. When the staple cereal is polished rice or cassava, special efforts need to be made to include legumes and/or nuts in the ration.

Niacin Deficiency Disorders

Deficiency of niacin is not usually observed since it can be synthesized in the body from tryptophan (an essential amino acid). Its deficiency, however, may occur in:

- People whose staple food is maize or sorghum (Jowar). These cereals are rich in leucine but are deficient in tryptophan; the amino acid imbalance affects tryptophan-niacin pathway, and in turn, reduces the biosynthesis of niacin (normally 60 mg tryptophan forms 1 mg niacin). Leucine itself also inhibits endogenous biosynthesis of niacin.
- Patients taking isonicotinic acid hydrazide (INH), an antitubercular drug (along with the deficiency of vitamin B_6).
- Patients with Hartnup's disease, which is due to a defect in tryptophan absorption.

Causes

There are two types of niacin deficiencies:

1. **Primary niacin deficiency:** Primary niacin deficiency occurs when a person does not take enough niacin or tryptophan. In regions of the world where maize, sometimes called Indian corn, is a major part of the diet, people may not get enough niacin. This is because the body cannot absorb niacin in maize unless it has been treated with alkali.
2. **Secondary niacin deficiency:** Secondary niacin deficiency occurs when another condition such as diarrhea, Hartnup disease, liver disease, or alcoholism interferes with the body's ability to absorb niacin. Other possible causes include prolonged treatment with the tuberculosis drug isoniazid.

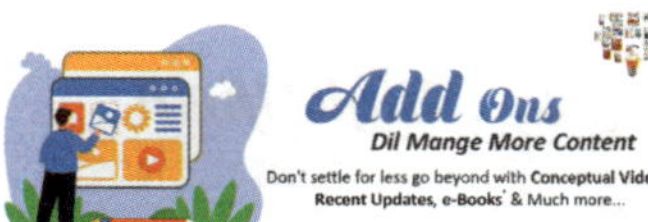

Signs and Symptoms

Deficiency of niacin leads to pellagra, a disease characterized by 3Ds, i.e., **D**ermatitis, **D**iarrhea and **D**ementia:

1. **Dermatitis:** It results in pain in those parts of the body which are exposed to sunlight, such as face, neck, hands and feet. These parts become bronze-colored resembling sunburn and later become thickened (Fig. 20.10).
2. **Diarrhea:** It is accompanied with anorexia and other abdominal discomforts.
3. **Dementia:** It is due to impaired ability of the brain to utilize carbohydrates. Symptoms like depression, confusion and psychosis are commonly observed, which are due to decreased synthesis of tryptophan-derived neurotransmitters.

   Prolonged deficiency of niacin may ultimately result in fourth D, i.e., Death.

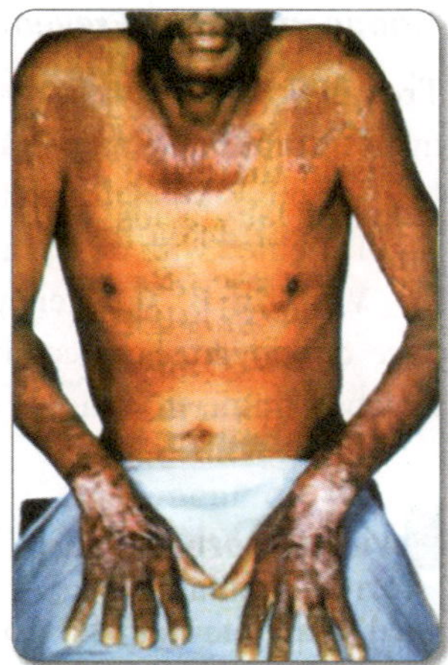

Fig. 20.10: Dermatitis on hands in pellagra

Management and Prevention

Pellagra can be reversed with niacin supplementation. Nicotinamide is usually used to treat niacin deficiency, because nicotinamide, unlike nicotinic acid (the most common form of niacin), does not cause flushing, itching, burning, or tingling sensations. Nicotinamide is given in doses of 250–500 mg orally daily.

Patients with pellagra should **avoid sun exposure and alcohol intake**.

Vitamin B_6 Deficiency Disorders

Vitamin B_6 is one of the central molecules in the cells of living organisms. As a coenzyme, B_6 is involved as a cofactor in over 100 enzymatic reactions including carbohydrate metabolism, amino acid metabolism, particularly homocysteine, gluconeogenesis, glycogenolysis and lipid metabolism. It also has a role in cognitive development through neurotransmitter synthesis, immune function with interleukin-2 (IL-2) production, and hemoglobin formation.

Causes

- Dietary vitamin B_6 deficiency, though rare, can develop because extensive processing can deplete foods of vitamin B_6.
- Secondary vitamin B_6 deficiency most often results from:
  - Protein-energy malnutrition
  - Malabsorption
  - Alcoholism
  - Use of pyridoxine-inactivating drugs (e.g., antiseizure drugs, isoniazid, cycloserine, corticosteroids, etc.).
  - Excessive loss during hemodialysis.

Signs and Symptoms

- Vitamin B_6 deficiency causes peripheral neuropathy and a pellagra-like syndrome, with seborrheic dermatitis, glossitis, and cheilosis, and, in adults, can cause depression, confusion, electroencephalogram (EEG) abnormalities and seizures.
- Normocytic, microcytic, or sideroblastic anemia can also develop.

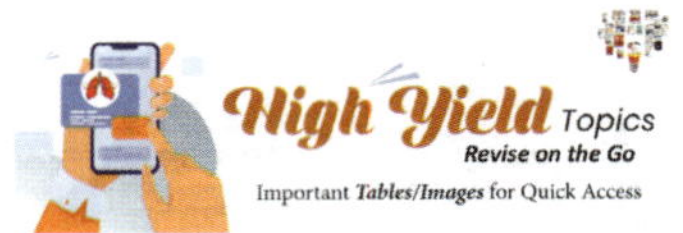

Management and Prevention

Treatment dosage is variable and depends on the severity of symptoms. The vitamin is available therapeutically in both oral and parenteral formulations. Neonates with B_6 deficiency seizures may require 10–100 mg intravenous (IV) for effective treatment of active seizures. Less serious or less acute presentations can be supplemented with doses ranging from 25 mg/day to 600 mg/day orally, depending on symptom complex.

Vitamin B_6 deficiency can be prevented, if supplementation is undertaken before severe deficits have developed. For secondary vitamin B_6 deficiency, causes (e.g., use of pyridoxine-inactivating drugs, malabsorption, etc.) should be corrected, if possible.

Folate Deficiency Disorders

Folate helps to make and repair DNA, and produce red blood cells. Since it is a water-soluble vitamin, not eating enough folate can lead to a deficiency in just a few weeks. Deficiency may also occur if one has a disease or genetic mutation that prevents the body from absorbing or converting folate to its active form.

Causes

Folate deficiency is not generally observed, as it can be synthesized by the intestinal flora. Causes of folate deficiency include:

- A diet low in fresh fruits, vegetables and fortified cereals is the main cause of folate deficiency.
- Stressful conditions, pregnancy and intestinal malabsorption (such as steatorrhea or due to antibiotic therapy).
- Use of certain compounds, which interfere with the metabolic functions of folic acid called folic acid antagonists. Most potent of these are **aminopterin** (4-aminofolic acid) and amethopterin (N^{10}-methylfolic acid or methotrexate), which are the competitive inhibitors of dihydrofolate reductase and are used as anticancer agents in childhood leukemias.

Signs and Symptoms

Deficiency of folate can result in:

- **Megaloblastic anemia**, which causes weakness and fatigue. It is characterized by the release of RBCs that are larger than normal and not fully developed due to impairment of the normal process of maturation of RBCs in the bone marrow.
- Folic acid deficiency also **impairs synthesis of white blood cells**, which are vital to immune response.
- Deficiency of folic acid is also, often, accompanied by **insomnia**, **depression**, **forgetfulness** and **irritability**.
- Heart palpitations and shortness of breath.
- Open sores in the mouth.
- Changes in skin, hair, or fingernail color.
- Pregnant women with a folate deficiency could result in their babies being born with **neural tube defects**, such as spina bifida.

Management and Prevention

- **Treatment** involves increasing the dietary intake/supplement of folate.
  - Folate is frequently combined with other B vitamins in supplements. These are sometimes called vitamin B complexes.

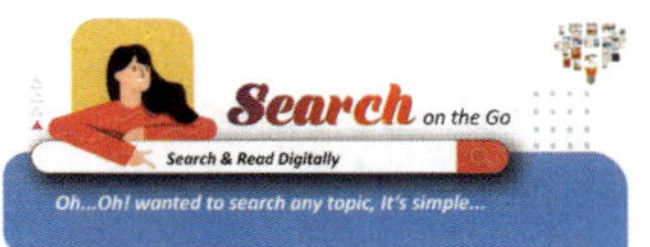

- Pregnant women should completely avoid alcohol. Besides, everyone else with a folate deficiency should decrease their alcohol intake.
- To prevent folate deficiency, one should eat a nutritious diet.
  Foods that contain high amounts of folate include green-leafy vegetables such as broccoli and spinach, Brussels sprouts, peas and citrus; fruits such as banana and melons; tomato juice, eggs and poultry, beans and legumes, etc.

Vitamin B_{12} Deficiency Disorders

Vitamin B_{12}, also called cobalamin, helps regulate the nervous system. It also plays a role in growth and red blood cell formation.

Causes

Dietary deficiency of vitamin B_{12} occurs among strict **vegans**, more common in **older people**, as a result of **impaired absorption**, usually, due to chronic inflammation of the stomach lining (atrophic gastritis) or lack of intrinsic factor (R-protein, the substance required for vitamin B_{12} absorption).

Signs and Symptoms

Vitamin B_{12} deficiency is a common cause of megaloblastic anemia, various neuropsychiatric symptoms, and other clinical manifestations. Vitamin B_{12} deficiency may lead to the following symptoms such as:
- **Pernicious anemia**, a condition where the bone marrow produces large (megaloblastic anemia) abnormally shaped red blood cells that do not function properly.
  - Weakness, tiredness or light headedness
  - Heart palpitations and shortness of breath
  - Pale skin
  - A smooth tongue
  - Constipation, diarrhea, loss of appetite or gas
  - Nerve problems like numbness or tingling, muscle weakness and problems walking
  - Vision loss
  - Mental problems like depression, memory loss or behavioral changes

Treatment and Prevention

Vitamin B_{12} deficiency is not generally observed, due to its widespread distribution in animal tissues such as kidney, egg, fish and milk, and its synthesis by the microbial flora.
- Individuals who had undergone geriatric surgery may be given 1 mg of oral vitamin B_{12} per day.
- Those who are strict vegetarians must be given supplementation, because plants do not synthesize vitamin B_{12}.

Most people can prevent vitamin B_{12} deficiency by eating enough meat, poultry, seafood, dairy products and eggs.
- To prevent vitamin B_{12} deficiency, vegans should take adequate amount of vitamin B_{12} supplements to make up for the shortage in their diet.
- For people who cannot absorb B_{12}, the condition cannot be prevented. However, once it is diagnosed, regular injections of vitamin B_{12} will prevent symptoms from returning.

VITAMIN C DEFICIENCY DISORDERS

Severe deficiency of vitamin C leads to a disease called scurvy, where connective tissue loses its ability to synthesize collagen. Deficiency symptoms include **bleeding from gums**, **poor wound healing**, and **damage to bone** and other tissues (Fig. 20.11).

Vitamin C deficiency can also lead to anemia, debility, exhaustion, spontaneous bleeding, pain in the limbs, and especially the legs, swelling in some parts of the body, and sometimes ulceration of the gums and loss of teeth.

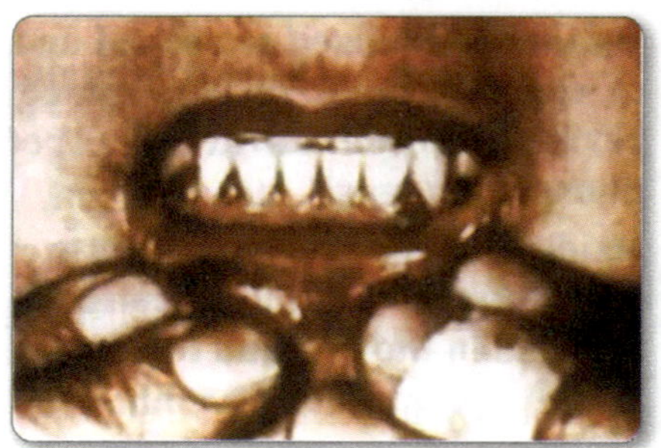

Fig. 20.11: Scurvy

Causes

- Vitamin C deficiency may be observed due to low intake of vitamin C rich foods such as amla, guava and citrus fruits.
- Other causes of vitamin C deficiency include smoking and old age.

Signs and Symptoms

- Prolonged deficiency of vitamin C causes **scurvy**, which is due to impaired collagen formation and poor blood vessel support. It is characterized by bleeding gums.
- In **infantile scurvy**, infants lose appetite and weight with painful tenderness of the extremities, and bleeding from gums and mucous membrane. In addition, long bones show cessation of osteogenesis.
- Because of the role of vitamin C in absorption, transport and storage of iron, deficiency of vitamin C may also lead to anemia, i.e., microcytic anemia.

Management and Prevention

- Management involves administering vitamin C supplements by mouth or by injection. The recommended dosage is:
  - 1–2 g/day for 2–3 days
  - 500 mg for the next 7 days
  - 100 mg for 1–3 months
- Within 24 hours, patients can expect to see an improvement in fatigue, lethargy, pain, anorexia and confusion. Bruising, bleeding, and weakness start to resolve within 1–2 weeks. After 3 months, a complete recovery is possible.
- Chronic gingivitis with extensive subcutaneous hemorrhage persists longer.
- In addition to immediate supplementation, educate the patient on lifestyle modifications to ensure adequate intake, and recommend cessation of alcohol and tobacco.
- **Vitamin C deficiency can be prevented** by making sure that you have a healthy, balanced diet that contains plenty of fruits and vegetables, including those high in vitamin C. As a rough guide, one large orange a day will provide with enough vitamin C.
- Vitamin C 75 mg orally once a day for women and 90 mg orally once a day for men prevents deficiency. Smokers should consume an additional 35 mg/day.

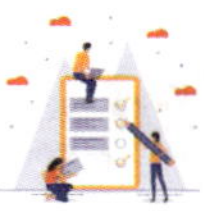
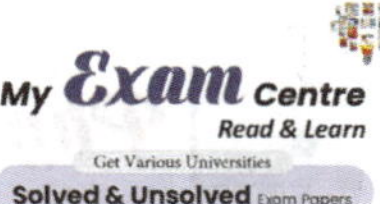

DEFICIENCY DISEASES OF MINERALS

DEFICIENCY DISEASES OF IRON

Deficiency of dietary iron leads to a condition called **anemia**, also referred to as **iron deficiency anemia**. Iron is required by the body to form hemoglobin, which is present in the red blood cells, in our body. The main function of hemoglobin is to transport oxygen from lungs to the various parts of body.

Iron deficiency anemia is most common in pregnant women, lactating mothers, infants, preschool children and adolescent girls. It adversely affects work output among adults, and learning ability in children. Patients suffering from anemia become pale, lose appetite and feel exhausted.

In India, among children, between the age of 6 and 59 months, a majority (70%) are anemic. Nearly, three-fourth (75%) of the women are anemic, with the prevalence of moderate to severe anemia, being highest (50%) among the pregnant women. It is estimated that nutritional anemia contributes to about 24% of the maternal deaths and is one of the important causes of low birth weight.

Anemia may be grouped as mild, moderate or severe (Table 20.2).

TABLE 20.2 Classification of anemia

Degree of anemia	Hemoglobin (g%)
Mild	10.0–10.9
Moderate	7–10
Severe	<7

Causes

Iron deficiency can be a result of injury, hemorrhage or some other illness, e.g., blood loss, hookworms or a GIT disease that interferes with iron absorption. Besides, iron deficiency may also be aggravated by an unbalanced diet, containing insufficient iron, protein, folate or vitamin C.

- Inadequate intake of iron
- Poor bioavailability and iron malabsorption
- Excessive loss of iron such as during menstruation, rapid pregnancies or hookworm infestations
- Malaria
- Gastrointestinal bleeding

Signs and Symptoms

Initially, iron deficiency anemia can be so mild that it goes unnoticed. But as the body becomes more deficient in iron, and anemia worsens, the signs and symptoms intensify. Signs and symptoms of iron deficiency anemia include:

- Extreme fatigue
- Weakness

- Pale skin
- Chest pain, fast heartbeat or shortness of breath
- Headache, dizziness or light headedness
- Cold hands and feet
- Inflammation or soreness of tongue
- Brittle nails
- Unusual cravings for non-nutritive substances such as ice, dirt or starch
- Poor appetite, especially in infants and children with iron deficiency anemia

Anemic children become dull, inactive, loose appetite and have poor growth. In females, deficiency of iron reduces their work capacity. It is also associated with reduced immune-competence (Fig. 20.12).

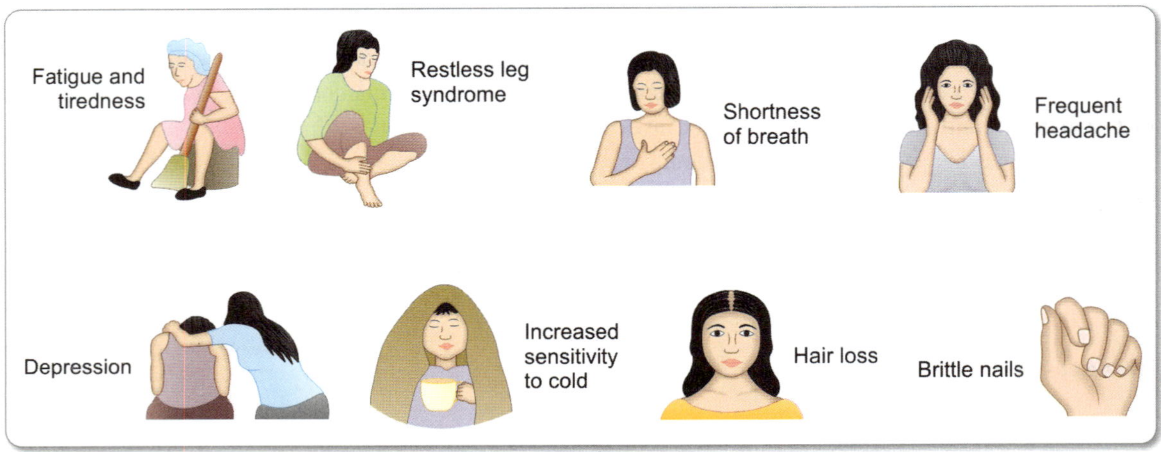

Fig. 20.12: Signs and symptoms of iron deficiency anemia

Management and Prevention

- Blood transfusion, in severe cases of anemia (<8 g/dL).
- **Treating the underlying cause of bleeding**.
- Iron tablets can help restore iron levels in the body, which preferably, should be taken empty stomach that helps the body absorb them better.
- **Diet:** The following foods can help treat or prevent iron deficiency:
  - Red meat
  - Dark green, leafy vegetables
  - Dried fruits
  - Nuts
  - Iron-fortified cereals
- **Vitamin C supplementation:** It helps body absorb iron.
- In the most severe cases, a blood transfusion can replace iron and blood loss quickly.
  When caused by inadequate iron intake, **iron deficiency anemia can be prevented** by eating a diet high in iron-rich foods and vitamin C.

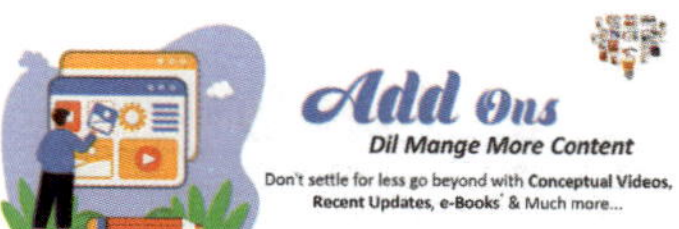

- **Preventing iron deficiency anemia in infants:** To prevent iron deficiency anemia in infants, breast-feed the baby for 6 months. After the age of 6 months, start feeding baby iron-fortified cereals or pureed meats at least twice a day to boost iron intake.
  - Iron and folic acid supplementation to pregnant women, lactating mothers and children under 12 years
  - Fortification of salt with iron
  - Food fortification with iron
  - Changing dietary habits
  - Control of parasites
  - Nutrition education and awareness

DEFICIENCY DISEASES OF IODINE

Iodine deficiency is due to lack of the trace element iodine. It leads to a wide range of disorders, referred to as **Iodine Deficiency Disorders (IDD)** that affects health of humans from fetal stage to adulthood, with serious health and social implications.

The IDD are prevalent worldwide. In India, IDD are very common among large sections of the population, in several parts of the country, particularly, in Himalayan region, known as goiter belt. About 167 millions of people are estimated to be living in IDD endemic areas.

About 90,000 still-births and neonatal deaths occur every year due to maternal iodine deficiency. Around 54 million persons are estimated to have goiter, 2.2 million have cretinism and 6.6 million suffer from mild psychomotor handicaps.

Causes

Deficient iodine intake may be due to:
- Consumption of foods with low iodine contents and the crops grown in the iodine depleted soil
- Increased demand for iodine by the body, such as during infancy, puberty, pregnancy and lactation.
- Presence of goitrogens (goiter producing substances that are naturally present in some foods, like cabbage, cauliflower, etc.) which interfere with iodine utilization.

Signs and Symptoms of Iodine Deficiency

Iodine deficiency causes **goiter** (enlargement of the thyroid gland in the neck), neonatal hypothyroidism, **cretinism** (among newborns), mental retardation, delayed motor development, stunting, deaf-mutism and neuromuscular disorders (Figs 20.13 and 20.14).
- Impaired mental functions and retardation
- Poor intellectual performance
- Lowered IQ
- Muscular disorders and impaired coordination, and sluggishness
- Delayed motor milestones, and hearing and speech defects
- Neuromuscular weakness

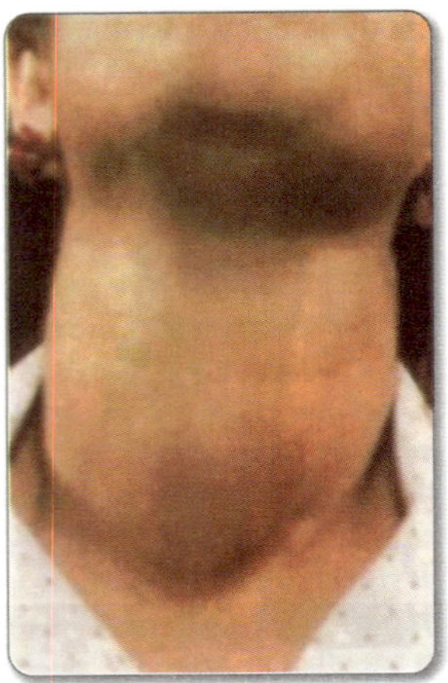

Fig. 20.13: Endemic goiter

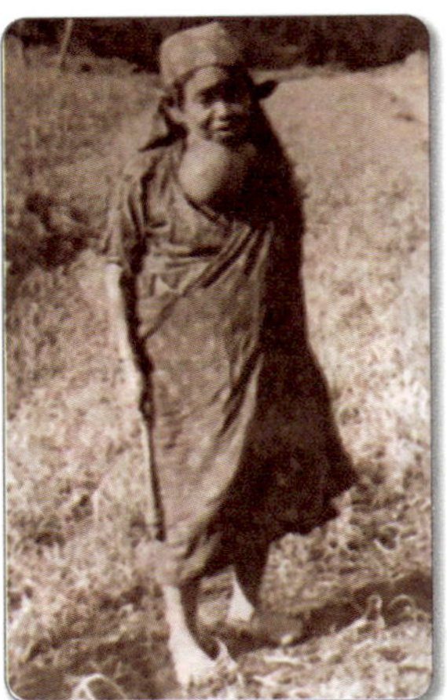

Fig. 20.14: Cretinism

- Endemic cretinism
- Intrauterine death
- In pregnancy, iodine deficiency causes spontaneous abortions, stillbirth and infant deaths.
- Deficiency of iodine in pregnant women interferes with brain development of the fetus and results in birth of the iodine deficient babies, who may be cretins, characterized by mental deficiency, hearing defects, squint and stunted growth.

Management and Prevention

- The best method of managing iodine deficiency is avoiding it in the first place. If deficiency develops, it can be treated with iodine supplementation and dietary modifications.
- Iodine deficiency is best corrected by a healthy diet. Mild cases may be managed by using iodized salt in daily food consumption.
- If diet alone is not supplying enough iodine, one may consider adding an iodine supplement containing potassium (potassium iodide and potassium iodate).
- People with myxedema require hospitalization to administer intravenous fluids and other stabilizing treatments. They will also be administered thyroid hormones to correct the condition.

Prevention includes:
- Consumption of iodized salt
- Iodine monitoring and surveillance
- Public awareness and education
- Increase intake of seafoods, green leafy vegetables, etc., which are rich in iodine

DEFICIENCY DISEASES OF CALCIUM

Calcium is a vital mineral. It is used by the body to build strong bones and teeth. Calcium is also important for your nerves, heart, and muscles function. Children who do not get enough calcium, may not grow to their full potential height as adults.

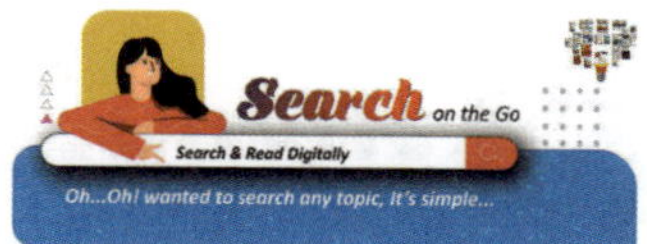

Causes

Some of the causes of calcium deficiency are:

- High alcohol or coffee consumption
- Hormonal disorders such as decline in estrogen levels (menopause)
- Disorder of calcium absorption, including low levels of vitamin D
- Kidney diseases
- Increase demand for calcium requirement by the body due to stages/phases such as puberty, breastfeeding, pregnancy, etc.
- Medication such as phenytoin, phenobarbital, rifampin, corticosteroids, diuretics and proton pump inhibitors
- Athletes who sweat a lot
- Massive blood transfusions
- Pancreatitis
- Thyroid diseases
- Elevated phosphorus level
- Lactose intolerant or people allergic to dairy products
- Genetic factors such as vitamin D resistance syndrome or inherited disorders of calcium and phosphate homeostasis
- Increase in age absorption of calcium gradually decreases
- Massive blood transfusions
- Removal of parathyroid gland tissue as part of surgery to remove the thyroid gland

Signs and Symptoms

Symptoms of hypocalcemia can vary and depend on cause of the deficiency. Some people may have no symptoms while others may experience a variety of symptoms.

Calcium deficiencies can affect all parts of the body, resulting in weak nails, slower hair growth, and fragile, thin skin. Calcium also plays an important role in both neurotransmitter release and muscle contractions. So, calcium deficiencies can bring on seizures in otherwise healthy people. In addition, symptoms of related vitamin D deficiency can include achiness or tenderness in the bones.

Severe symptoms of hypocalcemia include:

- Confusion or memory loss
- Muscle spasms and muscle cramps
- Numbness and tingling in the hands, feet, and face
- Depression
- Hallucinations
- Weak and brittle nails
- Easy fracturing of the bones
- **In addition:**
  - Inadequate intake of calcium, as well as inadequate intake of vitamin D, can lead to developing **rickets** in children. This condition results in bone deformities and growth retardation.
  - Calcium deficiency in adults can lead to softening of bones or **osteomalacia**.

- Hypocalcemia may also lead to **osteoporosis**, which is characterized by loss of bone matrix and progressive demineralization. Decreased calcium intake, particularly, during menopause, leads to increased fragility of bones, mainly, of extremities and pelvis.
- Hypocalcemia may also result in **tetany** of skeletal muscle. It is characterized by muscle twitching, leg cramps, muscle spasms and, eventually, convulsions.

Management and Prevention

Calcium deficiency can be corrected simply by ingesting more calcium and making sure that one is also getting enough vitamin D. Besides calcium and vitamin D supplements, it is also necessary to treat the underlying condition causing calcium deficiency.

Commonly recommended calcium supplements include:

- Calcium carbonate, which is the least expensive and has the most elemental calcium.
- Calcium citrate, which is the most easily absorbed.
- Calcium phosphate, which is also easily absorbed and does not cause constipation.

The best and easy way to prevent calcium deficiency is to switch to a calcium-rich diet. In addition, one must also take precautions and preventive measures to keep intact a healthy lifestyle, such as avoid excess alcohol consumption, smoking and eating too much of junk food. Also, exercise regularly and maintain healthy body weight. Eat food that is low in salt. Try to include fresh ingredients in your meal and keep away processed and preserved food. Have whole grains, vegetables, and fruits in fresh form. Limit your caffeine and carbonated drink intake.

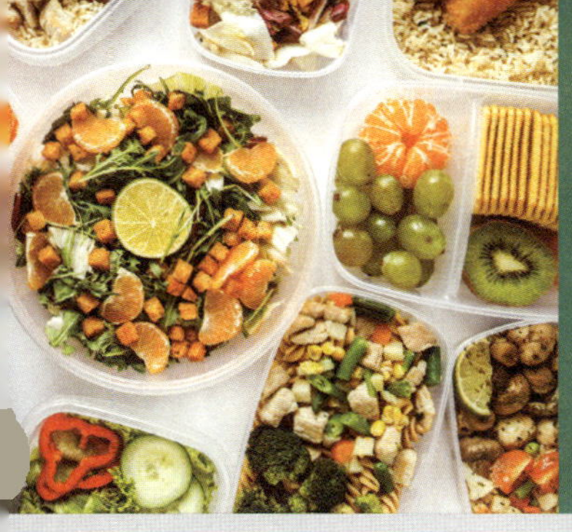

STUDENT ASSIGNMENT

LONG AND SHORT ANSWER QUESTIONS

1. Define protein energy malnutrition. Describe magnitude of the problem. Classify PEM with their features.
2. Describe severe acute malnutrition. Discuss its management and prevention.
3. What is childhood obesity? Describe its consequences, assessment, management and prevention.
4. **Describe briefly:**
   a. Vitamin A deficiency disorders
   b. Vitamin D deficiency disorders
   c. Vitamin B deficiency disorders
   d. Deficiency diseases of iron
   e. Deficiency diseases of calcium
   f. Deficiency diseases of iodine
5. **Differentiate between:**
   a. Kwashiorkor and marasmus
   b. Wet beriberi and dry beriberi
6. **Write notes on:**
   a. Body mass index
   b. Xerophthalmia
   c. Rickets
   d. Pellagra
   e. Scurvy

MULTIPLE CHOICE QUESTIONS

1. **Which of the following is the most essential nutrient for a woman during her initial stages of pregnancy to prevent birth defects?**
   a. Thiamine
   b. Folic acid
   c. Vitamin C
   d. Vitamin E

2. **Which of the following food sources has the highest levels of vitamin C?**
   a. Parsley
   b. Broccoli
   c. Black currants
   d. Orange

3. **Which of the following vitamin helps in blood clotting?**
   a. Vitamin A
   b. Vitamin C
   c. Vitamin D
   d. Vitamin K

4. **Which is the leading cause of blindness in children worldwide?**
   a. Glaucoma
   b. Cataract
   c. Color blindness
   d. Vitamin A deficiency

ANSWER KEY

1. b   **2.** c   **3.** d   **4.** d

Notes

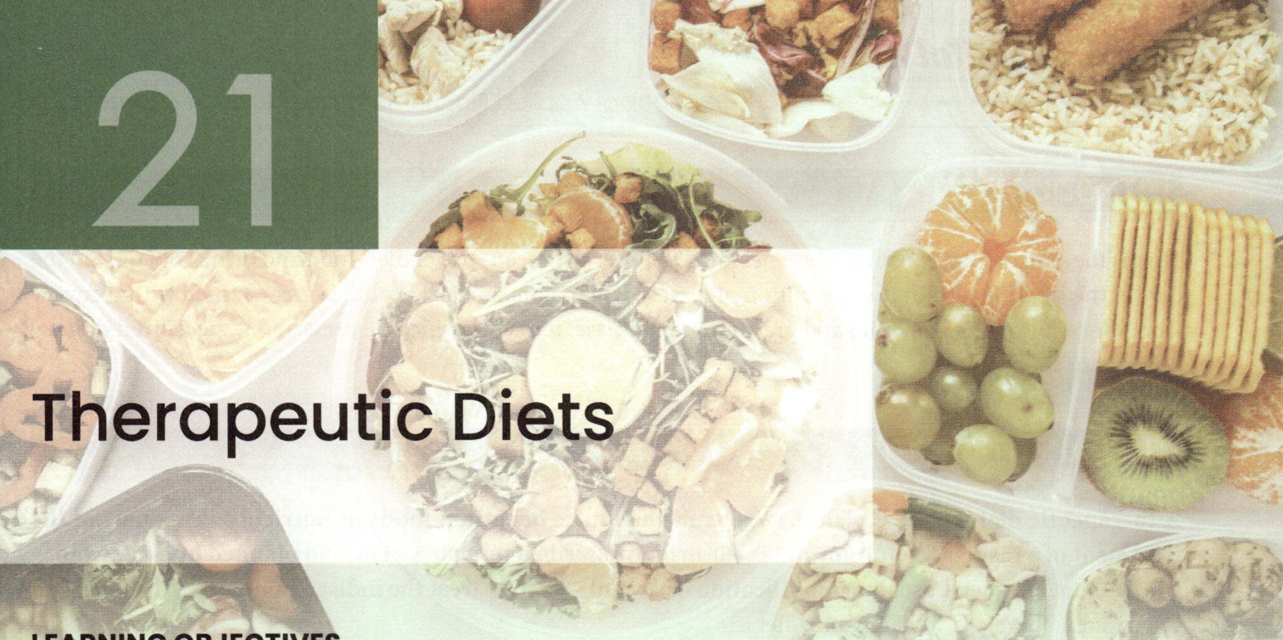

21

Therapeutic Diets

LEARNING OBJECTIVES

After the completion of the chapter, the readers will be able to:
- Apply nutrient and dietary modifications in caring patients.
- Explain the principles and practices of nutrition and dietetics.
- Identify the dietary principles for different diseases.
- Plan therapeutic diet for patients suffering from various disease conditions.

CHAPTER OUTLINE

- Introduction
- Therapeutic Diet
- Dietary Modifications
- Special Feeding Techniques
- Diet in Specific Diseases
- Diet during Pre- and Postoperative Period

KEY TERMS

Food intolerance: Digestive problems that occur after a certain food is eaten.

Nephrotic syndrome: A kidney disorder that causes the body to excrete too much protein in the urine; usually caused by damage to the nephrons that filter waste and excess water from the blood.

Preoperative nutritional therapy: Aims to store an adequate preoperative energy reserve to meet the functional requirements of the postoperative surgical stress.

Therapeutic diet: A meal plan that controls the intake of certain foods or nutrients. It is part of the treatment of a medical condition and are normally prescribed by a physician and planned by a dietician.

INTRODUCTION

Diet is the sum of food consumed by a person. **Diet therapy** means use of diet (food and drink) not only in the care of the sick, but also in the prevention of disease and maintenance of health. It is concerned with recovery from illness by giving good diet and prevention of disease. It may also include prescribing specialized **dietary regimes** or **meal plans**.

THERAPEUTIC DIET

A therapeutic diet is a **meal plan** that **controls the intake of certain foods or nutrients**. It is a **part of the treatment of a medical condition** and is, normally, **prescribed by a physician**, and **planned by a dietician**.

Therapeutic diet is usually a **modification of a regular diet, to treat the indiscriminate health state of an individual**. Therefore, a therapeutic diet is:

- Planned diet
- Modification of normal diet
- Used to supplement the medical or surgical treatment
- Prescribed by doctor
- Planned by dietician

Objectives

Therapeutic diets are formulated with the objective **to optimize the nutritional needs of the patient**, in order to treat a variety of diseases and disorders, or to improve the eating capabilities of a patient. Therefore, diet therapy is concerned with the **modification of normal diet to meet the requirements of the sick individual**.

Principles

The planning of therapeutic diet implied the ability to adopt the principle of normal nutrition to give the adequacy, economy and palatability of the food. The diet planned should be described according to the likes of patients. Care should be taken to modify the diet depending upon the nature of the disease. General principles of diet therapy are:

- To maintain a good nutritional status.
- To correct nutrient deficiencies, which may have occurred due to the disease.
- To afford rest to the whole body or to the specific organ affected by the disease.
- To adjust the food intake according to the body's ability to metabolize the nutrients during the disease.
- To bring about changes in body weight, whenever necessary.

DIETARY MODIFICATIONS

Dietary modifications are changes made during food preparation, processing and consumption, to increase bioavailability of micronutrients, and reduce micronutrient deficiencies in food at the commercial or individual/household level. Therapeutic diets can be modified in terms of quality and quantity.

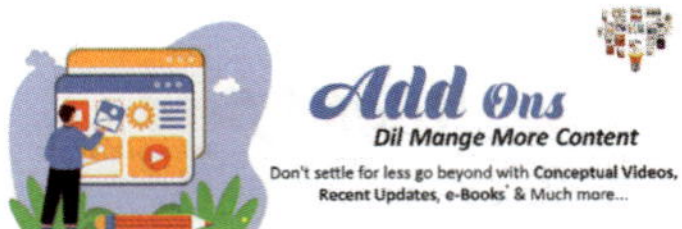

- **Qualitative modifications:**
  - Restriction of a nutrient, e.g., sodium in hypertension
  - Increase of a nutrient, e.g., in tuberculosis where increased protein and energy are required
- **Quantitative modifications:**
  - Change in consistency, e.g., clear liquid diet
  - Rearrangement of meals, e.g., increasing frequency of meals
  - Omission of foods, e.g., in allergy, which demands complete exclusion of the allergic food

Dietary Modifications Based on Consistency

Dietary modifications based on consistency may include:
- **Liquid diet:** It may be a:
  - **Clear liquid diet:** Clear liquid diet is free from any solid particles, e.g., clear soups, tea or coffee without cream, etc. This is given to the patient who cannot chew or swallow the food.
  - **Full liquid diet:** Full liquid diet is composed of solids, which are easily digestible, mixed in liquid. This diet is prescribed for patients, who are severely ill, not able to chew or swallow but need good calories. This diet is given in between a clear liquid diet and soft diet, e.g., eggs, vegetable soup, kheer, milk, etc.
- **Soft diet:** Soft diet is easy for chewing and is easily digestible. This diet contains all the required nutrients, especially proteins and carbohydrates. It is soft in consistency, easy to chew, made up of simple, easily digestible foods, containing limited fiber and does not contain rich or highly flavored foods.
- **Bland diet:** Bland diet is free from all spices and condiments, and is basically used to prevent peptic ulcers.

Dietary Modifications Based on Nutrients

Dietary modifications based on the nutrients may include:
- Decreased calories intake for weight reduction, or providing extra calories for weight gain
- Balance the amount of carbohydrates, fats or proteins
- High fiber diet
- Low fat and/or low cholesterol diet
- Decreased amount of a nutrient such as low sodium diet
- To exclude a particular food due to allergy or intolerance

SPECIAL FEEDING TECHNIQUES

Food consumption in the clients with different diseases, is altered. Different techniques used in hospitals for such patients, include:

Tube Feeding

Tube feedings (nutrition support) are used for people, who cannot take adequate food or fluid by mouth.

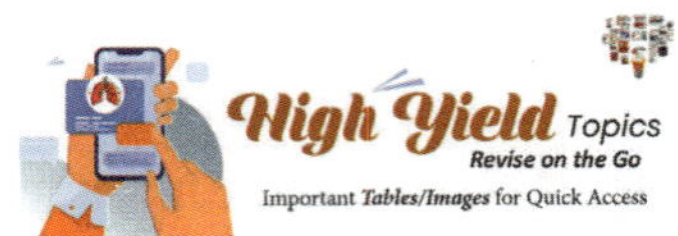

The tube may be passed through the nose into the stomach (nasogastric), duodenum (nasoduodenal) or jejunum (nasojejunal). When there is an obstruction in the esophagus, enteral feeding is done by passing a tube surgically through an incision in the abdominal wall into the stomach (gastrostomy), duodenum (duodenostomy) or jejunum (jejunostomy).

Food is given through the tube until the patient is able to eat by mouth. This is a simple method for helpless patients, who are not able to take the food orally. Full fluid diets or commercial formulas may be administered through this route.

Total Parenteral Nutrition (TPN)

The delivery of nutrients directly into the circulation through the peripheral or central vein is termed parenteral nutrition. This technique is used for long term purpose. In this method, a cannula is inserted in large veins to reach superior vena cava in the heart.

- **High fiber diet:** It is prescribed in the prevention or treatment of a number of gastrointestinal, cardiovascular and metabolic diseases. Increased fiber should come from a variety of sources, including fruits, legumes, vegetables, whole breads and cereals.
- **Low fat/low cholesterol diet:** It is low in total fat (limits to 50 g) and saturated fats, and contains approximately 250–300 mg of cholesterol. It is used to reduce fat levels and/or treat medical conditions that interfere with the use of body fat, such as diseases of the liver, gallbladder or pancreas.
- **Low sodium diet:** It has 2 g of sodium, e.g., sausage, cured meats, canned soups, salty seasonings, pickled foods, salted crackers, etc. It is used for people who have edema (may be holding water), or those who have high blood pressure, heart disease, liver disease or first stage of kidney disease.
- **Renal diet:** It is for people with a kidney disease and the laboratory tests are followed closely. The diet plan is individualized, depending on if the person is on dialysis. The diet restricts sodium, potassium, fluid and protein levels.
- **Food allergy modifications:** Food allergies are due to an abnormal immune response to an otherwise harmless food. The most common food allergens are milk, egg, soy, wheat, peanuts, tree nuts, fish and shellfish. Foods implicated with allergies are strictly eliminated from the diet and appropriate substitutions are made to ensure that the meal is adequate in nutrients. For example, a gluten-free diet includes the elimination of wheat, rye and barley, or corn and rice with potato, etc.
- **Food intolerance modifications:** The most common food intolerance is intolerance to lactose, called lactose intolerance due to milk sugar (lactose) because of a decreased amount of the enzyme lactase, in the body. Other common types of food intolerances include adverse reactions to certain products added to food, may be to enhance taste, color or protection against bacterial growth. Common symptoms involving food intolerances are vomiting, diarrhea, abdominal pain and headache.

DIET IN SPECIFIC DISEASES

Diet in Obesity

Prevention of obesity is most desirable and should start from infancy. Three essential principles to be remembered in diet therapy are:

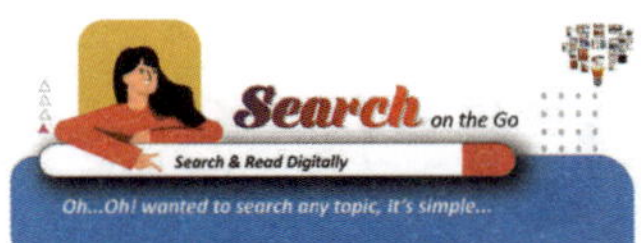

- Adherence to the diet plan
- Maintenance of the diet
- Maintenance of energy balance

Diet in obesity includes a low calorie diet, i.e., the diet restricted in carbohydrate and fat but with normal protein, vitamins and minerals (except sodium) with liberal intake of fluid and high in fiber is given.

- **Energy:** 20 kcal/kg ideal body weight is prescribed for a sedentary worker and 25 kcal for moderately active worker.
- **Proteins:** 0.8–1 g/kg body weight is prescribed for tissue repair.
- **Carbohydrates:** It is advised that obese individuals should consume foods rich in dietary fiber such as green leafy vegetable, whole grain cereals and whole fruits such as apple, oranges, etc. These food stuffs give a feeling of satiety and regulate bowel movement. They should avoid starch-rich foods like potatoes, rice, banana and mangoes, etc. They should also avoid consumption of refined sugar or sugar-containing beverages.
- **Fats:** To reduce the intake of calories, obese persons should also not consume deep-fried and fat-rich foods like whole milk or milk products made from whole milk. They should also avoid the consumption of nuts, oilseeds and trans fat. They should, preferably, consume low-fat skimmed milk, curd, etc.
- **Vitamins:** Due to prolonged consumption of low fat diet, it is likely that obese persons may suffer from the deficiency of fat soluble vitamins. It is therefore advised that they should take vitamins A and D supplements.
- **Minerals:** During obesity, one should also restrict the intake of sodium, since excess of sodium intake may predispose to fluid retention and cause edema.
- **Fluid:** With the restricted salt intake, obese individuals may take large amount of water or other low salt but sugar-free beverages.
- **High fiber:** As mentioned above in carbohydrates, obese individuals should consume diet rich in fiber, since such a diet is also low in calories. They may include whole grain cereals, pulses and legumes, green leafy vegetables, salad and fruits like apples and oranges, etc. High fiber diet has several advantages:
  - It not only reduces calories intake but also is low in sugar and fat.
  - High fiber diet also provides bulk to the feces and thus, prevents constipation and colon cancer.
  - It also helps in regulating blood glucose and cholesterol.
  - Due to the increased consumption of vegetables and some fruits, it also provides most of the vitamins and minerals.

Diet in Diabetes Mellitus

Diabetes mellitus is a group of diseases characterized by **high blood glucose concentration**, resulting from defects in insulin secretion and/or its action. Therefore, the **ideal diet for diabetic patient depends on the presence or absence of obesity, the response to a weight-reduction diet and the stage of progression of b-cell dysfunction**. Dietary modifications include:

- **Calories:** To lose weight, one need to eat fewer calories and replace less healthy foods with the food lower in calories, fat and sugar.
- **Carbohydrates:** Carbohydrates have a big impact on blood sugar level, so one needs to be smart about what type of carbohydrates to eat. Accordingly, one should limit refined carbohydrates, like white bread, pasta and rice, as well as soda, candy, packaged meals and snack foods. On the other hand, one should

focus on high-fiber complex carbohydrates. They are digested more slowly thus, prevent the body from producing too much insulin.

- **Proteins:** Persons with diabetes and normal renal function can have usual protein intake of 10% to 20% of energy. The protein consumed should, primarily, come from plant sources.
- **Fat:** Intake of fried foods and other foods high in saturated and trans-fat, should be limited.
- **Vitamins and minerals:** Whole grains and fruits and vegetables consumed by the diabetics can meet the required amount of vitamins and minerals.
- **Dietary patterns and food selection:** The goal of nutrition therapy for diabetes also emphasizes the role of lifestyle in improving glucose control, lipid and lipoprotein profiles, and blood pressure.

Diet in Cardiovascular Disease

As we know, a diet, particularly the calorie-rich diet increases blood sugar and lipids. Both of these blood constituents are related to dyslipidemia (disturbed lipid profile) and hence, the progression of atherosclerosis, the leading cause of cardiovascular disease (CVD). Dyslipidemia includes triglyceridemia, increased level of bad cholesterol (LDL-cholesterol) and reduced level of good cholesterol (HDL-cholesterol). Accordingly, it is suggested that these persons should consume foods that are low in calories contributed by sugar and fat. Dietary advice includes:

- **Carbohydrates, fiber and sugar: Complex carbohydrates (fiber)**, found in whole grains and vegetables, **are preferred** over those found in starchy foods, such as pastas, white-flour products and potatoes.
- **Most complex carbohydrates are high in fiber**, which is important for health. The recommended daily intake of dietary fiber for heart protection should be at least 25 g for women and 38 grams for men. Whole grains are extremely important for people with diabetes or those at risk for it. **Different fiber types** may have specific benefits. For example, **insoluble fiber** (found in wheat bran, whole grains, seeds, nuts, legumes, and fruits and vegetables) may **help achieve weight loss**. Consuming whole grains on a regular basis may lower the risk for heart disease and heart failure. **Soluble fiber** (found in dried beans, oat bran, barley, apples and citrus fruits) may **help achieve healthy cholesterol levels** and possibly reduce blood pressure.
- **Not >10% of daily calories should come from sugar. Naturally occurring sugars**, which are found in foods such as fruit (fructose) and milk (lactose), **should be preferred** over the added sugar or calories-rich sweeteners that are added to foods or beverages during processing or preparation (such as white sugar, brown sugar and honey as well as artificial sweeteners that are chemically manufactured).
- **Proteins:** In general, it is recommended that **proteins should provide 12–20% of daily calories**. Protein is found in animal-based products (meat, fish, and dairy) as well as vegetable sources such as beans, soy, nuts and whole grains. Fish is probably the best source of protein.
- When choosing protein, **opt for low-fat options** such as lean meats, skim milk or other foods with high levels of protein. **Avoid cheese** which adds protein, but also fat.
- **Fats and oils:** Patients with CVD should not consume diet rich in fat. Fat content of the diet should not exceed 20% of the total calories intake.
- Besides **limiting the total amount of fat** in the diet, more important is that they should **limit the fat intake of saturated and trans fat**. Foods such as whole milk, cream and butter, high fat meat, deep fried foods, etc., which are responsible for increased LDL and low HDL.

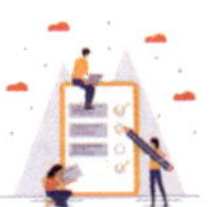
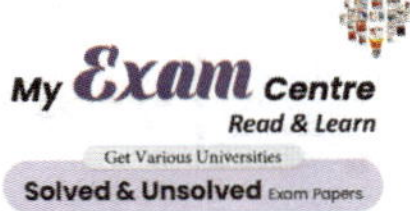

- Total dietary cholesterol intake should not exceed 200 mg/day. Accordingly, they should not consume cheese and butter, meat, egg yolk, etc.
- They should increase the intake of foods rich in ω-3 fatty acids which are good for heart, such as salmon and tuna fish, walnuts, and canola and soybean oils, etc.
- **Vitamins: Consume antioxidant vitamins** that help to protect the body from the formation and elimination of free radicals. These should include **vitamin E** (a fat soluble vitamin present in nuts, seeds, vegetable and fish oils, whole grains especially wheat germ, fortified cereals and apricots), **vitamin C** (a water soluble vitamin, present in citrus fruits and juices, green peppers, cabbage, spinach, broccoli, kale, cantaloupe, kiwi and strawberries) and **beta-carotene** (present in liver, egg yolk, milk, butter, spinach, carrots, squash, broccoli, yams, tomato, cantaloupe, peaches and grains).
- **Minerals:** Minerals of significance in diabetic diet are potassium, calcium and sodium.
- **A potassium-rich diet** can provide a small reduction in blood pressure. Potassium-rich foods include bananas, oranges, pears, prunes, cantaloupes, tomatoes, dried peas and beans, nuts, potatoes and avocados. For those using potassium-sparing diuretics (such as spironolactone) or have chronic kidney problems, potassium supplements may be very dangerous.
- **Magnesium supplements** may cause small but significant reduction in blood pressure.
- **Calcium** regulates the tone of the smooth muscles lining blood vessels.
- **Sodium (salt) increases blood pressure** because it holds excess fluid in the body and puts burden on the heart. Blood pressure rises with age, and eating less sodium will help to reduce the rise. Besides hypertension, low sodium intake also decreases the risk of other associated disorders such as stroke and renal diseases.

Dietary Approaches to Stop Hypertension (DASH)

Experts have recommended that DASH helps in lowering blood pressure, and has been shown to have several advantages in preventing a heart disease, such as stroke and heart failure. DASH contains high amount of dietary fiber besides all the essential nutrients. DASH recommends daily intake of 4700 mg of potassium, 1250 mg of calcium, 500 mg of magnesium and 2300 mg of sodium (salt). It also recommends that reduce saturated fat to not more than 6% of daily calories and total fat to 27% of daily calories, but include calcium-rich dairy products that are low in fat. When choosing fats, select monounsaturated oils, such as olive or canola oils. Choose whole grains over white flour or pasta products. Other daily nutrient goals include limiting carbohydrate intake to 55% of daily calories and dietary cholesterol to 150 mg. Patients should try to get at least 30 g of daily fiber.

Diet during Underweight

Nutrition therapy can also help eat more calories and gain weight. As one gains weight, health also improves. Meal planning tips include:

- **Foods which are not recommended** include **light, lite or diet foods** as these are low in calories as well as plain beverages which do not have calories or proteins. For example, one should avoid plain coffee, tea and diet soda.
- **Eat at least five small meals and snacks each day**. Drink healthy beverages that add calories, e.g., juice, milk or shakes.

- **Eat sweeten foods** and beverages with sugar, jam, jelly or honey. Choose high-calorie starchy vegetables, like potatoes, corn and peas. Add cream, butter, margarine, cheese sauce, olive oil, or salad dressing to get more calories. **Choose foods high in protein** such as milk, eggs, cheese, meat, fish, poultry and beans.
- **Add high-fat foods to meals** and snacks, e.g., butter, regular margarine, vegetable oils and peanut butter. Whole milk, high-fat meats and whole-milk cheese provide more calories than lean or low-fat types. Try to avoid relying on high-calorie foods full of saturated fat. These foods can increase body fat instead of lean body mass and increase risk of developing high levels of cholesterol.
  Aim to gain weight gradually until you reach a healthy weight.

Diet in Renal Diseases

Each kidney consists of approximately one million functioning units, called nephrons. The nephron consists of a glomerulus connected to a series of tubules. Each nephron functions independently in producing a contribution to the final urine. The main function of the kidney is to maintain homeostatic balance with respect to fluid, electrolytes and organic solutes. The majority of the solute load consists of nitrogenous wastes (urea, uric acid, creatinine and ammonia), largely the end products of protein metabolism. **Inability of the kidney to excrete daily load of the waste products leads to renal failure**. The kidney is also involved in the **control of blood pressure** by renin-angiotensin mechanism. The kidney also produces the hormone erythropoietin, which in turn **determines erythroid activity in the bone marrow**. Role of the kidney also includes **production of the active form of vitamin D** and elimination of both calcium and phosphorus.

Manifestations of renal disease include glomerular disease, tubular defects, acute renal failure and end-stage renal disease.

- **Nephrotic syndrome:** It comprises a heterogeneous group of diseases, whose common manifestations derive from a loss of the glomerular barrier to protein. Large protein losses in the urine lead to hypoalbuminemia with consequent edema, hypercholesterolemia, hypercoagulability and abnormal bone metabolism.
- The primary objectives of nutrition therapy are to manage the symptoms associated with the syndrome and maintain nutritional stores. The diet should attempt to provide **sufficient protein and energy**.
- **Protein** is essential to maintain a positive nitrogen balance and produce an **increase in plasma albumin concentration**, and **disappearance of edema**. To allow for optimal protein use, three-fourth of the protein should be taken from sources of **high biological value.**
- **Energy intake** should be about 35 kcal/kg/day for adults and 100–150 kcal/kg/day for children.
- **Sodium:** Edema is the most clinically apparent manifestation, hence there should be modest **sodium restriction** to approximately 3 g daily.
- **Cholesterol:** To reduce total cholesterol, LDL-cholesterol and triglycerides, the diet should be **low in cholesterol.**
- **End-stage renal disease:** It can result from a wide variety of diseases such as diabetes mellitus, glomerulonephritis, or hypertension. As renal failure slowly progresses, the level of the circulating waste products eventually leads to symptoms of uremia.
- Nutrition therapy is aimed to prevent deficiency and maintain good nutritional status through **adequate proteins, energy, vitamins** and **minerals intake.**
- **Electrolytes and fluid:** To control edema and electrolyte imbalance, **reduce sodium, potassium** and **fluid intakes.**

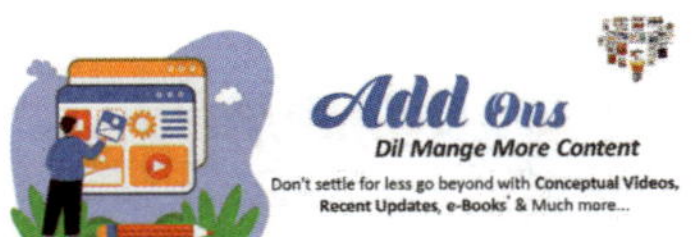

- Also **control calcium**, **phosphorus** and **vitamin D intakes** to prevent, or retard, development of renal osteodystrophy.

Diet in Hepatic Disorders

The liver is largest gland in the body, weighing about 1500 g. It has two main lobes, referred to as the right lobe and the left lobe. Important functions of the liver include metabolism of carbohydrates, proteins and fats; storage and activation of vitamins and minerals; formation and excretion of bile; conversion of ammonia into urea and metabolism of steroids.

Patients with a liver disease should be given **small but more frequent meals,** since they are better tolerated in such patients. Frequent feeding also improves nitrogen balance and prevents hypoglycemia.

- **Energy requirement** varies among patients with a liver disease. In patients with end-stage liver disease, energy requirement **is increased** by 120–140% of the resting energy expenditure. The body prefers lipid as an energy substrate, and lipolysis is increased with active mobilization of lipid deposits.

    There is also increased protein breakdown and inadequate resynthesis, resulting in depletion of visceral protein stores and muscle wasting. Accordingly, **protein requirement is also increased**.

- **Vitamins and minerals supplementation is also needed** in patients with end-state liver disease because of the role of liver in transport, storage and metabolism of these nutrients. **Deficiencies of fat soluble vitamins** have also been found in all types of liver failure. **Water soluble vitamins deficiencies** associated with alcoholic liver disease **include thiamine, niacin, pyridoxine, folate** and **vitamin B$_{12}$**.

- **Zinc and magnesium levels are low**, in part because of diuretic therapy. **Calcium, magnesium** and **zinc levels are also reduced** due to malabsorption associated with steatorrhea.

Diet during Constipation

Constipation is a state when one finds difficult to pass the stools. Dietary modifications include:

- **Carbohydrates:** Carbohydrates should be given in the form of fiber, e.g., fibrous fruits, vegetables, flour with bran, whole cereals, guava, apples, grapes, vegetables, salad, etc.
- **Proteins:** Protein foods like soybeans and legumes provide good dietary proteins.
- **Fat:** Fat should be given in reasonable amount to stimulate the flow of bile needed for digestion and keep the tract well lubricated. Spicy and fried foods irritate the tract.
- **Vitamins:** It is necessary to give B-complex vitamins, as it enhances muscular movement of the intestine.
- **Water:** Water is required for flushing out the body water. Person must consume 8-10 glasses of water.

One should have regular meal timings. Vegetables should be given in the form of salad, fruits with skin and seeds, besides whole pulses and sprouts. In addition, bulking agents such as Isabgol and other natural laxatives must be used.

Diet during Diarrhea

Diarrhea can be defined as frequent passage of stools. Dietary modifications include:

- **Energy:** The requirement of energy is increased to replace losses and can be met from foods like fruit juices, suji kheer, etc.

- **Proteins:** For proteins, foods that are easy to digest, e.g., washed moong dal, paneer, etc., can be given.
- **Fat:** Since GIT is not able to absorb high fat content in the diet, fat rich diet should not be given. These can be given after the condition is improved.
- **Vitamins:** As diarrhea can result in loss of water soluble vitamins, it is suggested that with the improvement in condition, they may be given fresh fruit juices.
- **Minerals:** Diarrhea also causes loss of electrolytes (sodium and potassium) and water, which in turn, may reduce appetite and cause generalized weakness with loss of muscle flexibility. These should be included in the diet may be in the form of fresh juices or other beverages such as lemon water, barley water, mineral water, etc.

Besides, small frequent meals should be given. Since milk is poorly tolerated, curd may be the better option. Strongly flavored foods, fried and fatty foods, and nuts and rich desserts should be avoided. Fiber intake should be restricted. Instead low fiber cereals and de-husked pulses should be included.

DIET DURING PRE- AND POSTOPERATIVE PERIOD

A person undergoing surgery, faces large physiologic and psychological stress. Subsequently, nutritional demands are greatly increased during this period. Therefore, careful attention must be given to a patient's nutritional status in preparation for surgery, as well as to the individual nutrition therapy needs that follow for wound healing and a more rapid recovery.

Preoperative Nutritional Care

When the surgery is elective, body nutrient stores can be built up to fortify a patient for the demands of the surgery and the period immediately following, when food intake may be limited. Particular needs are centered on protein, energy, vitamins and minerals for nutrient reserves.

- **Protein:** Protein deficiencies among surgical patients upon admission are common. Every patient facing surgery needs to be fortified with adequate body protein in tissue and plasma to counteract blood losses during surgery and prevent tissue breakdown in the immediate postoperative period.
- **Energy:** Sufficient energy always must be provided to maintain optimal glycogen stores in the liver as a necessary resource for immediate energy fuel, thus sparing protein for its tissue-building work.
- **Vitamins and minerals:** When increased protein and energy are necessary for any purpose, the appropriate intake of vitamins and minerals involved in protein and energy metabolism also must be supplied.

Postoperative Nutritional Care

Adequate nutritional support is necessary to aid recovery from surgery when nutrient losses are great. At the same time, food intake is greatly diminished or even absent for a period. To supply this additional nutritional support and nutrient needs for healing, several nutrients require particular attention.

- **Protein:** Optimal protein intake in the postoperative recovery period is of primary concern for all patients. Protein is needed to replace losses during surgery and supply the increased demands of the healing process, such as for building tissue, healing bone, controlling shock and edema, resisting infection

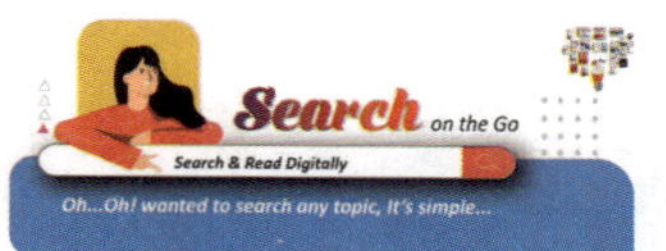

and transporting lipids. Because protein has many important functions during recovery from surgery, protein deficiency at this time can lead to many clinical problems.

- **Water:** Water balance after surgery is a constant concern. During the postoperative period, large water losses may occur from vomiting, hemorrhage fever, or excessive urination. Sufficient fluid intake is necessary to prevent dehydration, especially in elderly persons whose thirst mechanism may be depressed and cannot be depended on to ensure adequate fluid intake. In patients who have complications or are seriously ill and have extensive drainage, as much as 7 L of fluid may be necessary daily.

- **Energy:** As always, when increased protein is demanded for tissue building, enough non-protein calories must be supplied for energy to spare protein for its vital tissue-building function. The fuel sources, carbohydrate and fat, therefore, must be sufficiently supplied in the total diet. Because excess fat presents general health problems, carbohydrates become the major source of needed fuel.

- **Vitamins:** Several vitamins require particular attention in wound healing. **Vitamin C** helps to build connective tissue, new capillary walls and general tissue ground substance. As energy and protein intakes are increased, the B vitamins that have important coenzyme roles in protein and energy metabolism, especially **vitamin B$_1$**, **vitamin B$_2$** and **niacin**, also must be increased. Other B-complex vitamins, i.e., **vitamin B$_6$**, **pantothenic acid**, **folate** and **vitamin B$_{12}$**, also play important roles in building hemoglobin and thus, it must meet the demands of an increased blood supply and general metabolic stress.

- **Minerals:** Attention to mineral deficiencies is also essential, particularly electrolytes, phosphorus, iron and zinc. After surgery, when tissue is broken down, cell **potassium** and **phosphorus** are lost. Electrolyte imbalances of **sodium** and **chloride** also result from fluid losses. **Iron** deficiency anemia may develop from blood loss or faulty iron absorption. **Zinc** is also important in wound healing.

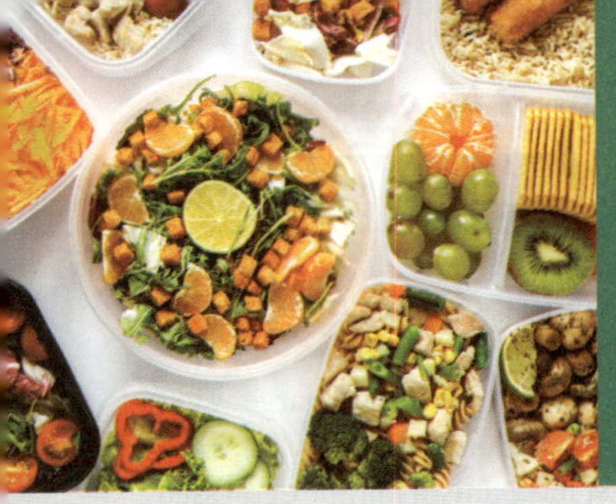

LONG AND SHORT ANSWER QUESTIONS

1. Define therapeutic diet. Describe its objectives and principles.
2. **Write notes on:**
   a. Therapeutic diet
   b. Dietary modifications
   c. Special feeding techniques
   d. Diet in obesity
   e. Diet during pre and postoperative period

MULTIPLE CHOICE QUESTIONS

1. **Which of the following is the therapeutic diet preferred in case of diarrhea?**
   a. Clear fluid diet
   b. Soft diet
   c. Bland diet
   d. Full fluid diet

2. **What is the primary goal of a therapeutic diet?**
   a. To enhance the flavor of meals
   b. To prevent or treat specific health conditions
   c. To promote rapid weight gain
   d. To standardize meal portions in hospitals

3. **Which therapeutic diet is commonly recommended for patients with hypertension?**
   a. Ketogenic diet
   b. Dietary approaches to stop hypertension (DASH) diet
   c. High-protein diet
   d. Gluten-free diet

4. **For which condition is a low-salt diet typically prescribed?**
   a. Diabetes
   b. Inflammatory bowel disease (IBD)
   c. Osteoporosis
   d. Hypertension

ANSWER KEY

1. b   2. b   3. b   4. b

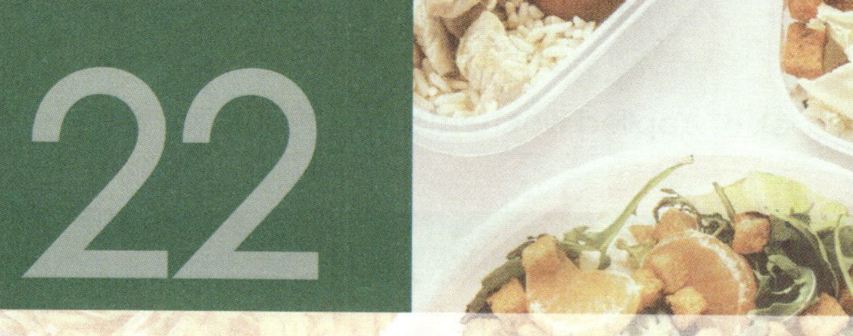

22

Cookery Rules and Preservation of Nutrients

LEARNING OBJECTIVES

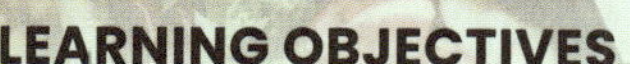

After the completion of the chapter, the readers will be able to:
- Explain how to prepare meals using different methods and cookery rules.
- Explain about food additives.
- Explain about food fortification, adulteration and food standards.

CHAPTER OUTLINE

- Introduction
- Principal Methods of Cooking
- Preservation of Nutrients
- Safe Food Handling
- Storage of Foods

- Food Additives
- Food Fortification
- Food Adulteration
- Food Standards

KEY TERMS

Food additives: Chemicals added to foods to keep them fresh or to enhance their color, flavor or texture.

Food fortification: The practice of deliberately increasing the content of one or more micronutrients (i.e., vitamins and minerals) in a food or condiment to improve the nutritional quality of the food supply and provide a public health benefit with minimal risk to health.

Food standards: A set of criteria that a food must meet if it is to be suitable for human consumption, such as source, composition, appearance, freshness, permissible additives, and maximum bacterial content.

Leavening: The process in which a substance such as baking soda is added to the fluor dough, which in turn causes it to swell and become lighter. For example in making cake, bread, etc.

Pasteurized milk: The milk which is heated to 70°C for 15–30 min and then quickly cooled to 10°C.

INTRODUCTION

Cooking is an art, which is linked with the dietary habits and cultural patterns of the people. Except some fruits and vegetables, used in salad, almost all foods need some form of cooking and processing. Although some amount of nutrient loss is inevitable, **cooking has many advantages**:

- Cooking increases palatability of food.
- It makes mastication easier and renders the food easy to digest.
- Cooking sterilizes food by killing microorganisms and parasite's ova and eggs. This, in turn also increases shelf-life of food due to destruction of organisms and denaturation of enzymes responsible for the spoilage of food.
- It lends a new flavor and, thereby stimulates digestive juices.
- Cooking improves appearance of food and increases its acceptability.
- Different types of dishes can be cooked from the same ingredients.

PRINCIPAL METHODS OF COOKING

Methods of cooking include dry heat methods, moist heat methods and combination methods.

Dry Heat Methods

Any cooking method that **does not use moisture** during cooking is referred to as dry heat cooking. It includes:

- **Grilling and broiling: Grilling** is a form of cooking that involves dry heat, applied to the surface of food, commonly, from above or below. Food is cooked on a grill (an open wire grid with a heat source above or below), using a grill pan (similar to a frying pan but with raised ridges).

  When the heat source for grilling comes from above, grilling is termed **broiling. This method is used only for tender foods**, e.g., cheese, tomato, brinjal, etc.
- **Roasting:** It is a method of cooking that uses dry heat, whether an open flame, oven or other heat source. For this purpose, food is smeared with a little fat and then exposed directly to heat or flame. Chicken or tender mutton is, generally, cooked by this method, also called **barbeque.**
- **Sauteing:** It is a method of cooking food that uses small amount of oil or fat, in a shallow pan, over relatively high heat. Ingredients are, usually, cut into pieces or thinly sliced, to facilitate fast cooking.
- **Deep-frying:** It is a method of cooking, where food is submerged in hot fat, e.g., oil. Deep frying is classified as **dry cooking**, because water is not used in this process. **Due to high temperature and high heat conduction of oil, it cooks food, extremely, quickly.**
- **Baking:** It is a technique of prolonged cooking of food by dry heat, normally, in an oven, but also in hot ash or on hot stones. **It is primarily used for the preparation of breads, cakes, pastries, etc.**

Moist Heat Methods

The cooking **method that uses moisture** as a cooking medium is referred to as moist heat method of cooking. These include:

- **Poaching:** It is the process of gently simmering food in liquid, generally, milk or vinegar. It is particularly **suitable for delicate foods**, such as eggs, fish and fruits.

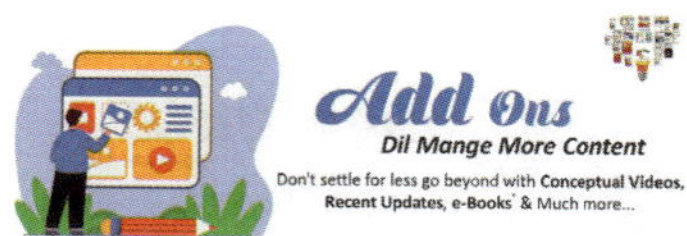

- **Simmering:** It is a technique in which foods are cooked in hot liquids, kept at or just below the boiling point of water (100°C), but higher than poaching temperature.
- **Boiling/Blanching:** Cooking in water at 100°C is called boiling. Rice, pulses, roots, tubers and other vegetables are cooked in this way. **Boiling in excess of water may result in loss of vitamins and minerals.** Therefore, it is a general rule that boiling should be done using minimum amount of water.
- **Steaming:** It is employed in a pressure cooker, in which food is cooked by the heat of direct steam. Temperature attained is higher than 100°C.

Combination Methods

These methods of cooking use, both, **dry heat as well as moisture**, and include:

- **Stewing:** This method of cooking includes boiling in small amount of liquid, for a longer time, at low degree of heat (about 80°C). In this method, a pan is used, which has well-fitted lid to prevent evaporation. Many **vegetable and fruit stews are prepared and used by individuals who have dentures, or by small children**, e.g., apple stew, amla stew, etc.
- **Pressure cooking:** Some foods that require long time to cook, e.g., dried beans, are put in a container along with water, and are cooked under pressure. Such utensils, called **pressure cookers,** cook food at high temperature, by means of steam under pressure, where the temperature of water is increased to above 100°C. In this process, the food cooks faster than boiling.

  Pressure method of cooking is a better method of cooking, since **it saves nutrients, fuel and time.** Pressure cooking **also kills bacteria** and, hence, the food cooked under pressure is safe, and hygienic, to eat. Rice, pulses, meat, potatoes, roots, beans and peas are, generally, cooked in pressure cooker.
- **Microwave ovens:** Another fast method of cooking uses microwaves (short radio waves) ovens. **Microwave ovens heat food, much faster** than gas or electric ovens. Microwave ovens are, **especially, useful for thawing frozen foods, and heating** soups, vegetables and leftovers.

PRESERVATION OF NUTRIENTS

Food provides the ideal mix of vitamins, minerals and other nutrients. However, the nutrients in foods begin to decrease as soon as the food article is picked and continued to decline until it is eaten. The various vitamins and minerals are susceptible to destruction by air, light, water, acid, alkali, heat, time and the action of enzymes in the foods themselves. Nevertheless, we can cut losses and significantly increase nutrient intake by the care in choosing, storing and cooking foods.

Lean meats, skinless poultry and low-fat dairy products have more nutrients per calorie than their fattier versions. Whole grains, e.g., whole wheat pasta, oatmeal, brown rice, etc., have more nutrients than foods made from refined grains, even if they are enriched. Whole grain foods leavened with yeast have less phytate, which can inhibit the absorption of minerals like calcium, iron and zinc. Parboiled, or converted white rice is more nutritious than regular white rice. Dark green-leafy vegetables and deep-yellow vegetables have more vitamin A than lighter-colored ones.

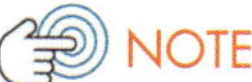 NOTE

The three R's for nutrient preservation include:
- Reduce the amount of water used in cooking
- Reduce the cooking time
- Reduce the surface area of the food that is exposed

Measures to Prevent Loss of Nutrients during Preparation

Longer cooking time and higher temperature, destroy the nutrients as most of the vitamins are sensitive to heat and air exposure. Prolonged exposure to water, heat, and light may cause some foods to lose nutritional value like vitamin B_1, vitamin C and polyphenols.

- Always wash the vegetables first and then chop them. Chopping first and then washing takes away the nutrition of your food.
- Do not chop vegetables into very small pieces as most of the nutrients will be destroyed when they come in contact with air. The best way is to chop the vegetable into larger chunks. As soon as you chop veggies, you should cook them as the vitamins and minerals remain secured in their cells, and once they are exposed to light and air, the nutrient contents can be destroyed.
- Waterless cooking, pressure cooking, steaming, stir-frying and microwaving are least destructive of nutrients.
- Cook vegetables in smaller amount of water. Boiling in too much water damages the nutrients. It is best advised to cook the veggies covered on low flame in their own water that is released.
- Do not throw away the excess water drained after boiling rice or vegetables. The excess water is loaded with nutrients and it can be used in preparing gravies, kneading dough or serve it as a refreshment drink.
- Root vegetables like potato, ginger, turnip and carrots should be boiled with skins and the peel should be removed after boiling. Boiling with peels helps the nutrients to migrate to the center of the vegetables which helps in better retention of its nutrients.
- Do not use baking soda when cooking vegetables. Although it helps in retaining color of the vegetables as well as speeds up the cooking process, but destroys the vitamin C content of the veggies.
- Avoid re-heating of food as it destroys the chemical structure of nutrients and vitamins.
- To reduce the loss of vitamins A and E, cook with very little oil, e.g., bake or broil vitamin A rich liver or vitamin D rich fish, oil-free instead of frying it.
- B-Vitamins leak out into cooking liquid or drippings. So, use the cooking liquid in soup or sauce. Do not over wash grains (rice) before cooking. Washing rice once, may take away as much as 25% of thiamine. Toast or bake cakes and bread only until the crust is light brown, to preserve heat-sensitive B vitamins.
- To reduce the loss of water soluble and oxygen sensitive vitamin C, cook fruits and vegetables in the least possible amount of water. Serve cooked vegetables quickly. After 24 hours in the fridge, vegetables lose one-fourth of their vitamin C while after two days, nearly half of it. Root vegetables (carrots, .potatoes and sweet potatoes) baked or boiled whole, with their skins, retain about 65 percent of their vitamin C.

SAFE FOOD HANDLING

Several precautions are required to be taken for safe food handling, to avoid the risk of food borne illnesses. These include **general precautions** and specific steps at different stages such as **during shopping, storage in the house, freeze or refrigerator; before, during** and **after cooking;** and **storage of the leftover food.**

- **General precautions for safe food handling**
  - Use of fresh ingredients and personal hygiene are the most important concepts of safe food. Food turns harmful, when dirty hands are used to serve cooked food.

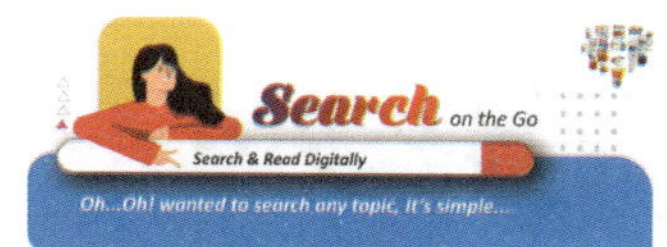

- Use of rotten and unwashed vegetables makes food unsafe. As physical and biological contaminants are the major hazards, raw foods should be thoroughly washed/cleaned, to make them free from physical contaminants and suitable for consumption.
- Cooked food, particularly, purchased from restaurants, eateries, take away, etc., is also considered to be unsafe, since one cannot be sure of the quality of ingredients, used in it. Moreover, since it is prepared in large quantity, it may not be possible to take full care during its preparation.
- Packed foods may be considered safer than the one that is kept in open and sold in eateries, since packets protect it from exposure to flies, insects and dust, etc. However, one cannot be certain about the ingredients used in it.

- **Safe food handling during shopping:** Selection of the right food is the first step to ensure safe and good quality diet. For this purpose:
  - Food items should be purchased from **reliable sources**, having a high turnover ensure their freshness.
  - We should purchase foods that carry **certification mark**, assuring good quality, e.g., AGMARK (Agriculture marketing) for honey and ghee; Fruit products order (FPO) for fruit and vegetable products, such as jams, squashes; and ISI (Bureau of Indian Standards) for food colors and essences, etc.
  - While purchasing packaged food, always look for its date of packaging, such as **best before** or **date of expiry**:
    - **Best before:** This term is appropriate for most foods. It relates to the quality of food and is an indication of the period for which a food can reasonably be expected to retain its optimal condition.
    - **Use by:** This term is appropriate for perishable foods. These foods present a microbiological risk to the consumer, if sold after the indicated date. It is an offence for shops to sell food that is after the use by date.
    - **Sell by:** Products may be labelled with sell by and display until dates, but these are not required by law and are used mainly for stock control premises.
  - Food grains purchased should be **free from infestation and foreign matter,** such as rodent excreta or insect remains, etc. Further, they should be of uniform size and should not be shrivelled, shrunken or mouldy.
  - Foodstuffs should be **free from artificial colors**.
  - **Fats/oils should not be purchased loose**, from unsealed containers, to avoid the risk of adulteration.
  - One must buy **pasteurized milk** in sachets from a reputed dairy, or from a reliable vendor, to avoid the risk of adulteration and contamination. Milk products, such as butter, ghee and khoa should also be purchased from reliable sources.
  - **Whole spices** should be preferred, which should be uniform in color, size and shape, since powdered spices are more likely to be adulterated. Also, always buy certified products.
  - **Fruits and vegetables** that show patches, physical damage with bruises or wilted and decayed with visible evidence of insects and moulds, should be avoided.
  - **Eggs** should be fresh and free from cracks.
  - **Meat or poultry** must be examined for characteristic color, odor and texture, and should be purchased fresh or frozen.
  - Freshness of fresh-water **fish** is indicated by a stiff body, bright, clear and bulging eyes, reddish gills, tight scales and absence of stale odor or discoloration. Fresh fish will not show any pitting on finger pressure.

- **Safe food handling while storing**
  - **Always refrigerate perishable food** within 2 hours (1 hour when the temperature is above 32°C). Check the temperature of refrigerator and freezer with a thermometer. The refrigerator should be at 4°C or below, and the freezer at −18°C or below. Perishable foods, such as meat and poultry, should be wrapped securely, to maintain quality and to prevent meat juices from getting onto other foods.
  - To maintain quality when freezing **meat and poultry** in its original package, **wrap the package again** with foil or plastic wrap or place the package on a plate so that their juices do not drip on other foods. Raw juices can contain bacteria. Cook or freeze fresh poultry, fish or meat within 2 days.
  - Always **keep eggs in the refrigerator**.
  - In general, **high-acid canned foods**, such as tomatoes, grapefruit and pineapple, **can be stored on the shelf** for 12–18 months. Low-acid canned foods, such as meat, poultry, fish and most vegetables can be kept for 2–5 years, if the can remains in good condition and has been stored in a cool, clean and dry place. Discard cans that are dented, leaking, bulging or rusted.

- **Safe food handling before cooking**
  - Always wash hands with warm water and soap for 20 seconds before and after handling food, using the bathroom, changing diapers or handling pets.
  - Since, kitchen towels, sponges and cloths can harbor bacteria, so, wash them often and replace sponges after every few weeks.
  - Do not cross contaminate food. Keep raw meat, poultry, fish and their juices away from other foods. After cutting raw meat, wash cutting board, utensils and countertops with hot and soapy water, or sanitize by using a solution of 1 tablespoon of unscented, liquid chlorine bleach in 1 gallon of water.
  - Thaw frozen food in the microwave or refrigerator. Do not thaw the items on kitchen counter, since it allows bacteria to grow in the outer layers of the food, before the inside thaws.
  - Refrigerator allows slow but safe thawing. Cook meat and poultry immediately after microwave thawing.
  - For faster thawing, place food in a leak proof plastic bag. Submerge in cold tap water and change the water every 30 minutes. Cook immediately after thawing.

- **Safe food handling during cooking**
  - Preferably, use fresh vegetables and wash them, thoroughly, by dipping in a container of water.
  - Cook the food thoroughly, since cooking kills harmful bacteria. Raw or partially cooked meat, poultry, fish or eggs may result in exposure to bacteria that can make one ill, e.g., Salmonella (bacteria), that causes food poisoning, can grow inside fresh unbroken eggs. This is, particularly important for children, pregnant women, the elderly and for those whose immune system is compromised.
  - Cook all raw beef, pork and lamb, chop and roast to a minimum internal temperature of 65°C (150°F), before removing it from the heat source. For safety and quality, allow meat to rest for at least three minutes before carving or consuming. Use a meat thermometer to ensure that meat and poultry are cooked to the appropriate temperature. Check the chart, at the end of the fact sheet, for the proper internal cooking temperatures, for various meats and poultry.
  - If food has been cooked ahead of time, divide large portions into small shallow containers and refrigerate. This ensures rapid and safe cooling.

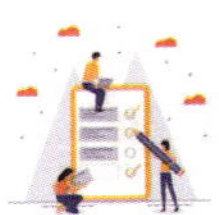
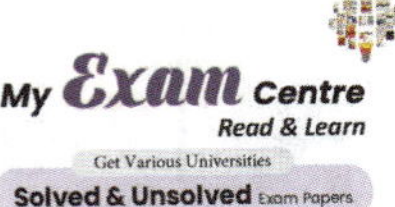

- Though the microwave oven is time saver, but it has food safety disadvantage. It sometimes leaves cold spots in the food and the bacteria may survive in these spots. Hence, be sure to cover food with a lid or plastic wrap. Leave a small section uncovered so that steam can escape. Do not let wrap touch the food. Stir and rotate food for even cooking. If there is no turntable in the oven, rotate the dish by hand, once or twice, during cooking.
- Observe the standing time, called for in a recipe or on package. During the standing time, food finishes cooking. Use an oven temperature probe, or a meat thermometer, to check that food is cooked and be sure to check several spots.

- **Safe food handling after cooking**
  - Keep cold food on ice, or refrigerated, until the time to replenish platters. If serving hot food, maintain it at 60°C, or divide into small serving platters, which can be refrigerated until time to warm them up for serving.
  - Always use clean dishes and utensils to serve food, not those which were used to prepare the raw food. If the food is being grilled, serve it on a clean plate, not on the one that held the raw meat, poultry or fish.
  - When serving food at a buffet, keep food hot with chafing dishes, slow cookers or warming trays. Keep food cold by nesting dishes in bowl of ice or use small serving trays and replace them often.
  - Perishable food should not be left out for >2 hours at room temperature (1 hour when the temperature is above 32°C). Bacteria, that can cause food poisoning, grow quickly at warm temperature.
  - Pack lunch in an insulated carrier, with a cold pack. Be sure not to leave lunch in direct sunlight or on warm radiator.
  - Carry picnic food in a cool pack carrier (cooler), with a cold pack. Try to keep the cooler in the shade and do not open the lid any more than it is necessary.

- **Safe food handling of the leftover food**
  - Discard any food left out at room temperature for >2 hours (1 hour, if the temperature is above 32°C). Also, discard any food with a strange color, or odor, immediately.
  - Divide large amount of leftovers into small shallow containers, for quick cooling in the refrigerator. With poultry or other stuffed meats, remove stuffing and refrigerate it in a separate container.
  - Bring sauces, soups and gravy to a boil. Heat other leftovers thoroughly to 74°C.
  - Microwave leftovers, using a lid or vented plastic wrap, to ensure thorough heating.
  - Use cooked leftovers within 4 days. Meat and poultry defrosted in the refrigerator may be refrozen before, or after, cooking. If thawed by other methods, cook before refreezing.
  - Discard any thawed food that has risen to room temperature and remained there for 2 hours or more.

STORAGE OF FOODS

Food storage refers to **food**, which is kept in the fridge, freezer, pantry, or in some instances, a warming receptacle. **Food** should be **stored** in clean, dry, sanitary **containers** that are airtight, if possible. This will help keep **food** for longer and reduce the risk of contamination.

Types of Storage of Foods

- **Regular canned foods:** This is usually, the practice, where people start with their food storage. The idea is that we buy a few extra cans of the goods we usually eat, when they go on sale. The idea about this is that, it is easy to use these types of food, since we are familiar with. It also saves time from rushing to the grocery store, in case of any emergency. However, this should not be a permanent solution to our food storage needs, due to the shelf-life limitations.
- **Dry bulk foods:** Dry bulk food is the old age policy of storing the food items, like wheat, rice, beans, sugar, rolled oats and other staples, packaged in large bags or large buckets.
- **Dehydrated foods:** Dehydrated food storage is a shelf-stable food that is processed using high heat. Basically, these are the items that have been dried for preservations. With the high temperature, it removes the moisture from the food, which allows for the extended shelf life.
- **Freeze-dried foods:** Freeze-dried food has been used since the space age, to provide the astronauts with food that is lightweight and compact, where dehydration uses evaporation to get the food out for use. The freeze-dried food uses high-end technology that removes the moisture, out of the food quickly, protecting all the natural nutrients, enzymes and taste. It is the best choice for long-term storage of food.

Food Preservation

The term food preservation refers to the **techniques used to prevent food from spoilage**.

Food preservation has become an increasingly important component of the food industry, as fewer people eat foods produced on their own, but the consumers who, generally, purchase and consume food, throughout the year.

Classification of Foods According to Duration of Preservation

There are a variety of foods, some of which get spoiled easily, while others may be stored for a longer duration. Accordingly, foods can be classified into three categories with respect to the duration of preservation. These include:

1. **Perishable foods:** These include the foods, which get spoiled very soon, e.g., milk and milk products, meat and meat products, and fruits and vegetables.
2. **Semi-perishable foods:** It includes the class of foods which can be stored for little longer, but under suitable storage conditions, e.g., onion, garlic, potatoes and eggs.
3. **Nonperishable foods:** These include food items, which have longer storage period (may be from months to years), e.g., cereal grains, pulses, nuts, sugar, oils, etc.

Causes of Food Spoilage

The vast majority of instances of food spoilage can be attributed to one of the two major causes:
- The **attack by pathogens (disease-causing microorganisms)**, such as **bacteria** and molds.
- **Oxidation** that causes destruction of the essential biochemical compounds and/or plant and animal cells.

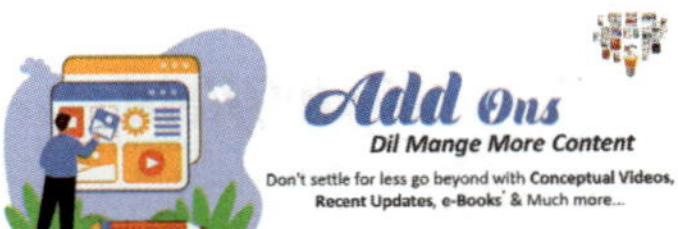

Methods of Food Preservation

Various methods that have been devised for preserving foods are designed to reduce, or eliminate, one and/or the other, above referred causative agents. For example, a simple and common method of preserving food is by **heating** it to some minimum temperature. This process prevents or retards spoilage because high temperature kills or inactivates most kinds of pathogens. The **addition of compounds**, such as ascorbic acid (vitamin C) or butylated hydroxytoluene (BHT), acts as antioxidants, thereby preventing chemical reactions, which cause the oxidation of food that results in its spoilage. All the techniques of food preservation are designed to extend the life of foods, by protecting the foods from spoilage, by anyone of the above two causes.

Traditional Methods of Food Preservation

- **Drying:** Since most of the disease-causing organisms require moist environment to survive and multiply, drying is a natural technique used for preventing spoilage. For example, leaving foodstuff out in the sun and wind, to dry is probably one of the earliest forms of food preservation.

  Drying removes water and prevents growth of microorganisms. Nowadays, host of dehydrating techniques is known, and is in use. However, the specific technique adopted for this purpose depends on properties of the food being preserved, e.g., drying in sun or by mechanical dryers, or by freeze-drying.

  Modern drying techniques use fans and heaters, in controlled environment. Vacuum drying, the form of preservation in which the food is placed in a large container from which air is removed, is also being practiced.

- **Curing:** The earliest form of curing was dehydration, or drying. Smoking and salting improve the drying process. This in turn, also acts as antimicrobial agents and aid in preservation. For example, **smoking** of food, deposits a number of products on it, including phenols and catechol; these chemicals inhibit the growth of microorganisms. **Salting** accelerates drying process using osmosis, and also inhibits the growth of several common strains of bacteria. More recently, nitrites are used to cure meat, contributing a characteristic pink color.

- **Cooling:** Cooling (refrigeration) preserves food, by slowing down the growth and reproduction of microorganisms, and the action of enzymes that cause the food to rot. Fruits and vegetables should be kept refrigerated at low temperature (1°–4°C). **Frozen foods** can be preserved for longer period, when stored at –18°C. **Chilling** temperature retards microbial growth and biochemical changes which affect color, texture, flavor and nutritive value.

- **Boiling:** Boiling, liquid food items can kill any existing microbes. For example, milk is boiled before storage to kill many microorganisms.

- **Addition of sugars:** The earliest cultures have used sugar as a preservative. It was also common to store fruits in honey. Sugar draws water from the microbes, which leaves the microbial cells dehydrated, and thus, kills them.

  Sugar is used to preserve fruits, either in antimicrobial syrup with fruit (such as apples, pears, peaches, apricots and plums) or in crystallized form, where the preserved material is cooked in sugar (to the point of crystallization) and the resultant product is then stored dry. Sugaring is also used in the production of jam and jelly.

- **Salting and pickling:** Salt is a preservative. By adding certain condiments and spices along with a lot of salt, certain foods like mango, lime, several vegetables and fish, may be stored in the form of pickle.

  Pickling is a method of preserving food, in an edible, antimicrobial liquid that inhibits the growth, or kills, bacteria and other microorganisms. Typical pickling agents include vinegar, salt and vegetable oil.

- **Canning:** Canning involves cooking food, sealing it in the sterilized cans or jars, and then boiling the containers to kill, or weakening growth of any remaining bacteria.

Modern Industrial Techniques of Food Preservation

- **Pasteurization:** According to WHO, pasteurization is defined as the process of heating milk to a fixed temperature, for a fixed period of time, to destroy pathogens that may be present in the milk, while causing minimal changes in its composition, flavor and nutritive value. In this process, milk is heated to about 70°C for 15–30 minutes, to kill the bacteria present in it, and cooling it quickly, to 10°C, to prevent the remaining bacteria from growing. After pasteurization, the milk is stored in sterilized bottles, or pouches, in cold places. This method was invented by Louis Pasteur in 1862.

- **Vacuum packing:** It involves storage of food in a vacuum environment, usually in an air tight bag or bottle. The vacuum environment strips bacteria of oxygen needed for survival. Vacuum packing is commonly used for storing nuts, to reduce loss of flavor from oxidization. A major drawback to vacuum packaging, at the consumer level, is that vacuum sealing can deform its contents and rob certain foods, such as cheese, of its flavor.

- **Addition of chemicals/preservatives:** It refers to the addition of certain preservatives to the food products, which are hazardous for microorganisms but not for the health of human beings, at the concentration used, e.g., benzoic acid, ascorbic acid, sulfur dioxide, nitrates, etc. Acetic acid (4% in water) is generally used for preserving vegetables (such as cauliflower, radish, green chilies, ginger, etc.).

  Artificial food additives also act as antimicrobials (that inhibit the growth of bacteria, fungi and mold) or antioxidants (which inhibit oxidation of food constituents). Common **antimicrobial preservatives** include sodium nitrite, sulfur dioxide, sodium bisulfite, potassium hydrogen sulfite, etc. **Antioxidants** include butylated hydroxyanisole (BHA) and butylated hydroxytoluene (BHT). Other preservatives include formaldehyde and glutaraldehyde, etc.

- **Irradiation:** Irradiation refers to the exposure of food to ionizing radiation. Multiple types of ionizing radiations can be used, including beta-particles (high-energy electrons) and gamma rays (emitted from radioactive sources, such as cobalt[60] or cesium[137]). Irradiation can kill bacteria, molds and insect pests, and reduce ripening and spoilage of fruits. Different doses of rays are selected for different foods.

- **Biopreservation (biological preservation):** It involves the use of natural or controlled microbes or antimicrobials as a way of preserving food and extending its shelf-life. In this process, enzymatic action involves alcoholic or acidic fermentation. Beneficial bacteria or the fermentation products, produced by these bacteria, are used in biopreservation, to control spoilage and render pathogens inactive in food. These microbes increase palatability, nutritive value and shelf-life of the food. For example, bread, wine, tea, coffee and alcoholic drinks are prepared and preserved by this technique.

FOOD ADDITIVES

Food additives are the substances, which are added to food, to preserve flavor or enhance its taste, appearance, or other qualities. Some additives have been used for centuries, such as vinegar and salt for preserving pickles. With the advent of processed foods in recent years, many more additives have been introduced, both, of natural and artificial origin.

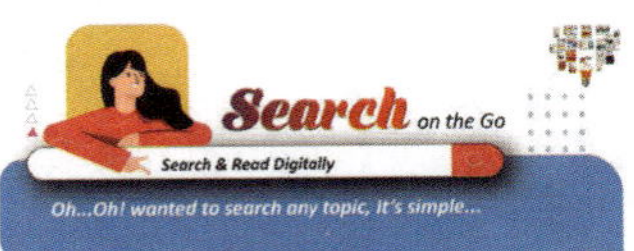

Identification of Food Additives by Number

Many countries have regulated the use of food additives and assigned unique number to each of them. To regulate the use of food additives and inform consumers, each additive is assigned a unique number, termed **E number**, which is used in **Europe** for all the approved additives. This numbering scheme has now been adopted and extended by the **Codex Alimentarius Commission**, to internationally identify all additives. For example, **acetic acid** is written as **E260** on products sold **in Europe,** but is simply known as **additive 260** in some other countries.

United States Food and Drug Administration (USFDA) lists these items as **G**enerally **R**ecognized **A**s **S**afe (GRAS). They are listed under, both, their Chemical Abstracts Service Number, and FDA regulation.

Categories of Food Additives

Food additives can be divided into several groups, although, there may be some overlap, because some additives exert more than one effect.

- **Acidity regulators:** Acidity regulators **(pH control agents)** are food additives used for controlling pH (to change or maintain pH, i.e., acidity or alkalinity) of foods for their stability, or to affect activity of enzymes. They can be **organic** or **mineral acids**, **bases**, **neutralizing agents**, or **buffering agents**. Typical agents include some of the acids or their sodium salts, e.g., ascorbic acid, acetic acid, benzoic acid, propionic acid, etc. Acidity regulators are indicated by their E numbers, such as E260 (acetic acid).
- **Antioxidants:** Antioxidants are compounds that inhibit oxidation, a chemical reaction that produces free radicals, which may damage cells of the organism.
  The term antioxidant is used for two groups of substances, i.e.:
  - **Industrial chemicals** that are added to products to prevent oxidation. They have diverse uses, such as acting as preservatives in food and cosmetics, or oxidation inhibitors.
  - **Naturally occurring compounds** that are present in foods and tissue, such as glutathione or enzymes (which are produced internally), or **dietary antioxidants,** such as vitamin C and vitamin E.
- **Bulking agents:** Bulking agents, such as starch, are additives that increase bulk of the food without affecting its taste.
- **Food coloring agents:** Food coloring or **color additive** is any dye, pigment or substance that is added to food to replace the color lost during preparation, or to make food look more attractive. They come in many forms, such as liquids, powders, gels or pastes. Food coloring agent is used, both, in commercial food production as well as in domestic cooking. Besides, color retention agents are used to preserve the food's existing color.
- **Fortifying agents:** They are added to increase nutritional value of food, e.g., vitamins, minerals, dietary supplements, etc.
- **Emulsifiers:** Emulsifiers, also known as an **emulgents**, are compounds, which typically have a polar, or hydrophilic (i.e., water soluble) part, and a nonpolar (i.e., hydrophobic or lipophilic) part, e.g., egg yolk (which has lecithin as the main emulsifying agent), or mono and diglycerides that are added in many food products, such as coffee creamers, icecreams, spreads and cakes, etc.
- **Flavoring agents:** Flavor is a quality of food that affects sense of taste. Flavoring agents (flavorants) are added to give food a particular taste or smell, and may be derived from natural ingredients or made artificially. For example, artificially flavored jellies, soft drinks or candies have various flavors, due to the use of different scents or fragrances.

Besides, **flavor enhancers**, such as monosodium glutamate (MSG), enhance existing flavor of the food. Some flavor enhancers have their own flavor that is independent of the food.

- **Preservatives:** A preservative is a substance or a chemical that is added to products, such as food, beverages, pharmaceutical drugs, biological samples, cosmetics, and many other products, to prevent decomposition by microbial growth or undesirable chemical changes. Preservatives include chemicals or physical agents:
    - **Chemical preservation** refers to the addition of certain chemical compounds to the product. They reduce the risk of food-borne infections, decrease microbial spoilage, but preserve nutritional quality.
    - **Physical techniques** of food preservation include dehydration, UV radiation, freeze-drying and refrigeration.
- **Sweeteners:** Sweeteners, (**sugar substitutes**) are food additives that provide sweet taste like that of sugar but provide significantly less calories. Most of them are not produced naturally and are also referred to as **artificial sweeteners**, saccharin, aspartame, etc.
- **Thickeners:** Thickener or **thickening agent** is a substance, which can increase viscosity of a liquid, without, substantially, changing its other properties. These are commonly used to thicken sauces, soups, and puddings, etc., without altering their taste.
- **Glazing agents:** They provide a shiny appearance or protective coating to foods.

Functions of Food Additives

- **To maintain product consistency:** Additives such as emulsifiers, stabilizers and thickeners are used to maintain consistency of food. For example, emulsifier such as peanut butter gives a consistent texture to the product and prevents it from separating. Stabilizers and thickeners are used in ice cream to give it a smooth and uniform texture.
- **To improve or maintain nutritional value:** Such additives are added to make up for the elements that are likely to be lacking in a diet, or replacing those which may be lost during processing. Such nutrients should be listed in the list of ingredients. For example, thiamine, riboflavin, niacin and iron in flours and cereals; vitamins A and D in milk, vegetable oils and ghee; or iodine in salt, etc.
- **To provide leavening or control acidity and alkalinity:** Leavening agents release acids, when heated, e.g., baking soda added to cakes, biscuits and other baked foods. It is added during baking to improve the texture. Some additives also modify acidity or alkalinity of the food.
- **To enhance flavor or impart desired color:** Many spices and flavoring agents enhance taste of the food. For example, color, dye, pigment, or any other substance that imparts color to a food, enhances appearance of food and make it more appealing.
- **To maintain palatability and wholesomeness:** Some preservatives retard spoilage of food, caused by mold, bacteria, fungi or yeast. Others, like antioxidants, are added to prevent fat (in baked and other foods) from becoming rancid and, thus, to develop bad flavor.

General Principles for Use of Food Additives

- Food additives (whether in use or being proposed for use) should have undergone, or should be subjected to, appropriate toxicological testing and evaluation. This should take into account (among other things) any cumulative, synergistic or potentiating effects of its use.

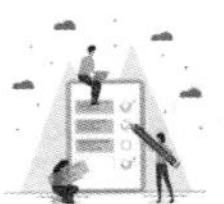
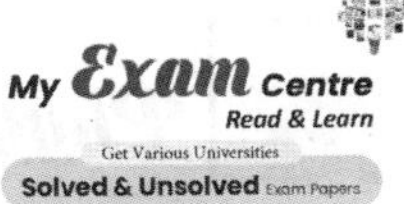

- Only those food additives should be endorsed for use, which can be judged on the basis of presently available evidences that are known to cause no health hazards, at the level of proposed use.
- Food additives should be kept under continuous observation and should be re-evaluated, whenever necessary, in the light of changing conditions of use and new scientific information.
- Food additives should, at all times, conform to approved specifications, e.g., the specifications of identity and purity recommended by the **Codex Alimentarius Commission**.
- The use of food additives should be justified and allowed only to serve one or more of the following purposes (given below from a to d) and that these purposes cannot be achieved by other means, which are economically and technologically practicable, and do not present a hazard to the health of the consumer:
  a. To preserve the nutritional quality of the food; an intentional reduction in the nutritional quality of a food would be justified in the circumstances dealt with in sub-paragraph b, and also in other circumstances where the food does not constitute a significant item in a normal diet.
  b. To provide necessary ingredients or constituents for foods manufactured for groups of consumers having special dietary needs.
  c. To enhance the keeping quality or stability of a food or to improve its organoleptic properties, provided that this does not change the nature, substance or quality of the food to an extent that it deceives the consumer.
  d. To provide aids in the manufacture, processing, preparation, treatment, packing, transport or storage of food, provided that the additive is not used to disguise the effects of the use of faulty raw materials or of undesirable (including unhygienic) practices or techniques during the course of any of these activities.
- Approval, or temporary approval, for the inclusion of a food additive in an advisory list or in a food standard should:
  - As far as possible be limited to specific foods for specific purposes and under specific conditions.
  - Be at the lowest level of use, necessary to achieve the desired effect.
  - As far as possible take into account any "Acceptable Daily Intake" or equivalent assessment, established for the food additive and the probable daily intake of it from all sources. Where the food additive is to be used in foods eaten by special groups of consumers, account should be taken of the probable daily intake of the food additive by consumers in those groups.

FOOD FORTIFICATION

Food fortification means addition of nutrients to a food, so that the quality is maintained or improved without the quantity being significantly increased. Food fortification can be important part of nutrition intervention strategy as a means of delivering nutrients to population.

The program of food fortification has been launched in India to overcome the widespread micronutrients deficiencies in the community, such as of iodine, vitamin A and iron. For example, iodination of common salt with potassium iodate (to eliminate iodine deficiency disorders). Similarly, delivery of iron through common salt was launched by National Institute of Nutrition (NIN) to mitigate the problem of anemia.

FOOD ADULTERATION

Food adulteration refers to the addition of some non-food material or inferior quality product to the food. A spoilt, stale or poor-quality food is made attractive and fresh, by adding harmful colors or other chemicals. Frequently adulterated food items include milk and milk products, cereals, pulses and their products, edible oils and spices.

- **Different classes of adulterants** include non-permitted colors (like metanil yellow), non-edible oils (like castor oil), cheaper agricultural produce (like various starches in milk powder), extraneous matter (like husk, sand and sawdust) and metal contaminants (like aluminum or iron filings).
- Consumption of adulterated foods **could lead to disease outbreaks** of epidemic proportions.
- **Buying food from a reliable and reputed source**, careful checking of foods before purchase and insisting on certified brands will all minimize the risk of food adulteration.

Prevention of Food Adulteration Act

To ensure protection of health of the consumers, **Government of India** enacted **Prevention of Food Adulteration Act (PFA)**, to consolidate the laws relating to food being administered by different ministries/departments. Since food is essential for the maintenance of health, the act was enacted with the object that the food available to the consumer should be nutritious, wholesome and pure.

According to PFA, **food** is described as any article that is used as food or drink for human consumption other than drugs and water, and includes:

- Any article, which ordinarily enters into or is used in the composition or preparation of human food
- Any flavoring matter or condiments
- Any other article, which the Central Government may be having regard to its use, nature, substance or quality, declare, by notification in the official gazette as food for the purpose of the PFA

On the other hand, an **adulterant** means any material, which is or could be employed for the purposes of adulteration.

Objectives of the PFA

Objectives of PFA include:

- To protect the public from poisonous and harmful foods
- To prevent the sale of substandard foods
- To protect the interests of the consumers by eliminating fraudulent practices

Rules and Standards of PFA

Rules and standards framed under the PFA act are uniformly applicable throughout the country.

- **Enforcement** of the food laws primarily rests **with the State/UTs**.
- The **implementation** of the Act in most of the States is under the administrative control of the **Directorate of Health Services**, whereas, in a few States, the implementation is being combined with Drugs Administration under the Joint Food and Drug Administration.
- The provisions under PFA Rules have been **amended nearly 360 times** and standards of around 250 articles of food, which are of mass consumption have been prescribed.

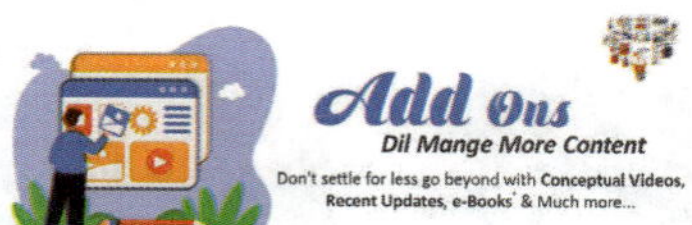

- By and large, in most of the States, implementation in corporation/municipal area rests with the **Local Bodies**, which employ their own **food inspectors**. Licensing of food industries/establishments is also left to them.
- There are **72 food laboratories** in the country at District/Regional or State level in addition to four Central Food Laboratories set-up by the Central Government.
- Almost **every State has got one or more laboratory** depending upon its need.
- About 12 of these laboratories are under the **administrative control** of the **local bodies** whereas the remaining ones are under the administrative control of the **State Government**.

FOOD STANDARDS

Food standard is a set of criteria that a food must meet, if it is to be suitable for human consumption such as source, composition, appearance, freshness, permissible additives and maximum bacterial content.

Food standards are the body of rules, directly governing foodstuffs, whether they are issued by official, semiofficial or factory authority. Food standards, such as those that specify the maximum allowable level of contaminants in food, or the amount of food additives permitted, are an important instrument for the assurance of food safety.

The food standards explain that:
- The **quality must meet the expectations of the consumer**,
- It must be as described and **not presented in a way that misleads the consumer**, and
- **Nothing may be added or removed that would make it harmful to be.**

Legislations and Regulations about Food Standards

Several organizations/countries have made legislations and regulations about food standards. Some of these include:
- **WHO** and **FAO**, in 1963, published the **Codex Alimentarius**, which serves as a **guideline to food safety**.
- In **Australia, food safety standards** place obligations on Australian food businesses, to produce food that is safe and suitable to eat, and also place health and hygiene obligations on food handlers.
- In **United Kingdom,** the **Food Standards Agency** is a non-ministerial Government Department of the Government of the United Kingdom, who is responsible for protecting public health in relation to food standards in England, Wales and Northern Ireland. It is led by a board appointed to act in the public interest with its headquarters in London.
- In **India**, the **Food Safety** and **Standards** Authority of India (**FSSAI**) has been created for laying down science-based standards for articles of food, and to regulate their manufacture, storage, distribution, sale and import, to ensure availability of safe and wholesome food for human consumption.

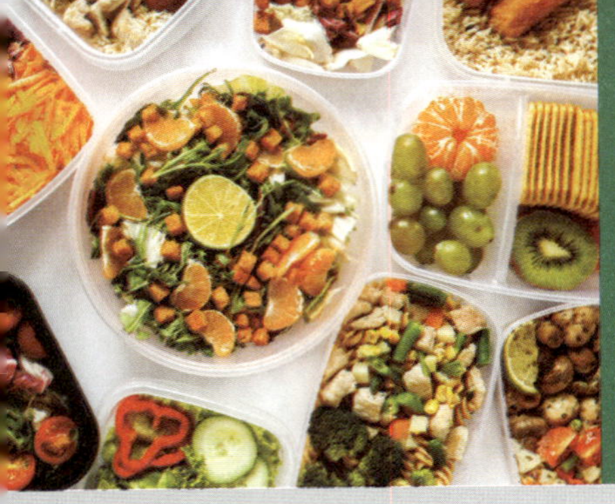

LONG AND SHORT ANSWER QUESTIONS

1. Define food preservation. Describe various methods of food preservation.
2. Describe various methods of prevention of loss of vitamins from foods.
3. What are food additives? Describe various categories of food additives.
4. **Describe briefly:**
   a. Principles of healthy cooking
   b. Principle methods of cooking
   c. Dry heat cooking methods
   d. Moist heat cooking methods
   e. Prevention of Food Adulteration Act (PFA)
5. **Write notes on:**
   a. Food storage
   b. Food preservation
   c. Classification of foods according to duration of preservation
   d. Curing of foods
   e. Pasteurization
   f. Vacuum packing of foods
   g. Biopreservation of foods
   h. Canning of foods
   i. Grilling
   j. Broiling
   k. Roasting
   l. Sauteing
   m. Deep-frying
   n. Baking
   o. Poaching
   p. Simmering
   q. Stewing

MULTIPLE CHOICE QUESTIONS

1. **Which cooking method is considered healthiest due to its ability to retain most nutrients?**
   a. Deep frying
   b. Boiling
   c. Steaming
   d. Grilling

2. **What is the best way to reduce unhealthy fats in cooking?**
    a. Use butter or lard for flavor
    b. Opt for oils high in saturated fats
    c. Use healthy fats like olive oil and limit their quantity
    d. Avoid using oils or fats altogether

3. **Which method of food preservation works by removing moisture to prevent the growth of microorganisms?**
    a. Canning
    b. Freezing
    c. Dehydration
    d. Pickling

4. **Which food preservation technique uses high acidity to prevent bacterial growth?**
    a. Fermentation
    b. Vacuum sealing
    c. Pasteurization
    d. Pickling

Notes

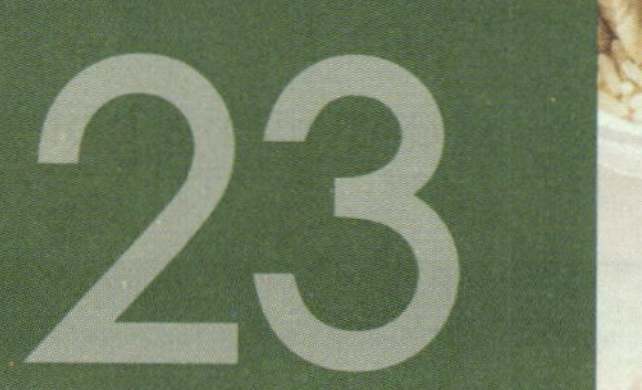

23

Nutrition Assessment and Nutrition Education

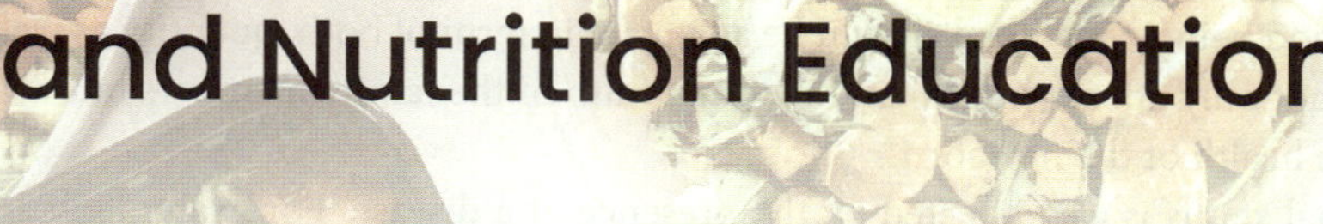

LEARNING OBJECTIVES

After the completion of the chapter, the readers will be able to:
- Explain objectives of nutritional assessment.
- Explain nutrition education—purposes, principles and methods.

CHAPTER OUTLINE

- Assessment of Nutritional Status
- Nutrition Education

KEY TERMS

Anthropometry: The systematic measurement of the physical properties of the human body, primarily dimensional descriptors of body size and shape.

Nutritional education: Any set of learning experiences designed to facilitate the voluntary adoption of eating and other nutrition-related behaviors conducive to health and well-being.

Nutritional status: An individual's health condition as it is influenced by the intake and utilization of nutrients.

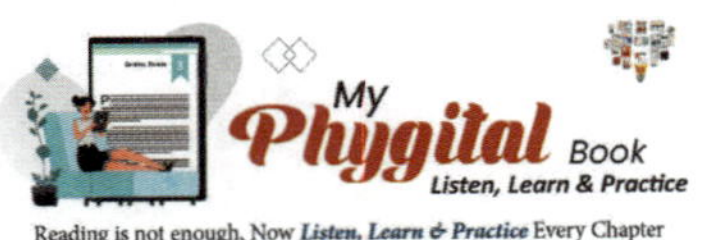

ASSESSMENT OF NUTRITIONAL STATUS

Assessment of nutritional status involves measurement of nutritional health of the body. It is a routine part of nutritional care of the individual, since both, undernutrition and overnutrition may affect health.

Nutritional status of an individual, family or community depends upon several factors, each one of which plays an important role, such as:

- **Consumption of food:** Availability and consumption of food is one of the most important factors to assess nutritional status. The food being consumed should be adequate in term of both, quantity as well as quality. Poor nutrition will not only affect physical and mental health of the family members but will also have adverse effects on the health of the newborn.
- **Presence of disease:** Nutritional status is also affected by the presence of a disease. For example, if an individual or family is suffering from some chronic disease such as coronary heart disease, hypertension or diabetes mellitus, the type of dietary restrictions, in turn, will affect nutrition status of the individual and the family.
- **Pregnancy:** Food intake during pregnancy affects health status of the newborn. For example, malnutrition during pregnancy affects health of the newborn such as low birth weight babies, disability or poor quality of life, and mortality, etc.

Thus, assessment of nutritional status of an individual, family and community are important for public health. Assessment of nutritional status helps the Government and policy makers to get information regarding the prevalence of nutritional disorders in the particular area or community. It can also help to identify high-risk groups and define epidemiological factors in the causation of the nutritional deficiency disorders.

Significance of Assessment of Nutritional Status

Assessment of nutritional status serves a variety of purposes:

- Nutrition assessment helps **to evaluate nutrition-related risks** that may affect current, or future, health of an individual.
- It is a routine part of **nutrition care of the hospitalized patients**, including effectiveness of treatment.
- Nutrition assessment helps **identify people in need of nutrition-related interventions** and to monitor effectiveness of such programs.
- It also determines **nutritional health of population**, to identify common health risks in a population group.

Methods of Assessment of Nutritional Status

Nutritional assessment can be done by using various methods, generally, referred to as **A**, **B**, **C** and **D**, i.e.:

A = **A**nthropometry

B = Laboratory and **B**iochemical assessment

C = **C**linical examination

D = Assessment of **D**ietary intake

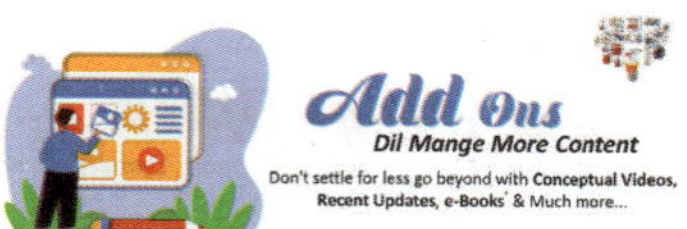

A - Anthropometry

The word **anthropometry** comes from two words, i.e., "**Anthropo**" means "**human**" and "**metry**" means **measurement**. Thus, anthropometry allows for assessment of different component parts of the human body, i.e., the anatomical make-up of the body in terms of bone, muscle, water and fat. Since a single measure cannot provide a comprehensive overview of an individual's condition, so, a number of measurements are done to make a reasonable assessment.

Anthropometric measurements include measurement of physical characteristics of the body, such as weight, length/height, mid upper arm circumference and skin fold thickness. In young children, head and chest circumference are also measured to assess patterns of growth and development.

- **Weight:** A weighing sling (spring balance), also called the **Salter scale,** is used for measuring weight of children under two years old, to the nearest 0.1 kg. In adults and children over two years, a beam balance is used and the measurement is done to the nearest 0.1 kg. Weight is a measure to assess child's growth, predict energy expenditure and protein needs, and determine body composition. Sudden change in weight in growing children reflects a disease, and also monitors progress in fat loss, e.g., in cancer or thyroid disorders.

- **Height:** It is measured with the child, or adult, in a standing position (usually, children who are two years old or more). For infants and young children, it is the measurement of recumbent length. The head should be in a position where the line passing from the external ear hole to the lower eye lid is parallel to the floor (referred to as the **Frankfurt position**) during measurement and the shoulders, buttocks and the heels should touch the vertical stand. Either a stadiometer or a portable anthropometer can be used for measuring the height and the measurements are recorded to the nearest millimeter. Comparison with the standard growth charts shows, how growth of the child is comparable to that of the others, of the same age and sex.

- **Upper mid arm circumference:** It is an accurate way to measure fat-free mass (muscle mass). It is the circumference of the upper arm at the midway, between the shoulder tip and the elbow tip on the left arm. The mid-arm point is determined by measuring the distance from the shoulder tip to the elbow and dividing it by two. A low reading indicates a loss of muscle mass.

  A special tape is used for measuring the mid upper arm circumference of a child. The tape has three colors, with the red, indicating severe acute malnutrition, the yellow, moderate acute malnutrition and the green, normal nutritional status.

- **Skin-fold thickness:** Measurement of skin-fold thickness is a method to estimate thickness of a fold of skin and subcutaneous fat, with a calliper. It provides an indication of fatness of the body, since a significant amount of body's fat store lies just beneath the skin.

- **Head circumference:** It refers to the measurement of the circumference of the head (along the forehead and the area on the back part of the head). It is measured in millimeters using a measuring tape. Measurement of head circumference is useful in assessing chronic nutritional problems in children below two years of age, the period of brain growth.

- **Body mass index (BMI):** It is obtained from the weight of a person (in kg) divided by his/her height (in meters square). An adult is considered to have a normal BMI, if it is in the range of 18.5–25.0. If an adult has BMI less than 16, he has very poor energy stores. If BMI is above 25, the person is said to be overweight.

B - Laboratory and Biochemical Assessment

Assessment of nutritional status by biochemical methods refers to laboratory estimations that measure the quantity of a particular nutrient, or its metabolite, in one or more body fluids, such as blood, urine or feces. For example, estimation of serum albumin concentration is an indicator of protein status of the body. Biochemical measurements of the metabolites, storage or transported compounds, or enzymes are better indicators of nutritional status, than directly measuring the blood level of a particular nutrient, such as vitamin A or calcium.

Biochemical investigations are extremely helpful in detecting early changes in body metabolism and nutritional status, before the appearance of overt clinical signs. In addition, the biochemical test results are precise, accurate and reproducible. Common laboratory investigations include:

- Estimation of routine blood parameters, such as hemoglobin (Hb), serum proteins and enzymes.
- Estimation of the level of specific nutrient in blood, such as vitamins, iron, amino acids, etc.

C - Clinical Examination

- Clinical observations mean assessment by evaluating characteristics of well-being that can be seen by physical examination. Some nonspecific clinical signs provide clue to nutrient deficiency, or excess, that can be confirmed, or ruled out, by biochemical tests, e.g., wasting of muscle or obesity.
- Clinical methods of assessing nutritional status involve checking signs and symptoms of deficiency at specific places on the body, or asking the patient whether he has any symptoms that might suggest nutrient deficiency. Clinical observations assess changes in skin color and health, hair texture, finger nail shape, eyes, lips, mouth, bones, muscles and joints. There may be some specific clinical findings depicting the deficiency of a particular nutrient, e.g., hemorrhages on the skin (indicative of vitamin C deficiency), cracking at the corners of mouth (suggestive of riboflavin, B6 and niacin deficiency), etc.
- **Clinical signs** of nutrient deficiency include pallor (on the palm of the hand or the conjunctiva of the eye), pitting edema, severe visible wasting, Bitot's spots on the eyes, or swelling on the neck, etc. (Table 23.1).

TABLE 23.1: Clinical signs and symptoms of some common nutritional problems

Nutritional deficiency disease	Signs/symptoms
• Anemia, may be due to the deficiency of iron, folic acid, vitamin B_{12}, copper, protein or vitamin B_6	• Pale palms, conjunctiva and tongue, gets tired easily, loss of appetite and shortness of breath
• Vitamin A deficiency	• Bitot's spots (whitish patchy triangular lesions on the side of the eye)
• Iodine deficiency disorder	• Goiter (swelling on the front of the neck)

- **Bitot's spots:** These are the signs of vitamin A deficiency. These spots are of creamy color and appear on the cornea (white portion) of the eye.
- **Goiter:** It is a swelling on the neck and is the only visible sign of iodine deficiency.
- Clinical examination also includes **assessment of the associated problems**, like tuberculosis, malabsorption syndrome, any infection or infestation, etc.

D - Assessment of Dietary Intake

- Assessment of dietary intake is a comprehensive evaluation to assess food consumption at national level, household level and an individual level.

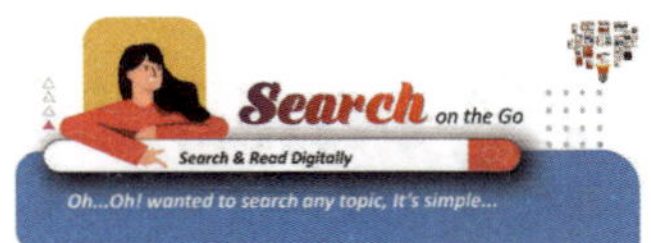

- **Objectives of the assessment of dietary intake:**
  - It provides information about dietary intake patterns
  - It also provides information about estimate nutrient intakes
  - It is helpful in planning health education activities
  - It also provides information about food habit and attitudes.

- **Methods of assessment of dietary intake:** Dietary intake can be assessed by subjective report and objective observation. Subjective assessment is possible using open-ended surveys such as dietary recalls or records, or using closed-ended surveys including food frequency questionnaires. Both the methods differ from each other with respect to the information received during the fixed duration of dietary intakes. Selection of the appropriate dietary assessment method, however, depends upon the group of participants and their lifestyles.

  - **Diet records/food diary:** Food diary or diet records method, of obtaining the information, is a type of survey where the record of the person with respect to the consumption of foods and beverages are made in a diary. To ensure the accuracy and reliability of the data obtained, detailed instructions regarding the collection of data about food diary and making diet records are provided to the individuals collecting the information. The record of all the ingredients used; methods of preparation of food, and the amount of the particular food consumed in one meal by the person is also made.

    Diet records/food diary may be prepared based on either **3 days** or **7 days record of** intake of nutrients. As diet records/food diary depend on the collection of data based on the memory of the person being interrogated, so if the study period is prolonged the study may not have much advantage.

  - **24-hour dietary recall method:** Twenty-four-hour dietary recall method describes food and beverages in detail that an individual consumed in the past 24 hours. The individual, to be interrogated, is asked to explain the kind and quantity of different foods and beverages consumed in 24 hours, on any day. For example, the person may be asked to recall the details of dietary intakes either starting from the beginning of the recalling day or starting with the current day and go backward. In routine, it requires about 15–20 minutes, depending upon the type of food consumed. The health care worker may request the individual to recall what he/she consumed by giving details of the time of consumption (such as in the morning, afternoon or at dinner, etc.) or by showing the food item, its picture, etc. It can be repeated again after some time and the data may be averaged to get better results.

    24-hour dietary recall is a quick and easy method to assess the average intake of the groups by applying standardized data collection methods with careful administration and with repeated assessments on more than one day. It has advantages as it is to administer and fast completion, with the major disadvantage being the needs of an experienced interviewer. Further, it is dependent upon the subject's short-term memory and may not be very accurate.

  - **Food frequency questionnaires:** A food frequency questionnaire (FFQ) **consists of a finite list of foods and beverages with response categories to indicate usual frequency of consumption over** a specified time. The subject is given a list of foods and asked to indicate intake per day, per week and per month. To assess the total diet, the number of foods and beverages queried, typically, ranges from 80 to 120. Completing a questionnaire aimed at capturing the total dietary intake usually requires 30–60 minutes.

    The FFQ examines how often someone eats certain foods, and sometimes the size of the portions. This method is **quick**, **inexpensive** and **easy to administer** but **under-reporting is common.**

However, it is **more accurate than the 24-hour dietary recall method**. Food frequency questionnaires have been mostly used to assess dietary intake in cancer studies. Being self-administered, FFQs are considered easy to use with practical application in cohort studies.

The FFQs consist of a list of specific foods or food types associated with frequency of consumption, which may be a disadvantage for prospective studies as hypotheses to be tested are limited by the list. They are termed semiquantitative if portions are included. FFQs need to be developed for specific population groups otherwise, important foods may be missed. FFQs may become outdated if the supply of foodstuffs changes.

NUTRITION EDUCATION

People in the community show their lack of knowledge about nutrition, when they make poor food choices. Nutrition education is a set of learning experiences designed to assist in healthy eating choices and other nutrition-related behavior. It includes any combination of educational strategies, accompanied by environmental supports conducive to health and well-being. It also critically looks at issues such as food security, food literacy and food sustainability.

Health professionals have a role in educating an individual in the clinic, community or long-term health-care facility. In these settings, **the dietician, nutritionist** or **nurse serves to assist or enable individuals to incorporate changes in eating patterns and behavior into their lives**. The major focus of this type of nutrition is not knowledge and facts, but rather the development of permanent behavioral changes.

Purposes of Nutrition Education

Nutrition education programs should include:

- **Significance of nutrition:** Public as well as policy makers should be apprised of the nutrition knowledge and its significance for health. They should be told about the role of nutrition in the maintenance of physical and mental health, daily requirements of various dietary nutrients, causes and prevention of nutritional disorders, food standards, food additives and safety.
- **Information about hygiene and safe food handling:** Besides providing the knowledge about nutrition and its role in health, education should also be provided about good hygienic practices, hand washing and cleanliness. Nutrition Educationist should also provide information regarding safe food handling at various stages from shopping to cooking and storage of the leftover food.
- **Food quality and diversity:** Nutrition education should also include information about the quality food, variety of food items and use of color combinations in daily needs. Education should also provide knowledge about locally grown and available food items, growing of seasonal vegetables, etc.

Nutrition education should include each of these components and provide detailed information about the significance of each. The person responsible for providing education should interact with the public and discuss their problems.

Principles of Nutrition Education

Nutrition education is a part of applied nutrition that focuses its resources toward learning, adaptation and acceptance of healthy eating habits, according to one's own food culture and scientific knowledge in

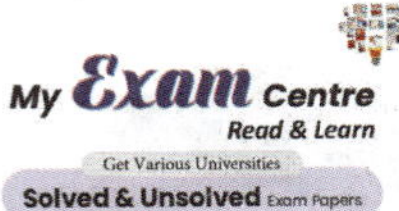

nutrition, all with the ultimate aim of promoting health of the individual or community. An effective nutrition intervention program should integrate good instructional design and learning principles, and use media that facilitates a high degree of individualization.

- **Identification of the target group:** It is important to identify the target group so that the person responsible for nutrition education can set the standard of the information to be given, accordingly.
- **Relevance of the subject:** The information to be given should be relevant and of interest to the audience, using local dialect and resources. For example, if one wants to address the school children, they should be told about the relevance of the particular nutrients with respect to their availability and usefulness. In school children, it will be more relevant to speak about anemia and its prevention with the help of locally grown vegetables, etc.
- **Discussion and feedback:** It is important to involve the audience in discussion and ask them to give feedback. Some local leaders and experienced people may also be requested for this purpose.
- **Encouragement and appreciation:** At the end of the talk or show, etc., it will be good to encourage the audience by giving them small gifts for their active involvement, such as distribution of some healthy foodstuff or pictures depicting nutrition and health, etc.

Methods of Nutrition Education

The first step in developing a lesson plan is to know the target audience, settings and contents. Focus on the learners and their interests, needs and motivations, and actively involve them in the process.

Common methods of education which can be practiced in nutrition education may include:

- **General lectures and discussions:** The person providing nutrition education must deliver the desired information in the form of lecture, which should not be too lengthy. The information should be delivered in simple language, preferably in local language. He/she should not use technical language, however, if necessary, some of the technical words may be explained in simple words with the aid of suitable diagrams or pictures. The person should create the interest of the audience and actively involve them in discussion.
- **Slide shows:** The information may also be conveyed in the form of slide show explaining the details, wherever required.
- **Nukkar nataks/small group presentations:** Local people may be involved to convey the message with acting so as to make it more useful and simple.
- **Movies:** Small movies regarding nutritional disorders and their prevention will help them in easily understanding the significance of health and nutrition. Also, information about hygiene, cleanliness and immunization may be conveyed by this method.
- **Small booklets and leaflets:** Some of the information may also be supplied in the form of small booklets and leaflets exhibiting some of the pictures of food components and their significance.
- **Posters and exhibitions:** Periodically, some interesting posters may be prepared and displayed at places such as main streets, bus stops, panchayat buildings, etc. Sometimes, exhibitions may also be arranged with the aim of providing information regarding nutrition and health.

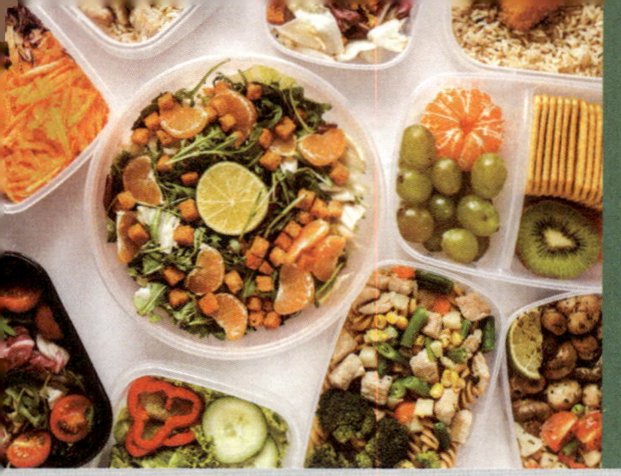

LONG AND SHORT ANSWER QUESTIONS

1. Explain objectives and methods of nutritional assessment.
2. Describe purposes, principles and methods of nutrition education.
3. **Briefly describe:**
   a. Anthropometry
   b. Assessment of dietary intake
   c. Principles and methods of nutrition education
4. **Write notes on:**
   a. Assessment of nutritional status
   b. Methods of assessment of nutritional status
   c. Significance of assessment of nutritional status
   d. Principles of Nutrition Education
   e. Food frequency questionnaire

MULTIPLE CHOICE QUESTIONS

1. **What is the primary purpose of nutrition education?**
   a. To promote the sale of dietary supplements
   b. To encourage people to eat only organic foods
   c. To improve knowledge and behavior related to healthy eating
   d. To teach people how to cook gourmet meals

2. **Which method helps to assess the effectiveness of a nutrition education program?**
   a. Observational study of eating habits after the program
   b. Guessing the level of knowledge retention
   c. Ignoring participant feedback
   d. Measuring the weight of participants before and after sessions

3. **What is the primary objective of nutritional assessment?**
   a. To promote the consumption of specific brands of food
   b. To determine an individual's dietary supplement needs
   c. To evaluate an individual's nutritional status and identify potential deficiencies
   d. To measure an individual's exercise capacity

4. **Which method of nutritional assessment involves the measurement of body weight, height, and body mass index (BMI)?**
   a. Biochemical assessment
   b. Dietary assessment
   c. Anthropometric assessment
   d. Clinical assessment

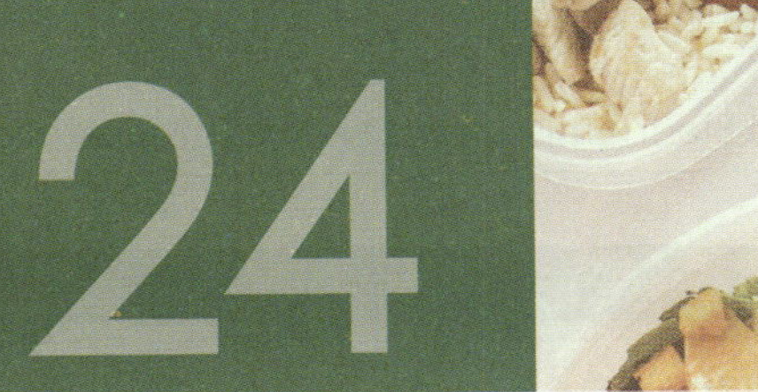

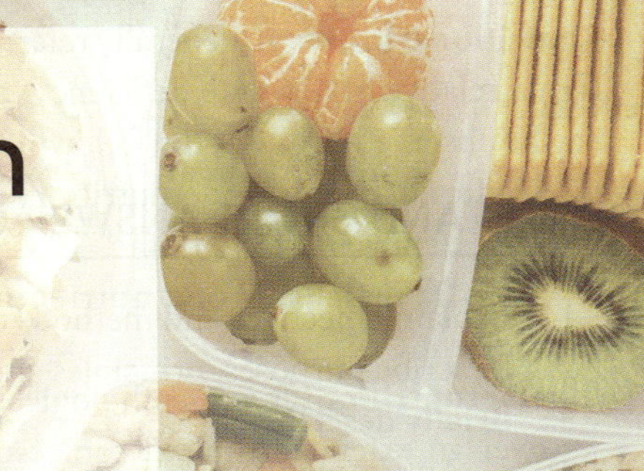

24

Nutritional Problems in India and National Nutritional Programs

LEARNING OBJECTIVES

After the completion of the chapter, the readers will be able to:
- Explain nutritional problems in India.
- Explain National Nutritional Policy.
- Explain national nutritional programs: Vitamin A supplementation.
- Explain Anemia Mukt Bharat Program.
- Explain Integrated Child Development Services.
- Explain Mid-day Meal Scheme.
- Explain National Iodine Deficiency Disorders Control Program.
- Explain weekly Iron Folic Acid Supplementation and others as introduced.
- Explain role of nurse in every program.

CHAPTER OUTLINE

- Nutrition Problems in India
- Low Birth Weight Babies
- Protein Energy Malnutrition
- Vitamin A Deficiency
- Nutritional Anemia
- Iodine Deficiency Disorders
- Endemic Fluorosis
- Problems Related to Overnutrition
- National Nutrition Policy
- National Programs Related to Nutrition
- Anemia Mukt Bharat Program
- Integrated Child Development Services
- Mid-day Meal Scheme
- National Iodine Deficiency Disorders Control Program
- Weekly Iron Folic Acid Supplementation
- National Program for Prevention and Control of Fluorosis
- Role of Nurse in National Nutritional Programs

KEY TERMS

Endemic fluorosis: Refers to that individuals living in a region characterized by high levels of fluoride in the drinking water.

Intrauterine growth retardation: When a baby in the womb (a fetus) does not grow as expected. The baby is not as big as would be expected for the stage of the mother's pregnancy.

Low birth weight baby: Defined by WHO as weight at birth of <2500 grams (5.5 pounds).

Truncal obesity: When a person has more fat concentrated around the center of their body, such as their stomach and abdomen, than their extremities.

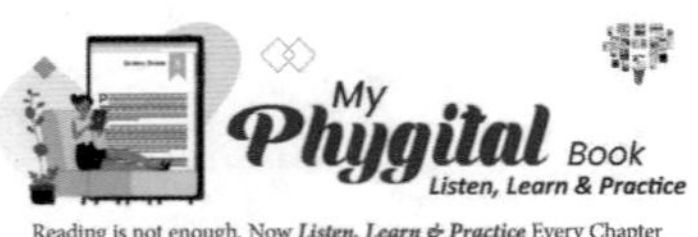

NUTRITION PROBLEMS IN INDIA

A **nutritional problem**, generally referred to as **malnutrition**, may be defined as a pathological state, resulting from a relative or absolute deficiency; or excess, of one or more essential nutrient(s). A nutritional problem may be observed in any of the following forms:

- **Undernutrition:** Undernutrition, or undernourishment, is a result of insufficient food, consumed over the extended period of time.
- **Specific deficiency of a nutrient:** It is a state resulting from the relative or absolute lack of a specific nutrient.
- **Overnutrition:** It is a pathological state resulting from the consumption of excessive quantity of food over an extended time. It can result in being overweight and obesity. Obesity can cause several non-communicable diseases, such as a cardiovascular disease, diabetes or cancer.

Undernutrition

Undernutrition, as discussed in Chapter 11, is a result of reduced intake of total food, including calories, protein, vitamins and minerals. Besides poor intake, other contributing factors to undernutrition include poverty, large family size, unhealthy atmosphere and lifestyle leading to repeated infections, ignorance about nutrition and faulty feeding practices.

Undernutrition is, generally, observed in people living in backward rural areas and urban slums. Population, mostly, affected include socially-backward persons belonging to the scheduled castes and schedule tribe groups, landless laborers and daily wage workers.

The effect of undernutrition starts as early as during conception resulting in low birth weight babies (birth-weight below 2500 g), and continues during childhood and adolescence (resulting in short stature and reduced work capacity, etc.), sometimes, may be during adulthood, as well.

High-Risk Groups

High-risk groups include:

- **Low birth weight babies:** A low birth weight newborn is any newborn with a birth weight of less than 2.5 kg, regardless of gestational age. Nearly one-third of the babies born in India are low birth weight babies (undernourished in the womb). They have a poor start of life cycle and are exposed to the increased risk of morbidity and mortality.
- **Preschool children:** They are most vulnerable to the effect of undernutrition because of rapid growth. A large population of children under five has protein energy malnutrition (PEM), which is a major nutritional health problem in India.
- **Adolescent girls:** Adolescence is a period of second decade of life (10–19 years). During this phase, significant physical, physiological, psychological and emotional changes occur. In females, adolescence marks the beginning of menstrual cycle or reproduction. Adolescents gain 50% of their adult weight and >20% of their adult height, in age group 10–19 years, which is called **growth spurt**. Chronic deprivation of food, particularly, during the period of growth and development, leads to short stature.
- **Pregnant and lactating women:** During pregnancy and lactation, nutritional requirements increase to support fetal and infant growth, and development, as well as maternal metabolism and tissue development

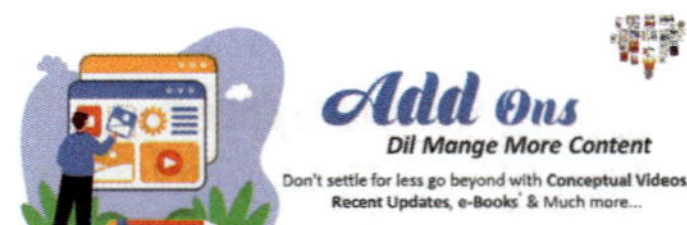

specific to reproduction. If the increased demand of calories, protein, vitamins and minerals is not met accordingly, undernutrition during pregnancy will result in low birth weight babies. Undernutrition during lactation will disturb maternal metabolism, leading to the stage of adaptation.

In India, as per reports of the experts, it has been observed that diets of women from the low socio-economic groups are essentially similar during prepregnant, pregnant and lactating periods. This, in turn, results in maternal malnutrition, leading to increased incidence of low birth weight babies with the increased maternal mortality. It is, therefore, essential to provide not only extra food but also additional healthcare and supervision during pregnancy and lactation.

- **Elderly socially-deprived persons:** Nearly one-third of adult population has various grades of chronic energy deficiency. The effects of undernutrition of childhood are carried over to adolescents and adults. Work capacity of adult goes down due to chronic malnutrition of long-standing. PEM may also occur in persons who are unable to absorb vital nutrients that are essential for healthy tissue formation and organ function.

Causes of Undernutrition

- **Socioeconomic status:** In general, those who are poor, are at risk for undernutrition, due to inadequate intake of food.
- **Lack of breastfeeding:** Lack of breastfeeding results in low birth weight of the baby. It may be a result of large family size, poor maternal health, failure of lactation or premature termination of breastfeeding, delayed supplementary feeding or use of over diluted milk.
- **Infections:** Infections, such as tuberculosis, gastroenteritis, measles, diarrhea, respiratory infections and intestinal worms cause malnutrition.
- **Food habits**: Being strictly vegan, sometimes, may result in protein malnutrition. It is due to the reason that the type of proteins present in cereals does not parallel to the proteins those are present in animal products.
- **Communicable diseases:** Diseases such as hepatitis, tuberculosis and malaria continue to plague India due to increased resistance to drugs. These diseases can be attributed to poor sanitation and inadequate safe drinking water.
- **Noncommunicable diseases (NCDs):** These include cardiovascular diseases (CVD), diabetes, chronic obstructive pulmonary disease (COPD), cancer, mental health disorders and injuries. Indians are particularly, at high risk for atherosclerosis and coronary artery disease. This may be attributed to genetic predisposition, metabolic syndrome and adverse changes in coronary artery vasodilation.
- **Poor environment and hygiene:** Poor sanitation, due to open air defecation, leads to the spread of disease and malnutrition, through parasitic and bacterial infections. Several million people in India suffer from multiple episodes of diarrhea or fall ill on account of Hepatitis A, enteric fever, intestinal worms, and eye and skin infections, which are caused by poor hygiene and unsafe drinking water. Insufficient maintenance of the environment around water sources, groundwater pollution, excessive arsenic and fluoride contents in drinking water also pose a major threat to health in India.

Prevention of Undernutrition

- Breastfeeding can reduce rates of malnutrition and death in children.
- In young children, providing food (in addition to breast milk) between six months and two years of age improves outcomes.

- Supplementation of micronutrients to women during pregnancy and to young children in the developing stage improves their health.
- Long-term measures include improving agricultural practices, reducing poverty, improving sanitation and the empowerment of women.

LOW BIRTH WEIGHT BABIES

The problem of low birth weight babies is widespread and multi-factorial:
- Low birth weight is associated with poor growth during infancy, and thereafter, throughout the childhood period.
- Retrospectively, low birth weight reflects poor nutritional and health status of women during pregnancy, during adolescence and during childhood period.

Causes of Low Birth Weight Babies

- Illness/infections
- Short maternal stature
- Very young age
- High parity
- Close birth intervals
- Intrauterine growth retardation
- Hard physical labor during pregnancy
- Maternal malnutrition
- Anemia
- Smoking

Prevention of Low Birth Weight Babies

- Increasing food intake of mother
- Supplementary feeding
- Distribution of iron and folic acid tablets
- Avoidance, if, smoking
- Improved sanitation methods
- Early detection and treatment of medical disorders, such as diabetes and hypertension
- Controlling infections, like urinary tract infection, rubella, syphilis, malaria, etc.

PROTEIN ENERGY MALNUTRITION

Protein energy malnutrition **(PEM)** also referred to as **protein calorie malnutrition** (PCM), refers to the form of malnutrition due to inadequate intake of calories and/or protein. WHO recommended three terms, i.e., stunting, underweight and wasting, for assessing the magnitude of malnutrition in children <5 years of age (Chapter 20).

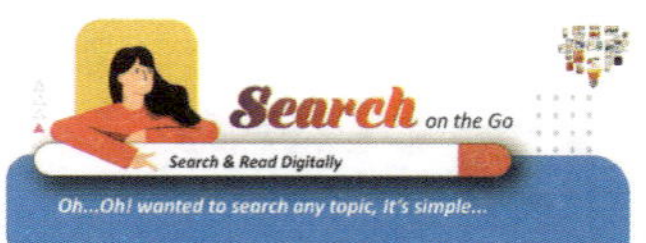

VITAMIN A DEFICIENCY

Vitamin A deficiency (VAD) is a lack of vitamin A, which in humans, produces night blindness, delayed dark adaptation, lowers resistance to infections and may produce blindness as a permanent disability.

Young children (below the age of 3 years), and pregnant and lactating women are most vulnerable to vitamin A deficiency. In India, nearly, 0.8–1.0% of preschool children shows signs of Bitot's spots and night blindness (Chapter 20).

Vitamin A deficiency also increases the risk of disease and death. Its deficiency is more prevalent in vegetarian and often occurs along with zinc deficiency.

Risk Factors

- Faulty feeding practices and weaning
- Infectious diarrhea
- Use of skimmed milk (totally devoid of vitamin A)
- PEM.

NUTRITIONAL ANEMIA

Nutritional anemia is a condition, where hemoglobin content of blood is lower than normal, as a result of a deficiency of one or more essential nutrients, particularly, iron. Iron is required by the body to form hemoglobin, present in the red blood cells, in our body. The main function of hemoglobin is to transport oxygen from the lungs to the various parts of the body.

Nutritional anemia is most common in pregnant and lactating mothers, infants, preschool children and adolescent girls. It adversely affects work output among adults and learning ability in children. Patients suffering from anemia become pale, lose appetite and feel exhausted.

In India, among children, between the ages of 6 and 59 months, a majority (70%) are anemic. Nearly, three-fourth (75%) of women are anemic, with the prevalence of moderate to severe anemia, being highest (50%) among pregnant women. It is estimated that nutritional anemia contributes to about 24% of maternal deaths, every year and is one of the important causes of low birth weight (Chapter 20).

IODINE DEFICIENCY DISORDERS

Iodine deficiency is a lack of the trace element iodine. It leads to a wide range of disorders, referred to as **iodine deficiency disorders (IDD)** that affects health of humans from fetal stage to adulthood, with serious health and social implications.

Iodine deficiency causes goiter (enlargement of thyroid gland in the neck), neonatal hypothyroidism, cretinism (among newborns), mental retardation, delayed motor development, stunting, deaf-mutism and neuromuscular disorders (Chapter 20).

ENDEMIC FLUOROSIS

Endemic fluorosis is due to excess intake of fluoride in drinking water. It has been observed in many parts of the world, where drinking water contains excessive amounts of fluoride (3–5 mg/L). It occurs, when excess fluoride is ingested during the years of tooth calcification, i.e., first 7 years of life. It is characterized by moulting of dental enamel, particularly, on the incisors of upper jaw.

Prevention

- Keep the drinking water fluorine level below 1 mg/L
- Prevent use of fluoride toothpaste in areas of endemic fluorosis. Fluoride supplements not prescribed for children consuming fluoridated water.
- Change the water sources
- Chemical defluorination

PROBLEMS RELATED TO OVERNUTRITION

Overnutrition means either too many calories or the wrong types of calories, such as saturated fats or highly processed sugar, that lead to diet-related chronic diseases, such as obesity and other lifestyle disorders.

India is passing through the phase of economic transition, where, although undernutrition continues to be a major problem, overnutrition, particularly, in the urban areas, is greatly increasing. As a result of overnutrition, problem of overweight and obesity is tremendously increasing. It is due to the increased consumption of energy-rich foods, particularly, junk foods which are rich in fat, sugar and salt. In addition, increased indoor sitting hours, sedentary lifestyle and decreased physical activity are the other contributory factors to overweight and obesity.

Overweight and Obesity

Overweight is defined as abnormal or excessive fat accumulation that presents a risk to health. A crude population measure of obesity is the body mass index. **Body mass index (BMI)** is computed by dividing the weight in kilograms by the square of the height in meters (Chapter 20).

A person with a BMI ≥25 is considered **overweight** while a person with a BMI of **30 or more** is, generally, considered **obese**.

The cut-off levels for categorizing overweight and obesity in children and adolescents are different. Since, growth spurt in boys and girls occurs in different age groups, age and gender specific BMI centiles of reference population is used to assess their nutritional status. Thus, children with BMI less than 5th centile are considered undernourished and those = 5th and <85th centiles are normal, and with = 85th and <95th centile are considered overweight. >95th centile is considered obese.

Obesity is one of the most prevalent nutritional problem, nowadays. Definition of obesity is based on the degree of excess fat. It may be defined as **increase in body weight by >20%** of the desirable weight.

The **waist circumference** and **waist-to-hip ratios** are useful for estimation of **central** and **truncal obesity**, respectively. More than a general accumulation, the distribution of fat around the abdomen, indicated by higher waist circumference, is considered to be more harmful than fat around the hips.

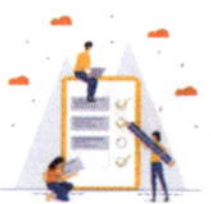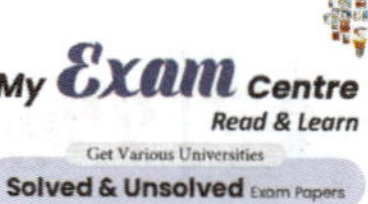

Several studies have shown that central obesity was directly correlated with chronic degenerative diseases, especially, metabolic syndrome. Waist-to-hip ratio of >0.9 among men and 0.8 in women, and waist circumference 90 cm for men and 80 cm for women, are associated with increased risk of several chronic diseases, especially, in Indians.

Overweight and obesity, in turn, leads to:

- Several disorders such as hypertension, type 2 diabetes and cardiovascular disease.
- Dyslipidemia, i.e., disturbed lipid profile resulting in reduced level of good cholesterol (HDL or high density lipoprotein-cholesterol) with increased concentration of bad cholesterol (LDL or low density lipoprotein-cholesterol).
- Hyperglycemia, abnormal glucose tolerance test (GTT) and reduced insulin secretion/action.

NATIONAL NUTRITION POLICY

The Government of India announced National Nutrition Policy (NNP) in 1993, which was adopted under the aegis of the Department of Woman and Child Development. The policy has identified key areas for action in various spheres like food production, food supply, education, information, health care, rural development, woman and child development, people with special needs, and monitoring and surveillance.

Aims of the National Nutrition Policy

The national nutrition goals, which were to be reached by 2000 AD, were as under:

- Reduction in moderate and severe malnutrition among pre-school children by half
- Reduction in chronic undernutrition and stunted growth in children
- Reduction in incidence of low birth weight to less than 10%
- Eliminate blindness due to vitamin A deficiency
- Reduction in iron deficiency anemia among pregnant women by 25%
- Universal iodization of salt for reduction of iodine deficiency disorders to 10%
- Giving due emphasis to geriatric nutrition
- Production of 250 million tons of food grains per year
- Improving household food security through poverty alleviation programs
- Promoting appropriate diets and healthy lifestyles.

NNP advocates a comprehensive intersectoral strategy for:

- Alleviating the multifaceted problem of malnutrition and achieving an optimal state of nutrition for all sections of the society.
- The policy seeks to strike a balance between the short-term measures like direct nutrition intervention and the long-term measures like institutional/structural changes and thus, create an enabling environment and necessary conditions for improving nutritional and health status.

Direct Short-term Interventions

- Expanding the nutrition intervention net (Integrated Child Development Services, Universal Immunization Program, Oral Rehydration Therapy) to have a considerable impact on child survival and extreme forms of malnutrition.

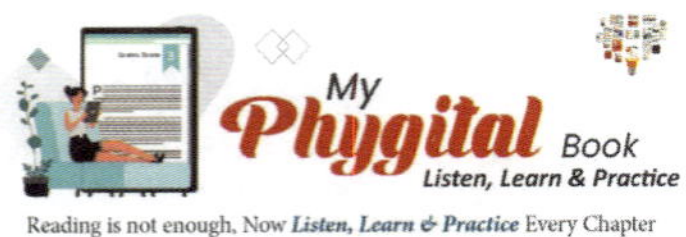

- Empowering mothers with nutrition and health education
- Reaching the adolescent girls
- Ensuring better coverage of expectant women
- Controlling micronutrients deficiencies
- Fortifying essential foods with nutrients.

Indirect Long-term Interventions

- Food security
- Improving dietary pattern
- Purchasing power
- Public food distribution system
- Land reforms
- Health and family welfare
- Information and communication
- Nutrition and health education
- Education and literacy
- Nutrition surveillance
- Community participation.

The overall strategy comprises increased awareness of energy and micronutrient deficiencies, and empowering households and communities to tackle these through existing resources.

NATIONAL PROGRAMS RELATED TO NUTRITION

Vitamin A Supplementation

Vitamin A is important for maintaining normal growth, regulating cellular proliferation and differentiation, controlling development and maintaining visual and reproductive functions. Prevalence of clinical and subclinical vitamin A deficiency in India is among the highest in the world. In view of the serious nature of the problem of blindness due to vitamin A deficiency, it was felt that the urgent remedial measures in the form of **massive dose vitamin A supplementation covering the entire population of susceptible children** should be undertaken.

In 1970, Ministry of Health and Family Welfare launched **vitamin A prophylaxis for prevention of nutritional blindness**, or **vitamin A deficiency program**, as a component of **National Program for Control of Blindness** (NPCB). Under this scheme, all children between ages of one and three years were to be administered 200,000 IU of vitamin A orally, once in six months.

Finally, in 2006, the age group of eligible children was broadened to include children between 6 months and 5 years after reconsidering recommendations of the WHO, UNICEF and Ministry of Women and Child Development.

Aim of Vitamin A Supplementation Program

To decrease the prevalence of vitamin A deficiency.

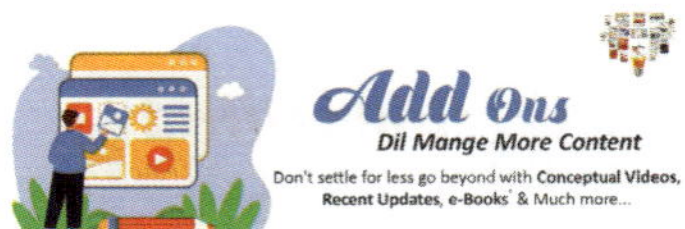

Objectives of the Vitamin A Supplementation Program

Prevention of Vitamin A Deficiency

- **Promoting consumption of vitamin A rich foods:** Promotion of regular dietary intake of vitamin A rich foods by all pregnant and lactating women and by children under 5 years of age by increasing local production and consumption of green leafy vegetables and other plant foods those are rich sources of carotenoids.

- **Creating awareness about the importance of preventing vitamin A deficiency:** Among the women's attending Antenatal clinics, immunization session, as well as women and children registered under ICDS program.

- **Prophylactic vitamin A** as per the following dosage schedule:
  - 100000 IU at 9 months, with measles immunization
  - 200000 IU at 16–18 months, with DPT booster
  - 200000 IU every 6 months, up to the age of 5 years.

  Thus, a total of 9 mega doses are to be given from 9 months of age up to 5 years.

Treatment of Vitamin A Deficient Children

- All children with xerophthalmia are to be treated at health facilities.
- All children having measles, to be given one dose of vitamin A, if they have not received it in the previous month.
- All cases of severe malnutrition to be given one additional dose of vitamin A.

ANEMIA MUKT BHARAT PROGRAM

Anemia is a condition in which the number of red blood cells or their oxygen-carrying capacity is insufficient to meet the body's physiological requirements, which vary by age, sex, altitude, smoking habits, and during pregnancy. The **manifestations of anemia** vary by its severity and range from **fatigue, weakness, dizziness** and **drowsiness** to impaired cognitive development of children and increased morbidity. Anemia in pregnancy is associated with post-partum hemorrhage, neural tube defects, low birth weight, premature births, stillbirths and maternal deaths. Anemia, like fever, is a manifestation, not a disease. It can be prevented and treated.

Iron deficiency anemia is the most common form of nutritional anemia **in pregnant and lactating mothers**, **infants**, **pre-school children** and **adolescent girls**. It occurs when iron intake is inadequate, insufficient iron is absorbed, bioavailability of dietary iron is reduced, need of iron is increased or there is chronic blood loss. Other nutritional deficiencies besides iron, such as **vitamin B$_{12}$, folate** and **vitamin A**, can cause anemia although the magnitude of their contribution is unclear. Infectious diseases, in particular **malaria**, **helminth infections**, **tuberculosis** and **hemoglobinopathies**, are other important contributory causes to the high prevalence of anemia (Chapter 20).

In 1970, National Nutritional Anemia Prophylaxis Program was launched by the **Ministry of Health and Family Welfare**, as a part of **National Family Planning Program** for the **Prevention of Nutritional Anemia** in Mothers and Children. The target beneficiaries included expectant and nursing mothers, acceptors of family planning methods (like IUCD users and tubectomised women) and pre-school children.

In 1991, the program was **renamed** as **National Nutritional Anemia Control Program**, and the beneficiaries were redefined as the program was extended to both anemic and non-anemic lactating and expecting mothers and, 1–5 years of age children. The dosages of iron given vary from 60 mg to 100 mg of elemental iron daily. **Since 2005**, the Program is **integrated** with **National Rural Health Mission (NRHM)**.

According to the National Family Health Survey-4 (NFHS-4), 2015/16, anemia prevalence across all ages is extremely high in India; varying from 30% to 69%.

The reduction of anemia is one of the important objectives of the **POSHAN Abhiyaan launched in March 2018**. Complying with the targets of POSHAN Abhiyaan and National Nutrition Strategy set by NITI Aayog, the **Anemia Mukt Bharat Program** was designed to bring about behavior change in people towards healthy living.

Anemia Mukt Bharat Strategy has been designed to reduce prevalence of anemia by three percentage points per year among children, adolescents and women in the reproductive age group (15–49 years), between the year 2018 and 2022.

Objectives of the Anemia Mukt Bharat Program

The **6 × 6 × 6** (i.e., **6-Beneficiaries**, **6-Interventions** and **6-Institutional Mechanisms**) **strategy** is estimated to reach out to 450 million beneficiaries with specific anemia prevalence targets for year 2022 to be achieved among various population groups, which include six groups of beneficiaries.

Beneficiaries of the Anemia Mukt Bharat Program

- Children, 6–59 months of age (At Village Health and Nutrition Day/Anganwadi Centers)
- Children, 5–9 years of age (At schools/Anganwadi Centers)
- Adolescent boys, 10–19 years of age (At schools); and Adolescent Girls, 10–19 years of age (At schools and Kishori Divas/Anganwadi Centers)
- Women of reproductive age, 20–24 years of age (Under Mission Parivar Vikas Yojna)
- Pregnant women (Any antenatal contact point)
- Lactating mothers, of 0–6 months, child (Any antenatal contact point)

Interventions of the Anemia Mukt Bharat Program

- Prophylactic iron and folic acid supplementation
- Deworming
- Intensified year-round Behavior Change Communication Campaign (solid body, smart mind) including ensuring delayed cord clamping in newborns
- Testing of Anemia using digital methods and point of care treatment
- Mandatory Provision of Iron Folic Acid fortified foods in Government-Funded Health Programs
- Addressing non-nutritional causes of anemia in endemic pockets, with special focus on malaria, hemoglobinopathies and fluorosis

Institutional Mechanisms of the Anemia Mukt Bharat Program

- National Anemia Mukt Bharat Unit

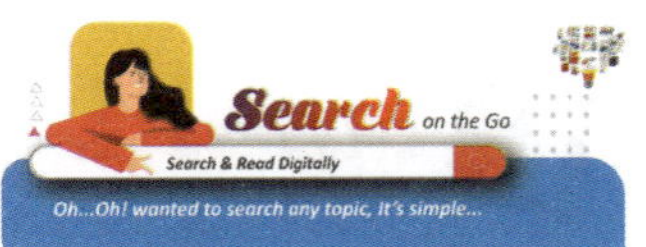

- Intra Ministerial Coordination
- Strengthening Supply Chain and Logistics
- Convergence with Other Ministries
- National Center of Excellence and Advanced Research on Anemia Control
- Anemia Mukt Bharat Dashboard and Digital Portal—One-Stop Shop on Anemia

INTEGRATED CHILD DEVELOPMENT SERVICES

Integrated Child Development Services (ICDS) scheme was **launched on 2nd October, 1975** (under 5th Five-year Plan), under **Ministry of Social Welfare**, in pursuance of the **National Policy for Children** in 33 experimental blocks. Success of the scheme led to its expansion to 2996 projects by the end of March 1994 and, subsequently, with the goal of universalization, throughout the country.

Administration of the scheme at the central level is **under** the **Department of Women and Child Development**, **Ministry of Human Resource Development**; at the **state level** under the **Department of Social Welfare**; and at the **district level** under **CDPO**, **Medical Officer**, **Mukhya Sevika**, **Multipurpose Health Worker** and **Anganwadi Worker**.

Aims of ICDS

- Improve the nutrition and health status of children, in the age group of 0–6 years
- Lay the foundation for proper psychological, physical and social development of the child
- Effective coordination and implementation of policy among the various departments
- Enhance the capability of the mother, to look after the normal health and nutrition needs, through proper nutrition and health education.

Beneficiaries of ICDS

- Children below 6 years
- Pregnant and lactating women
- Women in the reproductive age group (15–44 years)
- Adolescent girls (in selected blocks).

Services Covered under ICDS

- Supplementary nutrition, vitamin A, iron and folic acid
- Immunization
- Health check-ups
- Referral services
- Treatment of minor illnesses
- Nutrition and health education to women
- Pre-school education of children in the age group of 3–6 years
- Convergence of other supportive services, like water supply, sanitation, etc.

MID-DAY MEAL SCHEME

Mid-day Meal Scheme (MDMS), also known as **School Lunch Program**, is in operation since **1961**, with the objective to attract more children for admission to schools.

The program was initiated by the **Government of India** in 1962–63, as a follow-up measure of the **School Health Committee Report** (1961–62). The supplies for this were donated by the **Cooperative of American Relief Everywhere (CARE)**.

In this scheme Central Government provides a free supply of food grains through FCI. At least 300 kcal and 12 g protein is provided to all primary class students through this scheme.

Aim of the MDMS

To provide **food supplement to school going children** (age 6–11 years), to meet at least one-third of calories and half of the protein requirements for the day.

Beneficiary of the MDMS

School going children, age 6–11 years (classes 1–8th)

Services Covered under MDMS

Supplement to home diet—At least 1/3 of the energy and 1/2 of the protein requirements for the day (cereals 75 g, pulses 30 g, oils and fats 8 g, leafy vegetables 30 g and non-leafy vegetables 30 g/day/child).

NATIONAL IODINE DEFICIENCY DISORDERS CONTROL PROGRAM

Iodine is an essential micronutrient necessary for the synthesis of thyroid hormones, which regulate vital physiological processes, such as early growth and development of the brain and the body, in man. **Iodine deficiency** has serious consequences for human beings. In children, it results in impaired mental functions, poor intellectual performance, lowered IQ, muscular disorders, and impaired coordination and sluggishness. In pregnancy, iodine deficiency causes spontaneous abortions, stillbirth and infant deaths. Deficiency of iodine in pregnant women also interferes with brain development of the fetus and results in birth of iodine deficient babies, who may be cretins (i.e., those characterized by mental deficiency, hearing defects, squint and stunted growth).

Iodine deficiency disorders (IDD) are prevalent Worldwide. In India, IDD was earlier thought to be a problem in the sub-Himalayan region, however, surveys, carried out subsequently, showed that no state in the country is completely free from IDD. In 1994, it was estimated that around 1500 million people were at risk of IDD and that 225 million had goiter, 0.6 million were cretins and 20 million had mild neurological disorders.

Realizing the magnitude of the problem, **Government of India** launched **National Goiter Control Program (NGCP) in 1962**, and a policy decision of **universal iodization of edible salt** was taken **in 1984**. NGCP was **renamed** as **National Iodine Deficiency Disorders Control Program (NIDDCP), in August 1992**, taking into consideration the control of wide-spectrum of IDD, like mental and physical retardation, deaf mutism, cretinism, stillbirth, abortion, etc.

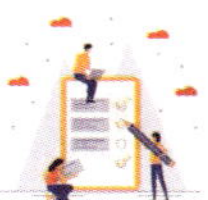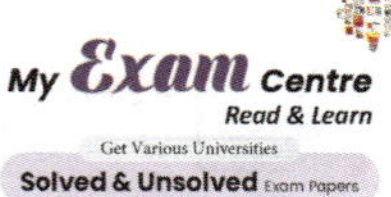

Aim of the NIDDCP

- Surveys to assess the magnitude of the IDD
- Universal iodization of salt and supply of iodized salt all over the country
- Resurvey after every 5 years to assess the extent of IDD and impact of iodized salt
- Laboratory monitoring of iodized salt and urinary iodine excretion
- Health education and publicity.

Services Covered under NIDDCP

- Replacement of common salt with iodized salt
- Use of iodized tablets to school children
- Use of iodized oil (1 mL injection of iodized oil to those suffering from IDD) for oral administration, as prophylaxis in IDD severe areas
- Mass communication for public awareness through mass media and public health programs.

WEEKLY IRON FOLIC ACID SUPPLEMENTATION

Weekly Iron and Folic Acid Supplementation (WIFS) Program, also known as WIFS-Blue campaign, was launched by The Ministry of Health and Family Welfare, to meet the challenge of high prevalence and incidence of anemia amongst adolescent girls and boys. The long-term goal is to break the intergenerational cycle of anemia, the short-term benefits is of a nutritionally improved human capital. The program, implemented across the country both in rural and urban areas.

Objective of WIFS

To reduce the prevalence and severity of anemia in adolescent population (10–19 years)

Target Groups of WIFS

School going adolescent girls and boys in 6th–12th class (10–19 years) enrolled in government/government aided/municipal schools, and out of school adolescent girls (10–19 years) in urban and rural areas.

Objectives of WIFS

- To ensure administration of IFA tablet (Iron-Folic Acid Supplements of 100 mg elemental iron and 500 µg folic acid) once per week (using a fixed day approach, preferably Monday) and Albendazole (400 mg) twice a year, for control of helminthic infestation.
- To inform adolescent boys and girls of the correct dietary practices for increasing iron intake.
- To disseminate information on preventing worm infestation among adolescences and encourage adoption of correct hygiene practices, including use of footwear to prevent worm infestation.

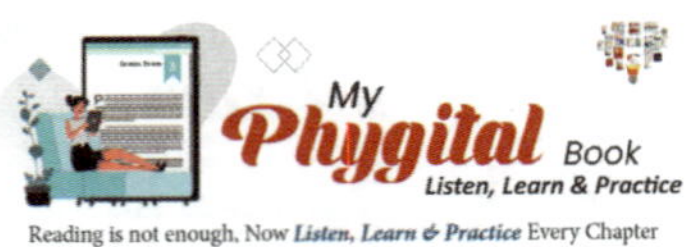

NATIONAL PROGRAM FOR PREVENTION AND CONTROL OF FLUOROSIS

Excess intake of fluoride in drinking water leads to a condition referred to as **endemic fluorosis**. Fluoride, once impregnated in tooth and bone, stays there for life time. This, in turn, affects all parts of the body, predominantly, skeletal system (skeletal fluorosis) and teeth (dental fluorosis). These are irreversible conditions and cannot be cured by any drug or medicine. Further, fluorosis produces crippling effects, permanent disability, discoloration and loss of teeth. Children under 10 years of age are most vulnerable.

Endemic fluorosis has been reported to be an important health problem in certain parts of the country, where drinking water contains excessive amount of fluoride. It is endemic in 19 states of India. Over 70–100% of the districts are affected in the state of Rajasthan, Gujarat and Andhra Pradesh, where the problem is very severe.

Realizing that there is no cure of skeletal and dental fluorosis, and that prevention is the only means to tackle the problem, Government of India initiated **National Program for Prevention and Control of Fluorosis (NPPCF)**, as a preventive measure against fluorosis, as a part of safe water supply. WHO has set the standard of fluoride in drinking water at 1.5 mg/L. These guidelines further state that climatic conditions, volume of water consumed and intake of fluoride from other sources are to be considered while setting national standards.

Aim of the NPPCF

Preventive measure against fluorosis, as a part of safe water supply.

Services Covered under NPPCF

Safe water supply.

ROLE OF NURSE IN NATIONAL NUTRITIONAL PROGRAMS

Nurses play several important roles in National Nutritional Programs:
- Collaborates with Government and Nongovernment agencies working for nutritional betterment of public sectors.
- Plays a role in school health programs, helps in identification of malnourished children and maintains growth charts.
- Create awareness among the public about nutritional supplementation programs.
- Conduct a nutritional surveillance of the community to know the health status of the community.
- Assess the nutritional status of the individual; family and community.
- Analyze the nutritional demands of the individuals.
- Encourage other health professionals to participate actively in the nutritional programs.
- Encourage women to grow kitchen gardens.
- Help them in choosing, storing and preparing the nutritionally rich foods.
- Maintain records and reports of nutritional surveys and identified cases of nutritional deficiencies.

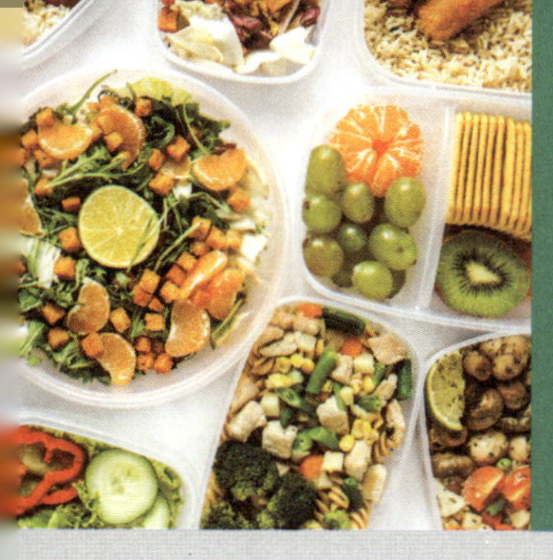

STUDENT ASSIGNMENT

LONG AND SHORT ANSWER QUESTIONS

1. Describe common nutritional problems in India.
2. What is undernutrition? Describe causes and prevention of undernutrition.
3. Describe various nutritional problems related to overnutrition.
4. **Differentiate between:**
   a. Undernutrition and overnutrition
   b. Overweight and obesity
5. **Write notes on:**
   a. Undernutrition
   b. Low birth weight babies
   c. Vitamin A deficiency
   d. Nutritional anemia
   e. Iodine deficiency disorders
   f. Fluorosis
   g. Overweight
   h. Obesity
6. **Describe briefly:**
   a. National Midday Meal Scheme
   b. Integrated Child Development Services (ICDS)
   c. National Program for Control of Blindness
   d. National Iodine Deficiency Disorders Control Program
   e. Anemia Mukt Bharat Program
   f. National program for prevention and control of fluorosis

MULTIPLE CHOICE QUESTIONS

1. **Which of the following is a prevalent micronutrient deficiency in India, particularly affecting children and women?**
   a. Vitamin A deficiency
   b. Iodine deficiency
   c. Iron deficiency (anemia)
   d. Vitamin D deficiency

2. **Which is a major nutritional issue in India caused by the excessive intake of calories and fats, leading to health complications?**
   a. Protein-energy malnutrition
   b. Obesity
   c. Rickets
   d. Kwashiorkor

3. **Which of the following is a common consequence of undernutrition in children?**
    a. Hypertension
    b. Stunted growth
    c. Type 2 diabetes
    d. Hyperlipidemia

4. **What is overnutrition primarily associated with?**
    a. Lack of essential vitamins and minerals
    b. Excessive calorie intake leading to overweight and obesity
    c. Insufficient protein consumption
    d. Dehydration

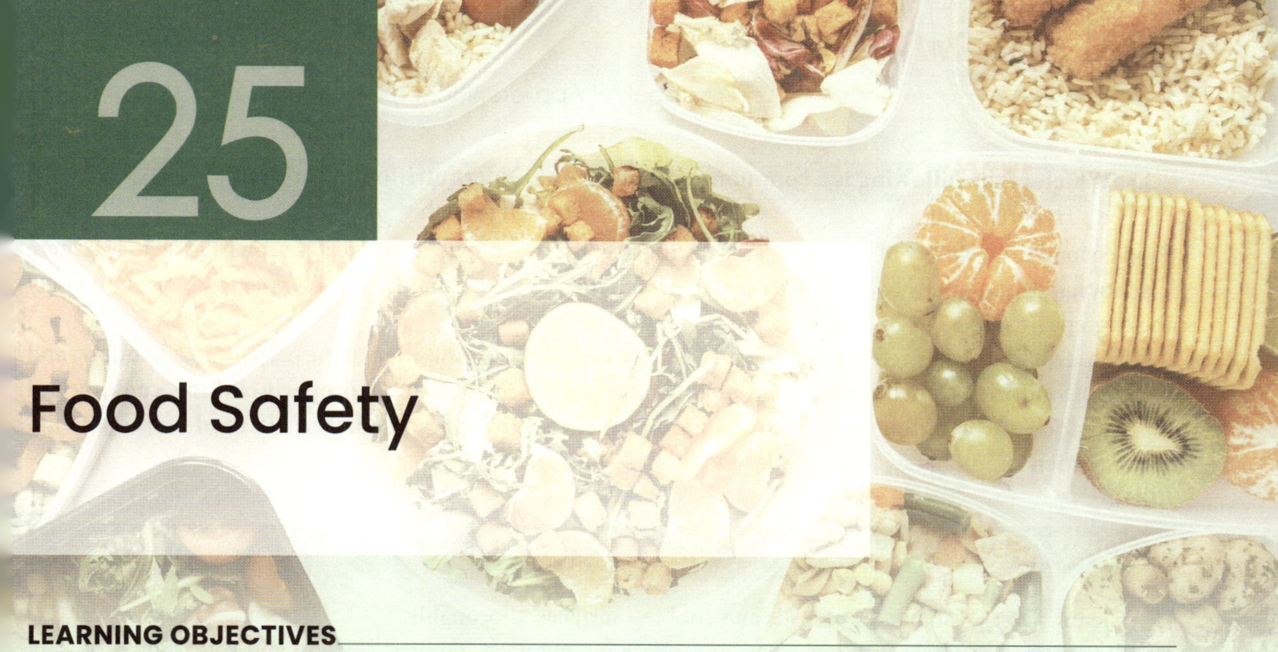

25

Food Safety

LEARNING OBJECTIVES

After the completion of the chapter, the readers will be able to:
- Learn food safety regulatory measures.
- Explain five keys to safer food.
- Learn essential steps in safe cooking practices.
- Learn how to store food.

CHAPTER OUTLINE

- Introduction
- Food Safety Considerations
- Food Safety Regulatory Measures
- Food Safety and Standards Authority of India
- Five Keys to Safer Food
- Food Storage
- Essential Steps in Safe Cooking Practices

KEY TERMS

Food safety: A scientific discipline describing handling, preparation, and storage of food in ways that prevent foodborne illness.

Persistent organic pollutants: Toxic chemicals that adversely affect human health and the environment around the world.

Safe cooking practices: Refers to the conditions and practices that preserve the quality of food to prevent contamination and foodborne illnesses.

INTRODUCTION

Food encounters a variety of health hazards during its journey from field (where it is grown) to factory (where it is processed) and finally to the actual user. To prevent these health hazards, it is essential to follow food safety and hygiene practices.

The term food safety refers to all the routine practices which are followed in the preparation, handling and storage of food, to prevent foodborne illnesses. Food hygiene is the **practice of properly chilling, cooking and cleaning food and avoiding cross-contamination to prevent the spread of bacteria in food.** Improper food hygiene when handling raw food may lead to food poisoning.

FOOD SAFETY CONSIDERATIONS

- **Cleanliness:** Wash hands, utensils and cooking surfaces, thoroughly.
- **Separation:** Separate different types of foods, e.g., raw meat, poultry, seafood and eggs should be kept separate from other foods, vegetables and fruits, at all the times such as during storage, cooking or serving. Also use different types of utensils for cooking and serving of different types of foods.
- **During shopping:** While shopping, do not buy open or broken cans or packs as the contents may be contaminated, particularly the frozen foods.
- **Storage:** All the perishable foods should be refrigerated appropriately, immediately after shopping, preparation and leftovers.

FOOD SAFETY REGULATORY MEASURES

Almost every country has its own regulatory body for the enforcement of food safety standards. It is also essential, in order to manufacture and market food products in the domestic as well as international standards. **Majority of the laws about food safety, all over the World, are based on** good hygienic practices that are supplemented by two approaches:

1. Hazard analysis and critical control point (HACCP), a systemic risk-based approach to prevent the biological, chemical and physical contamination of food during production, packaging and distribution.
2. Good manufacturing practices (GMP), which comprises of internationally recognised quality assurance guidelines for the production of food, beverages, cosmetics, pharmaceuticals, dietary supplements and medical devices.

Relevant Acts

- **In the European Union**, the food safety legislation has been described in detail in Regulation (EC) 852/2004.
- **In the United States**, the legal requirements for food safety have been described in Food Safety Modernization Act.
- **In India**, under the Food Safety and Standards Act 2006, Food Safety and Standards Authority of India (FSSAI) was established as a regulating body for laying down science-based standards for articles of food, and to regulate their manufacture, storage, distribution, sale and import.

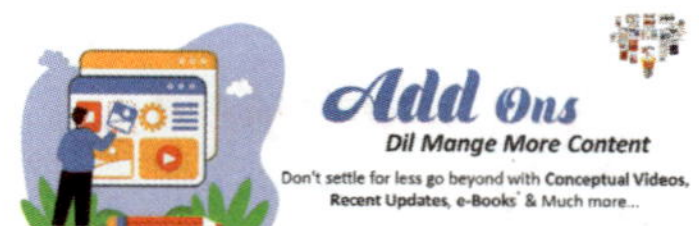

FOOD SAFETY AND STANDARDS AUTHORITY OF INDIA

Food Safety and Standards Authority of India (FSSAI) was established under the Food Safety and Standards Act 2006, as an autonomous body under the Ministry of Health and Family Welfare of the Government of India.

- It is a regulating body related to the issues of food safety and standards in India.
- It is also responsible for protecting and promoting public health through regulations and supervision concerning food safety regarding:
  - Agriculture and animal husbandry practices
  - Food manufacturing practices
  - Food additives
  - Novel foods
  - Genetically modified foods
  - Food labels, and
  - Food contamination

FIVE KEYS TO SAFER FOOD

To assist the Member States, WHO built Five Keys to Safer Food program, with tools that are easy to adopt and adapt in promoting safe food handling behaviors and educate all food handlers including consumers.

The core messages of the five keys to safer food are:

1. Keep clean
2. Separate raw and cooked
3. Cook thoroughly
4. Keep food at safe temperatures
5. Use safe water and raw materials

The poster to this effect has been translated into >87 languages and is being used to spread WHO's food hygiene message throughout the world.

FOOD STORAGE

Food storage refers to the conditions under which the food is stored as well as the types of storage containers.

In general, it is recommended that according to the type of the food (perishables or non-perishables), it should be stored at appropriate temperatures, may be in the refrigerator, freezer, pantry or warming receptacles. Raw food should be stored in clean and sanitary containers, which, preferably should be airtight. This, in turn, will help in storing the food for a longer duration and reduce the risk of contamination and thus, avoid foodborne illnesses (Chapter 22).

General Principles of Food Storage

- Always refrigerate perishable food within 2 hours (1 hour when the temperature is above 32°C. The refrigerator should be at 4°C or below while the freezer should be at −18°C or below.

- Perishable foods such as meat and poultry, should be wrapped securely, to maintain quality, and to prevent meat juices from getting onto other foods.
- To maintain quality, when freezing meat and poultry in its original package, wrap the package again with foil or plastic, or place the package on a plate, so that their juices do not drop on other foods as raw juices can have bacteria.
- Cook or freeze fresh poultry, fish or meat within 2 days.
- Always keep eggs in the refrigerator.
- High-acid canned foods such as tomatoes, grapefruit or pineapple can be stored on the shelf for 12–18 months.
- Low-acid canned foods such as meat, poultry, fish and most of the vegetables can be kept for 2–5 years, it can remains in good condition and has been stored in a cool, clean and dry place.
- Discard cans that are dented, leaking, bulging or rusted.

Role of Food Handlers in Foodborne Diseases

Foodborne illnesses are, usually, infectious or toxic in nature. They are caused by bacteria, viruses, parasites or chemical substances, which may enter the body through contaminated food or water.

- *Bacteria such as Salmonella, Campylobacter and Enterohemorrhagic Escherichia coli* are among the most common foodborne pathogens which affect human beings to a large extent. They may cause severe diarrhea or debilitating infections, including meningitis. *Listeria* infection can lead to miscarriage in pregnant women, or death of new born babies.

  Vibrio cholerae can cause abdominal pain, vomiting and profuse watery diarrhea that may lead to severe dehydration, and possibly death.
- Chemical contamination of food may be due to naturally occurring toxins, environmental pollutants (such as **persistent organic pollutants)** and heavy metals. Naturally occurring toxins include mycotoxins, marine biotoxins, cyanogenic glycosides and toxins found in poisonous mushrooms. **Persistent organic pollutants (POPs)** include dioxins and polychlorinated biphenyls (PCBs) which are unwanted by-products of industrial processes and waste incineration. Contamination by heavy metal (such as lead, cadmium or mercury) in food occurs, mainly, through pollution of air, water or soil. Chemical contamination can lead to acute poisoning or long-term diseases (such as cancer). Heavy metals can cause some neurological disease or kidney damage.

Personal Hygiene Practices for Food Handlers

Food hygiene is important as it ensures that the food one handles is safe for consumption. If personal hygiene practices are not maintained, consumers could become seriously ill with food poisoning and foodborne illnesses. Therefore, to protect the health of consumers, it is essential that the food handlers follow personal hygiene practices, e.g.:

- To ensure that no hairs fall into the food, the food handlers should keep their hairs tie all the time while handling food.
- To ensure that no germs from their hands are transferred to the food, they should wash hands with soap and hot water, before, during and after handling food and utensils.

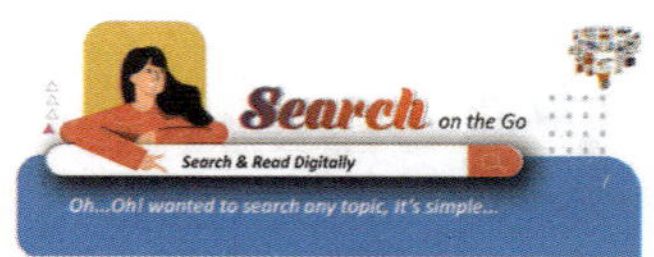

- To ensure that no germs are transferred from their clothes, they should wear clean clothes during work. While handling food they should also wear protective clothing such as hair restrains, gloves, apron, etc.
- After using the toilet, smoking, coughing, sneezing, blowing nose, touching body parts (face, nose, ears or mouth), handling rubbish or after performing cleaning duties (such as mopping), the food handlers should wash their hands using soap and warm running water. The hands should also be dried may be with the hand drier or disposable paper towels.
- If there is any wound, the bandage or dressing on any exposed part of the body should be covered with a waterproof covering.

ESSENTIAL STEPS IN SAFE COOKING PRACTICES

As mentioned above, biological and chemical contaminants are the major hazards in food. Food also becomes harmful when dirty hands are used to cook and serve cooked food. Cooked food, particularly purchased from restaurants, eateries or take away may also be unsafe as one may not be sure of the quality of the ingredients used in it. Moreover, since such a food is prepared in large quantity, it may not be possible to take full care during its preparation.

- Use of fresh ingredients and personal hygiene are the most important concepts of safe food. Food turns harmful, when dirty hands are used to serve cooked food.
- Use of rotten and unwashed vegetables makes food unsafe. As physical and biological contaminants are the major hazards, raw foods should be thoroughly washed/cleaned, to make them free from physical contaminants and suitable for consumption.
- Cooked food, particularly, purchased from restaurants, eateries, take away, etc., is also considered to be unsafe, since one cannot be sure of the quality of ingredients, used in it. Moreover, since it is prepared in large quantity, it may not be possible to take full care during its preparation.
- Packed foods may be considered safer than the one that is kept in open and sold in eateries, since packets protect it from exposure to flies, insects and dust, etc. However, one cannot be certain about the ingredients used in it.

Accordingly, safe food handling of the food is essential before, during and after cooking, as well as storage of the leftover food.

Safe Food Handling before Cooking

- Always wash hands with warm water and soap for 20 seconds before and after handling food.
- As kitchen towels, sponges and cloths can harbor bacteria, so it is advised that they should be washed regularly. Further replace sponges after every few weeks.
- Do not use rotten and unwashed vegetables, as they make food unsafe. Raw food should be thoroughly washed and cleaned to make it free from physical contaminants.
- Do not cross contaminate food. For example, keep raw meat, poultry and fish away from other foods. After cutting raw meat, wash cutting board, utensils and countertops with hot and soapy water, or sanitize by using a solution of chlorine bleach.
- Thaw frozen food in the microwave or refrigerator. Do not thaw these items on the kitchen counter, since it allows bacteria to grow in the outer layer of the food, till the inside layer thaws.

- Refrigerator allows slow but safe thawing. For faster thawing, place the food in a leak-proof plastic bag. Submerge in cold tap water and change the water after every 30 minutes. Cook immediately after thawing.

Safe Food Handling during Cooking

- Preferably, use fresh vegetables and wash them thoroughly, may be by dipping in a container of water.
- Cooking kills harmful bacteria, it is therefore advised that the food should be cooked thoroughly. Raw or partially cooked meat, poultry, fish or eggs may result in exposure to bacteria that can make cause foodborne disease compromised.
- Cook raw beef, pork and lamb, chops and roasts to a minimum internal temperature of 65°C, before removing it from the heat source. For safety and quality, allow meat to rest for at least three minutes before carving or consuming. If food has been cooked ahead of time, divide large portions into small shallow containers and refrigerate. This ensures rapid and safe cooling.
- Microwave oven though is time saver but it has food safety disadvantage. It sometimes leaves cold spots in the food and the bacteria may survive in these spots. Hence, be sure to cover food with a lid or plastic wrap. Leave a small section uncovered so that steam can escape.
- Observe the standing time, mentioned in the recipe or on package. During the standing time, food finishes cooking.

Safe Food Handling after Cooking

- Keep cold food on ice or refrigerated, until the time to replenish platters. If serving hot food, maintain it at 60°C, or divide into small serving platters, which can be refrigerated until time to warm them up for serving.
- Always use clean dishes and utensils to serve food, not those which were used to prepare the raw food. If the food is being grilled, serve it on a clean plate, not on the one that held the raw meat, poultry or fish.
- When serving food at a buffet, keep food hot with chafing dishes, slow cookers or warming trays.
- Keep food items cold by nesting dishes in bowl of ice or use small serving trays and replace them often.
- Perishable food should not be left out for more than 2 hours at room temperature (1 hour when the temperature is above 32°C). Bacteria, that can cause food poisoning, grow quickly at warm temperature.
- Pack lunch in an insulated container. Do not leave lunch in direct sunlight or on warm radiator.
- Carry picnic food in a cool pack carrier or with a cold pack. Try to keep the cooler in the shade and do not open the lid any more than it is necessary.

Safe Food Handling of the Leftover Food

- Discard any food left out at room temperature for >2 hours (1 hour, if the temperature is above 32°C). Also, discard any food with a strange color, or odor, immediately.
- Divide large amounts of the leftover into small shallow containers, for quick cooling in the refrigerator. With poultry or other stuffed meats remove stuffing and refrigerate it in a separate container.
- Bring sauces, soups and gravy to a boil. Heat other leftovers thoroughly to above 70°C.
- Microwave leftovers, using a lid or vented plastic wrap, to ensure thorough heating.

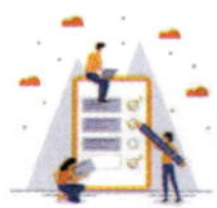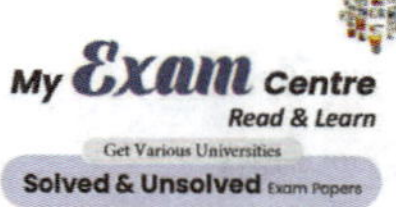

- Use cooked leftovers within 4 days. Meat and poultry defrosted in the refrigerator may be refrozen before or after cooking. If thawed by other methods, cook before refreezing.
- Discard any thawed food that has risen to room temperature and remained there for 2 hours or more.

Preservation of Nutrients during Storage

- In general, the longer food is stored in the refrigerator, freezer or cupboard, the greater the nutrient losses.
- Ripe fruits and vegetables are best kept cold until they are to be eaten.
- Ripe bananas can be stored in the refrigerator too.
- Orange juice can be kept refrigerated in a covered container for several days before vitamin C is lost.
- Wash produce quickly.
- Store potatoes, canned foods and grain foods in a cool, dark, dry place, but do not refrigerate potatoes.
- Milk and bread should be kept in an opaque container to prevent destruction of riboflavin and vitamins A and D.
- Frozen foods should be stored at or below 0 degrees.
- Refrigerate immediately all cooked foods that are not going to be eaten right away.
- Keep all fresh, cut and cooked foods well-wrapped to reduce exposure to air.
- Do not cap strawberries until they are ready to be eaten.

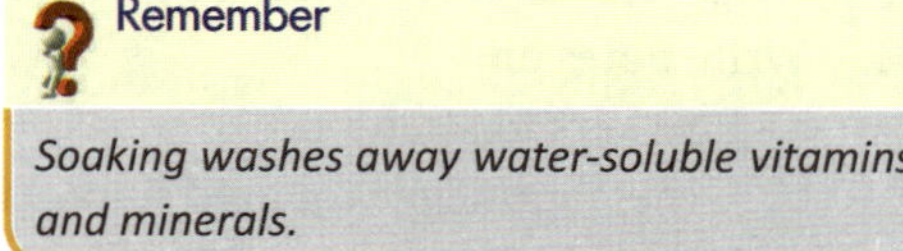

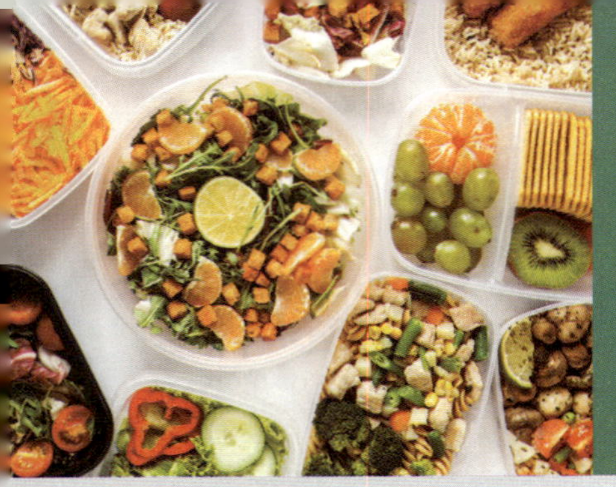

LONG AND SHORT ANSWER QUESTIONS

1. Define food safety. Describe food safety considerations and measures.
2. Discuss food safety regulatory measures in India and its relevant acts.
3. Define food storage. Describe general principles of food storage.
4. **Write notes on:**
   a. Five keys to safer food
   b. General principles of food storage
   c. Role of food handlers in food borne diseases
   d. Essential steps in safe cooking practices
   e. Food Safety Regulatory Measures
   f. Food Safety and Standards Authority of India
   g. Personal hygiene practices for food handlers
   h. Essential steps in safe cooking practices

MULTIPLE CHOICE QUESTIONS

1. **Which of the following is a critical measure to prevent foodborne illnesses?**
   a. Storing food at room temperature for extended periods
   b. Using the same cutting board for raw meat and vegetables
   c. Washing hands, utensils, and surfaces frequently
   d. Defrosting frozen food on the kitchen counter

2. **What is the recommended minimum internal cooking temperature for poultry to ensure safety?**
   a. 100°F (38°C)
   b. 145°F (63°C)
   c. 165°F (74°C)
   d. 180°F (82°C)

3. **Which regulatory body is primarily responsible for food safety and standards in India?**
   a. Indian Council of Medical Research (ICMR)
   b. Food Safety and Standards Authority of India (FSSAI)
   c. Ministry of Health and Family Welfare
   d. Bureau of Indian Standards (BIS)

4. **Under which act are the safety standards for food products regulated in India?**
   a. Prevention of Food Adulteration Act, 1954
   b. Food Safety and Standards Act, 2006
   c. Essential Commodities Act, 1955
   d. Consumer Protection Act, 1986

ANSWER KEY

1. c	2. c	3. b	4. b

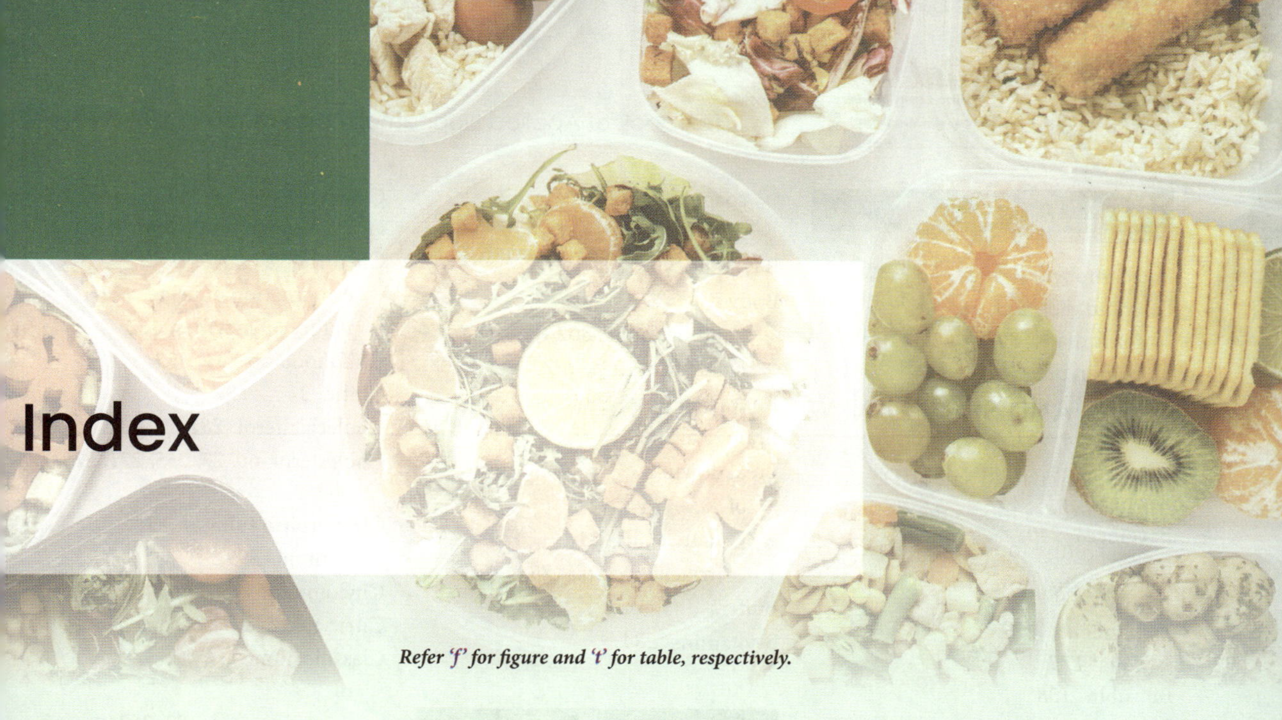

Index

Refer 'f' for figure and 't' for table, respectively.

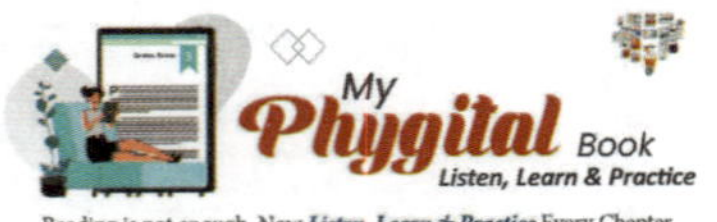

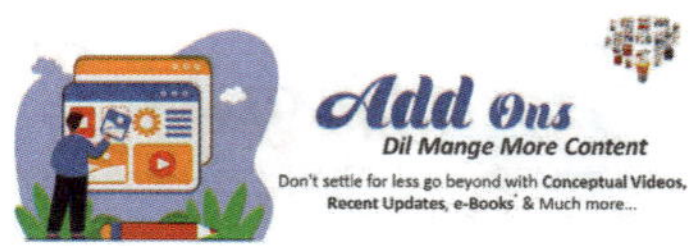

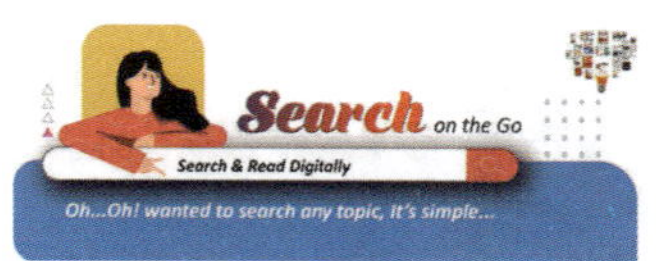

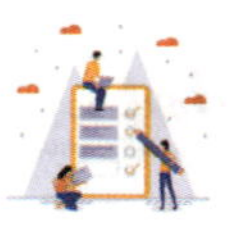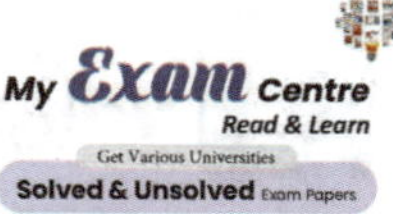

N

O

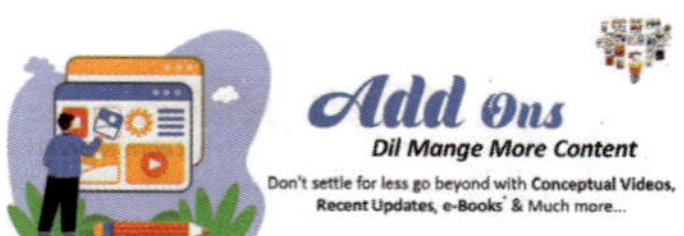

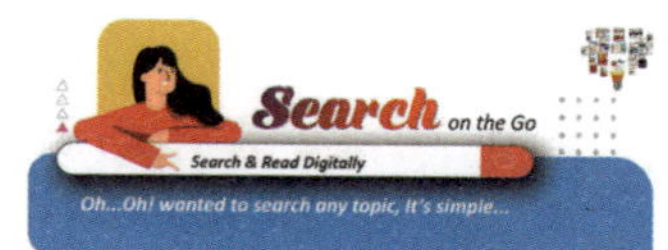

Notes